# Treatment-resistant mood disorders

While antidepressants have helped millions worldwide, a substantial proportion of patients fail to respond or remit. There is little published information available to clinicians for diagnosis and management of treatment-resistant depression, so they have to make difficult decisions about treatment options with very limited data.

The editors and their internationally distinguished team of contributors have set out to address this problem, giving a critical assessment of all aspects of treatment-resistant depression: causes, epidemiology, comorbidity, evaluation, and treatment.

This timely book will be invaluable to clinicians, neuroscientists, researchers, and graduate students.

**Jay D. Amsterdam** is Professor of Psychiatry and Director of the Depression Research Unit at the University of Pennsylvania Medical Center.

**Mady Hornig** is Adjunct Assistant Professor at the Emerging Diseases Laboratory, University of California at Irvine.

**Andrew A. Nierenberg** is Associate Director at the Depression Clinical and Research Program (Psychopharmacology Unit), Massachusetts General Hospital, and Associate Professor of Psychiatry at the Harvard Medical School.

# Treatment-resistant mood disorders

Edited by

**Jay D. Amsterdam**
University of Pennsylvania Medical Center

**Mady Hornig**
University of California at Irvine

and

**Andrew A. Nierenberg**
Massachusetts General Hospital and Harvard Medical School

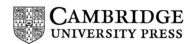

CAMBRIDGE
UNIVERSITY PRESS

CAMBRIDGE UNIVERSITY PRESS
Cambridge, New York, Melbourne, Madrid, Cape Town, Singapore, São Paulo

Cambridge University Press
The Edinburgh Building, Cambridge CB2 8RU, UK

Published in the United States of America by Cambridge University Press, New York

www.cambridge.org
Information on this title: www.cambridge.org/9780521593410

First published 2001
This digitally printed version 2007

*A catalogue record for this publication is available from the British Library*

*Library of Congress Cataloguing in Publication data*

Treatment-resistant mood disorders / edited by Jay D. Amsterdam,
Mady Hornig, Andrew A. Nierenberg.
   p.  cm.
Includes bibliographical references and index.
ISBN 0 521 59341 7
1. Depression, Mental – Treatment.   2. Depression, Mental – Chemotherapy.   I. Amsterdam, Jay D.
II. Hornig, Mady, 1957–   III. Nierenberg, Andrew A. (Andrew Alan), 1955–

RC537.T7435 2001
616.85'27 – dc21   00-064221

ISBN 978-0-521-59341-0 hardback
ISBN 978-0-521-04181-2 paperback

The colour figures 6.4 and 6.5 referred to within this publication have been removed for this digital
reprinting. At the time of going to press the original images were available in colour for download from
http://www.cambridge.org/9780521593410

This volume is dedicated to the memory of
our dear friend and colleague, Anna Sluzewska, MD,
whose infectious smile, laughter and enthusiasm
will always be remembered.

# Contents

# Contributors

**Jonathan E. Alpert**
Depression & Clinical Research Program
ACC 812
Massachusetts General Hospital
Boston, MA 02114
USA

**Jay D. Amsterdam**
University of Pennsylvania Medical Center
University City Science Center
3600 Market Street
8th Floor
Philadelphia
PA 19104-2649
USA

**David Bakish**
Psychopharmacology Unit
Royal Ottawa Hospital
1145 Carling
Ottawa, Ontario K1Z 7K4
Canada

**Claudia Baugh**
Department of Psychiatry and Behavioral
Sciences
Emory University School of Medicine
1639 Pierce Drive, Suite 4003
Atlanta, GA 30322
USA

**Christopher J. Bench**
Department of Psychiatry
Charing Cross and Westerminster Medical School
University of London
London, UK

**Kelly N. Botteron**
Departments of Psychiatry and Radiology
Washington University School of Medicine
3940 Children's Place
St Louis, MO 63110
USA

**William Boyer**
Emory University School of Medicine
1440 Clifton Road
Atlanta, GA 30322
USA

**Richard Bunt**
Emory University School of Medicine
1440 Clifton Road
Atlanta, GA 30322
USA

**Arthur Caplan**
University City Science Center
University of Pennsylvania
3401 Market Street, Suite 320
Philadelphia, PA 19104-3308
USA

**Linda L. Carpenter**
Butler Hospital
Department of Psychiatry and Human Behavior
345 Blackstone Boulevard
Providence, RI 02906
USA

**Kirk D. Denicoff**
Biological Psychiatry Branch, NIMH
Building 10, Room 3N212
10 Center Drive MSC-1272
Bethesda, MD 20892-1272
USA

**Robert J. DeRubeis**
Departments of Psychology and Psychiatry
University of Pennsylvania
3815 Walnut Street
Philadelphia, PA 19104
USA

**Jan Fawcett**
Department of Psychiatry
Rush Medical College
1725 West Harrison Street, Suite 955
Chicago, IL 60612
USA

**Antonio T. Fernando**
Auckland University School of Medicine
New Zealand

**Max Fink**
Long Island Jewish Medical Center
270-05 76th Avenue
New Hyde Park
New York, NY 11040
USA

**Mark A. Frye**
Biological Psychiatry Branch, NIMH
Building 10, Room 3N212
10 Center Drive MSC-1272
Bethesda, MD 20892-1272
USA

**Barbara Geller**
Washington University School of Medicine
3940 Children's Place
St Louis, MO 63110
USA

**Mark S. George**
Departments of Psychiatry, Radiology and
Neurology
Medical University of South Carolina
Charleston
South Carolina
USA

**Geralyn Groh-Szuba**
Emergency Department
Children's Hospital of Philadelphia, USA

**Stanley G. Harris, Sr**
Rush Institute for Mental Well-Being
Chicago, IL 60612
USA

**Cynthia L. Hooper**
Biomedical Research and Communications
56 Starwood Road
Nepean
Ontario K2G 1Z3
Canada

**Mady Hornig**
Emerging Diseases Laboratory
University of California
3109 Gillespie
Neuroscience Research Facility
Irvine
CA 92697-4292
USA

**Amy Hostetter**
Department of Psychiatry and Behavioral
Sciences
Emory University School of Medicine
1639 Pierce Drive, Suite 4003
Atlanta, GA 30322
USA

**Rita L. Hui**
Department of Pharmaceutical Economics &
Policy
School of Pharmacy
University of Southern California
Los Angeles, CA 90089-0911
USA

**Russell T. Joffe**
McMaster University Medical Center
Room 2E1, 1200 Main Street West
Hamilton
Ontario L8N 3Z5
Canada

**Terence A. Ketter**
Department of Psychiatry and Behavioral
Sciences
Stanford University School of Medicine
300 Pasteur Drive
Stanford, CA 94305
USA

**Tim A. Kimbrell**
Biological Psychiatry Branch
National Institute of Mental Health
Bethesda
Maryland
USA

**Isabelle T. Lagomasino**
Charles R. Drew University of Medicine and
Science
Department of Psychiatry
UCLA School of Medicine
Los Angeles, CA
USA

**Gabriele S. Leverich**
Biological Psychiatry Branch, NIMH
Building 10, Room 3N212
10 Center Drive MSC-1272
Bethesda, MD 20892-1272
USA

**Olivier Lipp**
Department of Psychiatry, University Clinics
Erasmus Hospital, Free University of Brussels
808 Route de Lennik
1070 Brussels
Belgium

**Alexis Llewellyn**
Department of Psychiatry and Behavioral
Sciences
Emory University School of Medicine
1639 Pierce Drive, Suite 4003
Atlanta, GA 30322
USA

**Jeffrey S. McCombs**
Department of Pharmaceutical Economics and
Policy
School of Pharmacy
University of Southern California
Los Angeles, CA 90089-0911
USA

**Pamela McCreary**
Department of Psychiatry and Behavioral
Sciences
Emory University School of Medicine
1639 Pierce Drive, Suite 4003
Atlanta, GA 30322
USA

**Isabelle Massat**
Department of Psychiatry
University Clinics
Erasmus Hospital, Free University of Brussels
808 Route de Lennik
1070 Brussels
Belgium

**Julien Mendlewicz**
Department of Psychiatry, University Clinics
Erasmus Hospital, Free University of Brussels
808 Route de Lennik
1070 Brussels
Belgium

**Paul A. Newhouse**
Department of Psychiatry
University of Vermont College of Medicine
1 South Prospect Street
Burlington, VT 05401
USA

**John P. O'Reardon**
Depression Research Unit
University of Pennsylvania School of Medicine
University Science Center, Room 840
3600 Market Street
Philadelphia, PA 19104
USA

**Robert M. Post**
Biological Psychiatry Branch, NIMH
Building 10, Room 3N212
10 Center Drive MSC-1272
Bethesda, MD 20892-1272
USA

**Lawrence H. Price**
Butler Hospital
Department of Psychiatry and Human Behavior
345 Blackstone Boulevard
Providence, RI 02906
USA

**Steven A. Rasmussen**
Butler Hospital
Department of Psychiatry and Human Behavior
345 Blackstone Boulevard
Providence, RI 02906
USA

**Victor I. Reus**
Department of Psychiatry
401 Parnassus Avenue
San Francisco
CA 94143-0984
USA

**Janusz Rybakowski**
Department of Adult Psychiatry
University of Medical Sciences
Szpltalrin 27/33
60-572 Poznan
Poland

**Jan Scott**
Department of Psychiatry
Gartnavel Royal Hospital
1055 Great Western Road
Glasgow G12 0XH
UK

**Adelita Segovia**
Washington University School of Medicine
3940 Children's Place
St Louis, MO 63110
USA

**Barbara B. Sherwin**
Department of Psychology
McGill University
1205 Dr Penfield Avenue
Montreal, Quebec H3A 1B1
Canada

**Jaskaran Singh**
Department of Psychiatry
University of Vermont College of Medicine
1 South Prospect Street
Burlington, VT 05401
USA

**Anna Sluzewska**
Department of Adult Psychiatry
University of Medical Sciences
Szpltalrin 27/33
60-572 Poznan
Poland

**Daniel Souery**
Department of Psychiatry, University Clinics
Erasmus Hospital, Free University of Brussels
808 Route de Lennik
1070 Brussels
Belgium

**Andrew M. Speer**
Biological Psychiatry Branch, NIMH
Building 10, Room 3N212
10 Center Drive MSC-1272
Bethesda, MD 20892-1272
USA

**Glen L. Stimmel**
Department of Clinical Pharmacy
School of Pharmacy and Department of
Psychiatry
University of Southern California
Los Angeles, CA 90089-0911
USA

**Zachary N. Stowe**
Department of Psychiatry and Behavioral
Sciences
Emory University School of Medicine
1639 Pierce Drive, Suite 4003
Atlanta, GA 30322
USA

**Martin P. Szuba**
Department of Psychiatry, University Science
Center
University of Pennsylvania School of Medicine
3600 Market Street
Philadelphia, PA 19104
USA

**Susan R.B. Weiss**
Biological Psychiatry Branch, NIMH
Building 10, Room 3N212
10 Center Drive MSC-1272
Bethesda, MD 20892-1272
USA

**T. Jeffrey White**
Department of Pharmaceutical Economics
& Policy
School of Pharmacy
University of Southern California
Los Angeles, CA 90089-0911
USA

**Owen M. Wolkowitz**
Department of Psychiatry
401 Parnassus Avenue
San Francisco
CA 94143-0984
USA

**Paul Root Wolpe**
University City Science Center
University of Pennsylvania
3401 Market Street, Suite 320
Philadelphia, PA 19104-3308
USA

# Preface

As many as 60–70% of depressed patients fail to achieve complete remission. In its broadest sense, treatment-resistant depression (TRD) characterizes the vast majority of depressed patients in therapy, and substantially contributes to the overwhelming morbidity and mortality associated with depressive illness. TRD is now recognized as a major public health problem which accounts for a disproportionate amount of physician treatment time, and as much as $50 billion in annualized healthcare expenditures (Greenberg et al., 1993).

The paucity of systematic data on TRD has led to inconsistent definitions and treatment approaches. While *ad hoc* definitions of TRD have been used to identify patients for specific treatment studies, the clinical applicability of these definitions is limited (Souery et al., 1999). Almost three decades after its initial description, TRD continues to be 'an important clinical problem that is surprisingly understudied. The decision regarding what to do for patients who fail to respond to an adequate trial of an antidepressant must be made by a clinician without the benefit of controlled studies that compare subsequent treatment strategies.' (Nierenberg, 1991).

The lack of response to initial antidepressant treatment has important clinical implications and results in considerable suffering and an increased risk of suicide. The recent demonstration of a 'therapeutic decrement,' whereby patients who have not responded to one antidepressant drug will have 20% less likelihood of responding to the next drug treatment (Amsterdam & Maislin, 1994) has critical treatment implications. It suggests that the current clinical practice of prescribing low doses of antidepressants for brief periods may, in itself, contribute to the development of TRD. This sobering possibility suggests that initial, aggressive antidepressant therapy is vital in order to prevent the progression of a therapeutic decrement and the development of TRD.

Because TRD is not a unitary clinical disorder, there has been no consensus on how to clinically define or identify it (O'Reardon & Amsterdam, 1998). This is partly the result of a paucity of information on the etiology of TRD, and a lack of understanding about what constitutes an 'adequate' antidepressant treatment trial. In this regard, many patients with TRD who are referred to specialty clinics are found not to have TRD, but rather to have received inadequate treatment (Thase & Rush, 1995). Thus, TRD remains an under-recognized, undertreated and underfunded health-care problem, with precious little in the way of controlled data to guide us in studying its etiology or treatment.

This volume builds upon earlier research experience presented at three International Conferences on Refractory Depression held in 1988 (Philadelphia), 1992 (Amsterdam) and 1995 (Napa), and at the European Consensus Meetings on TRD held between 1996 and 1998 in France and Belgium. It represents the thoughts and opinions of more than 30 internationally recognized researchers in the field of affective disorders.

The volume is composed of several Parts which include: The clinical problem; Biological basis of TRD; Treatment approaches; Special patient populations; and Treatment algorithms. The chapters in Part I present vital new information about the diversity of problems encountered in defining and diagnosing TRD. The diversity of syndromal definitions of TRD are reviewed, and operational criteria proposed to reduce definitional confusion. Other chapters address the economic impact of TRD and ethical issues involved in the treatment and study of patients with TRD. In Part II, authors review important new findings on the pathobiology of TRD including chapters on immunology, neuroendocrinology, brain imaging and sleep disorders. Part III on treatment approaches presents the latest findings on electroconvulsive therapy, pharmacotherapy (including drug combinations, hormonal augmentations, and cognitive/behavioral therapy. Part IV on TRD in special patient populations includes chapters on children and adolescents, the elderly, pregnancy and comorbid medical and psych disorders. Finally, the book concludes with a chapter on treatment algorithms in patients with refractory bipolar disorders.

In this book, we respectfully commit our thoughts and observations about TRD to paper. It is our aim to throw what precious light we can upon what often appears to be an insurmountable problem. In doing so, it is our sincere hope that we can, in some small way, contribute to progress in developing a more comprehensive understanding of TRD to benefit the lives of so many patients and their families.

**Jay D. Amsterdam, MD**
Philadelphia, PA

## REFERENCES

Amsterdam, J.D. & Maislin, G. (1994). Fluoxetine efficacy in treatment resistant depression. *Progress in Neuro-Psychopharmacology and Biological Psychiatry*, **18**, 243–61.

Greenberg, P.E., Stiglin, L.E., Finkelstein, S.N & Berndt, E.R. (1993). The economic impact of depression in 1990. *Journal of Clinical Psychiatry*, **54**, 405–18.

Nierenberg, A.A. (1991). Treatment choice after one antidepressant fails: a survey of Northeastern psychiatrists. *Journal of Clinical Psychiatry*, **52**, 383–85.

O'Reardon, J. & Amsterdam, J.D. (1998). Treatment-resistant depression – promises and limitations. *Psychiatry Annals*, **28**, 633–30.

Souery, D., Amsterdam, J.D., & de Montigny, C. (1999). Treatment resistant depression: methodological overview and operational criteria. *European Psychopharmacology*, **9**, 83–91.

Thase, M.E. & Rush, A.J. (1995). Treatment-resistant depression. In *Psychopharmacology: The Fourth Generation of Progress*, ed. F.E. Bloom & D.J. Kupfer, NY: Raven Press.

# Part I

## The clinical problem

# The characterization and definition of treatment-resistant mood disorders

Daniel Souery, Olivier Lipp, Isabelle Massat, and Julien Mendlewicz

## Introduction

Despite rapid development in the therapeutic management of mood disorders, with the introduction of new classes of antidepressants and mood stabilizers since the 1980s, in clinical practice the problem of treatment resistance continues to occupy a considerable amount of the physician's time. Resistance to treatment is observed across the various forms of mood disorders, but has been mainly described for unipolar depression and bipolar affective disorder.

The importance of the problem is underlined by the existence of the many treatment algorithms and strategies proposed for treatment-resistant depression (TRD). Numerous outcome studies have demonstrated that approximately one-third of patients treated for major depression do not respond satisfactorily to the first round of antidepressant pharmacotherapy. Furthermore, follow-up observations reveal that a considerable number of patients have a poor prognosis, with as many as 20% remaining unwell 2 years after the onset of the illness (Paykel, 1994). Even after multiple interventions, up to 10% of patients remain depressed (Nierenberg & Amsterdam, 1990). A poor outcome in 17–21% of unipolar patients at 2 years and 8–13% at 5 years was also noted by the National Institute of Mental Health (NIMH) study of the psychobiology of depression (Winokur et al., 1993). It is estimated that 20% of patients with bipolar affective disorder remain ill for at least one year (Keller et al., 1986b) and up to 10% for 5 years (Coryell et al., 1989). It is difficult, however, to evaluate the true levels of resistance for different mood disorders from these figures (i.e., treatment resistance in unipolar and bipolar affective disorders).

Although TRD appears to be relatively common in clinical practice, a major problem has been the inconsistent way in which it has been characterized and defined, limiting systematic research. The poor level of attention previously paid to any conceptual examination of TRD has resulted in unsystematic research and uncontrolled clinical trials, which in turn have led to a degree of confusion. An analysis of the existing publications on TRD highlights the absence of a standardized definition and operational criteria. In our review of a 10-year period of the literature (1985–1995), we observed the existence of more than 15 separate definitions (Schatzberg et al., 1983, 1986; Ayd, 1983; Fawcett & Kravitz, 1985; Feigner et al., 1985; Roose et al., 1986; Links & Akiskal, 1987; McGrath et al., 1987; Fink, 1991; Montgomery, 1991; Nelson & Dunner, 1993; Thase & Rush, 1995). Thus, a substantial number of definitions have been employed in clinical trials and have given rise to various treatment guidelines. This may explain why it remains difficult in clinical practice to treat resistant patients using the proposed systematic algorithms.

Recently, research in this field has focused on the more fundamental aspects of TRD. These aspects include methodological considerations, predictive factors, neurochemistry, and biological markers. Methodological advances have contributed to the achievement of a reasonable level of consensus on the general concept of resistance and they allow an improved understanding of the issues of characterization and definition. It is widely accepted that TRD does not represent a diagnosis or a syndrome *per se* (Dyck, 1994), but there is no consensus on the specific elements involved in its definition. The key parameters that characterize and define TRD include the basic criteria used to specify the diagnosis, the response to treatment, previous treatment trials, and the adequacy of treatment. Diagnostic aspects include the need to reach an accurate diagnosis; the various forms of treatment relating to other subtypes of depressive disorders; comorbidity with other psychiatric or personality disorders, and chronicity. The assessment of treatment response raises the problems of how to evaluate remission and the minimum length of remission required. Previous failed treatment trials remain a subject of controversy and refer to the number and type of adequate antidepressant treatment trials required by the patient before the question of resistance can be considered. Finally, treatment adequacy has to be considered in terms of dosage, duration, and compliance. The standardization of these criteria is essential if a more systematic approach to research is to be applied to the evaluation of specific strategies and new drugs in clinical trials. The interpretation and clinical application of research findings is only possible through a comparison of results obtained from studies that employ consistent definitions. Unfortunately, there is still no agreement on most of these items.

Such methodological issues have not been considered extensively in other resistant mood disorders, namely resistant bipolar disorders and 'resistant' dysthymia, where many of the conceptual definitions are derived from the approach used in unipolar major depression. Treatment-resistant bipolar disorder is largely unstudied, and many of the treatment strategies for bipolar depression are based on guidelines derived from studies on unipolar TRD. In this manner, when the methodological aspects of treatment resistance are examined, it is of necessity to use unipolar depression as a model for all mood disorders taking into account the limitations of this approach.

Reliable definition is necessary to examine the epidemiology of resistant mood disorders. Our current knowledge is based on naturalistic follow-up studies of the outcome of depressive disorders in general and relates both to the proportion of patients failing to respond satisfactorily to the available treatments and to factors associated with this poor outcome (Paykel, 1994). As a result of this approach it has been observed that approximately 30% of patients fail to respond to treatment. The literature on TRD generally quantifies this poorly responsive group conceptually, referring to relative treatment resistance, treatment resistance, and refractory depression (Thase & Rush, 1995). It is possible that the true proportion of poorly responsive patients has been overestimated as an unknown number of apparently resistant patients have been included who may have been inadequately treated, poorly compliant or affected by other conditions that prolong chronic depression. Examples of conditions presenting along with a chronic depressive disorder are associated medical conditions, comorbid Axis I psychiatric disorders, and personality disorders. Since there has been no control for these associated factors, the true rate of therapy resistance may be substantially lower than that suggested by the poor outcome observed in naturalistic follow-up studies. In addition, chronicity and double depression may affect the number of unresponsive patients (Keller & Shapiro, 1985). Double depression implies persistent residual or complete dysthymic symptoms in spite of adequate treatment of the major depressive episode.

In various treatment phases, some patients will have a different level of resistance to a given therapeutic strategy or agent, reflecting their response or resistance to acute treatment and their postrecovery maintenance or relapse. This observation should be taken into consideration and may assist in the differentiation of acute and long-term resistance.

Problems with the definition of therapy resistance vary according to the clinical and research perspectives. Research objectives are primarily concerned with the validation of a concept, suggesting operational criteria for the identification of predictive factors, biological investigations, or drug trials. From the clinical perspective, the definition of therapy resistance focuses more closely on recognition, diagnosis, and alternative forms of treatment.

This chapter will review the methodological considerations and current limitations involved in the characterization and definition of treatment resistant mood disorders, concentrating mainly on TRD and highlighting the advances that have been made towards consensus on this subject. The research and clinical implications, influencing the definition of treatment resistant mood disorders, will be discussed in light of recent knowledge.

## Methodological considerations in treatment-resistant depression

### Correct diagnosis and comorbidity

Diagnostic validity and the recognition of depression subtypes and comorbid conditions are crucial elements in the evaluation and management of TRD. Accurate diagnosis in major depression depends on the reliability and validity of the diagnostic instruments employed and on the diagnostic practices of the physician and will not be discussed here. Before any assumption about resistance is made, these factors must be considered. Misdiagnosis leads to the inclusion of heterogeneous groups of patients with pseudoresistant depression, who are then treated for resistant depression when, in fact, they are suffering from a primary psychiatric disorder other than depression. Such patients should not be included in the TRD category. Moreover, misdiagnosis is not associated with problems in defining treatment resistance, rather with the classic question of diagnostic accuracy, and this is addressed by employing reliable and valid diagnostic instruments.

The major subtypes of affective disorder respond in different ways to the available therapies, and the failure to recognize these subtypes is one of the most common factors contributing to non-response. Important differential diagnoses that may influence the treatment response in TRD are the primary–secondary classifications, melancholic depression, psychotic depression, atypical depression, and bipolar depression. Guscott and Grof (1991) conducted a comprehensive review of the overdiagnosis of primary affective disorders in patients who were defined as having resistant depression. Evidence exists to indicate that the misdiagnosis of primary non-affective disorders accounts for a substantial proportion of patients classified as having resistant depressive disorders (MacEwan & Remick, 1988; Levine, 1986; Nelsen & Dunner, 1995). Careful attention should be paid both to the identification and appropriate treatment of primary non-affective disorders. In these conditions, the pharmacological treatment of secondary depression can differ from that of primary depression in terms of dosage, duration, and onset of response. Melancholic depression, characterized by an absence of mood reactivity, severe neurovegetative symptoms, and psychomotor retardation, appears to show a greater degree of response to tricyclic antidepressants (TCAs) and electroconvulsive therapy (ECT) (Nelson et al., 1990) than to other antidepressant therapies. In atypical depression, which is characterized by mood reactivity, hypersomnia, hyperphagia, and increased sensitivity to environmental events and rejection, evidence supports the use of specific treatment choices. Adequate treatment of atypical depression should include a trial of a monoamine-oxidase inhibitor (MAOI) (Liebowitz et al., 1988; Zisook et al., 1985; Quitkin et al., 1991). In bipolar depression, the treatment of choice depends on whether psychotic symptoms are present and on the severity of depression. The first line of treatment in cases of severe psychotic bipolar depression remains ECT or a mood stabilizer, combined with an antidepressant and an antipsychotic. The use of antidepressants alone in less severe bipolar depressive episodes is not recommended (Thase & Kupfer, 1996). Specific forms of treatment that relate to affective disorder subtypes are reviewed elsewhere in more detail (Amsterdam & Hornig-Rohan, 1996).

The differential diagnosis is important not only in identifying the subtypes of depression but also in evaluating potential comorbid disorders. Comorbid psychiatric disorders that are often seen with mood disorders include substance abuse or dependence, personality disorders, eating disorders, obsessive-compulsive disorders, and panic or generalized anxiety disorders (Hirschfeld et al., 1988; Maser & Cloninger, 1990). In treatment failure, a thorough evaluation of these conditions should always be considered. Comorbidity entails the treatment of complex syndromes of which depression forms only a part. It has been observed that in depression, concomitant personality disorders reduce the efficacy of antidepressant treatments and may contribute towards treatment resistance (Pfohl et al., 1984; Black et al., 1988; Shea et al., 1990, 1992). It is not clear, therefore, whether the observed 'treatment resistance' relates to the depressive state or to the comorbid personality disorder (Thase, 1996). The complexity of the subject is illustrated by the extreme heterogeneous nature of the diagnosis in some published reports, involving patients whose diagnostic characteristics include a wide range of personality disorders.

A range of concurrent medical conditions may also contribute to treatment resistance in depression. Results from several studies have shown that thyroid dysfunction may be associated with TRD (Gold et al., 1981; Hatterer & Gorman, 1990; Howland, 1993). Other medical conditions have been implicated as organic causes of depression and require documentation and exclusion in TRD (Gruber et al., 1996; Levine, 1986). These conditions should be labeled as mood disorder due to a general medical condition according to the DSM-IV (American Psychiatric Association, 1994). Examples of such conditions are Cushing's syndrome, Parkinson's disease, neurological neoplasms, pancreatic carcinoma, connective-tissue disorders, vitamin deficiencies and certain viral infections. Several types of medication also, such as beta-blockers, immunosuppressants, steroids and sedatives may precipitate or contribute to chronic depression and adversely affect remission and response. Hence it is essential to elicit a thorough medical history when evaluating treatment resistance. Although some patients with major depression induced by a medical condition may respond to antidepressant treatment (Primeau, 1988), diagnosis of secondary depression is associated with a major factor of chronicity despite adequate treatments (Keller et al., 1985; Dinan & Mobayed, 1992).

In the field of research, the issues of diagnosis and comorbidity have important implications, and inclusion–exclusion criteria should reflect the effect of their clinical characteristics. A majority of studies excluded patients with severe concomitant Axis I, II, or III disorders (Thase & Rush, 1995). Excluding patients with comorbidity has the advantage of reducing heterogeneity, but conversely, the findings from such studies are generally less relevant clinically. Additionally, there is no clear consensus in studies on resistance on the merits of excluding a major depressive disorder that is secondary to other psychiatric or organic disease.

## Adequate treatment

At a clinical level, treatment adequacy in terms of dose, duration, and compliance remains one of the key issues in dealing with resistant patients. As many as 30–60% of patients referred for an evaluation of treatment resistance may have received inadequate trials of antidepressants (Keller et al., 1982; Scott, 1992). Furthermore, a significant proportion of cases referred to university settings for 'refractory depression' have not received even a single adequate antidepressant trial (Bridges, 1983). The same holds true for many research trials into antidepressant use in TRD (Quitkin, 1985). A systematic review of the adequacy of previous courses of treatment is required prior to any decision on the management of resistant cases. As indicated above, other essential factors relating to treatment, such as the accuracy of the diagnosis, comorbidity with other medical or psychiatric disorders, and patient compliance must be considered also before any assumption is made about resistance.

For major depressive disorders, specific recommendations on antidepressant dosage and the duration of treatment should be based on literature data and practice guidelines (Phillips & Nierenberg 1994; Amsterdam & Hornig-Rohan, 1996). In the course of time, the recommendation of adequate dosage has increased from 150 mg/day to 250–300 mg/day of imipramine or its equivalent (Ayd, 1983; Nierenberg et al., 1991). Indeed, the maximum tolerated dose should be used, according to dosage recommendations. Before treatment resistance is considered, the recommended daily doses of standard treatment that should be attained are 300 mg of imipramine, 90 mg of phenelzine or the equivalent therapeutic regimens with at least 4 weeks of treatment at the optimal dose (verified by blood levels where appropriate). For some antidepressants, the need to reach maximal doses to consider non-response is less clear. For instance, no greater subsequent response was observed when increasing dose from 20 mg to 60 mg of fluoxetine after non-response to 3 weeks of treatment as compared to maintenance on the original 20 mg (Schweizer et al., 1990). On the other hand, patients who had failed to respond to 8 weeks of treatment with fluoxetine 20 mg were analyzed in a double-blind randomized study (Fava et al., 1994). Patients treated with high doses of fluoxetine (40–60 mg) responded significantly better than patients treated with fluoxetine plus lithium and those treated with fluoxetine plus desipramine.

An insufficient duration of antidepressant trial is considered as a cause of non-response by several authors. The adequate duration of an antidepressant trial has also evolved over the years from 3 to 6 weeks (Quitkin, 1985; Quitkin et al., 1984). Some studies have suggested that prolonged trials of treatment, lasting more than 10 or 12 weeks (Greenhouse et al., 1987, Georgotas et al., 1989), can lead to a therapeutic response in certain resistant patients. However, there is a lack of evidence to support the advantage of prolonged trials over 8 weeks as compared to switching strategies. In current reports on TRD, the absence of a standardized pattern for dosage and duration of treatment is more a question of the study design and selection criteria than a conceptual inconsistency.

Most of the studies that explored the efficacy of the SSRIs, as compared with the TCAs, for severe depression found that these two classes of antidepressants were equivalent (Nierenberg, 1994). Imipramine, desipramine, and nortriptyline should be monitored using plasma levels, which have been demonstrated to relate accurately to clinical outcome (Roose & Glassman, 1994). Moreover, blood levels should be measured because a significant proportion of the general population are slow metabolizers of nortriptyline. For other antidepressants, plasma levels can be used to assess a patient's compliance with treatment. When appropriate, plasma levels should also be used for patients who do not respond to adequate doses of antidepressants, so that possible individual variations in pharmacokinetic characteristics can be documented. In such patients, dosage adjustments, based on blood levels, may produce a treatment response (Amsterdam et al., 1980; Glassman, 1994).

The efficacy of pharmacotherapy in mood disorders may vary according to the treatment phase. Treatment is generally divided into acute, continuation and maintenance phases (Thase & Kupfer, 1996). Adequate dosage and duration of treatment must be considered relative to the treatment phase. Thus, not only should resistance to the acute treatment phase be examined, but also to the continuation and maintenance phases of therapy. Some patients, who respond to the acute phase of pharmacotherapy, may be resistant to long-term treatment with high rates of recurrence, exhibiting 'continuation' or 'maintenance resistance.' As in the acute treatment phase, treatment adequacy should also be considered in the long-term treatment of depression. Recommendations on dosages and the duration of treatment are essential for a successful outcome in the continuation and maintenance phases. In particular, compliance should be assessed in maintenance resistance, since many patients reduce or end their treatment following remission of their symptoms.

It is crucial also to consider the use of psychosocial forms of treatment for patients with resistant depression. Specific psychotherapeutic interventions may be beneficial for selected groups of patients. For example, a combination of psychotherapy and somatic treatment should be considered in resistant patients with concomitant personality disorders.

## Treatment response

The criteria most widely applied for defining 'responders' and 'non-responders' are based on standardized rating scales, which are used to assess the severity of depression. In clinical trials, the criteria classically used to indicate response to treatment are the following: a minimum rating of 'much improved' on the Clinical Global Impression (CGI) scale; a minimum reduction of 50% on the Hamilton Depression Rating Scale (HRSD); a score of 9 or less on the Beck Depression Inventory scale and a score of 15 on the Montgomery–Asberg Depression Rating Scale (MADRS). Remission is also frequently defined as a score of 7 or less on the HAM-D. The process of defining these criteria in TRD is a complex one, due to the marked variability in the severity and morbidity of resistant depression as well as to variations in the therapeutic objectives. It is more likely that resistance to treatment will occur along a continuum, which could complicate the use of prespecified thresholds, particularly in very severe pretreatment major depression. In such cases, even with a 50% reduction in symptoms, significant residual symptoms may remain. A minimum reduction of 60% on the HAM-D was thus proposed in order to eliminate patients with only a partial response (Nierenberg et al., 1991). In the management of therapy resistance, the implication of this is whether or not to regard partial response or partial remission as indicators of treatment efficacy. A return to complete remission is not necessarily the same thing as a response to treatment and both can be considered as separate criteria. It is important also to define therapeutic objectives according to the patient's quality of life and in the context of subjective evaluation by the patient and other family members. A moderate improvement, as measured on a given rating scale for depressive symptoms, can be sufficient to give a noticeable improvement in the quality of life of some depressive patients. A moderate improvement in long-term and chronic resistant depression, as recorded on scales such as the CGI, HAM-D or MADRS, should be associated with an improved quality of life evaluation. The general rule in epidemiological studies and clinical trials, should be the joint use of thresholds (e.g. a score of 6 or less on the HAM-D) and percentages of improvement (e.g. a minimum 50% reduction in the baseline scores on the HAM-D). In addition to this, improvement should be assessed on more than one rating scale.

The advantage of using the HAM-D is that it covers the whole spectrum of depressive symptoms, while the MADRS and CGI are more sensitive to improvement, measuring change (Galinowski & Lehert, 1995). No appropriate instrument exists to examine specific symptoms in relation to the therapeutic response or to non-response. Discovering a solution to this last issue should be a major objective in TRD research. Finally, the minimum length of response required before remission can be considered to have been achieved must be established. In general, remission is defined as a response of at least 2 weeks' duration. In addition to the failure to respond to treatment, the duration of the episode without response has also been examined, with some definitions of TRD specifying a minimum two-year period for this (Feighner et al., 1985).

## Number and type of failed trials

In the literature on TRD, a controversial subject is the number and type of adequate antidepressant treatment trials required before the definition of TRD can be considered. The criteria range from a single adequate antidepressant treatment (McGrath et al., 1987) to at least one trial of ECT (Fink, 1991) to treatment with two tricyclic antidepressants (TCAs), a single monoamine oxidase inhibitor trial, a single ECT trial, a single lithium trial, and a single trial of the newer heterocyclics (Nelsen & Dunner, 1993). The classification of resistant depression in stages has also been proposed, based on the previous treatment response (Schatzberg et al., 1986; Nierenberg et al., 1991; Thase & Rush, 1995), where increasing resistance is equated with an increased failure to respond to the less common antidepressant treatments, such as augmentation strategies or ECT. For theoretical considerations, all of these definitions may be acceptable but do not provide an operational tool that can be easily applied to clinical practice and research. For instance, if ECT is essential to be eligible for resistance status, clinicians will be left with a large segment of the affectively ill population that are resistant to several drugs and augmentation strategies yet cannot be characterized. At the very minimum, it is possible for those currently involved in research to use each definition in a limited manner, but this in no way represents a widely accepted consensus. The use of stringent criteria in prospective studies would mean that only a small percentage of patients would be selected and followed up. It is still difficult to provide a definitive answer on the required number of failed therapeutic trials constituting TRD. Empirically derived criteria, which would need to be validated through careful therapeutic studies, could overcome this problem.

Another controversial issue is the requirement for consecutive trials of the same or different classes of drugs. With the TCAs, the benefits of switching treatment from one of the group members to another has not been supported by the available data (Charney et al., 1986, Reimherr et al., 1984). Conversely, there is emerging evidence that some patients who do not respond to a selective serotonin reuptake inhibitor (SSRI) may respond to a second trial with a different SSRI or to a trial with a TCA (Brown & Harrison, 1992). Although more controlled data are needed to document the effectiveness of TCAs in SSRI resistance, some studies suggest that this strategy is effective (Peselow et al., 1989). SSRI response in TCA resistant outpatients has been documented in several studies with response rates of between 30 and 70% (Delgado et al., 1988; Faravelli et al., 1988; Gagiano et al., 1993; Nolen et al., 1988; White et al., 1990).

## Terminology and stages of resistance

Various terms, based on the stages considered in several of the variables, have been suggested and employed in the literature to indicate treatment resistance. These variables include treatment dosage and duration, the number of failed antidepressant trials, and the classes of medication employed. The terms 'resistant,' and 'chronic depression' are often used synonymously to describe a failure to respond to an unspecified number of adequate trials, involving one or more courses of specific antidepressant treatment. Such terminology causes confusion and leads to the inclusion of a highly heterogeneous population in the study samples. According to the DSM-IV (American Psychiatric Association, 1994), a chronic specifier implies a major depressive episode continuously sustained for at least the past 2 years. Resistant and refractory depression implies some unsuccessful therapeutic trials, which differs from 'chronic depression' in which therapy has not necessarily been tried. The term refractory suggests a greater degree of treatment resistance and may be more closely associated with absolute or sustained resistance. Applied more narrowly, these terms allow for a more detailed description of the various stages of resistance; however, they also imply that a treatment history has been systematically acquired. Several instruments and interviews have been developed to assist in the standardization and improvement of data collection (Nierenberg et al., 1991). Were the use of such options shown to be valid, this could permit a very detailed classification of the stages of treatment resistance, based on the previous treatment response. Some authors propose such a process (Thase & Rush, 1995; Fawcett & Krantz, 1985, Nierenberg et al., 1991), but owing to its relative complexity, this area remains substantially limited to a few research trials. A more usual application of the stages of resistant depression was based on the concepts of relative and absolute treatment resistance. Relative resistance was defined as a failure to respond to an average minimum dose of antidepressant (150–200 mg/day of imipramine, 20 mg/day of fluoxetine or equivalent) taken for a minimum period of 4 weeks). While it is considered that absolute resistance cannot be defined using similar treatment characteristics, the use of the term relative resistance does imply that depressive patients exist who could respond to higher dosages and/or longer periods of treatment. This definition takes no account of the number of previous forms of treatment received. In a clinical context, therefore, such a definition is practical and limits treatment resistance to a specific antidepressant trial. Unfortunately, most of the previous research makes no distinction between those patients who are relatively unresponsive to an average antidepressant trial and those who are unresponsive to more aggressive treatment, including higher dosages and longer treatment periods or numerous courses of treatment. It is difficult, therefore, to identify the importance of true treatment resistance from the available research findings. The clinical implications of relative resistance are concerned with the problem of the undertreatment of depression. An illustration of this is the observation that as many as 60% of patients, who are defined as resistant to treatment and referred for alternative forms of treatment or for evaluation of resistance, may have been undertreated in terms of adequate dosage and duration of psychopharmacological treatment (Schatzberg et al., 1983). Some authors argue that relative resistance corresponds to a failure to respond to an inadequate drug trial, and that it is not logical, therefore, to consider a patient resistant if such treatment has been given (Nierenberg et al., 1991). In the context of research objectives, where strict criteria apply to the identification of treatment resistance, this last consideration may appear obvious; however, it is also apparent that relative resistance is a clinical reality. Treatment-resistant depression relates to trials lasting up to 8 weeks, with a confirmed daily dose compliance of 300 mg of imipramine or the equivalent. Absolute resistance refers to a failure to respond to the maximum non-toxic dose, received over an extended treatment period. Agreement on the use of a broad rather than a narrow distinction will benefit both the clinician, who will have guidelines available that can be applied to systematic treatment algorithms and the researcher who designs the clinical trials. A narrow definition is useful in defining a homogeneous group of absolute non-responders and the criteria relating to this are suitable for use in biological investigations, research on clinical characteristics, and predictive factors. The broader definition of resistance applies more appropriately to the clinical reality of treating patients with side effects, drug intolerance, and compliance difficulties, and allows a range of resistance severity to be considered.

## Predictive factors

The identification of predictors of non-response to antidepressant treatment is complicated by the different definitions used for resistance, including the methodological problems discussed above. Misdiagnosis, suboptimal treatment, and duration of illness remain among the more frequently encountered confounding variables. Data on treatment duration and dose are often difficult to assess from direct interviews and medical records. Despite these difficulties in defining TRD, there is evidence that both poor response and persistent depression can be predicted by specific variables.

A number of predictive factors primarily involve treatment issues, some of which have already been discussed above. For methodological reasons, it is important to differentiate between the types of treatment which may contribute to non-response and specific demographic or clinical predictors of resistance. Guscott and Grof (1991) comprehensively discussed the importance of treatment variables in understanding TRD, concluding that undertreatment of depression remains the major treatment factor associated with persistent depression and TRD.

Delay in initiating treatment is another important predictor of chronicity and non-response (Johnston, 1974; Deykin & DiMascio, 1972; Scott & Eccleston, 1991; Scott, 1992). The probability of responding to adequate antidepressant treatment is significantly reduced in untreated episodes of long duration. Scott et al. (1992) demonstrated that more than 40% of the variance in the length of illness episode can be predicted by estimating the time lapse between the onset of symptoms and the start of a therapeutic dose of antidepressant treatment.

Among the other treatment variables associated with non-response, there has to be proper recognition of compliance and tolerance. There is little research to date on compliance in psychiatry (Guscott & Groff, 1991), but this phenomenon may represent a significant factor in the assessment of treatment resistance. Compliance with antidepressant drugs involved several areas such as false beliefs, fears of addiction, and intolerance (Book, 1987; Sackett et al., 1991). In patients taking complex drug regimens, the question of antidepressant non-compliance should be carefully considered. Ayd (1972) observed that over 70% of depressed patients failed to take between 25 and 50% of their prescribed dosage on a four times daily regimen, while only 7% of patients omitted a once daily dose.

A number of patient variables have been identified as being indicators of non-response to antidepressants. Older age and female sex appear to be associated with a higher risk of non-response to antidepressant treatment (Keller et al., 1986b; Paykel et al., 1973). The illness characteristics that have been associated with poor response are unipolar illness, psychotic depression, neurotic premorbid personality, past thyroid dysfunction, familial predisposition to affective disorders, multiple loss events, and a low socioeconomic classification (Keller et al., 1986b; Scott, 1991, 1995; Scott & Eccleston, 1991; Burrows et al., 1994). It should be noted that these variables are based on the results of long-term prospective studies of chronic depression and may include a significant proportion of 'pseudo-resistant' cases. It is apparent that a greater number of controlled design studies, employing standardized criteria, are required to investigate the factors that predict TRD. The role of biological disturbances has also been investigated in

TRD. There is evidence to suggest that patients who are treatment resistant present with central adrenergic disturbances and serotonergic disturbances (Meltzer et al., 1995) and hypothalamic–pituitary–adrenocortical dysfunction (Amsterdam et al., 1995).

## Treatment resistance in bipolar affective disorder

Unipolar and bipolar affective disorders are two different diseases when considering genetic studies (Gershon et al., 1982; Mendlewicz, 1988; Winokur et al., 1995), course of illness (Winokur et al., 1993), and treatment response (Sachs, 1996; Cole et al., 1993). Only 50 to 60% of patients achieved and sustained symptomatic recovery 6 to 12 months after a manic episode (Tohen et al., 1990). In a recent study, lithium alone for 3 weeks reduced manic symptoms by over 50%, corresponding to a partial remission, in approximately 50% of patients (Bowden et al., 1994). In bipolar depression, mood stabilizers are usually effective, and antidepressant medication should be used only in case of severe and unresponsive depressive episodes. Furthermore, treatment-resistant unipolar and bipolar depression may differ on the issue of comorbidity. Unipolar patients exhibit more current comorbid diagnoses with significantly more anxiety diagnoses; in comparison, bipolar patients have more substance abuse diagnoses (Sharma et al., 1995). Concurrent medical conditions may also contribute, as organic causes of mania.

All the methodological considerations reviewed above should be specifically adapted for defining treatment resistant bipolar disorder. Due to the clinical polarity of the disease, treatment resistance can be observed in several forms (Sachs, 1996). Hence, treatment-resistant mania, treatment resistant bipolar depression and treatment resistant mood cycling needs to be properly defined and recognized.

According to DSM-IV, rapid cycling bipolar disorder is defined by the occurrence of at least four periods of depression or mania per year. Rapid cycling bipolar disorder has been often associated with lithium resistance. For depressive states occurring in the context of bipolar disorder, no agreement on how to apply TRD criteria derived from the study of unipolar depression has been reached. The same problem exists in considering the criteria used to define change points in course of illness and treatment outcome, for which consensus has been reached for unipolar depression (Frank et al., 1991). The extrapolation of these criteria to bipolar disorder may require adjustment, taking into account differences in episode duration and recovery from acute episodes between the two illnesses (Keck & McElroy, 1996). Keeping in mind these limitations, the criteria used for TRD can be generalized to treatment-resistant bipolar depression.

**Table 1.1.** Treatment-resistant bipolar disorder

*Treatment-resistant bipolar depression*
Depression without remission despite two adequate trials of standard antidepressant agents
(6–8 weeks each), with or without augmentation strategies.

*Treatment-resistant mania*
Manic episode without remission despite 6 weeks of adequate therapy with at least two
antimanic agents (lithium, neuroleptic, anticonvulsant) in the absence of antidepressant or
other mood-elevating agents.

*Treatment-resistant mood cycling*
Continued cycling despite maximal tolerated lithium in combination with valproate or
carbamazepine for a period of three times the average cycle length, or 6 months, whichever is
longer, in the absence of antidepressants or other cycle-promoting agents.

Reproduced from Sachs (1996).

In a recent review, working clinical definitions for treatment refractory bipolar illness have been suggested (Sachs, 1996). These definitions are proposed as a starting point and need validation through controlled studies, as well as for TRD criteria. Treatment-refractory bipolar depression (Table 1.1) is defined by the lack of remission of a depressive state despite two adequate trials of standard antidepressant agents (6 weeks each), with or without augmentation strategies. This last definition suffers the same limitations as the definition proposed for TRD. Moreover, adequate antidepressant trial for bipolar depression is not well defined, in particular about the use of mood stabilizers.

Treatment-refractory mania is defined as a manic episode without remission despite 6 weeks of adequate therapy with at least two antimanic agents (lithium, neuroleptic, anticonvulsant) in the absence of antidepressant or other mood-elevating agents. Treatment-refractory mood cycling may be defined as continued cycling despite maximal tolerated lithium in combination with valproate or carbamazepine for a period of three times the average cycle length, or 6 months, whichever is longer, in the absence of antidepressants or other cycle-promoting agents. The definitions of treatment-refractory mania and mood cycling should also be examined regarding all methodological considerations discussed above for TRD. Lastly, resistance to long-term treatment or 'maintenance resistance' can be of particular relevance in bipolar affective disorder.

## Treatment resistance in dysthymic disorder

Previously known as 'depressive neurosis', dysthymic disorder affects 3% to 6% (Kessler et al., 1994) of the general population. Dysthymia and major depression are observed together in 40% of patients with dysthymia, a condition known as double depression (Keller & Shapiro, 1985; Weissman et al., 1988). Patients with double depression pursue a highly recurrent course (Akiskal, 1994). Being viewed as a chronic and characterologic form of mood disorder, dysthymia is still a condition undertreated (Keller, 1993; Shelton et al., 1997). On the other hand, there are several double-blind studies showing the efficacy of antidepressants in dysthymic and 'neurotic' depression (for review see Howland, 1991). A recent randomized, placebo-controlled, double-blind trial was conducted in patients suffering from primary dysthymia without concurrent depression (Thase et al., 1996). Both sertraline and imipramine were effective in reducing the symptoms of this disorder in this study. Moreover, follow-up assessment of medication-treated dysthymia indicates that improvement is maintained over time (Hellerstein et al., 1996).

If dysthymia is 'treatable' in a significant proportion of patients, the issue of therapy resistance should also be considered in this disorder. Patients can be classified as responders and non-responders. However, several methodological problems are encountered when studying this condition. First, until now no clear definition of remission in dysthymia has been stated. Using criteria of 50% reduction in total HAM-D score or a HAM-D score of less than 8, patients are still dysthymic (Thase et al., 1996). Dysthymia is a chronic disorder, often present for many years. It is thus possible that the delay of onset of action of antidepressant is longer than for treating unipolar affective disorder. Prospective data on the evolution of response of patients during the course of antidepressant treatment are lacking to speculate on the 'adequate duration' of an antidepressant treatment in this condition. There are also little data on long-term treatment and on response to switching and augmentation strategies on dysthymic disorder. Harrison et al. (1986) observed in a randomized, placebo controlled, continuation study that antidepressant treatment should be maintained for at least 6 months.

## The rationale for operational criteria

Facing the unresolved issues discussed above in the different elements of TRD definition, it is of major concern to reach consensus on an operational definition of TRD for use in clinical practice, and in research into the characterization and treatment of the condition. In particular, research should include an examination of the conceptual aspects of TRD, in tandem with an investigation of treatment efficacy. Operational criteria should not be first considered as providing an absolute definition of TRD, but as logical instruments, capable of initiating research projects by virtue of their standardized nature. Studies, designed along these lines, could make a further contribution in validating the conceptual aspects and lead to clinical applications.

There must be documentation and control of the diagnostic and treatment variables associated with treatment resistance, such as misdiagnosis and inadequate treatment, prior to the inclusion of any patient in a TRD research protocol. The same consideration also applies when considering TRD in the clinical context. In terms of diagnostic variables, the accurate recognition of primary depression is of major importance. There is a need also to examine homogenous populations with regard to depressive subtypes. A systematic review of previous trials should include the choice of drug and a quantification of dosage, duration, and compliance in the acute and long-term treatment phases. Dosage should always reach the maximum recommended range for each antidepressant. A minimum period of 6 to 8 weeks of treatment should always be required for antidepressants.

The number of adequate treatment trials required to define resistance and comorbidity are among the remaining unresolved issues. Based on the current scientific knowledge of TRD, it is impossible to determine the number of failed adequate trials of antidepressant treatment that are required to indicate the presence of resistance. A possible basic starting point is to concentrate on the specific drug involved in the observed resistant depressive episode. A single resistant episode, occurring in an adequately treated patient, may provide sufficient evidence to indicate a future pattern of resistance. For example, non-response in a fully compliant patient, who has received an adequate course of treatment with an SSRI, could be taken as the starting point. Once this stage is reached, patients are classified as non-responders to the specific antidepressant therapy such as TCA, SSRI, serotonin and noradrenaline reuptake inhibitor (SNRI), noradrenaline reuptake inhibitor (NARI), monoamine-oxidase inhibitor (MAOI) or ECT.

In a prospective study, the next stage could be to treat this SSRI resistant depressive episode with a different antidepressant, or with augmentation strategy and to observe the clinical course. The drug used at this stage should preferably be a recognized reference treatment for depression, such as imipramine, clomipramine or fluoxetine. In a research context, this simple exercise may be sufficient to provide important information on non-response to a particular type of medication, in relation to the subsequent standard treatment. If this basic pattern is employed in controlled trials, it could also provide the framework for evaluating treatment response in alternative strategies. In the clinical context, this approach also fits with the available and generally recognized treatment algorithms for TRD. Regarding dysthymia, the same definitions could be proposed, either non-response to a specific antidepressant or treatment resistant dysthymia. However, as previously mentioned, there is little evidence on the adequate duration of an antidepressant trial and this invalidates both definitions.

Retrospective information on previous, resistant treatment episodes could be used to describe patient characteristics but should not be used to select cases nor to define TRD. The application of this principle could simplify the standardization of the number and type of adequate therapeutic treatment trials required, so that any potentially resistant episode would be considered sufficient for defining non-responding patients. Results from several studies have shown that there is a therapeutic advantage to be gained by switching from one antidepressant to another from a different class (Brown & Harrison, 1992). In a prospective follow-up study, failure to respond to two consecutive adequate pharmaco-therapeutic trials with different classes of antidepressants could be considered, therefore, as the first stage of TRD. In clinical research, it would be feasible to conduct two sequential drug trials to test the effect of switching. Conducting two drug trials allows controlled studies to be performed, using a crossover design with different drugs. The stages of TRD would correspond to the number of subsequent failed adequate trials of antidepressant treatment.

Since the above definition applies to acute treatment and does not cover prolonged episodes of treatment resistance, an additional concept, that of 'Chronic Refractory Depression' (CRD), is proposed, which takes account of the duration of the non-response episode. Chronic refractory depression can be defined as a resistant depressive episode whose duration exceeds 1 year and in which there have been multiple episodes of failed trials of adequate treatment, including augmentation strategies (Table 1.2). Assuming a mean adequate treatment of between 6 and 8 weeks' duration, CRD assessed after one year would correspond to about six consecutive treatment resistant episodes.

## Further research

As mentioned above, it is important to assess the validity of the diagnosis prior to labeling a patient as being treatment resistant. In a major depressive episode, possible diagnostic inclusion criteria include persistent depressive symptoms occurring in a primary unipolar recurrent depressive disorder or in a single major depressive episode. The selection of such criteria allows attention to be concentrated on resistance that is primarily associated with depression or with some of its characteristics. Although concomitant psychiatric and personality disorders can contribute to treatment resistance, for research purposes we recommend that the focus be on primary major depression, with no Axis I or Axis II comorbidity. The question of whether to include patients with severe concomitant Axis I and II disorders is addressed by very few studies in the available literature. However, in order to obtain valid results, it is important to limit the heterogeneous nature of the sample of patients. Studies should focus on the identification of a valid concept before proceeding to an examination of concomitant disorders and their possible effects on treatment response. The more complex aspects of patients who

**Table 1.2.** Stages of treatment resistance for depressive episode

| | |
|---|---|
| *Non-responder to* | TCA |
| | SSRI |
| | MAOI |
| | SNRI |
| | NARI |
| | ECT |
| | Other |

Non-response to one adequate antidepressant trial
Duration of trial: 6–8 weeks

*Treatment-resistant depression*
Resistance to two or more adequate antidepressant trials
Duration of trial: TRD1: 12–16 weeks
TRD2: 18–24 weeks
TRD3: 24–32 weeks
TRD4: 30–40 weeks
TRD5: 36 weeks – 1 year

*Chronic refractory depression*
Resistance to several antidepressant trials, including augmentation strategy
Duration of trial: at least 12 months

Resistance: Major depression with lack of response to an adequate antidepressant trial.

are potentially resistant can be considered separately, or defined by appropriate studies in the future. Classic exclusion criteria include concomitant delirium, dementia and other cognitive disorders, and substance abuse.

Future research on the conceptual aspects of TRD should include objectives that relate to the following areas. First, prospective epidemiological studies, to include clinical, socio-demographic and treatment outcome data, should address the question of the validity of the proposed criteria in TRD. Consensus should be sought and standardized criteria used, but the protocols should be sufficiently flexible to permit the examination of possible alternative definitions of TRD, by including valid optimal baseline evaluations. Secondly, research projects should examine comorbidity of depression with severe personality disorders, other psychiatric disorders and physical conditions, in order to clarify whether these disorders, should be included or excluded in subsequent studies dealing with the definition of TRD. This approach will focus on the primary mechanisms, associated with depression, which are involved in treatment resistance. Thirdly, controlled research projects on TRD should include predictive factors involving the study of biological markers such as neurotransmitters, receptors, brain imaging, pharmacological challenges, and molecular genetics. In addition, demographic, personality, and psychosocial variables should be examined. Finally, controlled studies should evaluate treatment strategies. In TRD, the most promising approach to achieving these objectives and exploring new therapeutic strategies appears to be the use of multi-centre collaborative studies, which in turn lead to the creation of a large, standardized epidemiological database.

Research on treatment resistance in bipolar and dysthymic disorders is also essential since both conditions have been poorly investigated in regard to definition of resistance. Furthermore, double-blind randomized studies are needed on the adequate duration of antidepressant trials and response to switching and augmentation therapy in dysthymic disorder, in order to develop preliminary criteria of resistance for this prevalent disease.

## Conclusions

The economic and social impact of TRD is of major concern in health service management. TRD is associated with significant levels of social morbidity (Keller et al., 1986b). Patients suffer from an illness that is chronic and debilitating, are highly demanding on their families, and often require major involvement by the health-care services. This leads to lengthy spells in hospital with significant human, family, and social costs. The levels of disability related to mood disorders were compared to the disability observed in common chronic medical conditions such as hypertension, heart disease, and arthritis (Wells et al., 1989). Depression was second only to heart disease in disability, morbidity, and impact on the patient's life. A frequent complication of depression is suicide. Longer depressive states may lead to higher suicide rates, but this hypothesis has not been properly investigated yet. Indeed, future research into TRD should also investigate the socio- and pharmaco-economic implications of this condition. Using the above figures, we can expect that the economic burden of TRD is important and constitutes a major public health problem.

The absence of consensus on a suitable definition for TRD is one of the main problems affecting the management of treatment-resistant patients and the comparison of clinical trials. Moreover, the difficulties involved in defining this condition make it impossible to accurately assess the frequency of true treatment resistance in depression. In this chapter, we have reviewed the methodological problems associated with the characterization and definition of TRD.

It is evident that a significant improvement in the understanding of TRD depends on the accurate recognition of a number of diagnostic and treatment variables, which are independent of the characteristics of patients. Misdiagnosis and the inadequate treatment of depression may constitute the most common causes of apparent treatment resistance encountered in both clinical practice and research. Diagnostic issues involve the accurate diagnosis of primary depression, and the recognition of depression subtypes, comorbidity with Axis I and II disorders, and concomitant medical conditions. Inadequate treatment may include subtherapeutic dosage regimes, treatment of insufficient duration or inappropriate forms of treatment that fail to recognize depression subtypes. Furthermore, the adequacy of treatment has to be considered as a function of the specific treatment phase to which it relates. In depression, although there is an emerging consensus on the reliability of the diagnoses reached and the adequacy of treatment given, it appears that a significant proportion of patients continues to be misdiagnosed and to receive suboptimal dosages of medication or inappropriate forms of treatment. Decisions on diagnosis and treatment are frequently unrelated to the characteristics of patients, reflecting the physician's theoretical knowledge of depression and attitudes towards antidepressant therapy. Establishing an accurate diagnosis and initiating treatment are critical first steps in the evaluation of treatment resistance.

Once the issues of diagnosis and treatment have been resolved, patient variables can be assessed to identify those factors related to apparent resistance and the specific factors associated with true resistance. Apparent resistance may result from the consequences of non-compliance, the intolerance of drug side effects or unusual pharmacokinetic characteristics. A number of specific predictive factors have been identified such as older age, female sex, unipolar rather than bipolar illness, psychotic depression, neurotic premorbid personality, past thyroid dysfunction, familial predisposition to affective disorders, multiple loss events, and socioeconomic class. The potential role of these factors, as well as that of biological markers, should be further investigated in the context of a standardized definition of TRD.

Despite an increasing interest in TRD, as illustrated by various reports proposing alternative treatment strategies and outlining general conceptual considerations and definitions, there remains a need for further study into the subject, based on a reliable definition. Based on current knowledge, it is apparent that difficulties exist in reaching an absolute definition of TRD.

In this context, the following criteria emerge as the most operational ones for TRD definition. These criteria are useful, combining an evaluation of treatment efficacy with the validation of the conceptual aspects of TRD. These criteria should not be considered as providing an absolute definition of TRD, but rather as a standardized and user-friendly tool. Following the first failed trial, patients would be classified as non-responders to the specific antidepressant treatment received (TCA, SSRI, SNRI, NARI, MAOI, or ECT). Treatment Resistant Depression is defined as the failure to respond to two separate, consecutive, adequate treatment trials with different classes of antidepressants, in major depression. The maximum tolerated dose of antidepressant should be used, with an optimal dose being received for at least 6 weeks, and each separate course of treatment should last from 6 to 8 weeks. Stages of TRD would relate to the number of failed, adequate trials of antidepressant treatment subsequently received, with stage 1 TRD corresponding to two failed trials, stage 2 TRD to three failed trials, up to a maximum of six failed trials, corresponding to stage 5 TRD. At this point, TRD could be regarded as chronic refractory depression, which is defined as a resistant depressive episode, lasting longer than one year and consisting of a minimum of six consecutive treatment resistant episodes, despite multiple adequate interventions.

## REFERENCES

Akiskal, H.S. (1994). Dysthymic and cyclothymic depression: therapeutic considerations. *Journal of Clinical Psychiatry*, **555** (4 Suppl.), 46–52.

American Psychiatric Association (1994). *Diagnostic and Statistical Manual of Mental Disorders.* 4th edn.

Amsterdam, J.D. & Hornig-Rohan, M. (1996). Treatment algorithms in treatment-resistant depression. *Psychiatric Clinics of North America*, **19**(2), 371–85.

Amsterdam, J.D., Brusnwick, D.J., & Mendels, J. (1980). The clinical application of tricyclic antidepressant pharmacokinetics and plasma levels. *American Journal of Psychiatry*, **137**, 653–62.

Amsterdam, J.D., Rosenzweig, M., & Mozley, P.D. (1995). Assessment of adrenocortical activity in refractory depression: steroid suppression with ketoconazole. In *Refractory Depression: Current Strategies and Future Directions*, ed. W.A. Nolen, J. Zohar, S.P. Roose, & J.D. Amsterdam. Chichester, UK: John Wiley.

Ayd, F.J. (1972). Patient compliance. *International Drug Therapy Newsletter*, **7**, 33–40.

Ayd, F.J. (1983). Treatment resistant depression. *International Drug Therapy Newsletter*, **18**, 25–7.

Black, D.W., Bell, S., Hubert, J. et al. (1988). The importance of axis II in patients with major depression. *Journal of Affective Disorders*, **14**, 115–22.

Book, H.E. (1987). Some psychodynamics of non-compliance. *Canadian Journal of Psychiatry*, **32**, 115–17.

Bowden, C.L., Brugger, A.M., Swann, A.C. et al. (1994). Efficacy of divalproex vs lithium, placebo in the treatment of mania. *Journal of the American Medical Association*, **271**, 918–24.

Bridges, P.K. (1983). '. . . and a small dose of an antidepressant might help'. *British Journal of Psychiatry*, **142**, 626–8.

Brown, W.A. & Harrison, W. (1992). Are patients who are intolerant to one SSRI intolerant to another. *Psychopharmacology Bulletin*, **28**, 253–6.

Burrows, G.D., Norman, T.R., & Judd, F.K. (1994). Definition and differential diagnosis of treatment-resistant depression. *Internal Clinical Psychopharmacology*, **9**(2), 5–10.

Charney, D.S., Price, L.H., & Heninger, G.R. (1986). Desipramine-yohimbine combination treatment of refractory depression: implications for the beta-adrenergic receptor hypothesis of antidepressant action. *Archives of General Psychiatry*, **43**, 1155–61.

Cole, A.J., Scott, J., Ferrier, I.N., & Eccleston, D. (1993). Patterns of treatment resistance in bipolar affective disorder. *Acta Psychiatrica Scandinavica*, **88**, 121–3.

Coryell, W., Keller, M.B., & Endicott, J. (1989). Bipolar II illness: course and outcome over a five year period. *Psychological Medicine*, **19**, 129–41.

Delgado, P.L., Price, L.H., Charney, D.S. et al. (1988). Efficacy of fluvoxamine in treatment-refractory depression. *Journal of Affective Disorders*, **15**, 55–60.

Deykin, E.Y. & DiMascio, A. (1972). Relationship of patient background characteristics to efficiency of pharmacotherapy in depression. *Journal of Nervous Mental Diseases*, **155**, 209.

Dinan, T.G. & Mobayed, M. (1992). Treatment resistance after head injury: a preliminary study of amitriptyline response. *Acta Psychiatrica Scandinavica*, **85**, 292–4.

Dyck, M.J. (1994). Treatment-resistant depression: a critique of current approaches. *Australian and New Zealand Journal of Psychiatry*, **28**, 34–41.

Faravelli, C., Albanesi, G., & Sessarego, A. (1988). Viqualine in resistant depression A double-blind, placebo-controlled trial. *Neuropsychobiology*, **20**, 78–81.

Fava, M., Rosenbaum, J.F., McGrath, P.J. et al. (1994). Lithium and tricyclic augmentation of fluoxetine treatment for major depression, a double-blind, contolled study. *American Journal of Psychiatry*, **151**, 1372–4.

Fawcett, J. & Kravitz, H.M. (1985). Treatment refractory depression. In *Common Treatment Problems in Depression*, ed. A.F. Schatzberg, Washington, DC: American Psychiatric Press.

Feighner, J.P., Herbstein, J., & Damlouji, N. (1985). Combined MAOI, TCA, and direct stimulant therapy of treatment-resistant depression. *Journal of Clinical Psychiatry*, **46**, 206–9.

Fink, M. (1991). A trial of ECT is essential before a diagnosis of refractory depression is made. In *Advances in Neuropsychiatry and Psychopharmacology*, ed. J.D. Amsterdam, Vol. 2. *Refractory Depression*, pp. 87–92. New York: Raven Press.

Frank, E., Prien, R.F., Jarrett, R. et al. (1991). Conceptualization and rationale for consensus definitions of terms in major depressive disorder. *Archives of General Psychiatry*, **48**, 851–5.

Gagiano, C.A., Muller, P.G.M., Gourie, J., & LeRoux, J.F. (1993). The therapeutic efficacy of paroxetine: (a) an open study in patients with major depression not responding to antide-pressants; (b) a double blind comparison with amitriptyline in depressed outpatients. *Acta Psychiatrica Scandinavica*, **80**, 130–1.

Galinowski, A. & Lehert, P. (1995). Structural validity of MADRS during antidepressant treatment. *International Clinical Psychopharmacology*, **10**, 157–61.

Georgotas, A., McCue, R.E., Cooper, G.L. et al. (1989). Factors affecting the delay of antide-pressant effect in responders to nortryptiline and phenelzine. *Psychiatry Research*, **28**, 1–9.

Gershon, E., Hamovit, J.H., Guroff, J.J. et al. (1982). A family study of schizoaffective bipolar I, bipolar II, unipolar, and normal control probands. *Archives of General Psychiatry*, **39**, 1157–67.

Glassman, A.H. (1994). Antidepressant plasma levels revisited. *International Clinical Psycho-pharmacology*, **9**(2), 25–30.

Gold, M.S., Pottash, A.L.C., & Extein, I. (1981). Hypothyroidism and depression. *Journal of the American Medical Association*, **245**, 1919–22.

Greenhouse, J.B., Kupfer, D.J., Franck, E. et al. (1987). Analysis of time to stabilization in the treatment of depression: biological and clinical correlates. *Journal of Affective Diseases*, **13**, 259–66.

Gruber, A.J., Hudson, J.I., & Pope, H.G. (1996). The management of treatment-resistant depression in disorders on the interface of psychiatry and medicine. *Psychiatric Clinics of North America*, **19**(2), 351–61.

Guscott, R. & Grof, P. (1991). The clinical meaning of refractory depression: a review for the clinician. *American Journal of Psychiatry*, **148**, 695–704.

Harrison, W., Rabkin, J., Stewart, J.W. et al. (1986). Phenelzine for chronic depression, a study of continuation treatment. *Journal of Clinical Psychiatry*, **47**, 346–9.

Hatterer, J.A. & Gorman, J.M. (1990). Thyroid function in refractory depression. In *Treatment Strategies for Refractory Depression*, ed. S.P. Roose & A.H. Glassman, pp. 171–91. Washington, American Psychiatry Press.

Hellerstein, D.J., Wallner Samstag, L., Cantillon, M. et al. (1996). Follow-up assessment of medication-treated dysthymia. *Progress in Neuro-Psychopharmacology and Biological Psychiatry*, **20**, 427–42.

Hirschfeld, R.M.A., Kosier, T., Keller, M.B. et al. (1988). The influence of alcoholism on the course of depression. *Journal of Affective Disorders*, **16**, 151–8.

Howland, R.H. (1991). Pharmacotherapy of dysthymia: a review. *Journal of Clinical Psychopharmacology*, **11**, 83–92.

Howland, R.H. (1993). Thyroid dysfunction in refractory depression: implications for pathophysiology and treatment. *Journal of Clinical Psychiatry*, **54**, 47–54.

Johnston, D.A.W. (1974). A study of the use of antidepressant medication in general practice. *British Journal of Psychiatry*, **125**, 186–92.

Keck, P.E. & McElroy, S.L. (1996). Outcome in the pharmacologic treatment of bipolar disorder. *Journal of Clinical Psychopharmacology*, **16**(2), suppl. 1, 15S–23S.

Keller, M.B. (1993). The difficult depressed patient in perspective. *Journal of Clinical Psychiatry*, **54** (Suppl), S4–S8.

Keller, M.B. & Shapiro, R.W. (1985). Double depression: surimposition of acute depressive episodes on chronic depressive disorders. *American Journal of Psychiatry*, **139**, 794–800.

Keller, M.B., Klerman, G.L., Lavori, P.W. et al. (1982). Treatment received by depressed patients. *Journal of the American Medical Association*, **248**, 1848–55.

Keller, M.B., Lavori, P.W., Coryell, W. et al. (1986a). Differential outcome of pure manic, mixed cycling, and pure depressive episodes in patients with bipolar illness. *Journal of the American Medical Association*, **255**, 3138–42.

Keller, M.B., Lavori, P.W., Rice, J. et al. (1986b). The persistent risk of chronicity in recurrent episodes of non-bipolar depressive disorder, a prospective follow-up. *American Journal of Psychiatry*, **143**, 24–8.

Kessler, R.C., McGonagle, K.A., & Zhao, S. (1994). Lifetime and 12-month prevalence of DSM-III-R psychiatric disorders in the United States: results from the National comorbidity Survey. *Archives of General Psychiatry*, **51**, 8–19.

Levine, S. (1986). The management of resistant depression. *Acta Psychiatrica Belgica*, **86**, 141–51.

Liebowitz, M.R., Quitkin, F.M., Stewari, J.W. et al. (1988). Antidepressant specificity in atypical depression. *Archives of General Psychiatry*, **45**, 129–37.

Links, P.S. & Akiskal, H.S. (1987). Chronic and intractable depressions: terminology, classification, and description of subtypes. In *Treating Resistant Depression*, ed. J. Zohar & R.H. Belmaker, pp. 1–22. New York: PMA Publishing.

MacEwan, W.G. & Remick, R.A. (1988). Treatment resistant depression: a clinical perspective. *Canadian Journal of Psychiatry*, **33**, 788–92.

McGrath, P.J., Stewart, J.W., Harrison, W. et al. (1987). Treatment of refractory depression with a monoamine oxidase inhibitor anti-depressant. *Psychopharmacology Bulletin*, **23**, 169–73.

Maser, J.D. & Cloninger, R.C. (1990). *Comorbidity of Mood and Anxiety Disorders*. American Psychiatric Press, Washington.

Meltzer, H.Y. Maes, M., & Elkis, H. (1995). The biological basis of refractory depression. In *Refractory Depression: Current Strategies and Future Directions*, ed. W.A. Nolen, J. Zohar, S.P. Roose, & J.D. Amsterdam.

Mendlewicz, J. (1988). Population and family studies in depression and mania. *British Journal of Psychiatry*, **153** (suppl. 3), 16–25.

Montgomery, S.A. (1991). Selectivity of antidepressants and resistant depression. In *Advances in Neuropsychiatry and Psychopharmacology*, ed. J.D. Amsterdam, Vol. 2. *Refractory Depression*, pp. 93–104. New York: Raven Press.

Nelsen, M.R. & Dunner, D.L. (1993). Treatment resistance in unipolar depression and other disorders. *Psychiatric Clinics of North America*, **16**(3), 541–66.

Nelsen, M.R. & Dunner, D.L. (1995). Clinical and differential diagnostic aspects of treatment-resistant depression. *Journal of Psychiatric Research*, **29**(1), 43–50.

Nelson, J.C., Mazure, C.M., & Jatlow, P.I. (1990). Does melancholia predict response in major depression? *Journal of Affective Disorders*, **18**, 157–65.

Nierenberg, A.A. (1990). Methodological problems in treatment resistant depression research. *Psychopharmacology Bulletin*, **26**, 461–4.

Nierenberg, A.A. (1994). The treatment of severe depression: is there an efficacy gap between SSRI and TCA antidepressant generations? *Journal of Clinical Psychiatry*, **55**, Suppl. A., 55–61, 98–100.

Nierenberg, A.A. & Amsterdam, J.D. (1990). Treatment-resistant depression: definition and treatment approaches. *Journal of Clinical Psychiatry*, **51**(6), 39–47.

Nierenberg, A.A., Keck, P.E., Samson, J. et al. (1991). Methodological considerations for the study of treatment-resistant depression. In *Advances in Neuropsychiatry and Psychopharmacology*, ed. J.D. Amsterdam, Vol. 2. *Refractory Depression*, pp. 1–12. New York: Raven Press.

Nolen, W.A., Van De Putte, J.J., Dijken, W.A. et al. (1988). Treatment strategy in depression, I: tricyclic and selective reuptake inhibitors in resistant depression: a double-blind partial crossover study on the effects of oxaprotiline and fluvoxamine. *Acta Psychiatrica Scandinavica*, **78**, 668–75.

Paykel, E.S. (1994). Epidemiology of refractory depression. In *Refractory Depression: Current Strategies and Future Directions*, W.A. Nolen, J. Zohar, S.P. Roose & J.D. Amsterdam, pp. 3–17. Chichester, UK: John Wiley.

Paykel, E.S., Prussoff, B., Klerman, G., Maskell, D., & DiMascio. (1973). A clinical response to amitriptyline among depressed women. *Journal of Nervous and Mental Diseases*, **156**, 149–65.

Peselow, E.D., Filippi, A.M., Goodnick, P. et al. (1989). The short- and long-term efficacy of paroxetine HCL, B: Data from a double-blind crossover study and from a year-long trial vs. imipramine and placebo. *Psychopharmacology Bulletin*, **25**, 272–6.

Pfohl, B., Stangl, D., & Zimmerman, M. (1984). The implications of DSM-III personality disorders for patients with major depression. *Journal of Affective Disorders*, **7**, 309–18.

Phillips, K.A. & Nierenberg, A.A. (1994). The assessment and treatment of refractory depression. *Journal of Clinical Psychiatry*, **55**(Suppl. 2), S20–S26.

Primeau, F. (1988). Post-stroke depression: a critical review of the literature. *Canadian Journal of Psychiatry*, **8**(33), 757–65.

Quitkin, F.M. (1985). The importance of dosage in prescribing antidepressants. *British Journal of Psychiatry*, **147**, 593–7.

Quitkin, F.M., Rabkin, G.J., Ross, D. et al. (1984). Duration of antidepressant treatment: what is an adequate treatment. *Archives of General Psychiatry*, **41**(3), 238–45.

Quitkin, F.M., Harrison, W., Stewart, J.W. et al. (1991). Response to phenelzine and imipramine in placebo non-responders with atypical depression. *Archives of General Pychiatry*, **48**, 319–23.

Quitkin, F.M., McGrath, P.J., Stewart, J.W. et al. (1996). Chronological milestones to guide drug change. When should clinicians switch antidepressants? *Archives of General Psychiatry*, **53**(9), 785–92.

Rabkin, J.G. & Klein, D.F. (1987). The clinical measurement of depressive disorders. In *The Measurement of Depression*, ed. A.J. Marsalla, R.M.A. Hirschfeld, & M.M. Katz, pp. 30–83. New York: The Guilford Press.

Reimherr, F.W., Woods, D.R., Byerley, B. et al. (1984). Characteristics of responders to fluoxetine. *Psychopharmacology Bulletin*, **20**, 70–2.

Roose, S.P. & Glassman, A.H. (1994). Treatment with tricyclic antidepressants: defining the refractory patient. In *Refractory Depression: Current Strategies and Future Directions*, ed. W.A. Nolen, J. Zohar, S.P. Roose, & J.D. Amsterdam. Chichester, UK: John Wiley.

Roose, S.P., Glassman, A.H., Walsh, T., & Woodring, S. (1986). Tricyclic non-responders: phenomology and treatment. *American Journal of Psychiatry*, **143**, 345–8.

Sachs, G.S. (1996). Treatment-resistant bipolar depression. *Psychiatric Clinics of North America*, **19**(2), 215–36.

Sackett, D.L., Haynes, R.B., Guyatt, G.H. et al. (1991). Helping patients follow the treatment you prescribe. In *Clinical Epidemiology: A Basic Science for Clinical Medicine*, 2nd edn. ed. D.L. Sackett et al., pp. 249–81. Boston, MA: Little Brown.

Schatzberg, A.F., Cole, J.O., Cohen, B.M. et al. (1983). Survey of depressed patients who have failed to respond to treatment. In *The Affective Disorders*, ed. J.M. Davis & J.W. Maas, pp. 73–85. Washington, DC: American Psychiatric Press.

Schatzberg, A.F., Cole, J.O., & Elliott, G.R. (1986). Recent views on treatment resistant depression. In *Psychosocial Aspects of Non-response to Antidepressant Drugs*, U. Halbreich & S.S. Feinberg, pp. 95–109. Washington. DC: American Psychiatric Press.

Schweizer, E., Rickels, K., & Amsterdam, J.D. (1990). What constitutes an adequate treatment trial for fluoxetine? *Journal of Clinical Psychiatry*, **51**, 8–11.

Scott, J. (1991). Epidemiology, demography and definitions. *International Clinical Psychopharmacology*, 6(Suppl. 1), L 1–12.

Scott, J. (1992). Are there different subtype of chronic primary major depression? A preliminary report. *Advances in Affective Disorders*, **7**, 6–7.

Scott, J. (1995). Predictors of non-response to antidepressants. In *Refractory Depression: Current Strategies and Future Directions*, ed. W.A. Nolen, J. Zohar, S.P. Roose, & J.D. Amsterdam, pp. 19–28. Chichester, UK: John Wiley.

Scott, J. & Eccleston, D. (1991). Prediction, treatment and prognosis of major depression. *International Clinical Psychopharmacology*, **6** (Suppl 1) 41–9.

Scott, J., Cole, A., & Eccleston, D. (1991). Dealing with persisting abnormalities of mood. *International Review Psychiatry*, **3**, 19–33.

Scott, J., Eccleston, D., & Boys, R. (1992). Can we predict the persistence of depression? *British Journal of Psychiatry*, **161**, 633–7.

Sharma, V., Mazmanian, D., Persad, E. et al. (1995). A comparison of comorbid patterns in treatment resistance unipolar and bipolar depression. *Canadian Journal of Psychiatry*, **40**, 270–4.

Shea, M.T., Pilkonis, P.A., Beckham, E. et al. (1990). Personality disorder and treatment outcome in the NIMH treatment of depression collaborative research program. *American Journal of Psychiatry*, **147**, 711–18.

Shea, M.T., Wuidiger, T.A., & Klein, M.H. (1992). Comorbidity of personality disorders and depression: implications for treatment. *Journal of Consulting and Clinical Psychology*, **60**, 857–68.

Shelton, R.C., Davidson, J., Yonkers, K.A. et al. (1997). The undertreatment of dysthymia. *Journal of Clinical Psychiatry*, **58**, 59–65.

Thase, M.E. (1996). The role of axis II comorbidity in the management of patients with treatment-resistant depression. *Psychiatric Clinics of North America*, **19**(2), 287–92.

Thase, M.E. & Kupfer, D.J. (1996). Recent developments in the pharmacotherapy of mood disorders. *Journal of Consulting and Clinical Psychology*, **64**(4), 646–59.

Thase, M.E. & Rush, A.J. (1995). Treatment-resistant depression. In *Psychopharmacology: The Fourth Generation of Progress*, ed. F.E. Bloom & D.J. Kupfer. New York: Raven Press Ltd.

Thase, M.E., Fava, M., Halbreich, U. et al. (1996). A placebo-controlled, randomized clinical trial comparing sertraline and imipramine for the treatment of dysthymia. *Archives of General Psychiatry*, **53**, 777–84.

Tohen, M., Waternaux, C.M., & Tsuang, M.T. (1990). Outcome in mania, a four year prospective follow-up of 75 patients utilizing survival analysis. *Archives of General Psychiatry*, **47**, 1106–11.

Wagner, S.G. & Klein, D.F. (1988). Treatment refractory patients, affective disorders. *Psychopharmacology Bulletin*, **24**, 69–74.

Weissman, M.M., Leaf, P.J., Bruce, M.L. et al. (1988). The epidemiology of dysthymia in five communities, rates, risks, comorbidity and treatment. *American Journal of Psychiatry*, **145**, 815–19.

Wells, K., Stewart, A., Hays, R. et al. (1989). The functioning and well-being of depressed patients: results from the medical outcomes study. *Journal of the American Medical Association*, **262**, 914–19.

White, K., Wykoff, W., Tynes, L.L., Schneider, L., & Zemansky, M. (1990). Fluvoxamine in the treatment of tricyclic-resistant depression. *Psychiatric Journal of the University of Ottawa*, **15**, 156–8.

Winokur, G., Corell, W., Keller, M. et al. (1993). A prospective follow-up of patients with bipolar and unipolar affective disorder. *Archives of General Psychiatry*, **50**, 457–65.

Winokur, G., Coryell, W., Keller, M. et al. (1995). Family study of manic-depressive (bipolar I) disease. *Archives of General Psychiatry*, **52**, 367–73.

Zisook, B., Braff, D.L., & Click, M.A. (1985). Monoamine oxidase inhibitors in the treatment of atypical depression. *Journal of Clinical Psychopharmacology*, **5**, 131–7.

# 2

# Overview of treatment-resistant depression and its management

John P. O'Reardon and Jay D. Amsterdam

## Introduction

Although the therapeutic armamentarium available for the clinician treating major depression has expanded substantially over the last decade, the percentage of patients with treatment-resistant depression (TRD) remains unchanged and continues to be an important clinical problem. In spite of aggressive pharmacological and psychotherapy approaches, 10–15% of patients will remain chronically depressed with a significant psychosocial morbidity and a mortality rate by suicide (Keller et al., 1992). Although this percentage represents the minority of patients who have minimal or no response to at least one adequate therapeutic trial of an antidepressant, this figure obscures the more general problem of partial response or 'relative' TRD in 50–70% of patients undergoing antidepressant treatment (Fawcett, 1994).

In this chapter, the concept of TRD will be defined and distinguished from 'pseudo-TRD' resulting from either misdiagnosis, unrecognized concurrent medical and psychiatric illnesses, inadequate antidepressant treatment or unrecognized pharmacokinetic factors interfering with adequate treatment. Thus in 'pseudo-TRD' the treatment is judged to be inadequate for specific reasons and could not have reasonably been expected to be successful. In this regard, the criteria for what constitutes 'adequacy' of treatment will be examined more closely. Finally, several approaches for optimizing treatment and minimizing resistance in depressed patients will be reviewed, as well as some suggested approaches for directly treating TRD.

## Definition of TRD

In its broadest form, TRD can be defined as a failure to respond completely to a treatment known to be effective for major depression. However, in clinical practice it is best understood as occurring along a continuum (rather than as an

**Table 2.1.** Proposed terminology for treatment-resistant depression (TRD)

*Treatment response*
A response that is good enough that a change in treatment plan is usually not called for (e.g. at least a 50% reduction in HRSD score, final HRSD score $< 7$, CGI-improvement score $\leqslant 2$)

*Treatment non-response*
A response that is poor enough that a change in treatment plan is called for (e.g. less than 50% reduction in HRSD score, CGI-improvement score $\leqslant 1$, minimal improvement only or worsening of condition)

*Treatment-resistant depression*
There has been only a partial response to treatment, patient meets criteria for non-response

*Treatment-refractory depression*
There has been no response to treatment, symptoms unchanged or worse

*Remission*
Attainment of a virtually asymptomatic state (e.g. HRSD score $\leqslant 7$) for 2 consecutive months

*Recovery*
Remission for at least 6 consecutive months

---

all-or-none phenomenon) ranging from partial response to complete treatment resistance. Thus TRD should be approached as a syndrome comprising a heterogeneous group of conditions with varying etiologies and varying levels of therapy resistance. In this context some pragmatic definitions of treatment response and resistance are outlined in Table 2.1.

In controlled clinical drug trials, an antidepressant response is generally considered to be a reduction in score of 50% or more of the Hamilton Rating Scale for Depression (HRSD) (Thase et al., in press). While this criterion may be very useful in identifying therapeutic efficacy of antidepressant drugs, it does not distinguish 'responders' from patients who achieve full remission of symptoms (i.e. 'remitters') due to treatment. In this context, the term treatment responder can impart to clinicians a false sense of optimism regarding antidepressant drug efficacy. Thus, in a controlled clinical drug trial, overall treatment response may be adjudged similarly in all patients. As a result, more severely ill patients with higher initial HDRS severity scores (e.g. 25 or more) may continue to exhibit significant residual depressive symptoms, even after 'successful' antidepressant response. Even though about 70% of patients may be judged to be responders by the criterion of a reduction in baseline HRSD score of at least 50%, only about 30% of patients will actually achieve remission during six weeks of antidepressant treatment. Therefore, whilst all 'remitters' can be regarded as 'responders', only about half of the 'responders' will actually achieve remission.

Similarly, remission is not necessarily the same as 'recovery', which is defined as the presence of a sustained or full remission of symptoms, for at least a minimum of two months (DSM-IV, 1994). In clinical practice, as in clinical drug trials, the frequently accepted therapeutic outcome of drug treatment is a clinically and statistically significant reduction in symptom severity, rather than full remission and recovery from depression. The presence of residual symptoms, however, is important in two major respects: (i) patients who do not achieve full remission will have a significantly higher likelihood of relapse, and (ii) incompletely re-covered patients will continue to exhibit substantial functional impairment result-ing from residual symptoms of depression (Thase & Kupfer, 1987).

## Staging TRD

In formulating a treatment approach to TRD, some type of illness measurement or 'staging' is useful as a measure of the level of severity of the disease. In this framework, several investigators have constructed algorithms for classifying pro-gressive degrees of TRD. A wide variety of staging systems depending on the criteria used have used, including: (i) subclassifications based on depressive subtypes (i.e. psychotic vs. non-psychotic, bipolar vs. unipolar depression) (Malizia & Bridges, 1992); (ii) failure to respond to adequate doses of a single tricyclic antidepressant (TCA) or (iii) monoamine oxidase inhibitor (MAOI) trial for a minimum of 4 weeks (Roose et al., 1986); (iv) duration of episode of at least 2 years with non-response to conventional treatment (Cassano et al., 1983); (v) failure to respond to therapy after three or more adequate trials of treatment, one of which must have been a TCA (Nierenberg et al., 1994); (vi) failure to respond to five or more 'adequate' treatments (Amsterdam & Berwish, 1987). As one might expect, the lack of clear definition and consensus has been more of a hindrance than a help to progress in the field. Unfortunately, in terms of selecting between the different approaches to defining TRD, none of these classifications have been systematically examined or verified for reliability or validated for predictive utility. In addition, any staging system based on treatments administered has the limita-tion of being dependent on the available treatment options as they evolve over time, rather than based on the underlying neurobiology of the condition. Despite these limitations staging systems do have merit and should be clearly described and have clinical ease of use and utility in order to maximize their usefulness as a clinical and research tools. An example of such a staging system, as proposed by Thase and Rush (1995), which outlines five levels of increasing treatment resis-tance, is illustrated in Table 2.2 and which, if adopted, will assist in stratifying the

**Table 2.2.** A simple system for staging antidepressant resistance

Stage 0 ('pseudo'): Any medication trials, to date, judged to be inadequate

Stage I: Failure of at least one adequate trial of one major class of antidepressants

Stage II: Failure of at least two adequate trials of at least two distinctly distinctly different classes of antidepressant

Stage III: Stage II resistance plus failure of an adequate trial of a TCA

Stage IV: Stage III resistance plus failure of an adequate trial of an MAOI

Stage V: Stage IV resistance plus a course of bilateral ECT

heterogeneous group of treatment non-responders and facilitate more valid comparisons between studies.

## Treatment of TRD

When approaching a case of TRD the first task of the clinician is to re-evaluate the diagnosis, and ensure that no relevant medical or psychiatric comorbidity has been missed and which may be primarily responsible for the lack of response to treatment. Once this issue has been addressed the next task is to thoroughly review the adequacy of treatment administered to date, and so determine the level of TRD one is dealing with.

## Medical contributors to TRD

Organic factors may cause or contribute to affective illness in 50% of patients (Hall et al., 1981). In a patient with TRD it is critical to rule out the presence of underlying medical disorders (Akiskal, 1982; MacEwan & Remick, 1988). Moreover iatrogenic depression, may result from the coadministration of medications for acute and chronic medical illnesses (Metzger & Friedman, 1994). A list of common medical contributors to TRD is presented in Table 2.3.

Amongst medical causes of depression the most frequent appear to be endocrine, in particular thyroid (Gold et al., 1981; Prange et al., 1990). Grade I, or clinically overt hypothyroidism will manifest depression in up to 40% of cases (Jain, 1972) but even subtler subclinical grades of hypothyroidism may also contribute. These are Grade II, where only TSH is elevated (with normal T4 and T3), and Grade III where T4, T3, and TSH are all normal and the only abnormality is a TSH rise above normal in response to a TRH stimulation test (Targum et al., 1984). Hyperthyroidism is a less common cause of depression (Gadde & Krishnan, 1994). Overall, uncontrolled studies suggest a high frequency of thyroid dysfunction in patients with TRD compared to unselected depressed populations (Howland, 1993). Hypothalamic–pituitary–adrenocortical axis dysfunction

**Table 2.3.** Common medical contributors to TRD

Endocrinopathies
   Thyroid disease
   Hypercortisolism (Cushing's syndrome)
Infectious
   Postviral syndromes (Epstein–Barr, Cytomegalovirus, influenza)
   Human Immunodeficiency Virus
   Tuberculosis
   Syphilis
   Borreliosis (Lyme disease)
Neoplastic syndromes
Neurologic
   Poststroke
   Parkinson's disease
   Sleep disorders
   Autoimmune diseases (SLE, MS)

with elevated cortisol is also frequently reported in depression followed by normalization of the axis after remission of depression (Gold et al., 1986, 1988). Moreover, Reus and Berlant (Reus & Berlant, 1986) estimated that 40–90% of patients with Cushing's syndrome will manifest affective disturbances – in particular, depression. Neurological disorders, both cortical and subcortical, have been associated with depression. An important cortical cause is poststroke depression, where vulnerability to depression seems to correlate with proximity of the lesion to the anterior part of the left hemisphere (Cumming, 1994). In some clinical situations the onset of depression may be a harbinger of a malignant process, as with pancreatic cancer where up to two-thirds of patients experience psychiatric symptoms prior to local symptoms of the tumor (Green & Austin, 1993).

## Psychiatric comorbidity considerations in TRD

Many studies have reported the association between the presence of comorbid psychiatric conditions and TRD (Coryell et al., 1988; Pfohl et al., 1984; Black et al., 1988; Fawcett & Kravitz, 1988). It is often unclear clinically which came first. Nevertheless the implications for treatment are to address both conditions simultaneously, regardless of the linkage in order to avoid consolidating a TRD condition.

Comorbid anxiety and depressive features are common in clinical practice, and anxiety disorders may increase the likelihood of a major depression eventuating in

TRD. For example, a prospective study of depressed patients found that panic attacks was correlated with a poor outcome (Coryell et al., 1988). There is some evidence that such patients do better with MAOIs. Likewise depressed patients with obsessive compulsive disorder may be more resistant to treatment, even with serotonin specific reuptake inhibitors (SSRIs) (Hollander et al., 1991).

Similarly, covert substance abuse is also common in depression (Akiskal, 1982; MacEwan & Remick, 1988) and a leading cause of TRD. Not only does comorbid substance abuse lead to TRD, with alcohol abuse, the presence of resulting hepatic disease alters antidepressant pharmacokinetics making these patients more difficult to treat (Ciraulo & Jaffe, 1981; Ciraulo et al., 1988; Mason & Kocsis, 1991). Comorbid personality disorders have long been associated with TRD and a poor response to antidepressant treatment. For example, Pfohl et al. (1984) observed only a 16% response rate in inpatients with comorbid depression and personality disorder compared to a 50% response rate in patients with pure depression. Similar results were reported by Black et al. (1988), where, with use of ECT in addition to a TCA, the response rate amongst those with a comorbid Axis II disorder was lower, 42% compared to a 60% recovery in those without Axis II pathology.

## Identifying 'pseudo-TRD'

Once medical and comorbid psychiatric factors have been addressed, the next task of the clinician is to review the adequacy of treatment to date and so separate 'pseudo-TRD' patients from those with true TRD. As indicated in Table 2.2, at each level of treatment resistance, it is required that an 'adequate' trial of an antidepressant be given. Less than optimal treatment must be considered to be at stage 0 of treatment resistance. This raises the critical question of how one defines an 'adequate' trial of treatment and is the basis of determining when a true or valid level of treatment resistance has been attained. Failure to provide 'adequate' treatment represents 'pseudo-TRD', where the patient is perhaps referred as a case of TRD but, on systematic clinical data gathering, it transpires that no objectively adequate treatment course was administered. In such cases, the patient is prematurely labeled as treatment resistant.

In the past, 'pseudo-TRD' has been confused with true TRD. At the World Psychiatric Association Symposium on Treatment Resistant Depression in 1974, it was proposed that the definition of TRD be divided into two categories: absolute and relative TRD. Absolute resistance was defined as a failure to respond to one adequate antidepressant trial, defined as at least 4 weeks of imipramine at 150 mg/day (or its equivalent); while relative treatment resistance was applied to patients who failed to respond to a less than adequate antidepressant trial

(Heiman, 1974). The latter definition is spurious as a patient's depression can only be considered resistant to treatment when an adequate antidepressant treatment has been administered and until such time is better categorized as 'pseudo-TRD' (Stage 0).

## Criteria for adequacy of antidepressant treatment

There is strong evidence suggesting that up to 60% of depressed patients initially classified as TRD fall into the category of 'pseudo-TRD', namely Stage 0. For instance, one study in the pre-SSRI era of 110 patients referred with TRD found that only a minority of antidepressant trials (40%) was judged to be adequate (Schatzberg et al., 1983). A clear majority of antidepressant treatments were inadequate and failed to meet minimal therapeutic requirements. In only a proportion (20%) did the treatment failure appear to be due to intolerance to the medication. Other factors such as undue conservatism in the upward titration of dose or failure to assure adequate plasma drug concentrations appeared to be more critical. In this regard community based surveys have revealed that less than 50% of patients actually receive either an adequate dosage or duration of antidepressant treatment (Nelson & Dunner, 1993). Moreover, this figure does not take into account the known high non-compliance rate for taking medication as prescribed. While the prescribing ease and safety of the SSRIs has been demonstrated and has resulted in more adequate antidepressant dosing strategies with greater patient compliance and tolerance, the overall percentage of patients with 'pseudo' and true TRD has not substantially diminished. As a result, the approach to a case of TRD has not dramatically changed with the introduction of the SSRIs.

The two major factors to be reviewed in determining trial adequacy are medication dosing and trial duration. Table 2.4 furnishes a suggested guide to 'adequacy' of dose and therapy duration.

With respect to dosing it appears that many depressed patients may actually receive an inadequate dose of antidepressant medication. Given that there is a 30-fold range of drug metabolism among individuals taking antidepressant medications it is not uncommon that at least some patients who fail to respond to antidepressant therapy may do so as a result of less than optimal plasma drug concentrations. For some antidepressants, a plasma level–clinical response relationship has been defined, and drug efficacy may be correlated with the presence of 'adequate' antidepressant plasma levels (Schweizer et al., 1990). Faced with an inadequate treatment response Table 2.4 furnishes a guideline for adequate dosing (and plasma levels).

Inadequacy of treatment duration is probably a common, although rarely recognized, cause of 'pseudo-TRD'. The commonly held concept that a 4- to

**Table 2.4.** Adequacy of antidepressant trials

|  | Definite (>8 weeks) | | Probable (>4 and <8 weeks) |
|---|---|---|---|
|  | Dose (mg) | Plasma level | Dose (mg) |
| Imipramine | ⩾ 250 | ⩾ 180 ng/ml | ⩾ 150, ⩽ 250 |
| Desipramine | ⩾ 200 | ⩾ 150 ng/ml | ⩾ 150, ⩽ 250 |
| Nortriptyline | ⩾ 100 | 50–150 ng/ml | ⩾ 50, ⩽ 100 |
| Amitriptyline | ⩾ 250 | ⩾ 180 ng/ml | ⩾ 150, ⩽ 250 |
| Doxepin | ⩾ 250 | ⩾ 180 ng/ml | ⩾ 150, ⩽ 250 |
| Prtotriptyline | ⩾ 40 | — | ⩾ 20, ⩽ 40 |
| Clomipramine | ⩾ 250 | — | ⩾ 150, ⩽ 250 |
| Trimipramine | ⩾ 200 | — | ⩾ 150, ⩽ 250 |
| Maprotiline | ⩾ 250 | — | ⩾ 150, ⩽ 250 |
| Phenelzine | ⩾ 60 | — | ⩾ 45, ⩽ 60 |
| Tranylcypromine | ⩾ 40 | — | ⩾ 20, ⩽ 40 |
| Trazodone | ⩾ 450 | — | ⩾ 250, ⩽ 450 |
| Fluoxetine | ⩾ 20 | — | ⩾ 10, ⩽ 20 |
| Sertraline | ⩾ 200 | — | ⩾ 10, ⩽ 20 |
| Paroxetine | ⩾ 40 | — | ⩾ 20, ⩽ 40 |
| Venlafaxine | ⩾ 300 | — | ⩾ 150, ⩽ 300 |
| Bupropion | ⩾ 400 | — | ⩾ 250, ⩽ 400 |
| Mirtazapine | ⩾ 45 | — | > 15, < 45 |

6-week medication trial is probably inadequate for many patients. In this regard one study (Georgotas et al., 1987) has reported that the mean time to clinical response for patients treated with nortriptyline was almost 6 weeks, and that patients with more severe depressive illness took even longer to respond. Similarly, another study by Greenhouse et al. (1987) observed a substantial increase in the rate of remission as patients continued to take imipramine (at adequate doses and plasma levels) beyond 4 weeks of treatment. At 4 weeks of therapy the remission rate was only 25%; but this rate rose to 50% by 3 months and increased to 89% at 6 months of therapy. With respect to fluoxetine, there are somewhat analogous findings. One study by Schweizer et al. (1990) has shown that there was no significant difference in response rates if non-responders to fluoxetine at 3 weeks were randomized to either fluoxetine 20 mg/day or 60 mg/day for a further 5 weeks (response rates of 49% vs. 50%, respectively). This indicates that, at least in the first 8 weeks of treatment with fluoxetine, 'tincture of time' may be more important than dosage increase.

## Managing TRD

Treatment of true TRD should entail a dual approach in which the clinician pursues a systematic comprehensive treatment algorithm whereby treatment is optimized and comorbid illness and other factors producing non-response are identified and corrected.

### Optimizing existing treatment

Many TRD patients come for consultation with an established, although ineffective, antidepressant treatment. The first step in treating TRD is to ensure that each medication trial is adequate. With the TCAs, individual pharmacokinetic factors should be taken into account by measuring TCA blood levels. There is a wide interindividual variation in hepatic metabolism and it not unusual to find that a patient who is on TCA dosages at the top end of the recommended range may be unresponsive to the TCA due to plasma levels that are barely therapeutic (Amsterdam et al., 1980). In TRD patients taking TCAs, plasma drug levels can be used to assess (i) compliance with dosing; (ii) attainment of threshold plasma levels; and (iii) as a guide to maximizing and optimizing dosage by assuring the presence of 'adequate' blood levels. For tertiary amine TCAs, like imipramine, the dose–response curve appears to be linear such that the goal is to get the plasma level to at least the threshold level, whereas with a secondary amine like nortriptyline the dose response curve is curvilinear with a therapeutic window plasma level of 50–150 ng/ml, whereby optimal clinical response appears to occur within the therapeutic window. Once the adequacy of dose and treatment duration has been administered, and comorbid illness excluded, the clinician may consider more aggressive treatment approaches if TRD persists.

### Switching strategies

For some patients with TRD switching from one antidepressant to another antidepressant from another drug class may often be more attractive than augmentation with lithium, thyroid hormones or another antidepressant. Switching between drugs can be simpler with less risk of drug–drug interactions.

#### After an SSRI treatment failure

Should the clinician consider switching from a failed SSRI treatment to a second SSRI or is it best to switch out of the class to either a 'novel' agent (like bupropion, nefazodone, mirtazapine or venlafaxine) or a TCA? In two recent studies at least, it appears there is a reasonable chance of patients responding to a second SSRI after an initial SSRI failure (Joffe et al., 1996; Zarate et al., 1996). When patients truly resistant to the first SSRI are considered, and patients simply intolerant excluded, the response rate is about 50%. In contrast, success with switching out of the class to a TCA may be a little better with a response rate of 73% in one crossover study (Peselow et al., 1989). There is no comparable systematic data yet with venlafaxine or other 'novel' agents. In conclusion, the jury is still out on what is the optimal strategy for patients who demonstrate TRD to an adequate SSRI therapy.

### Switching after a TCA treatment failure

Switching within the class from secondary amines (nortriptyline, desipramine, and protriptyline) to tertiary amine TCAs (such as imipramine, amitriptyline, clomipramine) may be a reasonable consideration in TCA failures. This could be of importance in patient management when TCA plasma levels are utilized. A patient who has failed to respond to an adequate duration or dose of nortryptiline may respond when switched to one of the tertiary amines with a linear dose–response relationship (Asberg, 1976). In addition, there is some uncontrolled data suggesting that patients who have not achieved an adequate response with a TCA might improve with clomipramine – an 'atypical' TCA with potent norepinephrine and serotonin blockade (Hale et al., 1987).

In contrast to the above within class strategies, there may also be merit in switching out of the class to another antidepressant class. There is a substantial literature on the efficacy of switching from a failed TCA treatment to MAOIs in certain subtypes of TRD. For instance, in atypical depression (patients with reactive mood and reversed neurovegetative features), a number of studies have shown superiority of phenelzine over imipramine (Quitkin et al., 1993). Switching from a failed TCA treatment to an SSRI may also be effective with a response rate in one study of 65% (Thase et al., 1995). There are also promising results with the use of venlafaxine in the setting of prior treatment failures. In one noteworthy study by Nierenberg et al. (1994) in TRD patients who had failed a minimum of three prior adequate treatments, one of which had to be a TCA, the response rate at 12 weeks to venlafaxine, at an average dose of 250mg, was 40%. While, as yet there are no systematic studies in TRD with other 'novel' agents, some clinicians do advocate switching between novel classes in their patients with TRD.

### Augmentation strategies

In contrast to switching, another strategy is to add an additional medication to the existing drug regiment as an augmentation strategy. In this fashion, the clinician seeks a synergistic interaction between agents such that the therapeutic some of the whole is greater than the parts. A range of augmentation options is available including lithium, T3, buspirone and pindolol among others. The most commonly studied augmentation strategy is the addition of lithium. Use of lithium to augment TCAs has been shown to be effective with an average response rate of 50–60% (Thase & Rush, 1995). However, the latency of the synergistic response is variable and has been reported to be as short as 48 hours in the original report to a more consistent range of 2 to 6 weeks in the work since then (Thase & Rush, 1995). It should be emphasized that lithium addition needs to be optimized with a lithium level of at least 0.6 mmol/l. With the advent of the SSRIs, many clinicians have utilized lithium augmentation in TRD. At least one study has shown benefit from lithium augmentation of fluoxetine (Fontaine et al., 1991), while another has found a similar response with fluvoxamine (Delgado et al., 1988), implying that even with the SSRIs there is room for further enhancement of serotonergic transmission.

Another augmentation strategy that has received widespread attention is the addition of either thyroxine (T4) or triiodothyronine (T3). Thyroid augmentation overall does not appear to be quite as effective as lithium with a response range of 25 to 60% (Thase & Rush, 1995). T3 appears to be much more effective than T4 (53% response rate vs. 19%). Some data (Targum et al., 1984) suggest that benefit from thyroid augmentation is limited to a subgroup of depressives with subclinical thyroid hypoactivity as reflected in abnormal TRH test results (an exaggerated TSH rise in response to TRH).

Pindolol and buspirone both seem to work through effects on blocking the serotonin 1A autoreceptors, which may exert a powerful feedback effect on shutting down further serotonin presynaptic release. Two uncontrolled studies have shown efficacy for buspirone augmentation of a failed SSRI trial (Bouwer & Stein, 1997; Joffe & Schuller, 1993). Pindolol has, so far, been used more in a combination fashion, with pindolol initiated at the same time as standard therapy rather than added on in the face of non-response. There is some evidence that this approach may be effective for some patients with TRD (Blier & Bergeron, 1996).

## Treatment matching

Finally, it is important for the clinician to take into account subtypes of TRD. In the setting of psychotic depression, an adequate trial of a combination of neuroleptic and antidepressant together is essential before one can deduce evidence of TRD, as the addition of a neuroleptic significantly enhances the therapeutic response (Spiker et al., 1985). In atypical depression there is good evidence for the superiority of MAOIs over TCAs (Quitkin et al., 1993). Interestingly, a recent study (Pande et al., 1996) showed equal efficacy between fluoxetine and phenelzine in atypical depression, suggesting that SSRIs may also have the advantage over TCAs in this clinical setting. In bipolar depression, some investigators have recommended that TCAs be avoided because of the risk of inducing treatment resistance and a rapid cycling course (Wehr & Goodwin, 1987). Others have suggested that bupropion may be more effective in bipolar TRD with less likelihood of inducing mood elevation (Sachs et al., 1994), but the evidence for this is still somewhat limited (Fogelson et al., 1992).

### ECT treatment

In the view of many, ECT remains an essential treatment option in TRD. Early uncontrolled studies implied that the presence of TRD had little impact on reducing the likely therapeutic benefit of ECT with response rates even in this population ranging from 61% to 88% (Mandel et al., 1977; Paul et al., 1981). However, these earlier studies were retrospective and the criteria for medication resistance were inadequate. More recent studies indicate that the presence of TRD reduces the response rate to 50% (Prudic et al., 1994). There is an emerging consensus at this juncture that up to 12 treatments must be provided in the setting of TRD for a course to be judged adequate. Given the work which has shown that unilateral treatment close to the seizure threshold may be ineffective (Sackeim et al., 1991) it is important that stimulus parameters be increased during the course of treatment, as ECT itself causes the seizure threshold to rise. Decline in duration of the seizure duration on the EEG tracing (below a norm of 25 seconds), or for that matter in the quality of the seizure as reflected in the amplitude and symmetry of the slow waves on the EEG (reflecting poor seizure generalization across the hemispheres), should trigger an increase in parameters. In the face of an inadequate clinical response by six unilateral treatments, a switch to bilateral treatments should be considered. In the future, other modalities of direct brain stimulation to treat TRD, namely transcranial magnetic stimulation (TMS) may become generally available. With TMS, a powerful magnetic coil is used to stimulate a localized region of the brain rather than the whole brain, usually the left prefrontal cortex, and without inducing a seizure such that side effects can be kept to a minimum. Specifically there is no cognitive impairment, and no general anesthesia or muscle relaxation are required to manage the seizure. Such ease of use would be quite attractive to clinicians and patients. However, the promising results from an earlier study in patients with TRD, with marked improvement in 11 out of 17 patient with TRD after 5 days' treatment (Pascual-Leone et al., 1996) have yet to be replicated and the future place of this modality in treating depression yet to be determined.

## Conclusions

In conclusion, our approach to TRD is to apply systematic algorithms in such a fashion as to assure adequacy of diagnosis and treatment. In this framework we suggest careful data gathering and clinical detective work to make a valid diagnosis of true TRD and the identification of comorbid medical and psychiatric conditions. In addition, using systematic treatment algorithms will ensure that the specific depression subtype is matched with the most likely effective treatment. Finally, a careful consideration and pursuit of all treatment options at each stage of TRD with ongoing diagnostic reevaluation will permit the clinician to handle the difficult syndrome of TRD more effectively.

## REFERENCES

Akiskal, H.S.(1982). Factors associated with incomplete recovery in primary depressive illness. *Journal of Clinical Psychiatry*, **43**, 266–71.

American Psychiatric Association (1994). *Diagnostic and Statistical Manual of Mental Disorders (DSM-IV)*, pp. 377–8. Washington, DC: APA.

Amsterdam, J.D. & Berwish, N. (1987). Treatment of refractory depression with combination reserpine and tricyclic antidepressant therapy. *Journal of Clinical Psychopharmacology*, **7**, 238–42.

Amsterdam, J.D., Brunswick, D.J., & Mendels, J. (1980). The clinical application of tricyclic antidepressant pharmacokinetics and plasma levels. *American Journal of Psychiatry*, **137**, 653–62.

Asberg, M. (1976). Treatment of depression with tricyclic drugs – pharmacokinetic and pharmacodynamic aspects. *Pharmacopsychiatry and Neuropsychopharmacology*, **9**, 18–26.

Black, D.W., Bell, S., Hulbert, J. et al. (1988). The importance of axis II in patients with major depression. *Journal of Affective Disorders*, **14**, 115–22.

Blier, P. & Bergeron, R. (1996). Effectiveness of pindolol with selected antidepressant drugs in the treatment of major depression. *Journal of Clinical Psychopharmacology*, **15**, 217–22.

Bouwer, C. & Stein, D.J. (1997). Buspirone is an effective augmenting agent of serotonin selective re-uptake inhibitors in severe treatment-refractory depression. *South Africa Medical Journal*, **87**(4 Suppl.), 534–7.

Cassano, G.B., Maggini, C., & Akiskal, H. (1983). Short-term sub-chronic and chronic sequelae of affective disorders. *Psychiatry Clinics of North America*, **6**, 55–68.

Ciraulo, D.A. & Jaffe, J.H. (1981). Tricyclic antidepressants in the treatment of depression associated with alcoholism. *Journal of Clinical Psychopharmacology*, **1**, 146.

Ciraulo, D.A., Barnhill, J.G., & Jaffe, J.H. (1988). Clinical pharmacokinetics of imipramine and desipramine in alcoholics and normal volunteers. *Clinical Pharmacology Therapy*, **43**, 535–8.

Coryell, W., Endicott, J., Andreasen, N.C. et al. (1988). Depression and panic attacks: the significance of overlap as reflected in follow-up and family study data. *American Journal of Psychiatry*, **145**, 293–300.

Cumming, J.L. (1994). Depression in neurologic diseases. *Psychiatry Annals*, **24**, 525–31.

Delgado, P.L., Price, L.H., Charney, D.S. et al. (1988). Efficacy of fluvoxamine in treatment refractory depression. *Journal of Affective Disorders*, **15**, 55–60.

Fawcett, J. (1994). Progress in treatment-resistant and treatment-refractory depression: we still have a long way to go. *Journal of Clinical Psychiatry*, **24**, 214–16.

Fawcett, J. & Kravitz, K.M. (1988). Anxiety syndromes and their relationship to depressive illness. *Journal of Clinical Psychiatry*, **44**, 8–11.

Fogelson, D.L., Bystritsky, A., & Pasnau, R. (1992). Bupropion in the treatment of bipolar disorders: the same old story? *Journal of Clinical Psychiatry*, **53**, 443–6.

Fontaine, R., Ontiveros, A., Elie, R. et al. (1991). Lithium carbonate augmentation of desipramine and fluoxetine in refractory depression. *Biological Psychiatry*, **29**, 946–8.

Gadde, K.M. & Krishnan, K.R.R. (1994). Endocrine factors in depression. *Psychiatry Annals*, **24**, 521–4.

Georgotas, A., McCue, R.E., Friedman, E. et al. (1987). The response of depressive symptoms to nortriptyline, phenelzine, and placebo. *British Journal of Psychiatry*, **151**, 102–6.

Gold, M.S., Potash, A.L.C., & Extein, I. (1981). Hypothyroidism in depression: evidence from complete thyroid function evaluation. *Journal of the American Medical Association*, **245**, 1919–22.

Gold, P.W., Loriaux, D.L., Roy, et al. (1986). Responses to corticotropin releasing hormone in the hypercortisolim of depression and Cushing's disease: pathophysiologic and diagnosis implications. *New England Journal of Medicine*, **314**, 1329–35.

Gold, P.W., Goodwin, F.K., & Chrousos, G.P. (1988). Clinical and biochemical manifestations of depression: relation to the neurobiology of stress. Part II. *New England Journal of Medicine*, **319**, 413–20.

Gorman, J.M. & Hatterer, J.A. (1994). The role of thyroid hormone in refractory depression. In *Refractory Depression: Current Strategies and Future Directions*, ed. W.A. Nolen, J. Zohar, S.P. Roose, & J.D. Amsterdam, pp. 121–8. Chichester: John Wiley.

Green, A.I. & Austin, C.P. (1993). Psychopathology of pancreatic cancer: a psychophysiologic probe. *Psychosomatics*, **34**, 208–21.

Greenhouse, J.B., Kupfer, D.J., Frank, E. et al. (1987). Analysis of time to stabilization in the treatment of depression: Biological and clinical correlates. *Journal of Affective Disorders*, **13**, 259–66.

Hale, A.S., Procter, A.W., & Bridges, P.K. (1987). Clomipramine, tryptophan and lithium in combination for resistant endogenous depression: seven case studies. *British Journal of Psychiatry*, **151**, 213–17.

Hall, R.C., Gardner, E.R., Popkin, et al. (1981). Unrecognized physical illness prompting psychiatric admission: a prospective study. *American Journal of Psychiatry*, **138**, 629–35.

Heiman, H. (1974). Therapy resistant depressions: symptoms and syndromes. *Pharmakopsychiatry and Neuropsychopharmacology*, **7**, 156–63.

Hollander, E., Mullen, L., DeCaria, C.M. et al. (1991). Obsessive compulsive disorder, depression, and fluoxetine. *Journal of Clinical Psychiatry*, **52**, 418–22.

Howland, R.H. (1993). Thyroid dysfunction in refractory depression: implications for pathophysiology and treatment. *Journal of Clinical Psychiatry*, **54**, 47–54.

Jain, V.K. (1972). A psychiatric study of hypothyroidism. *Psychiatric Clinics of North America*, **5**, 121–30.

Joffe, R.T. & Levitt, A.J. (1992). Major depression and subclinical (Grade II) hypothyroidism. *Psychoneuroendocrinology*, **17**, 215–21.

Joffe, R.T. & Schuller, D.R. (1993). An open study of buspirone augmentation of serotonin reuptake inhibitors in refractory depression. *Journal of Clinical Psychiatry*, **54**, 269–71.

Joffe, R.T., Levitt, A.J., Sokolov, S.T.H. et al. (1996). Response to an open trial of a second SSRI in major depression. *Journal of Clinical Psychiatry*, **57**, 114–15.

Keller, M.B., Lavori, P.W., Mueller, T.I. et al. (1992). Time to recovery, chronicity, and levels of psychopathology in major depression – a 5-year prospective follow up. *Archives of General Psychiatry*, **49**, 809–16.

MacEwan, W.G. & Remick, R.A. (1988). Treatment resistant depression: a clinical perspective. *Canadian Journal of Psychiatry*, **33**, 788–92.

Malizia, A.L. & Bridges, P.K. (1992). The management of treatment resistant affective disorder: clinical perspectives. *Journal of Psychopharmacology*, **6**, 145–55.

Mandel, M.R., Welch, C.A., Mieske, M. et al. (1977). Prediction of response to ECT in tricyclic-intolerant or tricyclic resistant depressed patients. *McLean Hospital Journal*, **4**, 203–9.

Mason, B.J. & Kocsis, M.D. (1991). Desipramine treatment of alcoholism. *Psychopharmacology Bulletin*, **27**, 155–61.

Metzger, E.D. & Friedman, R.S. (1994). Treatment-related depression. *Psychiatry Annals*, **24**, 540–4.

Nelsen, M.R. & Dunner, D.L. (1993). Treatment resistance in unipolar depression and other disorders: diagnostic concerns and treatment possibilities. *Psychiatry Clinics of North America*, **16**, 541–66.

Nierenberg, A.A., Feighner, J.P., Rudolph, R. et al. (1994). Venlafaxine for treatment-resistant unipolar depresssion. *Journal of Clinical Psychopharmacology*, **6**, 419–23.

Pande, A.C., Birkett, M., Fechner-Bates, S. et al. (1996). Fluoxetine versus phenelzine in atypical depression. *Biological Psychiatry*, **40**, 1017–20.

Pascual-Leone, A., Rubio, B., Pallardo, F. et al. (1996). Rapid rate transcranial magnetic stimulation of left dorsolateral prefrontal cortex in drug resistant depression. *Lancet*, **348**, 233–7.

Paul, S.M., Extein, I., Calil, H.M. et al. (1981). Use of ECT with treatment-resistant depressed patients at the National Institute of Mental Health. *American Journal of Psychiatry*, **138**, 486–9.

Peselow, E.D., Fillippi, A.M., Goodnick, P. et al. (1989). The short and long-term efficacy of Paroxetine HCL: Data from a double-blind crossover and from a year long trial vs. imipramine and placebo. *Psychopharmacology Bulletin*, **25**, 272–6.

Pfohl, B., Stangl, D., & Zimmerman, M. (1984). The implications of DSM-III personality disorders for patients with major depression. *Journal of Affective Disorders*, **7**, 309–18.

Prange, A.J., Mason, G.A., & Garbutt, J.C. (1990). Thyroid axis syndromes in depression: definitions and interpretations. In *Pharmacotherapy of Depression: Applications for the Outpatient Practitioner*, ed. J.D. Amsterdam, pp. 35–55. New York: Marcel Decker, Inc.

Prudic, J.M., Sackeim, H.A., & Rifas, S. (1994). Medication resistance, response to ECT, and prevention of relapse. *Psychiatry Annals*, **24**, 228–31.

Quitkin, F.M., Stewart, J.W., McGrath, P.J. et al. (1993). A subgroup of depressives with better response to MAOI than to tricyclic antidepressants or placebo. *British Journal of Psychiatry*, **163** (Suppl. 21) 30–4.

Reus, V.I. & Berlant, J.R. (1986). Behavioral disturbances associated with disorders of the hypothalamic–pituitary–adrenal system. In *Medical Memics of Psychiatric Disorders*, ed. I. Extein & M.S. Gols, pp. 111–30. Washington, DC: American Psychiatry Press.

Roose, S.P., Glassman, A.H., Walsh, B.T. et al. (1986). Tricyclic nonresponders: phenomenology and treatment. *American Journal of Psychiatry*, **143**, 345–8.

Sachs, G.S., Lafer, B., Stoll, A.L. et al. (1994). A double blind trial of bupropion versus desipramine for bipolar depression. *Journal of Clinical Psychiatry*, **55**, 391–3.

Sackeim, H.A., Devanand, D.P., & Prudic, J. (1991). Stimulus intensity, seizure threshold, and seizure duration: impact on the efficacy and safety of electroconvulsive therapy. *Psychiatric Clinics of North America*, **14**(4).

Schatzberg, A.F., Cole, J.O., Cohen, B.M. et al. (1983). Survey of depressed patients who have failed to respond to treatment. In *The Affective Disorders*, ed. J.M. Davis & J.W. Maas, pp. 73–85. Washington, DC: American Psychiatric Press.

Schweizer, E., Rickels, K., Amsterdam, J.D. et al. (1990). What constitutes an adequate antidepressant trial of fluoxetine? *Journal of Clinical Psychiatry*, **51**, 8–11.

Spiker, D.G., Weiss, J.C., Dealy, R.S. et al. (1985). The pharmacological treatment of delusional depression. *American Journal of Psychiatry*, **142**, 430–6.

Targum, S.D., Greenberg, R.D., Harmon, R.L. et al. (1984). Thyroid hormone and the TRH stimulation test in refractory depression. *Journal of Clinical Psychiatry*, **45**, 345–6.

Thase, M.E. & Kupfer, D.J. (1987). Characteristics of treatment-resistant depression. In *Treating Resistant Depression*, ed. J. Zohar & R.H. Belmaker, pp. 23–45. New York: PMA Publishing.

Thase, M.E. & Rush, J.A. (1995). Treatment-resistant depression. In *Psychopharmacology: The Fourth Generation of Progress*, ed. F.E. Bloom & D.J. Kupfer, pp. 1081–97. New York: Raven Press.

Thase, M.E., Keller, M.B., Gelenberg, A.J. et al. (1995). Double blind crossover antidepressant study: sertraline versus imipramine. *Psychopharmacology Bulletin*, **31**, 535.

Thase, M.E., Rush, A.J., Kasper, S. et al. (2000). Tricyclics and newer antidepressant medications: treatment options for treatment resistant depressions. *Depression* (in press).

Wehr, T.A. & Goodwin, F.K. (1987). Can antidepressants cause mania and worsen the course of affective illness? *American Journal of Psychiatry*, **144**, 1403–11.

Zarate, C.A. Jr, Kando, J.C., Tohen, M. et al. (1996). Does intolerance or lack of response with fluoxetine predict the same will happen with sertraline. *Journal of Clinical Psychiatry*, **57**, 67–71.

# Part II

## Biological basis

# 3

# Psychoneuroendocrine aspects of treatment-resistant mood disorders

Owen M. Wolkowitz and Victor I. Reus

## Introduction

Recent advances in our understanding of hormone action in the brain, coupled with growing evidence of hormonal dysregulation in affective disorders, have prompted the use of hormones and hormone antagonists as endocrinologically based treatments of depression. Since hormonally based treatments presumably act at sites distinct from those of traditional antidepressants, they may specifically benefit patients unresponsive to the latter drugs. Clinical applications of psychoneuroendocrinology are largely in their infancy, but certain strategies have already entered clinical practice and others appear promising. The following selective review begins with the more well-established hormonal therapies for treatment-resistant depression and concludes with less well-studied, but nonetheless biologically informed ones.

## Thyroid

Although interest in the role of thyroid hormones in the biology of mood disorders is longstanding, the prevalence of abnormalities and their pathophysiologic significance remains controversial (Fava et al., 1995; Howland, 1995). Some, but not all, investigators have found a higher rate of elevations in total $T_4$ and $FT_4$ in the depressed population than in controls (Joffe & Sokolov, 1994; Nader et al., 1995; Scherer, 1994). Alterations in $T_3$ level and an increased prevalence of antithyroid antibodies have also been reported (Reus & Freimer, 1990), as have low levels of CSF transthyretin (Sullivan et al., 1999). Frank hypothyroidism is rarely found upon routine screening of patients with major depression, but subtle alterations in basal TSH and TSH response to TRH infusion are quite common (Bunevicius et al., 1994, 1996). Overall, 7 to 10% of depressed patients appear to have subclinical hypothyroidism as defined by an elevated basal TSH or an augmented TSH response to TRH (Reus, 1993), while approximately one-quarter of depressed patients have a blunted TSH response to TRH, the meaning of which remains unclear. Serum TSH level in the upper quarter of the reference range may also serve as an indicator of severity of major depression (Berlin et al, 1999). In patients who have been treated for hyperthyroidism, as many as one-third will continue to experience significant symptoms of depression and anxiety even after achieving euthyroid status (Fahrenfort et al., 2000).

A few case series have suggested that such abnormalities are predictive of poor treatment response, while others have found no such relationship (Joffe, 1999). Gewirtz et al. (1988), for example, found an underlying thyroid disorder in approximately 40% of treatment-resistant patients studied, while Joffe and Levitt (1992) reported a response rate of 16% in patients with subclinical hypothyroidism as opposed to 54% rate in patients who had a normal basal TSH level. Subclinical hypothyroidism most commonly arises as a result of autoimmune thyroiditis, a condition affecting approximately 5% of the general population, and as many as 15 to 20% of women over the age of 60 (Reus, 1989). Because, by definition, subclinical hypothyroidism, euthyroid sick syndrome, and subclinical hyperthyroidism are relatively benign conditions, the issue as to whether such individuals should be given thyroid replacement or other specific treatment remains controversial (Utiger, 1995; Schlote et al., 1992). In the endocrinological literature some investigators have found that complaints of fatigue, malaise, and loss of energy respond to L-thyroxine replacement, suggesting that in patients with major depression who present with an elevation in basal TSH, replacement with $T_4$ is empirically indicated (Lindsay & Toft, 1997). Whether the hormonal supplement will be sufficient in ameliorating the mood complaints or whether adjunctive treatment with an antidepressant is necessary, remains unknown at present.

The majority of thyroid disorders are autoimmune in origin and may evade identification until cellular destruction and apoptosis progress to a critical stage (Baker, 1992; Champion et al., 1992; Williams, 1997). This is a process that may take many years, but the ongoing immune alterations themselves may affect behavior and treatment response independent of peripheral thyroid status (Malek-Ahmadi, 1996). The molecular basis of thyroid hormone action is, however, increasingly understood and has helped to guide current recommendations on thyroxine therapy (for extensive reviews, see Toft, 1994, Brent, 1994 and Spitzweg et al., 2000).

## Effect of antidepressant treatments on thyroid hormones

Central noradrenergic neurons influence pituitary–thyroid regulation and, in turn, are affected by thyroid status (Cardinali et al., 1986). It is not surprising, therefore, that changes in thyroid hormone have been correlated with alterations in clinical state, or that antidepressant treatments affect thyroid parameters.

Southwick et al. (1989) found that changes in $FT_4$ and total $T_4$ levels within the normal range had clinical significance, and that movement from either high or low initial levels towards the mid range was associated with good recovery during standard antidepressant treatment. Animal studies (Martin et al., 1987) have indicated that the beneficial response to antidepressants in a behavioral despair paradigm is markedly attenuated in hypothyroid rats and significantly hastened in euthyroid rats given adjunctive $T_3$. Hypothyroidism has been found to depress metabolism in limbic forebrain, and limbic brainstem relay nuclei in rats (Dow-Edwards et al., 1988), a finding consistent with a recent positron emission tomography study of cortical blood flow in medication-free patients with major depression (Marangell et al., 1997b). In this latter report peripheral TSH, the best marker of thyroid status, was found to be inversely related to global and regional cortical blood flow and cerebral glucose metabolism. Although this suggests that the relationship between thyroid states and cerebral activity could be of clinical importance, the findings reported thus far of the specific effects of antidepressant medications on thyroid hormones remain difficult to integrate. In the animal studies reported, tricyclic antidepressants have been reported to decrease brain $T_3$ (Massol et al., 1990; Dow-Edwards et al., 1988) or have no effect on brain $T_3$ (Joffe et al., 1993). The latter group reported a significant decrease in plasma $T_4$ while others have found a significant enhancement of brain 5' II-D enzyme activity in hippocampus (Campos-Barros & Baumgartner, 1994). Chronic desipramine treatment has also been shown to upregulate the alpha-2 adrenoreceptors which modulate TSH secretion (Jaffer et al., 1987), while having no specific effect on brain TRH concentration (Przegalinski & Jaworska, 1990). In humans, baseline free thyroxine index and baseline TSH do decrease after desipramine treatment, suggesting a down regulation of the thyroid axis at the hypothalamic level (Brady & Anton, 1989). A similar decrease in FTI, $T_4$, and $T_3$ occurs with imipramine, the changes in thyroid indices being significantly correlated with parallel improvements in behavioral ratings of depression and global change, but not with serotonergic antidepressants such as fluvoxamine (Brady et al., 1994). In contrast, Shelton et al. (1993) reported that desipramine caused a small but significant increase in total $T_4$ over 6 weeks while fluoxetine, but not desipramine, caused a decline in $T_3$ levels. Other groups have linked a reduction in total $T_4$, after treatment with either maprotiline or fluvoxamine, with a reduction in body temperature, and with an increase in plasma TSH, but have been unable to link such alterations to differences in treatment response (Höflich et al., 1992). In contrast again, Duval and colleagues (1996) were able to relate reductions in $FT_4$ and $FT_3$ and increases in plasma TSH to beneficial response over time, but were unable to link the change to the direct effect of a specific antidepressant.

Other classes of antidepressants have also been examined. In rats, the increase in wheel running induced by monoamine oxidase inhibitor treatment was attenuated in hypothyroid relative to euthyroid rats (Duncan & Schull, 1994), while in humans, short-term phenelzine treatment was not found to be associated with any significant alteration in plasma thyroid hormone level (Joffe & Singer, 1987). Carbamazepine has been shown to decrease $T_4$ significantly over the course of treatment, but not to alter resting metabolic rate (Herman et al., 1991). Haloperidol induces a significant rise in TSH (Magliozzi et al., 1989) and trifluoperazine, an inhibition of TRH secretion (Fleckman et al., 1981).

The effects of electroconvulsive therapy (ECT) on thyroid function parameters have been less well studied, and the results reported thus far are conflicting. ECT was found to increase TSH in one series (Taubøll et al., 1987), while decrease it in another cohort (Nerozzi et al., 1987). No change in $T_4$ was found by Taubøll et al. (1987), but a significant drop in free thyroxine was reported by Scott et al. (1990). Rats that received $T_3$ while undergoing electroconvulsive shock did, however, perform better in tests of retrograde and antergrade amnesia than rats that received placebo (Stern et al., 1995).

Non-pharmacological treatments have also been examined for their effects on thyroid hormone level. Cognitive behavior therapy resulted in decreases in total $T_4$ in individuals who responded to the treatment while increasing it in non-responders (Joffe et al., 1996); in studies of light therapy, changes in $T_4$ level have either been significantly related to improvement in mood (Baumgartner et al., 1996) or not (Kasper et al., 1988).

In summary, some studies of clinical response to pharmacologic and non-pharmacologic antidepressant treatment have suggested that change in peripheral thyroid hormone status may be of therapeutic relevance. Whether this reflects a non-specific and indirect measure of improvement or reflects a more etiological effect induced by treatment remains unclear. The empirical animal literature thus far supports the clinical belief that diminished thyroid function at baseline impedes therapeutic response to antidepressant treatment.

## Thyroid hormones in the treatment of affective disorders

The usage of thyroid hormones to potentiate antidepressant treatment derives from the work of Prange and coworkers who reported that 25 µg of $T_3$ accelerated the therapeutic response of unipolar depressed females to 150 mg of imipramine. Males were much less likely to show evidence of clinical benefit (reviewed in Prange et al., 1984; Stein & Avni, 1988). The usage of triiodothyronine ($T_3$) to potentiate tricyclic response in individuals apparently resistant to the drug appeared first in a report by Earle (1970), who found that supplemental $T_3$ produced a response in 14 our of 25 female patients. Over the next 15 years, approximately a dozen papers appeared, each finding that 25 to 50 µg of $T_3$ produced a positive response in 50 to 75% of previously treatment-resistant patients (Coppen et al., 1972; Swartz, 1982; Price, 1989; Aronson, et al., 1996). Goodwin et al. (1982) in the first double-blind controlled study reported that eight out of 12 individuals responded to either 25 or 50 µg of $T_3$, and showed that the improvement could not be related to an indirect change in plasma tricyclic level.

The question as to whether responders to adjunctive $T_3$ could be predicted on the basis of subtle thyroid abnormalities at baseline was not systematically addressed in these reports. Whybrow and colleagues (1972) showed that women who had indirect evidence of decreased thyroid function achieved more benefit from $T_3$ supplementation than those who did not. In similar vein Wheatley (1972) found that women who had indices of thyroid activity in the low normal range were more likely to respond to $T_3$ supplementation than others. Targum et al. (1984) provided additional support, observing a positive response in five out of six patients who were judged to be subclinically hypothyroid on the basis of an augmented TSH response to TRH, but in only two out of 15 individuals who were euthyroid by these same criteria. Despite these data the antidepressant efficacy of $T_3$ alone has been relatively unexamined. In one controlled investigation reviewed by Prange et al. (1984) depressed women receiving $T_3$ in doses ranging from 25 to 62.5 µg showed a positive antidepressant response, although doses of $T_3$ above 50 µg produced anxiety and aversive side effects. Individual data regarding baseline thyroid status, however, were not presented. If likelihood of response is determined by the presence of subclinical hypothyroidism at baseline, the argument could be made that thyroxine ($T_4$) would be preferable to $T_3$ as an ongoing adjunctive treatment (Russ & Ackerman, 1989). In a study of euthyroid unipolar depressed patients, i.e. who did not have evidence of elevated basal TSH and who had previously failed trials of imipramine or desipramine, Joffe & Levitt (1993) gave 37.5 µg of $T_3$ or 150 µg of $T_4$ for three weeks. Fifty-three percent of the patients responded to $T_3$ compared to only 19% to $T_4$, but the length of the trial (3 weeks) strongly favored the pharmacokinetic profile of $T_3$ as opposed to $T_4$. Although the literature pertaining to thyroid hormone augmentation therapy has been generally positive, negative studies have appeared and the overall clinical impression is that thyroid augmentation is underutilized amongst clinicians. Whether this relates to a general lack of success in routine clinical practice or clinician discomfort with hormonal interventions remains unclear. Gitlin and colleagues (1987) assigned 16 patients (nine men and seven women) to either 25 µg of $T_3$ or placebo for 2 weeks, in addition to their ongoing imipramine therapy in a double-blind, random, cross-over design. No benefit was found for adjunctive $T_3$, although it is questionable whether the patients studied should have been truly judged treatment-resistant after only 2 weeks of therapy. However, Thase and colleagues (1989) studied individuals who had been non-responsive after 12 weeks of imipramine and reported in an open label trial that 25 µg of T$_3$ did not result in any greater degree of improvement than simple continued treatment with imipramine alone. High dose T$_4$ (150 to 300 µg/day) has recently been reported to have an antidepressant effect in more than 50% of previously treatment-resistant patients with chronic depression or dysthymia (Rudas et al., 1999).

In addition to the reports with tricyclics, T$_3$ has also been used successfully to supplement the monoamine oxidase inhibitor, phenelzine, in individual cases of treatment-resistant depression (Hullett & Bidder, 1983; Joffe, 1988b), and patients who received a nightly 50 µg dose of T$_3$ in the course of ECT had an accelerated antidepressant response and diminished amnestic side effects (Stern et al., 1991).

Animal models have attempted to shed some light on the positive clinical findings (Barsano et al., 1994). To determine whether T$_3$'s benefits in euthyroid patients is through the induction of subclinical hyperthyroidism, rats were given doses of T$_3$ sufficient to suppress T$_4$ and serum TSH over a 10-week period. Upon sacrifice, multiple parameters of metabolic status both in brain and in the periphery were found to be consistent with euthyroidism. Pretreatment with T$_3$ did, however, reverse escape and avoidance deficits associated with inescapable foot shock in rats evaluated in a learned helplessness paradigm (Martin et al., 1985).

A few studies have explored the possible benefit of T$_3$ potentiation in other diagnostic groups and the possible role of TSH or TRH in ameliorating depression. In one pilot study, Stein and Udhe (1990) failed to find evidence for adjunctive T$_3$ being of benefit in patients with panic disorder who had failed to respond to tricyclic antidepressant treatment.

Subcutaneous administration of TRH can reduce the deficits associated with behavioral despair and potentiate the benefits of desipramine in rats (Drago et al., 1990), but a series of clinical investigations in the 1970s, exploring the utility of 200 to 500 µg of TRH administered either IV or orally, failed to find a significant antidepressant response. More recently, Marangell and colleagues (1997a) reported a rapid mood enhancing response to 500 µg of TRH in treatment-resistant depressed patients. There is limited evidence that TSH, like T$_3$, may speed up antidepressant response, but it appears to have no distinctive antidepressant effect by itself.

In addition to demonstrable efficacy in unipolar disorder, thyroid supplementation has a clear role in the treatment algorithm of rapid cycling bipolar disorder, defined most commonly as the presence of four or more manic or depressive episodes per year. Approximately 15% of bipolar patients have such a course, the majority of whom are women. Individuals who experience rapid cycling have a poorer response to lithium and a higher prevalence of clinical or subclinical hypothyroidism in their history (Reus, 1989). On a purely empirical basis, Stancer and Persad (1982) treated ten rapid cycling patients in an open trial with high doses of thyroxine or $T_3$, added to ongoing neuroleptic therapy. Complete remission was noted in five women, although one man failed to respond. In the years since, a series of individual case reports and case series have supported the positive results of this original report (Balldin et al., 1987; Bernstein, 1992; Leibow, 1983). In the most well-controlled study to date, Bauer and Whybrow (1990) saw a marked improvement in manic symptoms in 10 of 11 patients treated with high dose L-thyroxine in addition to their ongoing mood stabilizer therapies. Treatment response did not depend upon previous thyroid status. Although the doses were quite large, ranging from 0.15 to 0.4 mg per day, side effects during the acute phase of treatment were minimal, with no evidence of tachycardia or weight loss. A follow-up study of individuals maintained on L-thyroxine treatment for a minimum of 18 months showed no increased incidence of osteoporosis over controls as measured by bone densitometry (Gyulai et al., 1997). In the patients who did respond, the free thyroxine index rose to approximately 150 to 200% above normal. High dose $T_4$ may also be useful in treating intractable non-rapid cycling bipolar disorder. Baumgartner et al. (1994) gave 250 to 500 µg of $T_4$ as a supplement to ongoing mood stabilizer treatment and followed patients for an average of 28 months. The mean number of relapses and mean duration of hospitalization significantly decreased for each patient compared to their pretreatment history. In some bipolar patients, however, supplemental thyroid treatment may trigger mania (Evans et al., 1986).

The mechanism for the beneficial response seen remains hypothetical (Whybrow et al., 1972). Bauer and Whybrow (1990) suggest a relative central thyroid hormone deficiency resulting from either a decreased $T_4$ transport into the brain or an alteration in $T_4$ to $T_3$ conversion within the brain. Alternative theories emphasize a possible relationship between rapid cycling and abnormalities in circadian oscillator regulation. Abnormal cycles in behavior and metabolism have been experimentally produced through partial thyroidectomy in animal models (Richter et al., 1959), while lithium can reverse thyroidectomy-induced deficits in circadian rhythm (Schull et al., 1988).

## Technical aspects of thyroid hormone supplementation

Although it seems clear that thyroid hormone supplementation is effective in certain cases of treatment resistance, its relative place in the algorithm of therapy remains uncertain. The evidence thus far would suggest that the clinical likelihood of a positive response is significantly higher in women and in individuals who have a basal TSH level in the high normal to elevated range. The presence of a thyroid diagnosis in past history may also increase likelihood of response. Most reports of triiodothyronine treatment have utilized doses of 25 to 50 µg. The side-effects associated with the lower dosage are generally acceptable, but higher doses may induce anxiety, tachycardia, and insomnia, as well as produce EKG abnormalities. A positive response should generally be observed within 2 to 3 weeks. If benefit is noted, it is unclear how long supplementation should be maintained. Continuation of triiodothyronine after 2 to 3 months is problematic, because of effects on endogenous thyroid hormone regulation, and consideration should be given either for discontinuation or for transition to $T_4$. The comparative efficacy of $T_4$ to $T_3$ in initial augmentation treatment remains unresolved.

## Estrogen

There have been relatively few systematic trials of the usage of estrogen either alone or in combination with traditional antidepressants in the treatment of treatment-resistant depression (Epperson et al., 1999). There is some evidence that estrogen replacement therapy has beneficial effects on mood on menopausal women, but it is unclear whether depressed postmenopausal women who are not taking supplemental estrogen have a greater resistance to traditional antidepressant interventions (Palinkas & Barrett-Connor, 1992). In a retrospective analysis, Schneider et al. (1997) examined the clinical response of elderly depressed women who were enrolled in a placebo-controlled trial of fluoxetine. A significant interaction between estrogen status and treatment effect was found, with patients who received fluoxetine in addition to their ongoing estrogen showing significantly greater improvement in Hamilton depression scores than either placebo patients or fluoxetine-treated patients who did not receive estrogen replacement therapy. In a classic study involving severely depressed premenopausal as well as postmenopausal women (Klaiber et al., 1979), subjects were randomly assigned to either conjugated estrogen (15 to 25 mg) or placebo, and followed for 3 months. Estrogen treatment significantly improved depression scores, although complete remission was rare. More recent uncontrolled studies are also supportive (Carranza-Lira & Valentino-Figuero, 1999).

Other investigators have explored the adjunctive benefits of estrogen. Prange et al. (1976) found that estrogen significant accelerated response to imipramine, while Shapira et al. (1985) reported a lack of efficacy of estrogen supplementation to imipramine in treatment-resistant female depressives. The doses used in this latter study, however, were much less (3.75 mg per day), and the duration much shorter (21 days) than Klaiber et al. (1979). A few case reports reporting possible benefit of the addition of oral contraceptives to antidepressants have appeared since, but methodologic problems compromise the conclusions that can be drawn (Amsterdam et al., 1999). Although the Klaiber et al. study (1979) has not been replicated, one recent double-blind placebo-controlled investigation and a case report have shown that transdermal or sublingual estrogen can be an effective treatment for postpartum depression (Ahokas et al., 1998; Gregoire et al., 1996). If estrogen were to be found effective, a number of plausible mechanisms of action could be put forward. Estrogen has a number of modulatory effects on catecholamine and indoleamine systems, and it inhibits monoamine oxidase (Joffe & Cohen, 1998). Direct effects on transcription and protein synthesis and neuronal electrical activity are also well established (Sherwin, 1991). Estrogen also increases the synthesis of thyroid binding globulin and interacts with thyroid hormone to regulate behavior (Dellovade et al., 1996).

In summary, the possible benefits of supplemental estrogen in treatment-resistant depression must remain speculative, particularly in premenopausal women. In postmenopausal women who demonstrate a resistance to traditional antidepressant therapy, an adjunctive trial of estrogen replacement treatment may be empirically warranted.

## Adrenocortical hormones

### Cortisol

Hypothalamic–pituitary–adrenal (HPA) axis overactivation is the most common biological abnormality in major depression, yet its pathophysiologic significance and treatment implications are unclear (APA Task Force on Laboratory Tests in Psychiatry, 1987; Amsterdam et al., 1989; Ribeiro et al., 1993). Hypercortisolemia (assessed basally or following the dexamethasone suppression test (DST)), does not necessarily predict acute antidepressant response (APA Task Force on Laboratory Tests in Psychiatry, 1987), although response to placebo is less common in hypercortisolemic depressed patients (APA Task Force on Laboratory Tests in Psychiatry, 1987; Ribeiro et al., 1993). Within the context of depression and other psychiatric illnesses, hypercortisolemia may be associated with more severe symptoms such as insomnia, psychosis, cognitive impairment, anxiety, agitation and suicidality (Reus, 1982; Schatzberg et al., 1985; Wolkowitz et al., 1990; Winokur et al., 1987). In addition, patients who have already failed several treatment trials are more likely to demonstrate enhanced HPA axis activity compared with patients with non-treatment-resistant depression (Amsterdam et al., 1994).

Various authors have suggested that the hypercortisolism seen in many patients with depression is secondary to the stress accompanying depression or to the primary neurotransmitter or neuropeptide imbalances which are independently responsible for the depressive symptoms (e.g. Gold & Chrousos, 1985). It is likely, however, that once hypercortisolism is established, it will further contribute to depressive symptomatology, exacerbating, perpetuating or altering the presentation of the depressive mood state (Checkley, 1992; Dinan, 1994; Murphy, 1991;

Murphy & Wolkowitz, 1993; Van Praag, 1996; Kathol, 1985; Reus, 1984; Wolkowitz, 1992; Wolkowitz & Reus, 1999).

To study the direction of causality between hypercortisolism and depressive illness, several research groups have assessed the temporal relationship between the appearance or resolution of this hormonal abnormality and the onset or remission of depressive symptoms. Holsboer et al. (1982) noted that decreases in post-dexamethasone cortisol levels preceded depressive remission by an average of 3.4 weeks, and that clinically remitted patients developed DST non-suppression approximately 1–2 weeks prior to the onset of depressive relapse. Greden et al. (1983) also reported that normalization of non-suppression in the DST typically precedes or coincides with, rather than follows, clinical recovery, and that failure to normalize on the DST portends poorly for clinical outcome (Greden et al., 1983; APA Task Force on Laboratory Tests in Psychiatry, 1987). Consistent with these earlier reports, Ribeiro et al. (1993) performed a meta-analysis of 144 articles related to the DST and concluded that DST non-suppression following treatment is strongly associated with early relapse and poor outcome on follow-up, and they hypothesized an etiologic role for hypercortisolemia in the genesis and maintenance of depression. Based on such findings, it may be that, at least in some depressed patients, normalization of HPA axis activity is a precondition for successful clinical response (Barden et al., 1995; Murphy, 1991; Murphy & Wolkowitz, 1993; Ribiero et al., 1993).

Given what is known about corticosteroid effects on brain, it is not surprising that these hormones influence mood and behavior (Wolkowitz, 1992; McEwen et al., 1992; Holsboer, 1989). Corticosteroids affect brain function via several general mechanisms. Interactions with the genome result in the regulation of transcription of specific genes such as those coding for monoaminergic synthetic and degradative enzymes as well as those coding for behaviorally active neuropeptides, G proteins, alpha-2 and beta- adrenergic receptors and norepinephrine (NE) receptor-linked adenylate cyclase (Holsboer, 1989). Some of these actions may counteract antidepressant drug effects on NE receptor responsiveness (Holsboer, 1989). Serotonin system responsivity is also under corticosteroid control, although these effects are complex (Van Praag, 1996; Chauloff, 1993; McKittrick & McEwen, 1995). As one example of such effects, in an animal model of depression, high corticosterone levels reduced serotonin system responsivity and successful adaptation to stress, whereas corticosterone-inhibiting drugs (e.g. metyrapone) facilitated serotonin system responsivity and hastened behaviorally adaptive responses (Kennett et al., 1985). In addition to such genomically mediated effects, cortico-steroids and their metabolites may have rapid (non-genomic) effects on brain excitability and on synaptic transmission via direct interactions with neuronal cell membranes and membrane receptors (e.g. the $GABA_A$ receptor) (McEwen et al., 1992; Holsboer, 1989; Majewska, 1987). Finally, chronic exposure of animals and possibly of humans to high levels of corticosteroids may induce morphological changes and even cell death in certain vulnerable neurons, e.g. hippocampal CA3 neurons (Sapolsky et al., 1986; Sheline et al., 1996), although corticosteroids may have trophic effects in other hippocampal regions, e.g. dentate gyrus (McEwen et al., 1992).

### Antiglucocorticoid treatments in depression and treatment-resistant depression

To the extent endogenous hypercortisolism does contribute to depressive symptomatology, two predictions should be borne out: (i) effective antidepressant medication should decrease HPA system activity; and (ii) treatments that directly decrease HPA system activity should have antidepressant effects. Evidence for the first prediction has already been reviewed (Holsboer, 1989; Greden et al., 1983; APA Task Force on Laboratory Tests in Psychiatry, 1987; Ribiero et al., 1993). In light of the fact that a substantial proportion of depressed patients shows evidence of defective glucocorticoid negative feedback, it is noteworthy that antidepressant medications increase levels of glucocorticoid receptors, rendering individuals more responsive to glucocortoid feedback inhibition. A body of literature, recently reviewed by Barden et al. (1995), and by Peeters et al. (1994) suggests that these effects are shared by many currently employed antidepressants, and that the time course of these changes parallels that of clinical antidepressant responses. They hypothesized that a primary and common mechanism of action of antidepressants is stimulation of hypothalamic and pituitary corticosteroid receptor expression leading to enhanced negative feedback and lowered HPA axis activity, leading to lowered levels of corticotropin releasing hormone (CRH), which itself increases depression (Holsboer, 1989). Effects secondary to lowered cortisol activity would be a lessening of the expression of genes which are under cortico-steroid regulatory control (e.g. those related to biogenic amine neurotransmission) (Wolkowitz, 1992). This conceptualization of antidepressant action opens up new mechanistic insights which may lead to the development of novel antidepressant drugs, as discussed below.

The prediction that drugs that directly lower HPA axis activity should have antidepressant effects has been widely studied in patients with Cushing's syndrome (for review see Wolkowitz & Reus, 1999) but only recently in psychiatric patients with major depression. Cushing's syndrome is associated with a high incidence of fatigue, decreased energy, irritability, decreased memory and concentration, depressed or labile mood, decreased libido, insomnia and crying; such symptoms are directly correlated with plasma cortisol levels (Starkman et al., 1981). Depressive and cognitive symptoms in Cushing's syndrome typically resolve with treatment of the hypercortisolemia, often in direct relationship to the reductions in circulating cortisol levels (Starkman & Schteingart, 1983; Starkman et al., 1986). At least 28 reports (the majority of which are reviewed in: Murphy & Wolkowitz, 1993; Reus et al., 1997; Murphy, 1997; Kiraly et al., 1997) have documented decreased depression and cognitive impairment, even complete psychiatric remission, in Cushing's syndrome patients who received either surgical or medical (e.g. ketoconazole, metyrapone, aminoglutethimide or RU-486) treatment aimed a lowering cortisol levels. Even patients resistant to traditional antidepressant medication have responded to this strategy (e.g. Sonino et al., 1986).

Studies of antiglucocorticoid treatment in patients with major depression have also been promising, but the majority have been small scale and/or open labeled. To date, 11 studies have reported positive effects of antiglucocorticoid drug treatment (used alone) in the treatment of some patients with depression and four studies have noted positive results of antiglucocorticoid augmentation of antidepressant medication or of other psychotropics in major depression, bipolar depression, atypical depression, severe obsessive-compulsive disorder and schizophrenia or schizoaffective disorder. Illustrative studies of antiglucocorticoid treatment in psychiatric patients are briefly reviewed below. For further review of this approach, see Murphy & Wolkowitz, 1993; Reus et al., 1997; Murphy, 1997; Wolkowitz & Reus, 1999.

Murphy et al. (1991, 1992) and Ghadirian et al. (1995) administered the antiglucocorticoid drugs, aminoglutethimide, metyrapone or ketoconazole, in an open-label manner for 2 months to 20 treatment-resistant patients with major depression. Eleven of 17 patients completing the 2-month protocol had 'complete remission' (defined as greater than 50% reduction in rated depressive symptoms) and an additional two had 'partial remission' (20–50% reduction in rated symptoms). They also noted that, in eight of the initial ten patients who improved, the improvement was sustained for an average of greater than 8 months following drug discontinuation. The authors cited this as evidence against a placebo effect and suggested that a 're-setting' of the HPA axis may lead to lasting remissions (Murphy et al., 1991). Of the six responders that had positive (i.e. non-suppressing) DSTs before starting therapy, five had reverted to normal suppression when tested 1–2 weeks following cessation of antiglucocorticoid therapy; the one patient who did not revert to normal suppression suffered an early relapse (Murphy, 1994). Baseline serum cortisol levels, however, did not predict treatment response, and treatment-associated decreases in serum cortisol levels were inconsistent and not statistically significant. No major differences were noted between the three antiglucocorticoid drugs they used, although ketoconazole was associated with a higher response rate (86%) than was aminoglutethimide (67%) or combinations with metyrapone (50%). These percentages should be interpreted cautiously, however, due to the small sample sizes.

Wolkowitz et al. (1993) reported that seven unmedicated hypercortisolemic depressed patients completing a 3- to 6-week open-label trial of ketoconazole (400–800 mg per day) demonstrated significant antidepressant responses. Four o'clock (pm) serum cortisol levels decreased by an average of 26% with ketoconazole treatment; decreases in serum cortisol levels were significantly correlated with decreases in Beck depression ratings.

Amsterdam et al. (1994) studied extremely treatment-resistant depressed patients and noted only partial or moderate responses in half, although ketoconazole augmentation of tranylcypromine resulted in dramatic improvement in one extremely treatment-resistant patient.

Anand et al. (1995), in one of only three double-blind reports, noted clinically significant improvements in depression and memory with ketoconazole treatment of one treatment-resistant patient. There was a close correlation between treatment-associated decreases in cortisol levels and decreases in depression ratings. The patient remained in remission through 12 additional weeks of open-label treatment and relapsed upon ketoconazole discontinuation.

O'Dwyer et al. (1995) treated eight depressed patients with metyrapone (plus 'replacement' doses of hydrocortisone) vs. placebo in single-blind manner in a 2-week per arm cross-over design, and noted significant decreases in depression ratings as well as in serum cortisol levels. After discontinuation of metyrapone, depression ratings remained low despite return of cortisol to baseline levels, supporting Murphy and colleagues (1991) report of persistent antidepressant effects following antiglucocorticoid treatment.

Sovner and Fogelman (1996) reported two cases of persistent atypical major depression that responded to open-label ketoconazole and remained in remission through periods ranging from 15 to 24 months of continued ketoconazole treatment. Both patients had previously been intolerant of, or unresponsive to, traditional antidepressants.

Thakore and Dinan (1995) treated eight non-treatment-resistant depressed patients with ketoconazole for 4 weeks and noted significant antidepressant effects as well as significant decreases in serum cortisol levels. They had postulated that elevated cortisol activity might provoke or maintain depressive symptoms via the induction of serotonin system subsensitivity. They based their hypothesis partially on observations that baseline cortisol levels in depressed patients are inversely related to the magnitude of serum prolactin (PRL) responses to serotonin agonists such as D-fenfluramine (a putative test of serotonin system sensitivity). To test this hypothesis, they administered D-fenfluramine to their depressed subjects at baseline and again after four weeks of ketoconazole treatment. Ketoconazole normalized the PRL response to D-fenfluramine (i.e. increased the response relative to baseline), and these increases in PRL responses were significantly correlated with reductions in depression ratings. These findings are consistent with the notion that hypercortisolemia downregulates serotonin system sensitivity, and that anti-glucocorticoid treatments may have antidepressant effects via normalization of serotonin sensitivity.

Ravaris et al. (1994) successfully treated a previously treatment-resistant bipolar II depressed patient with ketoconazole added to the prior regimen of lithium and phenelzine. Improvement was correlated with decreases in urinary-free cortisol (UFC) levels, and discontinuation of ketoconazole resulted in relapse which was preceded by increasing UFC levels. Chouinard et al. (1996) reported a case of severe treatment-resistant obsessive-compulsive disorder successfully treated by adding aminoglutethimide to the previously ineffective fluoxetine. This patient remained significantly improved for the entire 4 years he was on this combination but relapsed when either drug was discontinued. The authors suggested that serotonergic potentiation by aminoglutethimide might explain this combination's efficacy. Antiglucocorticoid augmentation of neuroleptics in schizophrenic and schizoaffective disorder patients also significantly decreased depression ratings in a small scale double-blind study by Marco et al. (in review).

Lastly, in the only other double-blind series to date, 20 unmedicated depressed patients were randomized to ketoconazole (mean dose = 655.6 mg per day) vs. placebo treatment for 4 weeks (Wolkowitz et al., 1999a). Among the hypercor-tisolemic patients ($n = 8$), but not among the eucortisolemic ones ($n = 12$), ketoconazole treatment was significantly superior to placebo in reducing depress-ion ratings. In the hypercortisolemic group, ketoconazole was associated with a 48% improvement in rated symptoms, compared to 6.6% with placebo. This study is limited by its small sample size, but reinforces the hypothesis that antiglucocorticoid drugs have more prominent antidepressant effects in the pres-ence of adrenocortical activation.

## Choice of specific antiglucocorticoid drugs

Since all of the available antiglucocorticoid drugs have shown some degree of efficacy in the above-reviewed studies, the choice of any specific one may be guided by side effects, tolerability and metabolic site of action (Murphy & Wolkowitz, 1993). However, the use of antiglucocorticoids in treating depression remains experimental at this time. Most available antiglucocorticoid drugs inhibit various cytochrome P-450 enzymes. (i) Ketoconazole is considered by some the drug of choice for pharmacological lowering of cortisol levels in Cushing's syndrome (Miller & Tyrrell, 1995; Orth et al., 1992). Ketoconazole (at doses $\geqslant 400$ mg/day, resulting in plasma levels of 1–5 mcg/dl) inhibits cholesterol side-chain cleavage, 17, 20-lyase, 11-$\beta$-hydroxylase, and, to a lesser extent, 17- and 18-hydroxylase. These effects result in decreased cortisol, androgen (androstenedione, DHEA, DHEA-S, testosterone) and aldosterone synthesis and in elevated levels of pregnenolone, 17-$\alpha$-hydroxypregnenolone, progesterone, 17-$\alpha$-hydroxyprogesterone and 11-deoxycortisol. In addition to inhibiting cortisol biosynthesis, ketoconazole acts at the receptor level as a glucocorticoid antagonist (Feldman, 1986; Loose et al., 1983), but this effect may be minimal in vivo at commonly achieved plasma levels. Ketoconazole may also be effective by directly decreasing basal and CRH-stimulated ACTH release at the level of the pituitary (Berselli et al., 1987; Stalla et al., 1989) although this is controversial. In any event, ketoconazole (as opposed to metyrapone and aminoglutethimide) treatment of Cushing's syndrome is not associated with a compensatory increase in ACTH release. Side effects of ketoconazole include nausea, diarrhea, menstrual irregularities, abdominal discomfort, headache, reversible increases in serum transaminase levels, and, less commonly, vomiting, sedation, decreased libido and reversible gynecomastia and impotence. Hepatotoxicity and hypoadrenalism are rare but serious complications which mandate frequent laboratory monitoring. (ii) Metyrapone inhibits 11-$\beta$-hydroxylase, leading to decreased cortisol and increased 11-deoxycortisol levels. Side effects include nausea, headache, sedation and rash. Compensatory increases in ACTH secretion are commonly observed with metyrapone; these often override the cortisol biosynthesis inhibition and necessitate combination drug therapy or increasing metyrapone doses. Further, metyrapone increases androgenic and mineralocorticoid precursors, occasionally resulting in acne, hirsutism and hypertension. (iii) Aminoglutethimide inhibits cholesterol side-chain cleavage, the enzyme which converts cholesterol to pregnenolone. It also affects hydroxylation at C11 and C18. Estrogen as well as cortisol synthesis is curtailed. The resulting decrease in cortisol synthesis, however, is partially overcome by increases in ACTH release. Most patients treated with aminoglutethimide develop transient generalized pruritic rashes. Other side effects include somnolence, dizziness, fever, headache, and more rarely, goiter, hyperthyroidism, cholestasis, bone marrow suppression and aldosterone deficiency. Significant side effects are seen in two-thirds of patients treated with aminoglutethimide. (iv) RU-486 (mifepristone) does not inhibit steroid biosynthesis but blocks progesterone and, at higher doses, cortisol receptors. Circulating cortisol levels may double secondary to receptor blockade (Berselli et al., 1987; Stalla et al., 1989). Its use for other than acute administration has been inadequately assessed and has been associated with prominent rashes in some subjects. Since it also blocks the effects of exogenous corticosteroids, it would be difficult to acutely treat any side effects resulting from glucocorticoid deficiency. (v) Less commonly employed antiglucocorticoid drugs include mitotone and etomidate, which would not be appropriate due to their adrenolytic and sedative properties, respectively.

**Dexamethasone**

In what seems a diametrically opposite approach to altering steroidal activity in depressed patients, Arana and colleagues (Arana, 1991; Arana et al., 1991, 1995; Beale & Arana, 1995) reported antidepressant effects of high dose dexamethasone. In this paradigm, dexamethasone was administered intravenously as a one-time bolus of 4–8 mg or orally as 4 mg per day for 4 days. Results of the open-label intravenous dexamethasone trial indicated 56% improvement within 10 days in 75% of depressed subjects, including five of seven treatment-resistant ones who had failed at least two prior antidepressant trials. In the blinded oral dexamethasone trial, dexamethasone was associated with only a 27.5% improvement in depression ratings compared with a 13.6% decrease with placebo. A significantly greater number of dexamethasone-treated subjects responded to treatment (defined as a $\geq 50\%$ decrease in depression ratings or a final Hamilton depression score of $\leq 14$) compared with placebo-treated subjects. The authors suggested that the beneficial effect of dexamethasone was secondary to regulation of CRH receptors, increased serotonergic activity or other genomically mediated changes in neurotransmission.

Similar results were obtained by another group using an open-label design. Dinan et al. (1997) studied ten depressed patients who had not responded to sertraline or fluoxetine, and added dexamethasone, 3 mg p.o. daily for 4 days, to the ongoing antidepressant regimen. By the following day (day 5), three of the six sertraline patients and three of the four fluoxetine patients demonstrated significant (50% reduction in depression ratings) antidepressant responses. Remarkably, this initial improvement was maintained through day 21, the last assessed day. Cortisol changes in response to dexamethasone treatment were not reported, but baseline morning serum cortisol levels were directly correlated with antidepressant responses (i.e. higher baseline cortisol was associated with better responses to dexamethasone). The dexamethasone was relatively well tolerated, but several patients reported sleep disruption, nausea and/or anxiety during dexamethasone treatment.

In one additional small-scale study, Goodwin et al. (1992) noted that an acute cortisol infusion transiently improved self-rated mood in 12 depressed patients. These patients were not hypercortisolemic at baseline.

Finally, Wolkowitz et al. (1996) reported negative results in a very small, double-blind replication study. Five depressed patients received one-time intravenous infusions of 6 mg of either dexamethasone or placebo and were evaluated 10 days later. The three subjects who received dexamethasone all fared more poorly than the two who received placebo; two of the three dexamethasone-treated subjects actually worsened following treatment. The one dexamethasone-treated subject who showed a mild antidepressant effect had the lowest baseline serum cortisol concentration of the group.

The preliminary evidence reviewed here suggests that modifications of HPA axis activity may have antidepressant effects in a subgroup of depressed patients. Interestingly, some patients resistant to traditional antidepressants have shown dramatic responses to such strategies. The existing database, however, is over-represented with small scale and open-label studies, and few studies have yet clarified the mechanisms by which these drugs may be effective or predictors of response. Thus, use of these strategies remains largely experimental at this time.

### Dehydroepiandrosterone (DHEA)

Although much has been written about the possible role of cortisol in depressive illness, this steroid is but one of approximately 150 steroids produced either by synthesis within the adrenal or by metabolism of these steroids elsewhere (Murphy & Wolkowitz, 1993). Several of these steroids may also play roles in affective regulation (c.f. Majewska, 1987; O'Dwyer et al., 1995; Raven et al., 1996; Wolkowitz et al., 2000). One such steroid receiving increasing attention is dehydro-epiandrosterone.

DHEA together with its sulfated metabolite, DHEA-S, is the most plentiful adrenal corticosteroid in humans, yet its physiologic role (other than serving as a sex steroid precursor) is unknown. Yet a role in central nervous system regulation is likely, since DHEA(S) is synthesized *de novo* in brain, since brain levels are to some extent regulated independently from those in plasma, and since DHEA(S) has intrinsic activity at brain GABA$_A$ and other receptors (c.f. Majewska, 1987; Wolkowitz et al., 2000). Relevant to the preceding discussion, DHEA(S) also has cortisol-antagonist effects in several models (Leblhuber et al., 1992). DHEA(S) levels decrease with aging and with chronic stress, and people with relatively lower DHEA(S) levels are reported to have poorer performance in activities of daily living (Rudman et al., 1990; Berkman et al., 1993), less amount, frequency and enjoyment of leisure activities (Fava et al., 1992), lower 'dominance' and 'expansive personality' ratings (Gray et al., 1991; Hermida et al., 1985), lower 'sensation seeking' attributes (Klinteberg et al., 1992) and greater perceived stress (Labbate et al., 1995).

Naturalistic studies in depressed patients are equivocal, with some reporting increased (Hansen et al., 1982), decreased (Goodyer et al., 1996) or unaltered (Reus et al., 1993) DHEA(S) levels compared to non-depressed controls. Nonetheless, treatment studies (most of which are open-label or small scale) suggest DHEA may have mood-enhancing and antidepressant effects.

Clinical trials in the 1950s suggested that DHEA improved energy, mood, self-confidence, occupational functioning, apathy and withdrawal in 'schizo-phrenic' or 'inadequate personality' patients (Strauss et al., 1952; Sands & Chamberlain, 1952; Strauss & Stevenson, 1955). A recent double-blind trial, in which healthy middle-aged and elderly subjects were given DHEA (50 mg p.o.

daily) or placebo for 3 months each, reported significant DHEA-induced improvements in self-rated well-being (Morales et al., 1994).

Two studies have so far evaluated DHEA treatment in major depression. The first, an open-label trial of 30–90 mg DHEA per day for 4 weeks found significant antidepressant and cognition-enhancing effects in six middle-aged or elderly depressed patients (Wolkowitz et al., 1997, 2000). The DHEA doses used in this study increased initially low plasma DHEA(S) levels to the middle or upper normal range (DHEA: 160–800 ng/dl; DHEA(S): 100–450 mcg/dl [males], 60–255 mcg/dl [females]). One woman in that study received DHEA (60–90 mg/d) in an open-label manner for 6 months and demonstrated antidepressant and cognition-enhancing effects which were greater at the 90 mg dose than at the 60 mg dose and which were significantly correlated with treatment-associated plasma DHEA(S) levels (Wolkowitz et al., 1997).

A recent double-blind, placebo controlled trial of DHEA in major depression was consistent with these findings (Wolkowitz et al., 1999b). Twenty-two depressed patients, some of whom were medication-free and the rest of whom remained depressed despite being on stabilized antidepressant regimens, were treated with DHEA, up to 90 mg/day ($n = 11$), or placebo ($n = 11$) for 6 weeks. On DHEA, Hamilton depression ratings decreased an average of 30.5%, compared to an average decrease on placebo of 5.3% ($P < 0.04$). Using a response criterion of a $\geqslant 50\%$ improvement in depression ratings plus an end-point Hamilton rating of $\leqslant 10$, 5/11 DHEA-treated patients responded, compared to 0/11 placebo-treated patients.

Lastly, a recent double-blind, placebo-controlled study examined the efficacy of DHEA in patients with mid-life onset dysthymia (Bloch et al., 1999). As was the case in patients with major depression (Wolkowitz et al., 1999b), dysthymic patients showed a significant antidepressant response, with about 60% of patients showing clinically significant improvement.

While these results suggest DHEA may have antidepressant effects, enthusiasm for this approach must remain tempered until more and larger controlled trials are completed.

Side-effects of DHEA are largely androgenic in nature (but considerably milder than those seen with testosterone or anabolic steroids) and include acne, hirsutism, male-pattern hair loss, and possibly prostatic hypertrophy and menstrual irregularities. As with other steroids, DHEA may alter the contraceptive efficacy of birth control pills, but this has not been well studied. DHEA, by virtue of its partial metabolism to testosterone and its subsequent aromatization to estrogen, has theoretical potential to induce or exacerbate hormone-sensitive tumors (e.g. breast, uterine, ovarian or prostate cancer or malignant melanoma), although – to our knowledge – no reports of such in humans have yet appeared, with possibly one exception (Jones et al., 1997). It seems prudent for patients with histories of such cancers to avoid DHEA, and for other patients contemplating long-term DHEA ingestion to have periodic mammograms, Pap smears, prostate exams and/or prostate-specific antigen levels measured. Finally, anecdotal evidence suggests that supraphysiologically elevated serum DHEA(S) levels may provoke anxiety, panic, manic reactions or psychosis in certain patients (Howard III, 1992). Several authors, including ourselves, believe that too little is yet known about the risk:benefit ratio of chronic DHEA use (e.g. > a few months) to warrant its clinical use.

## Treatment algorithm

It is advisable that all depressed patients, especially those resistant to initial pharmacotherapies, be evaluated for hormonal dysfunction that might be contributing to their depression. A simple initial test with a relatively high 'hit' rate is the ultrasensitive TSH assay and $FT_4$ measurement; it should be borne in mind that even TSH levels at the low or high end of the 'normal' range may represent a relative hyper- or hypothyroid state for an individual patient. Further endocrine tests which might be performed, depending on the clinical circumstances, include estradiol, FSH, testosterone, plasma or urinary-free cortisol, the DST and, more speculatively, serum DHEA(S) levels. An example of such an approach is illustrated in Fig. 3.1.

## Conclusions

It is apparent from this review that various hormones have significant effects on neurochemistry and on mental functioning and mood regulation. The role of hormones as psychotropic medications, however, remains to be adequately evaluated. Of the putative treatments reviewed here, thyroid augmentation in treatment-resistant depression and in rapid cycling bipolar affective disorder has received the greatest empirical support, followed by estrogen replacement therapy or estrogen augmentation in postmenopausal women. Strategies directly targeting the HPA axis (e.g. antiglucocorticoids, dexamethasone, DHEA) are being actively investigated but, to date, have not received sufficient empirical support to enter into routine clinical practice. For individual treatment-resistant patients who have exhausted other options, however, empirical trials with informed consent and with attention to possible side-effects, seem reasonable. We can expect that, with further delineation of the effects of hormones on mental functioning, therapeutic advances will rapidly accrue, and new classes of hormonally-active psychotropics will become available.

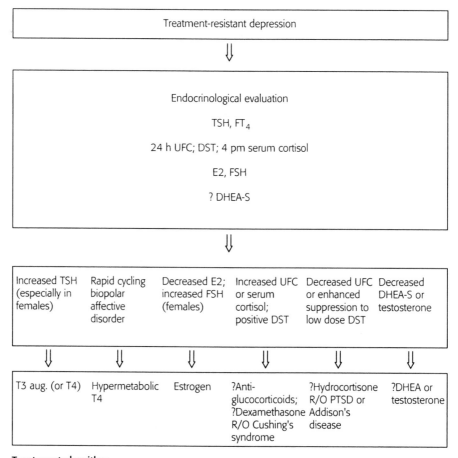

Fig. 3.1     Treatment algorithm.

## Acknowledgments

This work was supported in part by grants from the National Association for Research in Schizophrenia and Affective Disorders (NARSAD), the National Alliance for the Mentally Ill (NAMI) and The Scottish Rite Foundation to Owen Wolkowitz. James Kerns, Natasha Page Carroll and Dolores Cruz prepared the manuscript.

## REFERENCES

Ahokas, A.J., Turtiainen, S., & Alto, M. (1998). Sublingual oestrogen treatment of postnatal depression. *The Lancet*, **351**, 109.

Amsterdam, J.D., Maislin, G., Gold, P., & Winokur, A. (1989). The assessment of abnormalities in hormonal responsiveness at multiple levels of the hypothalamic–pituitary–adrenocortical axis in depressive illness. *Psychoneuroendocrinology*, **14**, 43–62.

Amsterdam, J., Mosley, P.D., & Rosenzweig, M. (1994). Assessment of adrenocortical activity in refractory depression: steroid suppression with ketoconazole. In *Refractory Depression*, ed. W. Nolan, J. Zohar, S. Roose, & J. Amsterdam, pp. 199–210. Chichester, UK: John Wiley.

Amsterdam, J., Garcia-Espana, F., Fawcett, J. et al. (1999). Fluoxetine efficacy in menopausal women with and without estrogen. *Journal of Affective Disorder*, **55**, 11–17.

Anand, A., Malison, R., McDougle, C.J., & Price, L.H. (1995). Antiglucocorticoid treatment of refractory depression with ketoconazole: a case report. *Biological Psychiatry*, **37**, 338–40.

Angeli, A. & Frairia, R. (1985). Ketoconazole therapy in Cushing's disease. *Lancet*, **i**, 821.

APA Task Force on Laboratory Tests in Psychiatry (1987). The dexamethasone suppression test: An overview of its current status in psychiatry. *American Journal of Psychiatry*, **144**, 1253–62.

Arana, G.W. (1991). Intravenous dexamethasone for symptoms of major depressive disorder. *American Journal of Psychiatry*, **148**, 1401–2.

Arana, G.W. & Forbes, R.A. (1991). Dexamethasone for the treatment of depression: a preliminary report. *Journal of Clinical Psychiatry*, **52**, 304–6.

Arana, G.W., Santos, A.B., Laraia, M.T., McLeod-Bryant, S., Beale, M.D., & Rames, L.J. (1995). Dexamethasone for the treatment of depression; a randomized, placebo-controlled double-blind trial. *American Journal of Psychiatry*, **152**, 265–7.

Aronson, R., Offman, H.J., Joffe, R.T. et al. (1996). Triiodothyronine augmentation in the treatment of refractory depression. *Archives of General Psychiatry*, **53**, 842–8.

Baker, J.R. Jr (1992). Immunologic aspects of endocrine diseases. *Journal of the American Medical Association*, **25**, 2899–903.

Balldin, J., Berggren, U., Rybo, E. et al. (1987). Treatment-resistant mania with primary hypothyroidism: a case of recovery after levothyroxine. *Journal of Clinical Psychiatry*, **48**, 490–1.

Barden, N., Reul, J.M.H.M., & Holsboer, F. (1995). Do antidepressants stabilize mood through actions on the hypothalamic–pituitary–adrenocortical system? *Trends in Neuroscience*, **18**, 6–11.

Barsano, C.P., Garces, J., & Iqbal, Z. (1994). Metabolic implications of low-dose triiodothyronine administration in rats. Relevance to the adjunctive use of triiodothyronine in the treatment of depression. *Biological Psychiatry*, **35**, 814–23.

Bauer, M.S. & Whybrow, P.C. (1990). Rapid cycling bipolar affective disorder. II. Treatment of refractory rapid cycling with high-dose levothyroxine: a preliminary study. *Archives of General Psychiatry*, **47**, 435–40.

Baumgartner, A., Bauer, M., & Hellweg, R. (1994). Treatment of intractable non-rapid cycling bipolar affective disorder with high-dose thyroxine: an open clinical trial. *Neuropsychopharmacology*, **10**, 183–9.

Baumgartner, A., Volz, H-P., Campos-Barros, A. et al. (1996). Serum concentrations of thyroid hormones in patients with nonseasonal affective disorders during treatment with bright an dim light. *Biological Psychiatry*, **40**, 899–907.

Beale, M.D. & Arana, G.W. (1995). Dexamethasone treatment of major depression in patients with bipolar disorder. *American Journal of Psychiatry*, **152**, 959–60.

Bender, K.J. (1997). Evidence of estrogen benefit in dementia and cognition. Supplement to *Psychiatric Times*, 20–2.

Berkman, L.F., Seeman, T.E., Albert, M. et al. (1993). High, usual and impaired functioning in community-dwelling older men and women: findings from the MacArthur Foundation Research Network on Successful Aging. *Journal of Clinical Epidemiology*, **46**, 1129–40.

Berlin, I., Payan, C., Corruble, E. et al. (1999). Serum thyroid-stimulating-hormone concentration as an index of severity of major depression. *International Journal of Neuropsychopharmacology*, **2**, 105–10.

Bernstein, L. (1992). Abrupt cessation of rapid-cycling bipolar disorder with the addition of low-dose L-tetraiodothyronine to lithium. *Journal of Clinical Psychopharmacology*, **12**, 443–4.

Berselli, M.E., Tagliaferri, M., Vignati, F., & Loli, P. (1987). Effect of ketoconazole on CRH-induced ACTH and cortisol release in patients with Cushing's disease. *Hormone and Metabolism Research*, 16 (suppl.), 58–59.

Birge, S.J. (1996). Is there a role for estrogen replacement therapy in the prevention and treatment of dementia? *Journal of the American Geriatric Society*, **44**, 865–70.

Bloch, M., Schmidt, P.J., Danaceau, M.A., Adams, L.F., & Rubinow, D.R. (1999). Dehydroepiandrosterone treatment of mid-life dysthymia. *Biological Psychiatry*, **45**, 1533–41.

Brady, K.T. & Anton, R.F. (1989). The thyroid axis and desipramine treatment in depression. *Biological Psychiatry*, **25**, 703–9.

Brady, K.T., Lydiard, R.B., Kellner, C.H. et al. (1994). A comparison of the effects of imipramine and fluvoxamine on the thyroid axis. *Biological Psychiatry*, **36**, 778–9.

Brent, G.A. (1994). The molecular basis of thyroid hormone action. *The New England Journal of Medicine*, **331**, 847–53.

Bunevicius, R., Kazanavicius, G., & Telksnys, A. (1994). Thyrotropin response to TRH stimulation in depressed patients with autoimmune thyroiditis. *Biological Psychiatry*, **36**, 543–7.

Bunevicius, R., Lasas, L., Kazanavicius, G. et al. (1996). Pituitary responses to thyrotropin releasing hormone stimulation in depressed women with thyroid gland disorders. *Psychoneuroendocrinology*, **21**, 631–9.

Campos-Barros, A. & Baumgartner, A. (1994). Effects of chronic desipramine treatment on thyroid hormone concentrations in rat brain: dependency on drug dose and brain area. *Biological Psychiatry*, **35**, 214–16.

Cardinali, D.P., Romeo, H.E., Boado, R.J. et al. (1986). Early inhibition and changes in diurnal rhythmicity of the pituitary–thyroid axis after superior cervical ganglionectomy of rats. *Journal of the Autonomic Nervous System*, **16**, 13–21.

Carranza-Lira, S. & Valentino-Figuero, M.L. (1999). Estrogen therapy for depression in postmenopausal women. *International Journal of Gynaecology and Obstetrics*, **65**, 35–8.

Champion, B.R., Cooke, A., & Rayner, D.C. (1992). Thyroid autoimmunity. *Current Opinion in Immunology*, **4**, 770–8.

Chaouloff, F. (1993). Physiopharmacological interactions between stress hormones and central serotonergic systems. *Brain Research Reviews*, **18**, 1–32.

Checkley, S. (1992). Neuroendocrine mechanisms and the precipitation of depression by life events. *British Journal of Psychiatry*, **160**, 7–17.

Chouinard, G., Belanger, M.C., Beauclair, L., Sultan, S., & Murphy, B.E. (1996). Potentiation of fluoxetine by aminoglutehimide, an adrenal steroid suppressant, in obsessive-compulsive disorder resistant to SSRIs: a case report. *Progress in Neuropsychopharmacology Biological Psychiatry*, **20**, 1067–79.

Coppen, A., Whybrow, P.C., Noguera, R. et al. (1972). The comparative antidepressant value of L-tryptophan and imipramine with and without attempt potentiation by liothyronine. *Archives of General Psychiatry*, **26**, 234–41.

Dellovade, T.L., Zhu, Y-S., Krey, L. et al. (1996). Thyroid hormone and estrogen interact to regulate behavior. *Proceedings of the National Academy of Sciences*, **93**, 12581–86.

Dinan, T.G. (1994). Glucocorticoids and the genesis of depressive illness: a psychobiological model. *British Journal of Psychiatry*, **164**, 365–71.

Dinan, T.G., Lavelle, E., Cooney, J. et al. (1997). Dexamethasone augmentation in treatment-resistant depression. *Acta Psychiatrica Scandinavica*, **95**, 58–61.

Dow-Edwards, D.L., Elowitz, E.H., Freed, L.A. et al. (1988). Cerebral metabolic interactions between thyroid state and imipramine in the rat. *The Journal of Pharmacology and Experimental Therapeutics*, **244**, 463–7.

Drago, F., Pulvirenti, L., Spadaro, F. et al. (1990). Effects of TRH and prolactin in the behavioral despair (swim) model of depression in rats. *Psychoneuroendocrinology*, **15**, 349–56.

Duncan, W.C. & Schull, J. (1994). The interaction of thyroid state, MAOI drug treatment, and light on the level and circadian pattern of wheel-running rats. *Biological Psychiatry*, **35**, 324–34.

Duval, F., Mokrani, M-C., Crocq, M-C. et al. (1996). Effect of antidepressant medication on morning and evening thyroid function tests during a major depressive episode. *Archives of General Psychiatry*, **53**, 833–40.

Earle, B.V. (1970). Thyroid hormone and tricyclic antidepressants in resistant depression. *American Journal of Psychiatry*, **126**, 1667–9.

Epperson, C.N., Wisner, K.L., & Yamamoto, B. (1999). Gonadal steroids in the treatment of mood disorders. *Psychosomatic Medicine*, **61**, 676–97.

Evans, D.L., Strawn, S.K., Haggerty, J.J. et al. (1986). Appearance of mania in drug-resistant bipolar depressed patients after treatment with L-triiodothyronine. *Journal of Clinical Psychiatry*, **47**, 521–2.

Fahrenfort, J.J., Wilterdink, A.M.L., & van der Veen, E.A. (2000). Long-term residual complaints and psychosocial sequelae after remission of hyperthyroidism. *Psychoneuroendocrinology*, **25**, 201–11.

Fava, M., Littman, A., Lamon-Fava, S. et al. (1992). Psychological, behavioral and biochemical risk factors for coronary artery disease among American and Italian male corporate managers. *American Journal of Cardiology*, **70**, 1412–16.

Fava, M., Labbate, L.A., Abraham, M.E. et al. (1995). Hypothyroidism and hyperthyroidism in major depression revisited. *Journal of Clinical Psychiatry*, **56**, 186–92.

Feldman, D. (1986). Ketoconazole and other imidazole derivatives as inhibitors of steroidogenesis. *Endocrine Review*, **7**, 409–20.

Fleckman, A., Erlichman, J., Schubart, U.K. et al. (1981). Effect of trifluoperazine, D600, and phenytoin on depolarization- and thyrotropin-releasing hormone-induced thyrotropin release from rat pituitary tissue. *Endocrinology*, **108**, 2072–7.

Gewirtz, G.R., Malaspina, D., Hatterer, J.A., et al. (1988). Occult thyroid dysfunction in patients with refractory depression. *American Journal of Psychiatry*, **145**, 1012–14.

Ghadirian, A.M., Englesmann, F., Dhar, V. et al. (1995). The psychotropic effects of inhibitors of steroid biosynthesis in depressed patients refractory to treatment. *Biological Psychiatry*, **37**, 369–75.

Gitlin, M.J., Weiner, H., Fairbanks, L. et al. (1987). Failure of $T_3$ to potentiate tricyclic antidepressant response. *Journal of Affective Disorders*, **13**, 267–72.

Gold, P.W. & Chrousos, G.P. (1985). Clinical studies with corticotropin releasing factor: implications for the diagnosis and pathophysiology of depression, Cushing's disease, and adrenal insufficiency. *Psychoneuroendocrinology*, **10**, 401–19.

Goodwin, F.K., Prange, A.J. Jr., Post, R.M. et al. (1982). Potentiation of antidepressant effects by L-triiodothyronine in tricyclic nonresponders. *American Journal of Psychiatry*, **139**, 34–8.

Goodwin, G.M., Muir, W.J., Seckl, J.R. et al. (1992). The effects of cortisol infusion upon hormone secretion from the anterior pituatary and subjective mood in depressive illness and in controls. *Journal of Affective Disorders*, **26**, 73–83.

Goodyer, I.M., Herbert, J., Altham, P.M., Pearson, J., Secher, S.M., & Shiers, H.M. (1996). Adrenal secretion during major depression in 8- to 16-year-olds, I. Altered diurnal rhythms in salivary cortisol and dehydroepiandrosterone (DHEA) at presentation. *Psychological Medicine*, **26**(2), 245–56.

Gray, A., Jackson, D.N., & McKinlay, J.B. (1991). The relation between dominance, anger, and hormones in normally aging men: results from the Massachusetts Male Aging Study. *Psychosomatic Medicine*, **53**, 375–85.

Greden, J.F., Gardner, R., King, D., Grunhaus, L., Carroll, B.J., & Kronfol, Z. (1983). Dexamethasone suppression tests in antidepressant treatment of melancholia: the process of normalization and test-retest reproducibility. *Archives of General Psychiatry*, **40**, 493–500.

Gregoire, A.J.P., Kumar, R., Evertt, R. et al. (1996). Transdermal oestrogen for treatment of severe postnatal depression. *Lancet*, **347**, 930–3.

Gyulai, L., Jaggi, J., Bauer, M.S. et al. (1997). Bone mineral density and L-thyroxine treatment in rapidly cycling bipolar disorder. *Biological Psychiatry*, **41**, 503–6.

Hansen, C.R. Jr, Kroll, J., & Mackenzie, T.B. (1982). Dehydroepiandrosterone and affective disorders. *American Journal Psychiatry*, **139**, 386–7.

Herman, R., Obarzanek, E., Mikalauskas, K.M. et al. (1991). The effects of carbamazepine on resting metabolic rate and thyroid function in depressed patients. *Biological Psychiatry*, **29**, 779–88.

Hermida, R.C., Hallberg, F., & Del Pozo, F. (1985). Chronobiologic pattern discrimination of plasma hormones, notably DHEA-S and TSH, classifies an expansive personality. *Chronobiologia*, **12**, 105–36.

Höflich, G., Kasper, S., Danos, P. et al. (1992). Thyroid hormones, body temperature, and antidepressant treatment. *Biological Psychiatry*, **31**, 859–62.

Holsboer, F. (1989). Psychiatric implications of altered limbic–hypothalamic–pituitary–adrenocortical activity. *European Archives of Psychiatry and Neurological Science*, **238**, 302–22.

Holsboer, F., Liebl, R., & Hofschuster, E. (1982). Repeated dexamethasone suppression test during depressive illness: normalization of test result with clinical improvement. *Journal of Affective Disorder*, **4**, 93–101.

Holsboer, F., Steiger, A., & Maier, W. (1983). Four cases of reversion to abnormal dexamethasone suppression test response as indicator of clinical relapse: a preliminary report. *Biological Psychiatry*, **18**, 911–16.

Howard, J.S. III (1992). Severe psychosis and the adrenal androgens. *Integrative Physiological and Behavioral Science*, **27**, 209–15.

Howland, R.H. (1995). Thyroid function in mood disorder. *Biological Psychiatry*, **37**, 63–5.

Hullett, F.J. & Bidder, T.G. (1983). Phenelzine plus triiodothyronine combination in a case of refractory depression. *The Journal of Nervous and Mental Disease*, **171**, 318–20.

Jaffer, A., Russell, V.A., & Taljaard, J.J.F. (1987). Effect of chronic desipramine treatment on neurotransmitter-thyrotropin releasing hormone – thyrotropin interactions in the rat. *Neurochemical Research*, **12**, 1013–17.

Joffe, H., & Cohen, L.S. (1998). Estrogen, serotonin, and mood disturbance: where is the therapeutic bridge? *Biological Psychiatry*, **44**, 798–811.

Joffe, R.T. (1988a). T₃ and lithium potentiation of tricyclic antidepressants. *American Journal of Psychiatry*, **145**, 1317–18.

Joffe, R.T. (1988b). Triiodothyronine potentiation of the antidepressant effect of phenelzine. *Journal of Clinical Psychiatry*, **49**, 409–10.

Joffe, R.T. (1999). Peripheral thyroid hormone levels in treatment resistant depression. *Biological Psychiatry*, **45**, 1053–5.

Joffe, R.T. & Levitt, A.J. (1992). Major depression and subclinical (grade 2) hypothyroidism. *Psychoneuroendocrinology*, **17**, 215–21.

Joffe, R.T. & Levitt, A.J. (1993). The thyroid and depression. In *The Thyroid Axis and Psychiatric Illness*, ed. R.T. Joffe & A.J. Levitt, pp. 195–253. Washington, DC: American Psychiatric Press, Inc.

Joffe, R.T. & Singer, W. (1987). Effect of phenelzine on thyroid function in depressed patients. *Biological Psychiatry*, **22**, 1033–5.

Joffe, R.T. & Sokolov, S.T.H. (1994). Thyroid hormones, the brain, and affective disorders. *Critical Reviews in Neurobiology*, **8**, 45–63.

Joffe, R.T., Nobrega, J., Kish, S. et al. (1993). Desipramine reduces plasma but not brain thyroxine levels. *Biological Psychiatry*, **33**, 292–4.

Joffe, R.T., Segal, Z., & Singer, W. (1996). Change in thyroid hormone levels following response to cognitive therapy for major depression. *American Journal of Psychiatry*, **153**, 411–13.

Jones, J.A., Nguyen, A., Straub, M. et al. (1997). Use of DHEA in a patient with advanced prostate cancer: a case report and review. *Urology*, **50**, 784–8.

Kasper, S., Sack, D.A., Vehr, T.A. et al. (1988). Nocturnal TSH and prolactin secretion during sleep deprivation and prediction of antidepressant response in patients with major depression. *Biological Psychiatry*, **24**, 631–41.

Kathol, R.G. (1985). Etiologic implications of corticosteroid changes in affective disorder. *Psychiatric Medicine*, **3**, 135–62.

Kennett, G.A., Dickinson, S.L., & Curzon, G. (1985). Central serotonergic responses and behavioral adaptation to repeated immobilisation: the effect of the corticosterone synthesis inhibitor metyrapone. *European Journal of Pharmacology*, **119**, 143–52.

Kiraly, S.J., Ancil, R.J., & Dimitrova, G. (1997). The relationship of endogenous cortisol to psychiatric disorder: a review. *Canadian Journal of Psychiatry*, **42**, 415–20.

Klaiber, E.L., Broverman, D.M., Vogel, W. et al. (1979). Estrogen therapy for severe persistent depression in women. *Archives of General Psychiatry*, **36**, 550–4.

Klinteberg, B., Hallman, J., Oreland, L., Wirsen, B., Levander, S.E., & Schalling, D. (1992). Exploring the connections between platelet monoamine oxidase activity and behavior. II. Impulsive personality without neuropsychological signs of disinhibition in air force pilot recruits. *Neurospsychobiology*, **26**, 136–45.

Labbate, L.A., Fava, M., Oleshansky, M., Zoltec, J., Littman. A., & Harig, P. (1995). Physical fitness and perceived stress. Relationships with coronary artery disease risk factors. *Psychosomatics*, **36**, 555–60.

Leblhuber, F., Windhager, E., Neubauer, C., Weber, J., Reisecker, F., & Dienstl, E. (1992). Antiglucocorticoid effects of DHEA-S in Alzheimer's disease. *American Journal of Psychiatry*, **149**, 1125–6.

Leibow, D. (1983). L-thyroxine for rapid-cycling bipolar illness. *American Journal of Psychiatry*, **140**, 1255.

Lindsay, R.S. & Toft, A.D. (1997). Hypothyroidism. *Lancet*, **349**, 413–17.

Loose, D.S., Stover, E.P., & Feldman, D. (1983). Ketoconazole binds to glucocorticoid receptors and exhibits glucocorticoid agonist activity in cultured cells. *Journal of Clinical Investigation*, **72**, 404–8.

McEwen, B.S., Angulo, J., Cameron, H. et al. (1992). Paradoxical effects of adrenal steroids on the brain: protection versus degeneration. *Biological Psychiatry*, **31**, 177–99.

McKittrick, C.R. & McEwen, B.S. (1996). Regulation of serotonergic function in the CNS by steroid hormones and stress. In *CNS Neurotransmitters and Neuromodulators: Neuroactive Steroids*, ed. T.W. Stone, pp. 37–76. CRC Press: Boca Raton FL.

Magliozzi, J.R., Gold, A., & Laubly, J.N. (1989). Effect of oral administration of haloperidol on plasma thyrotropin concentrations in men. *Psychoneuroendocrinology*, **14**, 125–30.

Majewska, M.D. (1987). Steroids and brain activity. *Biochemical Pharmacology*, **36**, 3781–8.

Malek-Ahmadi, P. (1996). Neuropsychiatric aspects of cytokines research: an overview. *Neuroscience and Biobehavioral Reviews*, **20**, 359–65.

Marangell, L.B., George, M.S., Callahan, A.M. et al. (1997a). Effects of intrathecal thyrotropin-releasing hormone (protirelin) in refractory depressed patients. *Archives of General Psychiatry*, **54**, 214–22.

Marangell, L.B., Ketter, T.A., Geroge, M.S. et al. (1997b). Inverse relationship of peripheral thyrotropin-stimulating hormone levels to brain activity in mood disorders. *American Journal of Psychiatry*, **154**, 224–30.

Marco, E., Wolkowitz, O.M., Vinogradov, S., Poole, J., Lichtmacher, J. & Reus, V.I. (2000). Double-blind antiglucocorticoid treatment of schizophrenia and schizoaffective disorder. In review.

Martin, P., Brochet, D., Soubrie, P. et al. (1985). Triiodothyronine-induced reversal of learned helplessness in rats. *Biological Psychiatry*, **20**, 1023–5.

Martin, P., Massol, J., Belon, J.P. et al. (1987). Thyroid function and reversal by anti-depressant drugs of depressive-like behavior (escape deficits) in rats. *Neuropsychobiology*, **18**, 21–6.

Massol, J., Martin, P., Chatelain, F., et al. (1990). Tricyclic antidepressants, thyroid function, and their relationship with the behavioral responses in rats. *Biological Psychiatry*, **28**, 967–78.

Miller, W.L. & Tyrrell, J.B. (1995). The adrenal cortex. In *Endocrinology and Metabolism*, ed. P. Felig, J.D. Baxter, & L.A. Frohman, pp. 555–712. 3rd edn. New York: McGraw-Hill, Inc.

Morales, A.J., Nolan, J.J., Nelson, J.C., & Yen, S.S.C. (1994). Effects of replacement dose of dehydroepiandrosterone in men and women of advancing age. *Journal of Clinical and Endocrinological Metabolism*, **78**, 1360–7.

Murphy, B.E.P. (1991). Steroids and depression. *Journal of Steroid Biochemistry and Molecular Biology*, **38**, 537–59.

Murphy, B.E.P. (1994). Experience with antiglucocorticoid strategies in major depression. *Neuropsychopharmacology*, **10**, 637S.

Murphy, B.E.P. (1997). Antiglucocortoid therapies in major depression: a review. *Psychoneuroendocrinology*, **22**, S125–32.

Murphy, B.E.P. & Wolkowitz, O.M. (1993). The pathophysiologic significance of hypercorticism: antiglucocorticoid strategies. *Psychiatric Annals*, **23**, 682–90.

Murphy, B.E.P., Dhar, V., Ghadirian, A.M., Chouinard, G., & Keller, R. (1991). Response to steroid suppression in major depression resistant to antidepressant therapy. *Journal of Clinical Psychopharmacology*, **11**, 121–6.

Murphy, B.E.P., Dhar, V., Ghadirian, A.M., Filipini, D., Keller, R., & Chouinard, G. (1992). Endocrine and psychiatric responses to inhibitors of steroid biosynthesis in patients with antidepressant-resistant major depression. Presented at the XXIII Congress of the International Society of Psychoneuroendocrinology, Madison, Wisconsin, August 16–20, 1992.

Nader, S., Warner, D., Doyle, S. et al. (1995). Euthyroid sick syndrome in psychiatric inpatients. *Biological Psychiatry*, **40**, 1288–93.

Nerozzi, D., Graziosi, S., Melia, E. et al. (1987). Mechanism of action of ECT in major depressive disorders: a neuroendocrine interpretation. *Psychiatry Research*, **20**, 207–13.

O'Dwyer, A.M., Lightman, S.L., Marks, M.N., & Checkley, S.A. (1995). Treatment of major depression with metyrapone and hydrocortisone. *Journal of Affective Disorders*, **33**, 123–8.

Orth, D.N., Kovacs, W.J., & DeBold, C.R. (1992). The adrenal cortex. In *Williams Textbook of Endocrinology*, ed. J.D. Wilson & D.W. Foster, pp. 489–620. W.B. Saunders Company, Harcourt Brace Jovanavich, Inc., Philadelphia.

Palinkas, L.A. & Barrett-Connor, E. (1992). Estrogen use and depressive symptoms in post-menopausal women. *Obstetrics and Gynecology*, **80**, 30–6.

Peeters, B.W.M.M., Van Der Heijden, R., Gubbels, D.G., & Vanderheyden, P.M.L. (1994). Effects of chronic antidepressant treatment on the hypothalamic–pituitary–adrenal axis of Wistar rats. *Annals of the New York Academy of Sciences*, **746**, 449–52.

Prange, A.J. Jr, Wilson, I.C., Breese, G.R. et al. (1976). Hormonal alteration of imipramine response: a review. In *Hormones, Behavior, and Psychopathology*, ed. E. J. Sachar, pp. 41–67. New York: Raven Press.

Prange, A.J. Jr, Loosen, P.T., Wilson, I.C., et al. (1984). The therapeutic use of hormones of the thyroid axis in depression. In *The Neurobiology of the Mood Disorders*, ed. J.C. Ballenger & R.M. Post, pp. 311–22, Baltimore: Williams and Wilkins, Company.

Price, L.H. (1989). Thyroid hormone potentiation of tricyclic antidepressants. In *Treatment of Tricyclic-Resistant Depression*, ed. I.L. Extein, pp. 29–47. Washington, DC: American Psychiatric Press, Inc.

Przegalinski, E. & Jaworska, L. (1990). The effect of repeated administration of antidepressant drugs on the thyrotropin-releasing hormone (TRH) content of rat brain structures. *Psychoneuroendocrinology*, **15**, 147–53.

Ravaris, C.L., Brinck-Johnsen, E.B., & Elliot, B. (1994). Clinical use of ketoconazole in hypercortisoluric depressives. *Biological Psychiatry*, **35**, 679.

Raven, P.W., O'Dwyer, A.M., Taylor, N.F., & Checkley, S.A. (1996). The relationship between the effects of metyrapone treatment on depressed mood and urinary steroid profiles. *Psychoeuroendocrinology*, **21**, 277–86.

Reus, V.I. (1982). Pituitary–adrenal disinhibition as the independent variable in the assessment of behavioral symptoms. *Biological Psychiatry*, **17**, 317–25.

Reus, V.I. (1984). Hormonal mediation of the memory disorder in depression. *Drug Development Research*, **4**, 489–500.

Reus, V.I. (1989). Behavioral aspects of thyroid disease in women. *Psychiatric Clinics of North America*, **12**, 153–64.

Reus, V.I. (1993). Psychiatric aspects of thyroid disease. In *The Thyroid Axis and Psychiatric Illness*, ed. R.T. Joffe & A.J. Levitt, pp. 183–208. Washington, DC: American Psychiatric Press, Inc.

Reus, V.I. & Freimer, N. (1990). Antithyroid antibodies: behavioral significance. In *Neuropsychopharmacology*, ed. W.E. Bunney Jr, H. Hippius, G. Laakmann, & M. Schmauss, pp. 362–70. Berlin: Springer-Verleg.

Reus, V.I., Wolkowitz, O.M., Roberts. E. et al. (1993). Dehydroepiandrosterone (DHEA) and memory in depressed patients. *Neuropsychopharmacology*, **9**, 66S.

Reus, V.I., Wolkowitz, O.M., & Frederick, S. (1997). Antiglucocorticoid treatments in psychiatry. *Psychoneuroendocrinology*, **22**, S121–4.

Ribeiro, S.C.M., Tandon, R., Grunhaus, L., & Greden, J.F. (1993). The DST as a predictor of Outcome in depression: a meta-analysis. *American Journal of Psychiatry*, **150**, 1618–29.

Richter, C.P., Jones, G.S., & Biswanger, L. (1959). Periodic phenomena and the thyroid. *Archives of Neurology and Psychiatry*, **81**, 117–39.

Rudas, S., Schmitz, M., Pichler, P. et al. (1999). Treatment of refractory chronic depression and dysthymia with high-dose thyroxine. *Biological Psychiatry*, **45**, 229–33.

Rudman, D., Shatty, K.R., & Mattson, D.E. (1990). Plasma dehydroepiandrosterone sulfate in nursing home men. *Journal of the American Geriatric Society*, **38**, 421–7.

Russ, M.J. & Ackerman, S.H. (1989). Antidepressant treatment response in depressed hypothyroid patients. *Hospital and Community Psychiatry*, **40**, 954–6.

Sands, D.E. & Chamberlain, G.H.A. (1952). Treatment of inadaquate personality in juveniles by dehydroisoandrosterone. *British Medical Journal*, **2**, 66.

Sapolksy, R.M., Krey, L.C., & McEwen, B.S. (1986). The neuroendocrinology of stress and aging: the glucocorticoid cascade hypothesis. *Endocrine Review*, **7**, 284–301.

Schatzberg, A.F., Rothschild, A.J., Langlais, P.J., Bird, E.D., & Cole, J.O. (1985). A corticosteroid/dopamine hypothesis for psychotic depression and related states. *Journal of Psychi-

*atric Research*, **19**, 57.

Scherer, J. (1994). The prevalence of goiter in psychiatric outpatients suffering from affective disorder. *American Journal of Psychiatry*, **141**, 453–4.

Schlote, B., Schaaf, L., Schmidt, R., et al. (1992). Mental and physical state in subclinical hyperthyroidism: investigations in a normal working population. *Biological Psychiatry*, **32**, 48–56.

Schneider, L.S., Small, G.W., Hamilton, S.H., et al. (1997). Estrogen replacement and response to fluoxetine in a multicenter geriatric depression trial. Fluoxetine Collaborative Student Group. *American Journal of Geriatric Psychiatry*, **5**, 97–106.

Schull, J., McEachron, D.L., Adler, N.T., et al. (1988). Effects of thyroidectomy, parathyroidectomy and lithium on circadian wheelrunning in rats. *Physiology of Behavior*, **42**, 33–9.

Scott, A.I.F., Milner, J.B., Shering, A. et al. (1990). Fall in free thyroxine after ECT: real effect or an artefact of assay? *Biological Psychiatry*, **27**, 784–6.

Shapira, B., Oppenheim, G., Zohar, J. et al. (1985). Lack of efficiency of estrogen supplementation to imipramine in resistant female depressives. *Biological Psychiatry*, **20**, 576–9.

Sheline, Y.I., Wang, P.W., Gado, M.H., Csernansky, J.G., & Vannier, M.W. (1996). Hippocampal atrophy in recurrent depression. *Proceedings of the National Academy of Science*, USA, **93**, 3908–13.

Shelton, R.C., Winn, S., Ekhatore, N. et al. (1993). The effects of antidepressants on the thyroid axis in depression. *Biological Psychiatry*, **33**, 120–6.

Sherwin, B.B. (1991). Estrogen and refractory depression. In *Advances in Neuropsychiatry and Psychopharmacology, Volume 2: Refractory Depression*, ed. J.D. Amsterdam, pp. 209–18. New York: Raven Press, Ltd.

Sonino, N., Boscaro, M., Ambroso, G., Merola, G., & Mantero, F. (1986). Prolonged treatment of Cushing's disease with metyrapone and aminoglutethimide. *IRCS Medical Science*, **14**, 485–6.

Southwick, S., Mason, J.W., Giller, E.L. et al. (1989). Serum thyroxine change and clinical recovery in psychiatric inpatients. *Biological Psychiatry*, **25**, 67–74.

Sovner, R. & Fogelman, S. (1996). Ketoconazole therapy for atypical depression. *Journal of Clinical Psychiatry*, **57**, 227–8.

Spitzweg, C., Heufelder, A. & Morris, J. (2000). Thyroid iodine transport. *Thyroid*, **10**, 321–30.

Stalla, G.K., Stalla, J., von Werder, K. et al. (1989). Nitroimidazole derivatives inhibit anterior pituitary cell function apparently by a direct effect on the catalytic subunit of the adenylate cyclase holoenzyme. *Endocrinology*, **125**, 699–706.

Stancer, H.E. & Persad, E. (1982). Treatment of intractable rapid-cycling manic-depressive disorder with levothyroxine. *Archives of General Psychiatry*, **39**, 311–12.

Starkman, M.N. & Schteingart, D.E. (1983). Cushing's syndrome: changes in psychiatric symptomatology and hormone levels with treatment. *Psychosomatic Medicine*, **45**, 83.

Starkman, M.N., Schteingart, D.E., & Schork, M.A. (1981). Depressed mood and other psychiatric manifestations of Cushing's syndrome: relationship to hormone levels. *Psychosomatic Medicine*, **43**, 3–18.

Starkman, M.N., Schteingart, D.E., & Schork, M.A. (1986). Cushing's syndrome after treatment: changes in cortisol and ACTH levels and amelioration of the depressive syndrome. *Psychiatry*

*Research*, **19**, 177–88.

Stein, D. & Avni, J. (1988). Thyroid hormones in the treatment of affective disorders. *Acta Psychiatrica Scandinavica*, **77**, 623–36.

Stein, M.B. & Uhde, T.W. (1990). Triiodothyronine potentiation of tricyclic antidepressant treatment in patients with panic disorder. *Biological Psychiatry*, **28**, 1061–4.

Stern, R.A., Nevels, C.T., Shelhorse, M.E. et al. (1991). Antidepressant and memory effects of combined thyroid hormone treatment and electroconvulsive therapy: Preliminary findings. *Biological Psychiatry*, **30**, 623–7.

Stern, R.A., Whealin, J.M., Mason, G.A. et al. (1995). Influence of L-triiodothyronine on memory following repeated electroconvulsive shock in rats: implications for human electroconvulsive therapy. *Biological Psychiatry*, **37**, 198–201.

Strauss, E.B. & Stevenson, W.A.H. (1955). Use of dehydroisoandrosterone in psychiatric practice. *Journal of Neurology Neurosurgery and Psychiatry*, **18**, 137–44.

Strauss, E.B., Sands, D.E., Robinson, A.M., Tindall, W.J., & Stevenson, W.A.H. (1952). Use of dehydroisoandrosterone in psychiatric treatment: a preliminary survey. *British Medical Journal*, **2**, 64–6.

Sullivan, G.M., Hatterer, J.A., Herbert, J. et al. (1999). Low levels of transthyretin in the CSF of depressed patients. *American Journal of Psychiatry*, **156**, 710–15.

Swartz, C.M. (1982). Dependency of tricyclic antidepressant efficacy on thyroid hormone potentiation: case studies. *The Journal of Nervous and Mental Disease*, **170**, 50–2.

Targum, S.D., Greenberg, R.D., Harmon, E.L. et al. (1984). Thyroid hormone and the TRH stimulation test in refractory depression. *Journal of Clinical Psychiatry*, **45**, 345–6.

Taubøll Gjerstad, L., Stokke, K.T. et al. (1987). Effects of electroconvulsive therapy (ECT) on thyroid function parameters. *Psychoneuroendocrinology*, **12**, 349–54.

Thakore, J.H. & Dinan, T.G. (1995). Cortisol synthesis inhibition: a new treatment strategy for the clinical and endocrine manifestations of depression. *Biological Psychiatry*, **37**, 364–8.

Thase, M.E., Kupfer, D.J., & Jarrett, D.B. (1989). Treatment of imipramine-resistant recurrent depression: I. An open clinical trial of adjunctive L-triiodothyronine. *Journal of Clinical Psychiatry*, **50**, 385–8.

Toft, A.D. (1994). Thyroxine therapy. *The New England Journal of Medicine*, **331**, 174–80.

Utiger, R.D. (1995). Altered thyroid function in non-thyroidal illness and surgery. *The New England Journal of Medicine*, **333**, 1562–3.

Van Praag, H.M. (1996). Faulty cortisol/serotonin interplay. Psychopathological and biological characterisation of a new, hypothetical depression subtype (SeCA depression). *Psychiatry Research*, **65**, 143–57.

Wheatley, D. (1972). Potentiation of amitriptyline by thyroid hormone. *Archives of General Psychiatry*, **26**, 229–33.

Whybrow, P.C. & Prange, A.J. Jr. (1981). A hypothesis of thyroid-catecholamine-receptor interaction. *Archives of General Psychiatry*, **38**, 106–13.

Whybrow, P.C., Coppen, A., Prange, A.J. Jr et al. (1972). Thyroid function and the response to liothyronine in depression. *Archives of General Psychiatry*, **26**, 242–5.

Williams, N. (1997). Thyroid disease: a case of cell suicide? *Science*, **275**, 926.

Winokur, G., Black, D.W., & Nasrallah, A. (1987). DST nonsuppressor status: relationship to specific aspects of the depressive syndrome. *Biological Psychiatry*, **22**, 360–8.

Wolkowitz, O.M. (1992). Prospective controlled studies of the behavioral and biological effects of exogenous corticosteroids. *Psychoneuroendocrinology*, **19**, 233–55.

Wolkowitz, O.M. & Reus, V.I. (1999). Treatment of depression with antiglucocorticoid drugs. *Psychosomatic Medicine*, **61**, 698–711.

Wolkowitz, O.M., Reus, V.I., Weingartner, H. et al. (1990). Cognitive effects of corticosteroids. *American Journal of Psychiatry*, **147**, 1297–303.

Wolkowitz, O.M., Reus, V.I., Manfredi, F., Ingbar, J., & Brizendine, L. (1993). Ketoconazole administration in hypercortisolemic depression. *American Journal of Psychiatry*, **150**, 810–12.

Wolkowitz, O.M., Reus, V.I., Manfredi, F., Chan, T., Ormiston, S., & Johnson, R. (1996). Dexamethasone for depression. *American Journal of Psychiatry*, **153**, 1112.

Wolkowitz, O.M., Reus, V.I., Roberts, E. et al. (1997). Dehydroepiandrosterone (DHEA) treatment of depression. *Biological Psychiatry*, **41**, 311–18.

Wolkowitz, O.M., Reus, V.I., Chan, T. et al. (1999a). Antiglucocorticoid treatment of depression: double-blind ketoconazole. *Biological Psychiatry*, **45**, 1070–4.

Wolkowitz, O.M., Reus, V.I., Keebler, A. et al. (1999b). Double-blind treatment of major depression with dehydroepiandrosterone (DHEA). *American Journal of Psychiatry*, **156**, 646–9.

Wolkowitz, O.M., Brizendine, L., & Reus, V.I. (2000). The role of dehydroepiandrosterone (DHEA) in psychiatry. *Psychiatric Annals*, **30**, 123–8.

# 4

# Estrogen and depressive illness in women

Barbara B. Sherwin

One of the most consistent findings in the epidemiology of mental disorders is the higher prevalence of depressive illness in women than in men. Several recent national and international studies have confirmed the increased prevalence of depression in women including the Epidemiologic Catchment Area Study (Regier et al., 1988), the National Comorbidity Study (Kessler et al., 1993) and others (Paykel, 1991; Weissman et al., 1993; Weissman & Klerman, 1977; Wittchen et al., 1972). In these studies, the prevalence of depressive illness among women is approximately 1.5 to 3 times that among men. Moreover, it has been established that this sex difference in the prevalence of depression is not due to genetic transmission of the disorder (Merikangas et al., 1985), to sex differences in help-seeking behavior (Dohrenwend & Dohrenwend, 1977), to experience and reaction to stressful life events (Kessler et al., 1979), or to differential exposure to the factors related to depression (Radloff & Rai, 1979). Nor is the sex difference in the prevalence of depressive illness attributable to the tendency for physicians to detect more psychiatric illness in women than in men (MacIntyre & Oldman, 1977).

In the face of a sex difference in the prevalence of any medical disorder, investigating the possible influence of the sex steroid hormones in its pathogenesis is frequently a sensible and useful strategy. It is clear that some women are at greater risk for the development of a depressive episode subsequent to a change in their circulating levels of the sex steroids during various reproductive events. For example, at the time that estradiol and progesterone levels reach a nadir premenstrually, 35% of women report moderate affective and physical symptoms and 3% experience severe, incapacitating symptoms (Andersch et al., 1986). Second, subsequent to the 100-fold decrease in circulating levels of estradiol and progesterone following childbirth, 50 to 70% of women experience a mild, transient mood disturbance between the third and tenth postpartum day, 10 to 21% develop a major depressive episode within the first 3 months, and 0.1 to 0.2% develop postpartum psychosis (Kendell et al., 1976). Finally, during the perimenopausal years when estradiol levels are declining drastically, 79% of women who seek medical care have physical symptoms and 65% have varying degrees of depression (Anderson et al., 1987).

Although reports of a mood-enhancing effect of estrogen first appeared more than 60 years ago (Hawkinson, 1938), these early findings were received with much skepticism. This may have been due to the lack of evidence at that time that estrogen could influence central nervous system function.

Neurological effects of estrogen that have been elucidated since the 1980s provide a scientific basis for possible biological mechanisms of action of this sex steroid on affective states and are reviewed here. In addition, clinical studies of estrogenic effects on mood in non-clinical and in clinical populations, although relatively few in number, also are discussed with regard to the therapeutic use of estrogen in depressive disorders in women.

## Neurobiology of estrogen

Estrogen can be called a neurosteroid since it can be synthesized from testosterone in various regions of the brain. Moreover, it is a neuroactive steroid since it influences neural tissue.

Estrogen has both inductive and direct effects on neurons. This hormone induces ribonucleic acid (RNA) and protein synthesis via genomic mechanisms, which, in turn, cause changes in levels of specific gene products, such as neurotransmitter synthesizing enzymes (Luine et al., 1975). Other prolonged neuronal regulatory effects include the expression of gonadal hormone receptors in specific brain areas. Estrogen is also capable of exerting non-genomic effects on brain function, which appear to take place more rapidly than genomic effects. For example, estrogens can alter the electrical activity of neurons in the hypothalamus (Kelly et al., 1977).

Electrophysiological evidence suggests that membrane actions of estrogen on certain target cells might regulate second messenger formation. For estradiol, depolarization of hypothalamic neurons involves cyclic AMP and also attenuates potassium conductance; in pituitary, estradiol inhibits GTPase activity whereas in stiatum, estradiol suppresses calcium currents (McEwen, 1994).

Autoradiographic studies have shown that estrogen receptors are found in large concentrations in specific areas of the brain including the hypothalamus, pituitary, amygdala, basal forebrain, hippocampus and the cerebral cortex (McEwen et al., 1995). Moreover, a number of neurotransmitter systems, including serotonergic, cholinergic, dopaminergic, GABAergic, adrenergic, and opioid systems, have been suggested to be responsive to estrogen, although not all of these effects have been demonstrated in vivo or at physiological conditions (McEwen et al., 1995).

There is increasing evidence of abnormal indoleamine metabolism in depressed patients, manifested by a reduced level of 5-hydroxytryptamine (5HT) and 5-hydroxyindole-acetic acid (5HIAA) in the brain and decreased levels of 5HIAA in the cerebrospinal fluid (Murphy et al., 1978; Coopen & Wood, 1982). In accordance with Schildkraut's biogenic amine hypothesis of depression (Schildkraut, 1965), a decrease in 5HT levels centrally may precipitate depression. There are at least two ways in which estrogen may influence neurotransmitter amine levels. First, it has been demonstrated in the rat that exogenous estrogen decreases monoamine oxidase (MAO) activity in the amygdala and hypothalamus (Luine et al., 1975). Since MAO is the enzyme that catabolizes 5HT, the net effect of estrogen administration would be to maintain higher brain 5HT levels. There is clinical evidence to support this theory. In normal premenopausal women, mean levels of plasma MAO activity before the thermal nadir (when estradiol levels are high) were lower than levels measured after the thermal nadir (postovulation) when estradiol levels had decreased (Klaiber et al., 1971). In healthy untreated postmenopausal women, plasma MAO activity was greater and estradiol levels lower compared to enzyme and hormone values observed during the luteal phase of the cycle in regularly menstruating women. Moreover, premenopausal depressed women with regular menstrual cycles had higher levels of plasma MAO activity compared to non-depressed women (Klaiber et al., 1972). Briggs and Briggs (1972) likewise reported that, in healthy women with regular menstrual cycles, plasma MAO activity was negatively correlated with estradiol concentrations. To the extent that similar events occur centrally, brain 5HT levels would increase as a function of higher estradiol levels.

There is also some evidence that in depressed, regularly cycling women, exogenous estrogen has a beneficial impact on both plasma MAO levels and mood. Klaiber et al. (1972) administered 5 mg of conjugated equine estrogen (Premarin) from days 1 to 25 and 10 mg medroxyprogesterone acetate (Provera) from days 21 to 25 to 14 depressed women whose mean age was 28.7 years. During the portion of the cycle when only estrogen was being taken, plasma MAO activity was significantly lower by the third and fourth treatment cycles compared to pretreatment levels. Although changes in affect were not quantified in this controlled study, patients spontaneously reported improvement in mood after estrogen treatment. Take together, these studies suggest that the estrogenic influence on MAO levels documented in rat brain (Luine et al., 1975) also occur in the plasma of human females.

Recent findings suggest that there is a positive correlation between serum estradiol levels and whole blood serotonin levels. First, blood serotonin levels were lower in amenorrheic, and in naturally and surgically postmenopausal women than in 30-year-old women with regular menstrual cycles, and blood serotonin levels increased when postmenopausal women were given exogenous estrogen (Gonzales & Carrillo, 1993).

A second mechanism that may explain the effect of estrogen on mood is that tryptophan, the precursor of 5HT, is displaced from its binding sites to plasma albumin by estrogens in vitro and in vivo (Aylward, 1973), thereby increasing free tryptophan in the brain. In 1976, Aylward found a significant negative correlation between depression scores and free plasma tryptophan levels in bilaterally oophorectomized women and an amelioration in their depression scores subsequent to estrogen administration. In a double-blind study, nine women taking lithium were given either conjugated equine estrogen 1.25 mg or placebo daily for 3 months, following which they were crossed-over to the other treatment for an additional 3 months (Coopen & Wood, 1978). There was a significant increase in the level of free plasma tryptophan when the patients were receiving estrogen compared to placebo. However, the mild affective morbidity of these patients was unaffected by either treatment.

When perimenopausal women with mild depressive symptoms were compared to a similar group whose depression scores were within the normal range, platelet 5HT content was significantly lower in the depressed group and in the subgroup of women who had experienced previous depressive episodes compared to the controls (Guicheney et al., 1988). However, plasma free tryptophan levels did not differ between groups, and a positive correlation between estradiol and platelet 5HT levels was evident only in the euthymic control group. In four women with depressive symptoms, platelet and blood 5HT levels increased moderately after 3 months of estrogen and progestin therapy (doses not reported) coincident with a decrease in their depression scores. The fact that the concentration of plasma-free tryptophan did not account for the low platelet 5HT values in the depressed group before treatment suggests that reduced 5HT levels in depression may be partially attributable to reduced platelet 5HT uptake. It should be noted that the failure to standardize the hormone replacement regimen in this study complicates the interpretation of its findings.

Finally, recent evidence suggests that estrogen influences the production of tryptophan hydroxylase, the rate-limiting enzyme in the synthesis of serotonin. Using in situ hybridization, estrogen induced tryptophan hydroxylase mRNA expression in serotonin neurons in the dorsal raphe of female rhesus monkeys (Pecins-Thomson et al., 1996).

## Effects on neurotransmitter receptors

Estrogen enhances central norepinephrine availability (Paul et al., 1979) and sensitizes dopamine receptors (Chiodo & Caggiula, 1983). Chronic estrogen treatment reduces $\beta$-adrenergic receptors in rats cortex (Wagner et al., 1979), an effect similar to that observed with chronic antidepressant treatment. Moreover, 72 hours after estrogen was administered to ovariectomized rats, there was an increase in muscurinic acetylcholine receptors in ventromedial and anterior hypothalamic nuclei (Rainbow et al., 1980).

The demonstration that long-term antidepressant treatment induces consistent changes in adrenergic and serotonergic receptor sensitivities suggests that modulation of receptor sensitivity may be a mechanism of action common to tricyclic antidepressants, MAO inhibitors, and electroconvulsive therapy (Charney et al., 1981). To the extent that estrogen has antidepressant effects, its involvement in the regulation of 5HT receptors would help to explain the phenomenon. When ovariectomized rats received estradiol, followed 48 hours later by progesterone, increased 5HT uptake and content were observed in brain raphe nuclei (Cone et al., 1981). Another study found biphasic effects on the density of 5HT receptors throughout the brain of ovariectomized female rats who were given estrogen (Biegon & McEwen, 1982). One to 2 hours after estradiol injection, an acute reduction in 5HT receptor density was evident throughout the brain. However, by 72 hours postinjection, there was a selective increase in 5HT receptor density in brain regions known to contain estrogen receptors, namely, the hypothalamus, preoptic area, and amygdala.

Kendall et al. (1982) reported an estrogen-dependent decrease in $5HT_2$ receptor binding in rat frontal cortex during long-term imipramine administration. Castration abolished this decline, which was reversed by estrogen or testosterone but not by the non-aromatizable androgen, dihydrotestosterone. This suggests that the receptor responses to some antidepressant drugs are dependent, at least in part, on the hormonal state of the animal. Thus, estrogen may have a facilitatory role in drug-resistant depressive patients similar to that proposed for lithium carbonate (de Montigny et al., 1981).

Yet another mechanism whereby estrogen may influence mood is related to the presence of tritiated imipramine binding sites in rat and human brain and platelets (Raisman et al., 1979). These binding sites are thought to modulate the presynaptic uptake of 5HT in both tissues (Paul et al., 1984). Many investigators have found a decrease in the density ($B_{max}$) but no change in the affinity ($K_d$) of these binding sites in brain and platelets of depressed patients (Raisman et al., 1982; Surany-Cadotte et al., 1983), and the density of platelet tritiated imipramine binding sites in now widely regarded as a biological correlate of depression. It has been reported that tritiated imipramine binding and tritiated 5HT uptake increased by 20 to 30% in the frontal cortex and hypothalamus of ovariectomied rats following 12 days of treatment with estradiol (Rehavi et al., 1987).

Recent evidence suggests that estrogenic enhancement of the $B_{max}$ of tritiated imipramine binding sites may be dose-dependent. Whereas changes in binding site density did not occur in association with fluctuating estradiol levels during normal menstrual cycles (Poirier et al., 1986) or following treatment of postmenopausal women with physiological doses of estradiol (Best et al., 1989), a significant increase in the density of tritiated imipramine binding sites on platelets was apparent in oophorectomized women given pharmacological doses of estradiol (Sherwin & Suranyi-Cadotte, 1990).

The psychotropic and neurobiological properties of progesterone also are important in the study of estrogenic influences on mood. Progesterone is an important component of oral contraceptive preparations and also is administered frequently to postmenopausal women in association with estrogen in order to prevent endometrial hyperplasia. Whereas estrogen increases the electrical excitability of the brain, progesterone decreases it, acting as an anticonvulsant (Bäckström, 1977). Progesterone also has sedative and hypnotic effects (Arafat et al., 1988) and, at high doses, induces deep sleep (Merryman et al., 1954). Furthermore, whereas estradiol reduces plasma MAO activity, progestins increase it (Klaiber et al., 1971).

## Clinical studies in non-psychiatric populations

Several studies of non-psychiatric populations of postmenopausal women have reported on changes in affect as a function of circulating estradiol levels. In a prospective investigation, premenopausal women received either an estrogen-androgen combined drug (E–A), estrogen-alone (E), androgen-alone (A), or placebo (PL) for 3 months following bilateral oophorectomy and were randomly crossed over to another treatment for an additional 3 months after a 1-month intervening placebo phase (Sherwin & Gelfand, 1985). Women who underwent hysterectomy but whose ovaries were retained served as an additional control group (CON). In both treatment phases, women who received PL had higher depression scores on the Multiple Affect Adjective Checklist compared to those of the hormone-treated groups, to the CON group, and to their own preoperative scores in association with their lower plasma levels of estradiol and testosterone.

A second study investigated otherwise healthy surgically menopausal women who had undergone hysterectomy and bilateral oophorectomy for benign disease approximately 4 years before their recruitment (Sherwin, 1988). Those who had been receiving either an E–A or an E preparation long term (one injection per month for the previous 2 years) had more positive moods and higher levels of plasma estradiol than an untreated oophorectomized control group. Women who were given estradiol plus testosterone felt more composed, elated, and energetic than those who were given E alone. These findings confirmed that mood covaries with circulating estradiol and testosterone levels in healthy, non-depressed women.

Thus, both of these studies (Sherwin & Gelfand, 1985; Sherwin, 1988) suggest a positive relationship between mood and estradiol levels in non-psychiatric populations treated with physiological doses of the hormone. The discrepancy between these results and those of other studies may be due to their failure to control for endocrine status (Strickler et al., 1977), psychiatric illness and the use of psychotropic drugs (Dennerstein et al., 1979), and malignant disease (Chakravarti et al., 1977). Nine of ten postmenopausal women whose pretreatment scores were less than 18 on the Beck Depression Inventory (BDI) improved with conjugated equine estrogen 1.25 mg daily, whereas six of the ten women who had pretreatment scores above 20 at baseline actually became more depressed with the same treatment (Schneider et al., 1977b). Taken together, these findings suggest that the administration of estrogen in doses conventionally used to treat menopausal symptoms enhances mood in dysphoric women but is therapeutically ineffective with respect to mood disturbances of a clinical magnitude when the hormone is given alone.

Recently, a meta-analysis of the effect of hormone replacement therapy on depressed mood in postmenopausal women was undertaken on 26 such studies (Zweifel & O'Brien, 1997). In most studies, subjects were dysthymic and few used women who would have met diagnostic criteria for a major depressive disorder. In these investigations which had pretreatment to post-treatment comparisons and treatment to control comparisons, estrogen replacement therapy (ERT) exerted a moderate to a large effect on depressed mood in these dysthymic postmenopausal women; the overall effect size for ERT was 0.68, which indicated that the average treatment patient had lower levels of depressed mood than 76% of the control patients.

Results of a cross-sectional study of middle-aged and healthy women suggested that ERT might actually prevent episodes of depression in older women. Between 1984 and 1987, over 1100 white upper middle-class women from Rancho Bernardo, California over the age of 50 years were administered the BDI (Feild et al., 1979). A cut-point of 13 on the BDI was used to define cases of mild to severe depression on 18 scale items. In estrogen non-users, mean depressive symptom scores increased steadily and significantly with age whereas depression scores remained stable with increasing age in the women who took estrogen. It cannot be determined to what degree a self-selection bias in this sample may have influenced these findings.

## Estrogen and treatment-resistant depression

Although there have been surprisingly few systematic investigations of the use of estrogen in treatment-resistant depression, several controlled studies and case reports serve to provide some (albeit inconsistent) evidence of its effects. The reports in the literature pertain (a) to the administration of estrogen alone to women with treatment-resistant depression, (b) to the use of estrogen as an adjunct to antidepressant treatment, and (c) to the use of both estrogen and progestin as adjuncts to a variety of psychotropic drugs.

Only one study in which depressed patients were given sex steroids but no other medication could be located (Klaiber et al., 1979). The women who participated were inpatients diagnosed as having recurrent unipolar major depressive disorders that had been resistant (for at least the 2 preceding years) to conventional treatments for depression available in the mid-1970s such as tricyclic antidepressant drugs, electroshock therapy, and psychotherapy. Over 60% of the women had a history of suicidal attempts, and all expressed suicidal thoughts at the time of their recruitment. Fifteen of the 23 women randomly assigned to the estrogen group were premenopausal, as were 12 of the 17 women in the placebo group. The other subjects were postmenopausal. Of the 23 women who received estrogen, five were given (after daily increases) a maximum dose of 15 mg conjugated equine estrogen (Premarin) per day, six received a maximum daily dose of 20 mg, and 12 were given a maximum daily dose of 25 mg Premarin. In addition, premenopausal patients had 2.5 mg medroxyprogesterone acetate (Provera) added to the Premarin from days 21 to 25 of each treatment month to induce menses. Hamilton Depression Rating Scale scores decreased significantly by the third month in the estrogen group, whereas depression scores maintained stability across time in the placebo-treated group. Although the improvement in mood scores was statistically significant, post-treatment scores still indicated moderate depression. Plasma MAO activity also decreased with estrogen but not with placebo treatment. The considerable variability in response to estrogen administration in these women with treatment-resistant depression was apparently not related to the fact that some also received a progestin, since neither menopausal status nor age were significantly related to amount of improvement.

Considering that the results of this study constitute an impressive demonstration of the antidepressant effect of estrogen, it should be acknowledged that they were achieved with very large pharmacological doses of the hormone. We have reported recently that, although 0.625 mg Premarin induced physiological levels of estradiol and estrone, circulating hormone levels following ingestion of 1.25 mg Premarin were supraphysiological (Sherwin & Gelfand, 1989). It will be recalled that, in the Klaiber et al. (1979) study, daily doses of Premarin ranged from 15 to 25 mg per day, which is 12 to 20 times the recommended dose for postmenopausal hormone replacement therapy.

In 1976, Prange et al. investigated whether estrogen might enhance the antidepressant effect of imipramine. Thirty women with unipolar depression randomly received either placebo ($n = 10$), 150 mg imipramine and placebo ($n = 10$),

150 mg imipramine and 50 µg ethinyl estradiol ($n = 5$), or 150 mg imipramine and 25 µg ethinyl estradiol ($n = 5$). After 1 week of treatment, women who received 50 µg ethinyl estradiol and imipramine were substantially improved, but by day 14, they showed signs of toxicity similar to those reported with imipramine overdosage (e.g. hypotension, drowsiness, coarse tremor, dry mouth). On the other hand, patients who received 25 µg ethinyl estradiol and imipramine improved slightly (although non-significantly) faster then patients who received only imipramine while showing no enhanced toxicity.

A second study investigated the interaction between imipramine and conjugated equine estrogen in 11 women between the ages of 26 and 74 years whose depression had been resistant to treatment with antidepressant drugs (Shapira et al., 1985). After 2 weeks on 200 mg imipramine/day, half were given Premarin and half were given placebo for one treatment cycle and were then crossed over to the other treatment for another month. Premarin was given in incremental doses of 1.25 mg/day for 2 days, 2.5 mg/day on days 3 and 4, and 3.75 mg/day on days 5 to 21. The dose was then decreased in similar fashion during the next 5 days. On day 26, norethistrone acetate 10 mg/day was given to the three premenopausal women for 5 days to induce menses. Overall, no improvement in depression (as measured by the Hamilton Depression Rating Scale) occurred with either estrogen or placebo. However, one patient improved strikingly after 1 week estrogen, and her depression remitted completely after 2 weeks. Another women with bipolar disease developed a manic episode 9 days after the addition of estrogen. Possible order effects of treatments were not controlled for by the statistical analyses. No toxic effects of the supraphysiological doses of conjugated equine estrogens added to imipramine were seen in these patients.

Several case reports suggest possible beneficial effects of adding oral contraceptives (containing both estrogen and progestin) to antidepressants for the treatment of treatment-resistant depression. A 35-year-old woman with bipolar illness who had experienced two manic and four depressive episodes in the previous year while being treated with 200 mg imipramine/day experienced a considerable improvement in depressive symptoms when Ortho-Novum 1/50 (1 mg norethindrone and 0.5 mg mestranol) was added to the antidepressant (Price & Giannini, 1985). She remained euthymic on this regimen by the ninth month of follow-up. In another report, the addition of Ovral (0.5 mg norgestrel and 50 µg ethinyl estradiol) to lithium, L-tryptophan, and Premarin 1.25 mg, resulted in the abatement of a treatment-resistant depressive episode in a 56-year-old women (Chouinard et al., 1987). A new depressive episode that began when the oral contraceptive was changed to a lower dose combination (0.15 mg norgestrel and 30 g ethinyl estradiol) was only slightly improved with the reinstitution of Ovral but remitted completely with the addition of medroxyprogesterone acetate 5 mg/

day. Similarly, a 49-year-old woman with bipolar illness whose depressive episode was resistant to lithium and L-tryptophan became euthymic after Ovral and haloperidol were added (Chouinard et al., 1987). The discontinuation of haloperidol and the replacement of Ovral by Premarin 1.25 mg precipitated a manic episode. Her mood was subsequently stabilized by treatment with clonazepam, lithium, tryptophan, Ovral, and medroxyprogestrone acetate 5 mg/day.

In a recent, multicenter trial of fluoxetine 20 mg/day, 72 of these older women with a unipolar major depression were estrogen users and 286 women were non-users (Schneider et al., 1997a). All women were > 60 years of age (mean age 67.9 years). The estrogen users had a significantly greater responsiveness to fluoxetine than the depressed non-users. In large part, the differences between the groups in their responsiveness to the antidepressant were due to the significantly lower responsiveness to placebo in subjects who were estrogen users. These subjects did not have treatment-resistant depression; indeed, a history of non-response to at least two different antidepressant drug classes or electroconvulsive therapy within 12 months prior to recruitment was a subject exclusion criterion. However, the fact that the placebo response in estrogen-users was significantly lower than in non-users raises the possibility that postmenopausal women who develop a depressive episode while receiving estrogen may have a particularly persistent form of illness.

## Conclusions

By means of a multitude of mechanisms, estrogen acts to increase the concentration and the availability of serotonin in the brain. There is evidence that physiological doses of estrogen improve depressive symptoms in dysthymic women but not in those with a major depressive disorder. Whereas pharmacological doses of estrogen may result in a significant decrease in depression scores in women with treatment-resistant depression when administered alone, hormonal treatment does not result in clinical remission. There is also some suggestion that estrogen may provide some protection against depressive episodes in elderly women.

It would seem then, that the clinical utility of prescribing estrogen to post-menopausal women with treatment-resistant depression may reside in its ability to potentiate the effects of an antidepressant drug. There is currently one report in the literature of the efficacy of estrogen as an adjunct to an antidepressant in which the addition of ethinyl estradiol to imipramine for the treatment of depressed women resulted in a decreased latency of responsiveness to the antidepressant (Prange et al., 1976). However, ethinyl estradiol is a potent synthetic estrogen that may inhibit hepatic microsomal enzymes causing impaired metabolism of imipramine (Feild et al., 1979) and resulting in imipramine toxicity (Luscombe & John, 1980). Although this interaction is likely dose related since lower doses of ethinyl estradiol did not cause imipramine toxicity (Prange et al., 1976), no such interactions have been found with other classes of estrogens such as conjugated equine estrogen (Shapira et al., 1985). This suggests that estrogen preparations other than ethinyl estradiol should be used in combination with antidepressant drugs.

Second, there are several reports of the precipitation of manic episodes in women with bipolar illness when estrogen was added to their antidepressant regimens for the treatment of a treatment-resistant depressive episode (Shapira et al., 1985; Chouinard et al., 1987). Rapid cycling also occurred in a 72-year-old woman with treatment-resistant depression but no history of bipolar illness 5 days after 4.375 mg Premarin was added to an antidepressant drug (dibenzepin, 480 mg/day) (Oppenheim, 1984). In a study using transdermal estradiol as an adjunct to nortriptyline 20 mg/day, one subject had her first lifetime episode of hypomania during the initial week of treatment (Meyers & Moline, 1997). On the other hand, in two women, with bipolar illness, cycling was abolished and a stable euthymic state was induced when an oral contraceptive was administered or when medroxyprogesterone acetate was given in addition to estrogen and antidepressant drugs (Chouinard et al., 1987). These reports suggest that progestins may obviate mood cycling in women with bipolar illness being treated with estrogen for a depressive episode. Why the administration of progestins in association with estrogens seems to induce a stabilizing effect on mood in patients with bipolar disease is not clear. It is tempting to speculate that the opposite effect of estrogen and progestin on brain electrical excitability (Bäckström, 1977) and on MAO levels (Kleiber et al., 1971) may provide one possible explanation. Moreover, $3\alpha$–$5\alpha$ tetrahydroprogesterone (THP), a neurosteroid that is a major metabolite of progesterone, modulates the GABA–benzodiazapine receptor complex (GBRC) by enhancing benzodiazapine binding and increasing chloride ion flux (Peters et al., 1988). It is the progesterone metabolite THP which mediates the sedative and anesthetic effect of this hormone by facilitating GABA action on $GABA_A$ receptors (Korneyev & Costa, 1996).

Although these various lines of evidence provide reason to believe that estrogen may be an effective adjunct to antidepressants in women with treatment-resistant depression, the critical supportive studies have not yet been done. Prospective controlled studies are needed to investigate whether the addition of estrogen to an antidepressant causes a faster and/or a more profound response than that to the antidepressant alone. Second, in a population of postmenopausal women with treatment-resistant depression it should be determined whether the addition of estrogen enhances responsiveness to the antidepressant drug. Finally, in view of the fact that so many of its mechanisms of action affect the serotonergic system, information on estrogen interactions with selective serotonin reuptake inhibitors would be especially useful.

## REFERENCES

Andersch, B., Wendestam, C., Hahn, L. & Ohman, R. (1986). Premenstrual complaints. I. prevalence of premenstrual symptoms in a Swedish urban population. *Journal of Psychosomatic Obstetrics and Gynaecology*, **5**, 39–49.

Anderson, E., Hamburger, S., Liu, J.H., & Rebar, R.W. (1987). Characteristics of menopausal women seeking assistance. *American Journal of Obstetrics and Gynecology*, **156**, 428–33.

Arafat, E.S., Hargrove, J.T., Maxson, W.S., Desiderio, D.M., Wentz, A.C., & Anderson, R.N. (1988). Sedative and hypnotic effects of oral administration of micronized progesterone may be mediated through its metabolites. *American Journal of Obstetrics and Gynecology*, **159**, 1203–1209.

Aylward, M. (1973). Plasma tryptophan levels and mental depression in postmenopausal subjects: Effects of oral piperazine-oestrone sulfate. *IRCS Medical Science*, **1**, 30–4.

Aylward, M. (1976). Estrogens, plasma tryptophan levels in perimenopausal patients. In *The Management of the Menopause and Postmenopausal Years*, ed. S. Campbell, pp. 135–7. Baltimore: University Park Press.

Bäckström T. (1977). Estrogen and progesterone in relation to different activities in the central nervous system. *Acta Obstetrica et Gynaecoliga in Scandinavica*, **66**, 1–17.

Best, N.R., Barlow, D.H., Rees, M.P., & Cowan, P.J. (1989). Lack of effect of estradiol implant on platelet imipramine and 5-HT$_2$ receptor binding in menopausal subjects. *Psychopharmacology*, **98**, 561.

Biegon, A. & McEwen, B.S. (1982). Modulation by estradiol of serotonin receptors in brain. *Journal of Neuroscience*, **2**, 199–205.

Briggs, M. & Briggs, M. (1972). Relationship between monoamine oxidase activity and sex hormone concentration in human blood plasma. *Journal of Reproduction and Fertility*, **29**, 447–50.

Chakravarti, S., Collins, W.P., & Newton, J.R. (1977). Endocrine changes and symptomatology after oophorectomy in premenopausal women. *British Journal of Obstetrics and Gynaecology*, **84**, 769–75.

Charney, D.S., Menkes, D.B., & Heninger, G.R. (1981). Receptor sensitivity and the mechanism of action of antidepressant treatment. *Archives of General Psychiatry*, **38**, 1160–80.

Chiodo, L.A. & Caggiula, A.R. (1983). Substantia nigra dopamine neurons: alterations in basal discharge rates and autoreceptor sensitivity induced by estrogen. *Neuropharmacology*, **22**, 593–9.

Chouinard, G., Steinberg, S., & Steiner, W. (1987). Estrogen-progesterone combination: another mood stabilizer? *American Journal of Psychiatry*, **144**, 826.

Cone, R.I., Davis, G.A., & Coy, R,W. (1981). Effects of ovarian steroids on serotonin metabolism within grossly dissected and microdissected brain regions of the ovariectomized rat. *Brain Research Bulletin*, **7**, 639–44.

Coopen, A. & Wood, K. (1978). Tryptophan and depressive illness. *Psychological Medicine*, **8**, 49–57.

Coopen, A. & Wood, K. (1982). 5-Hydroxytryptamine in the pathogenesis of affective disorders. In *Serotonin in Biological Psychiatry*, ed. B.T. Ho, J.C. Schoolar, & E. Usdin, pp. 249–59. New York: Raven Press.

de Montigny, C., Grunberg, F., Mayer, A., & Deschenes, J.P. (1981). Lithium induces rapid relief of depression in tricyclic antidepressant drug non-responders. *British Journal of Psychiatry*, **138**, 252–6.

Dennerstein, L., Burrows, G.D., & Hyman, G.F. (1979). Hormone therapy and affect. *Maturitas*, **1**, 247–59.

Dohrenwend, B.P. & Dohrenwend, B.S. (1977). Reply to Grove and Tudor's coment on sex differences in psychiatric disorder. *American Journal of Sociology*, **82**, 1136–45.

Feild, B., Lu, C., & Hepner, G.W. (1979). Inhibition of hepatic drug metabolism by norethindrone. *Clinical and Pharmacological Therapy*, **25**, 196–8.

Gonzales, G.F. & Carrillo, C. (1993). Blood serotonin levels in postmenopausal women: effects of age and serum oestradiol levels. *Maturitas*, **17**, 23–9.

Guicheney, P., Léger, D., Barrat, J. et al. (1988). Platelet serotonin content and plasma tryptophan in peri- and postmenopausal women: variation with plasma estrogen levels and depressive symptoms. *European Journal of Clinical Investigation*, 297–304.

Hawkinson, L.F. (1938). The menopausal syndrome: a thousand consecutive patients treated with estrogen. *Journal of the American Medical Association*, **111**, 390–3.

Kelly, M.J., Moss, R.L., Dudley, C.A., & Fawcett, C.P. (1977). The specificity of the response of preoptic-septal area neurons to estrogen: 17-$\beta$-estradiol vs. 17-$\alpha$-estradiol and the response of extrahypothalamic neurons. *Experimental Brain Research*, **30**, 43–52.

Kendell, R.E., Wainwright, S., Hailey, A., & Shannon, B. (1976). The influence of childbirth on psychiatric morbidity. *Psychological Medicine*, **6**, 297–302.

Kendall, D.A., Stancel, G.M., & Enna, S.J. (1982). The influence of sex hormones on antidepressant-induced alterations in neurotransmitter receptor binding. *Journal of Neuroscience*, **2**, 354–60.

Kessler, R.C., Reuter, J.A., & Greenley, J.R. (1979). Sex differences in the use of psychiatric outpatient facilities. *Social Forces*, **58**, 557–71.

Kessler, R.C., McGonagla, K.A., Swartz, M., Blazer, D.G., & Nelson, C.B. (1993). Sex and depression in the National Comorbidity Survey: I Lifetime prevalence, chronicity and recurrence. *Journal of Affective Disorders*, **29**, 85–96.

Klaiber, E.L., Kobayashi, Y., Broverman, D.M., & Hall, F. (1971). Plasma monoamine oxidase activity in regularly menstruating women and in amenorrheic women receiving cyclic treatment with estrogens and a progestin. *Journal of Clinical and Endocrinol Metabolism*, **33**, 630–8.

Klaiber, E.L., Broverman, D.M., Vogal, W., Kobayashi, Y., & Moriarty, D. (1972). Effects of estrogen therapy on plasma MAO activity and EEG driving responses of depressed women. *American Journal of Psychiatry*, **128**, 1492–8.

Klaiber, E.L., Broverman, D.M., Vogel, W., & Koboyashi Y. (1979). Estrogen therapy for severe persistent depression in women. *Archives of General Psychiatry*, 36, 550–4.

Korneyev, A. & Costa, E. (1996). Allopregnanalone (THP) mediates anesthetic effects of progesterone in rat brain. *Hormone Behavior*, 30, 37–43.

Luine, V.N., Khylchevskaya, R.I., & McEwen, B. (1975). Effect of gonodal steroids on activities of monoamine oxidase and choline acetylase in rat brain. *Brain Research*, 86, 293–306.

Luscombe, D.K. & John, V. (1980). Influence of age, cigarette smoking and the oral contraceptive on plasma concentrations of clomipramine. *Postgraduate Medical Journal*, 56(Suppl. 1), 99–102.

McEwen, B.S. (1994). Steroid hormone action on the brain: when is the genome involved? *Hormone Behavior*, 28, 396–405.

McEwen, B.S., Gould, E., Orchinik, M., Weiland, N.G., & Wooley, C.S. (1995). Oestrogen and the structural and functional plasticity of neurons; implications for memory, aging and neurodegenerative processes. *Neurology*, 48, 52–73.

MacIntyre, S. & Oldman, D. (1977). Coping with migraine. In *Medical Encounters*, ed. A. Davis & G. Horobin, pp. 61–72. London: Croom Helm.

Merikangas, K.R., Weissman, M.M., & Pauls, D.L. (1985). Genetic factors in the sex ratio of major depression. *Psychological Medicine*, 15, 63–9.

Merryman, W., Boiman, R., Barnes, L., & Rothchild, I. (1954). Progesterone 'anesthesia' in human subjects. *Journal of Clinical and Endocrinological Metabolism*, 14, 1567–9.

Meyers, B.A. & Moline, M.L. (1997). The role of estrogen in late-life depression: opportunities and barriers to research. *Psychopharmacological Bulletin*, 33, 289–91.

Murphy, D.L., Campbell, I., & Costa, J.L. (1978). Current status of the indoleamine hypothesis of affective disorders. In *Psychopharmacology: A Generation of Progress*, ed. M.A. Lipton, A. DiMascio, & K.F. Killam, pp. 1235–47. New York: Raven Press.

Oppenheim, G. (1984). A case of rapid mood cycling with estrogen: Implications for therapy. *Journal of Clinical Psychiatry*, 45, 34–5.

Palinkas, L.A. & Barrett-Connor, E. (1992). Estrogen use and depressive symptoms in post-menopausal women. *Obstetrics and Gynecology*, 80, 30–6.

Paul, S.M., Axelrod, J., Saaveda, J.M., & Skolnick, P. (1979). Estrogen-induced afflux of endrogenous catecholamines from the hypothalamus in vitro. *Brain Research*, 178, 479–505.

Paul, S.M., Rehavi, M., Skolnick, P., & Goodwin, F.K. (1984). High affinity binding of antidepressants to biogenic amine transport sites in human brain and platelet: studies in depression. In *Neurobiology of Mood Disorders*, ed. R.M. Post & J.C. Ballenger, pp. 846–53. Baltimore: Williams & Wilkins.

Paykel, E.S. (1991). Depression in women. *British Journal of Psychiatry*, 158 (Suppl. 10), 22–9.

Pecins-Thompson, M., Brown, N.A., Kohama, S.G., & Bethea, C.L. (1996). Ovarian steroid regulation of tryptophan hydroxylase mRNA expression in rhesus macaques. *Journal of Neuroscience*, 16, 7021–9.

Peters, J.A., Kirkness, E.F., Collachan, H., Lambert, J.J., & Turner, A.J. (1988). Modulation of the $GABA_A$ receptor by depressant barbiturates and steroids. *British Journal of Pharmacology*, 94, 1257–69.

Poirier, M.F., Benkelfat, C., Galzin, A.M., & Langer, S.Z. (1986). Platelet $^3$H-imipramine binding and steroid hormone concentrations during the menstrual cycle. *Psychopharmacology*, **88**, 86–9.

Prange, A.J. Jr, Wilson, I.C., Breese, G.R., & Lipton, M.A. (1976). Hormonal alteration of imipramine response: a review. In *Hormones, Behavior and Psychopathology*, ed. E.J. Sachar, pp. 41–67. New York: Raven Press.

Price, W.A. & Giannini, A.J. (1985). Antidepressant effects of estrogen. *Journal of Clinical Psychiatry*, **46**, 506.

Radloff, L.S. & Rai, D.S. (1979). Susceptibility and precipitating factors in depression: Sex differences and similarities. *Journal of Abnormal Psychology*, **88**, 174–81.

Rainbow, T.C., DeGroff, G., Luine, V.N., & McEwen, B.S. (1980). Estradiol-17 $\beta$ increases the number of muscarinic receptors in hypothalamic nuclei. *Brain Research*, **198**, 239–43.

Raisman, R., Briley, M., & Langer, S.Z. (1979). Specific tricyclic antidepressant binding sites in rat brain. *Nature*, **281**, 148–50.

Raisman, R., Briley, M.S., Bouchami, F., Sechter, D., Zarifian, E., & Langer, S.Z. (1982). $^3$H-Imipramine binding and serotonin uptake in platelets from untreated depressed patients and control volunteers. *Psychopharmacology*, **77**, 332–5.

Regier, D.A., Boyd, J.H., Rurke, J.D. et al. (1988). One-month prevalence of mental disorders in the United States: Based on five Epidemiologic Catchment Area sites. *Archives of General Psychiatry*, **45**, 977–86.

Rehavi, M., Sepcuti, H., & Weizman, A. (1987). Upregulation of imipramine binding and serotonin uptake by estradiol in female rat brain. *Brain Research*, **410**, 135–9.

Schildkraut, J.J. (1965). The catecholamine hypothesis of affective disorders: a review of supporting evidence. *American Journal of Psychiatry*, **122**, 509–22.

Schneider, M.A., Brotherton, P.L., & Hailes, J. (1977). The effect of exogenous oestrogens on depression in menopausal women. *Medical Journal of Australia*, **2**, 162–3.

Schneider, L.S., Small, G.W., Hamilton, S.H., Bystritsky, A., Nemeroff, C.B., Meyers, B.S. and the Fluoxetine Collaborative Study Group. (1997). Estrogen replacement and response to fluoxetine in a multicenter geriatric depression trial. *American Journal of Geriatric Psychiatry*, **5**, 97–106.

Shapira, B., Oppenheim, G., Zohar, J., Segal, M., Malach, D., & Belmaker, R.H. (1985). Lack of efficacy of estrogen supplementation to imipramine in resistant female depressives. *Biological Psychiatry*, **20**, 576–9.

Sherwin, B.B. (1988). Affective changes in estrogen and androgen replacement therapy in surgically menopausal women. *Journal of Affective Disorders*, **14**, 177–87.

Sherwin, B.B. & Gelfand, M.M. (1985). Sex steroid and affect in the surgical menopause: a double-blind, crossover study. *Psychoneuroendocrinology*, **10**, 325–35.

Sherwin, B.B. & Gelfand, M.M. (1989). A prospective one-year study of estrogen and progestin in postmenopausal women: effects of clinical symptoms and lipoprotein lipids. *Obstetrics and Gynecology*, **73**, 759–66.

Sherwin, B.B. & Suranyi-Cadotte, B.E. (1990). Up-regulatory effect of estrogen on platelet $^3$H-imipramine binding sites in surgically menopausal women. *Biological Psychiatry*, **28**, 339–48.

Strickler, R.C., Borth, R., Cecutti. A. et al. (1977). The role of oestrogen replacement in the climacteric syndrome. *Psychological Medicine*, **7**, 631–9.

Suranyi-Cadotte, B.E., Wood, P.L., Schwartz, G., & Nair, P.V.N. (1983). Altered platelet $^3$H-imipramine binding in schizoaffective and depressive disorders. *Biological Psychiatry*, **18**, 923–7.

Wagner, H.R., Crutcher, K.A., & Davis, J.N. (1979). Chronic estrogen treatment decreases β-adrenergic responses in rat cerebral cortex. *Brain Research*, **71**, 147–51.

Weissman, M.M. & Klerman, G.L. (1977). Sex differences and the epidemiology of depression. *Archives of General Psychiatry*, **34**, 98–111.

Weissman, M.M., Bland, R., Joyce, P.R., Newman, S., Wells, J.E., & Wittchen, H.U. (1993). Sex differences in rates of depression: Cross-national perspectives. *Journal of Affective Disorders*, **29**, 77–84.

Wittchen, H.U., Essau, C.A., von Zerssen, D., Krieg, J.C., & Zaudig, M. (1972). Lifetime and six-month prevalence of mental disorders in the Munich follow-up study. *European Archives of Psychiatry and Clinical Neuroscience*, **241**, 247–58.

Zweifel, J.E. & O'Brien, W.H. (1997). A meta-analysis of the effect of hormone replacement therapy upon depressed mood. *Psychoneuroendocrinology*, **22**, 189–212.

# 5

# Sleep abnormalities in treatment-resistant mood disorders

Martin P. Szuba, Antonio T. Fernando, and Geralyn Groh-Szuba

Oh Sleep! It is a gentle thing,
Beloved from pole to pole...
    Samuel Taylor Coleridge

The close inter-relationship between mood and sleep, has led some to suggest that sleep–wake cycle alterations are central to these disorders (Goodwin & Jamieson, 1990). In this chapter, we will review the existing literature on the relationship between sleep and mood disorders, in particular, treatment-resistant disorders.

(i) We will begin by reviewing the subjective and objective changes in sleep that occur in depressive and manic episodes and describe how these sleep findings may be predictive of treatment-resistant states.
(ii) We will then go on to describe the various manipulations, either deliberate or accidental, of the sleep–wake cycle which can either improve treatment-resistant depressive states, or conversely, contribute to treatment-resistant manic states.
(iii) We will then discuss the relationship between primary sleep disorders and treatment-resistant mood states.

## Normal Sleep

Normal sleep consists of alternating REM (rapid eye movement) and non-REM epochs. Non-REM sleep is divided into four stages. During Stages 1 and 2, individuals are easily awakened and can be partially aware of environmental events, such as someone entering the room. Thus, a person in these shallower stages, though asleep, may experience himself or herself as being awake. In contrast, the arousal threshold for Stages 3 and 4 (delta) sleep is much higher. Data suggest that this deeper sleep is the restorative period of the sleep cycle. Thus, in the absence of adequate delta sleep, one awakens feeling tired and unrefreshed.

The electroencephalographic characteristics of REM sleep bears similarities to Stage 1 and the waking stage, being predominated by low voltage, fast activity.

However, in contrast to other sleep stages, REM is characterized by paroxysms of rapid eye movements, muscle atonia, and high autonomic variability. The first REM sleep period usually begins about 70–100 minutes after sleep onset. There are three to five REM periods in a night, separated by about 70–120 minutes, with each REM period lasting about 20–30 minutes. As the night progresses, the REM periods become longer, with the bulk of the REM time occurring during the second half of sleep (Gillin et al., 1984).

## Sleep findings and treatment-resistant depression

Unfortunately, a full night of refreshing sleep rarely comes for most depressed patients. Over 90% of patients in major depressive episodes (MDE) report sleep problems, making it the single most frequent complaint of patents with depression. (Goodwin & Jamieson, 1990). Clinical lore supports the notion that sleep problems are integral to major mood episodes. While evaluating a patient for possible MDE, would not most clinicians experience doubt about that diagnosis if the patient reports *no* change in sleep? Of all patients complaining of sleep disturbance, approximately 85% complain of insomnia, whereas 15% complain of hypersomnia. The latter are predominately bipolar and younger patients. Insomnia, in particular, can be so distressing that patients often first seek help for the sleep problem rather than the mood episode. In a multi-center study, Buysse et al. (1994) found that of patients presenting to sleep disorders centers with a chief complaint of insomnia, 'sleep disorder associated with mood disorder' was the primary diagnosis in one-third. As will be seen, patients' subjective reports of sleep often parallel the findings of objective sleep measures. See Table 5.1 for an overview of the subjective and objective changes in sleep found during depressive and manic episodes.

Depressive sleep is shallow. Polysomnography (PSG) reveals more relative Stages 1 and 2, reduced Stages 3 and 4, and a decrease in arousal threshold (i.e., in response to an audible tone, individuals are more likely to awaken during Stages 1 and 2 sleep, than during delta sleep) (Gillin et al., 1984; Kupfer, 1995). During Stages 1 and 2, the depressed person appears asleep to observers, such as bed partners or inpatient nursing staff. Yet, the next morning, the patient can often recall and describe activities and events (of the bed partner or inpatient nursing staff) having occurred in the room during the night. The retention of environmental awareness during these lighter stages may account for this seeming paradox. The loss of delta sleep may contribute to the non-refreshing nature of depressive sleep.

Depressive sleep is fragmented. The depressed patient often complains of frequent awakenings during the night. PSG research has shown that there is an

**Table 5.1.** Summary of sleep symptoms and laboratory findings in depressive and manic episodes

| Mood episode | Sleep feature | Symptom (patient's subjective report) | Laboratory finding (NPSG) |
|---|---|---|---|
| *Depression* | Duration[a] | Shortened (85%) | Reduced |
|  |  | Excessive (15%) |  |
|  | Depth | Light sleep | Stages 1 and 2 increased |
|  |  | Easily awakened | Stages 3 and 4 reduced |
|  |  |  | Easily aroused |
|  | Continuity | Multiple awakenings | Frequent arousals |
|  | Restorative effects | Daytime sleepiness | Normal or minimally reduced alertness based on MSLT |
|  | REM related | Excessive dreaming | Shortened latency |
|  |  | Elaborate and/or disturbing dream content | Increased REM density |
| *Manic* | Duration | Normal | Shortened |
|  |  | Sometimes acknowledged as shortened | Early morning awakening |
|  | Depth | Normal or reduced | Stages 3 and 4 relatively preserved |
|  | Continuity | Normal or reduced | Disrupted |
|  | Restorative effects | Excellent | Data N/A |
|  | REM related | Data N/A | Shortened latency |
|  |  |  | Increased REM density |

[a]While positively correlated, patient reports of sleep duration are consistently lower than what is observed in the laboratory.
Nofzinger et al., 1991.

increase in intermittent wakefulness, decrease in total sleep efficiency and increase in the shifting between sleep stages (Gillin et al., 1984; Neylan, 1995). Among unipolar depressives, sleep continuity is poor (Kupfer, 1995).

Depressive sleep is shortened. The depressed patient often complains of problems falling asleep and/or awakening well before their appointed rising time (see Table 5.1). PSG studies confirm these patient reports. While patients sometimes overestimate the degree of insomnia, PSG results and self-reports are well correlated. Patients have a shorter total sleep time, a delay in sleep onset (increased sleep latency), and early morning awakening (Gillin et al., 1984; Benca et al.,

1992). Among atypical and bipolar depressives, total sleep time and daytime sleepiness may be increased (Neylan, 1995).

REM sleep is also altered during depressive episodes. Dreams, or at least dream recall, may be different, as depressed patients often report more frequent and more disturbing dreams, compared to their euthymic states. The fragmented sleep of depressed patients may contribute to these patient reports. Dreams are more likely to be consolidated into memory and recalled the next day if one awakens shortly following the dream. Objective confirmation of increased dream recall in depressed patients is lacking.

In the 1970s, a series of studies suggested certain features of the sleep of patients with MDE, shortened REM latency, increased REM density and sleep fragmentation might make PSG a useful diagnostic tool for MDE. Subsequent studies have shown however, that these same findings occur in patients with eating disorders, obsessive-compulsive disorder, schizoaffective illness, and even mania. Shortened REM latency has also been observed in borderline personality disorder, schizophrenia and narcolepsy (Benca et al., 1992). Thus, the specificity of these findings was thrown into question. Many now believe that computerized analysis of sleep EEG measures may well prove useful in the differential diagnosis of MDE. It does appear that in mood disorders, and not in other psychiatric disorders, REM sleep is more pronounced. REM is increased in the first half of the night and reduced during the latter half of the sleeping period (Gillin et al., 1984; Kupfer, 1995; Neylan, 1995). According to Benca in her meta-analysis in 1992, only in affective disorders is there an increase in duration of the first REM period. Percent time spent in REM is increased only in affective disorders and in alcoholism (Benca et al., 1992). This work may ultimately show that computerized analysis of sleep microarchitecture can be useful as a marker of mood disorders.

Data on sleep in treatment-resistant depression are difficult to glean from the literature. The use of different criteria by different authors for establishing 'treatment resistance' makes it difficult to generate concrete generalizations. Among an ECT population of treatment-resistant cases and/or severely depressed individuals with psychotic features, the 'characteristic' PSG findings are more prominent than in other depressive populations (Grunhaus et al., 1996). The ECT patients tend to manifest profound sleep disruption with numerous arousals, early awakenings, very short REM latency, sleep onset REM periods (first REM period within 20 minutes of falling asleep) and high REM density (Grunhaus et al., 1996). After ECT, all but one of these altered sleep parameters resolved (Grunhaus et al., 1997). Total sleep time, sleep maintenance factors, REM latency and REM density all returned to normal ranges post-ECT course. However, the prevalence of sleep onset REM periods was unchanged. The presence of sleep onset REM periods post-ECT was associated with poor response and a high relapse rate vs. patients without post-ECT sleep onset REM (Grunhaus et al., 1997). These intriguing results suggest that the presence of sleep-onset REM periods might predict treatment resistance to ECT. Further study of this area is needed since the findings may have prognostic values for many patients.

Others have found that subjective and objective findings of poor sleep before treatment of depression predicts a poorer response to medications, cognitive therapy and interpersonal therapy (Dew et al., 1997; Thase et al., 1996).

## Sleep findings and treatment-resistant vs. pseudotreatment-resistant mania

The hallmark sleep–wake cycle change in manic episodes is a decreased need for sleep. Patients in manic episodes sleep significantly less than they do during euthymic periods. Patients who usually need 7 to 8 hours of sleep during euthymia will only require 3–4 hours, or less, when manic, yet feel quite refreshed the next day. In contrast to depressives, manics do not feel the need to sleep, as they feel energized even with minimal sleep. Our experience suggests that manic patients overestimate their total sleep time. Thus, unless the clinician has access to an outside observer, such as a relative or inpatient nursing staff, that clinician may be led to believe that the sleep is adequate. Given the intimate link between mania and decreased sleep need, time asleep is often used as a target symptom in management of mania. Thus, the misinformation, due to a lack of outside observer input, can seriously and adversely impede proper management. The clinician may then decide *not* to adjust medications, as the patient may appear better than is actually the case. Thus, should the discrepancy between patient report of sleep and their actual sleep not be uncovered by the clinician, the condition may seem 'treatment resistant,' when optimizing the current line of pharmacotherapy may produce further benefit.

The few studies published on PSG in mania confirm observer reports that sleep is fragmented and shortened in mania. The REM features of mania are similar to those of depression; REM latency is reduced and REM density is increased. However, in contrast to depressive episodes, delta sleep is relatively preserved in manic episodes (Hudson et al., 1988; Linkowski et al., 1986, 1994). Given the restorative nature of delta sleep, the preservation of these deeper stages may account, at least in part, for the manic patient feeling rested and refreshed after brief sleeps. While studies of sleep in mania are rare, studies in treatment-resistant manias are non-existent. The importance of studying sleep in treatment-resistant manic states will become clearer in the later section on sleep induction treatment of mania.

## Sleep manipulations and treatment-resistant depression

Deliberate sleep deprivation produces an antidepressant effect in ~60% of all MDE patients. Bipolars respond much more frequently than unipolars (70% vs. 42%, respectively) (Szuba et al., 1991). Total sleep deprivation involves awakening the patient at 7 a.m. and then assisting them in maintaining wakefulness until 9 p.m. the next evening (approximately 36 hours of deprivation). Partial sleep deprivation in the early morning hours involves awakening the patient at 2 a.m. and assisting them in maintaining wakefulness until 9 p.m. that evening (19 hours of deprivation). This seemingly paradoxical effect of deliberate sleep restriction rapidly ameliorating depression was first described in modern medical literature by Schülte (1966) and Pflüg (1976). Some of the earliest reports included cases of depressed health care workers who underwent extended periods of sleep loss due to job requirements and for whom this led to antidepressant effects. Dozens of studies, from around the world since then have confirmed the antidepressant effects of sleep deprivation (for review, see Wirz-Justice & Van den Hoofdakker, 1999 for review).

Despite the large number of studies of sleep deprivation in depression, the role of sleep deprivation in improving treatment-resistant depression is not well known as few authors identify their depressed patients as treatment resistant or non-treatment resistant. In a series of patients previously treatment resistant to antidepressants, Dessauer (1985) found that repeated sleep deprivation induced a positive response even while the patient continued their previously unhelpful medication. Our own data indicate that amongst those subjects who failed at least two antidepressant medication trials, sleep deprivation produced an antidepressant effect in 55% (M.P. Szuba, unpublished data).

## Sleep deprivation and treatment-resistant mania

While acute sleep deprivation can be beneficial for symptoms of depression, like any effective therapy, there are side effects. For some depressed individuals, sleep deprivation simply induces fatigue (Kloss et al., 2000). However, for some bipolar depressed people, sleep deprivation can be problematic as it can induce hypomanic or even manic states. While estimates of hypomania/mania induction via deliberate sleep deprivation vary widely (Gillin, 1987; Wehr, 1987), our experience suggests the rate of mania is rare, except perhaps in postpartum depressions (Strousse et al., 1992).

Wehr (1987) has proposed that, in vulnerable individuals with bipolar disorder, various triggers to manic episodes share a common pathway – sleep disruption (see Fig. 5.1.) Within this model, triggers such as a newborn in the house, acute

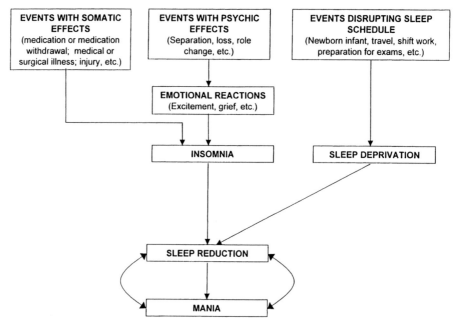

Fig. 5.1     Potential role of sleep disruption in mania induction and propagation. (Adapted with permission from Wehr, 1987.)

medical illness, etc. produce insomnia. This sleep disruption triggers hypomania or mania and since a hallmark symptom of hypomania or mania is insomnia, a self-reinforcing mechanism may be established. This model raises crucial questions regarding the mechanism of initiation and maintenance of manic episodes. Sound studies are now emerging to support this hypothesis (Malkoff-Schwartz et al., 1998). Two separate groups have found a significant relationship between sleep duration on a given night and subsequent hypomania/mania (Leibenluft et al., 1996; Barbini et al., 1996). In a purported animal model of mania, recent work suggests that sleep deprivation induced in rats may produce an agitated, hyper-sexual, and aggressive state that is attenuated by pretreatment with lithium (with serum levels 0.7–1.0 meq/l) (Gessa et al., 1995).

## Sleep induction and treatment-resistant mania

Clinicians often prescribe sedating benzodiazepines or sedating antipsychotics in early stages of mania. Wehr's model, described above, raised questions within our group about whether the cycle of mania leading to sleep loss resulting in worsening of mania could be interrupted by sleep induction. Could one modulate mania symptomatology through sleep induction? At least one study suggests that this may be the case (Finch et al., 1994). In our clinical practice, we were struck by the observation that some manic patients experienced a rapid resolution upon admission to an inpatient unit. What seemed common to all the patients was the fact that all had been extremely agitated, necessitating sedation with benzodiazepines and/or antipsychotic medications. After the medication, these rapid responders then slept for extended periods. Upon awakening they were markedly better and sustained this improvement for days, often with no further medication doses.

This led us to examine, in a naturalistic study, 27 consecutively admitted manic patients. Rapid responders were identified as those who showed moderately or markedly improved symptoms in mania within 1–2 days of admission. When the clinical and demographic characteristics were compared between the rapid and non-rapid responders, four significant differences emerged.

(i) rapid responders slept almost twice as long as the non-rapid responders on the first night in the hospital (7.7 vs. 4.1 hours),
(ii) rapid responders were significantly more likely to be in a first manic episode,
(iii) rapid responders were significantly more likely to have experienced a major life stressor prior to admission, and
(iv) rapid responders spent less time in the hospital (7 vs. 15 days).

The results of this study are consistent with Post's hypothesis that bipolar disorder becomes more treatment-resistant over time (Post, 1992). Furthermore, while the issue of causality remains in question, the data are consistent with the hypothesis that sleep induction, however achieved, can induce improvement in manic symptoms. A review of miscellaneous organic therapies tried during this century for psychiatric disorders indicated that those therapies that induce sleep are helpful in mania. Dauerschlaf (use of barbiturates to induce a 1–2 week sleep); continuous sleep therapy (often bromide salts were used); insulin coma therapy (producing extreme hypoglycemia with intent of inducing coma), atropine coma therapy; nitrous oxide therapy (which produces sleep), all worked best in manic and agitated patients (Hartman, 1968; Campbell, 1985).

## Primary sleep disorders and treatment-resistant mood episodes

Do primary sleep disorders predispose individuals to a treatment-resistant MDE? That is, do individuals who suffer from MDE and obstructive sleep apnea or MDE and narcolepsy respond poorly to antidepressant interventions? Surprisingly, few studies have examined these issues.

A depressed patient who is not responding fully to treatment warrants an investigation of possible organic factors (Amsterdam & Hornig-Rohan, 1996). In some cases, a primary sleep disorder produces a clinical picture similar to depression (Tiberge, 1995). Many of the major sleep disorders are characterized by depressive-like symptoms; including mood alterations (irritability, anxiety), apathy, fatigue, psychomotor slowing, and impaired cognitive function (Zammit et al., 1999; Roth & Ancoli-Israel, 1999; Engelman et al., 1997); in addition to sleep disruption. In a study by Mosko in 1989, 67% of patients who presented to their sleep disorder center reported an episode of depression within the previous 5 years, and 26% described themselves as depressed at presentation. Patients with disorders of excessive somnolence such as obstructive sleep apnea (OSA), narcolepsy, or sleep-related periodic leg movements average high rates of self-reported depressive symptomatology (Mosko et al., 1989). This finding suggests there may be a relationship between mood disorders and disorders of excessive somnolence that warrant examination.

Obstructive sleep apnea is estimated to occur in 2–4% of the population. Excessive daytime somnolence, heavy snoring, and choking and apneic spells while sleeping characterize this syndrome. Studies demonstrating a link between sleep apnea and depression are growing. Engleman, in 1997, studied 16 patients diagnosed with obstructive sleep apnea, to measure the effects of CPAP on neurobehavioral function. He measured sleepiness and emotional well being as well as cognitive performance (Engelman et al., 1997). CPAP produced significant improvements in depression ratings. In a larger study by Millman of 55 patients with obstructive sleep apnea, 25 had significant depression that improved with CPAP treatment (Millman et al., 1989). Ramos Platon in Spain found similar results; after a year's treatment with CPAP, significant improvements in psychopathology, particularly depression was observed in 23 patients (Ramos Platon & Espinar Sierra, 1992). In our experience, severe apneics sometimes present with major depressive disorders that do not respond to antidepressant therapy. Many have been referred for ECT without evaluation for primary sleep pathology. When properly diagnosed with OSA and appropriately treated with CPAP, most patients experience improvement in their snoring, excessive daytime sleepiness, and depressive symptoms. In cases of chronic or treatment-resistant depression, obstructive sleep apnea should be considered.

Narcolepsy is a relatively uncommon condition characterized by excessive daytime sleepiness, cataplexy, sleep paralysis and hypnagogic hallucinations. Studies suggest that narcolepsy and depressive illness may be linked. Reynolds et al. (1983) found that 20% of a narcoleptic sample met Research Diagnostic Criteria for a history of major or recurrent intermittent depression. A similar percentage of comorbid depression among narcoleptics was observed in a study comparing depression in narcolepsy and hypersomnia. Roth and Nevsimalova (1975) found that depression occurred in 29% of narcoleptics without the classic symptoms of cataplexy, sleep paralysis and hypnagogic hallucinations, and in 17% among narcoleptics with cataplexy, sleep paralysis and hypnagogic hallucinations. In most cases, he found a parallel clinical course between the manifestation of depressive symptoms and the hypersomnolence. Though the above studies suggest a possible relationship between narcolepsy and depression, the exact nature of this association still needs to be examined. Abnormalities in the cholinergic and monoamine systems have been explored as possible causes of narcolepsy and may play a role in depression (Mefford, 1981). Very recent work implicates a defect in the orexin gene as the cause of narcolepsy in animals and humans (Chemelli et al., 1999; Lin et al., 1999; Nishino et al., 2000). Whether there are common neuro-biological underpinnings between narcolepsy and depression remains to be eluci-dated. Since orexin regulates sleep, appetite and feeding behaviors; disturbances of which are common in depressive disorders; this relationship between depression and narcolepsy should be further explored. Further exploration of orexin's neur-obiological roles may help elucidate these issues.

Strikingly little literature has addressed the prevalence of primary sleep dis-orders in individuals presenting with treatment-resistant depression. To our knowledge, only one study was specifically designed to examine sleep disorders in treatment-resistant depression. James described PSG findings in ten patients who had failed at least one adequate trial of a tricyclic antidepressant and one adequate trial of a MAO inhibitor (James et al., 1990). Though limited by the lack of a comparison group, subjects appeared to manifest no changes in REM sleep latency, REM density, or sleep latency. Nevertheless, the sleep of these subjects was shallow and fragmented; 4.8% of total sleep time was spent in delta sleep, there were multiple awakenings during the night, and sleep efficiency averaged only 78%. These results vary greatly from other groups' reports within healthy popula-tions.

Perhaps most remarkably, seven of the ten subjects were diagnosed by NPSG with a primary sleep disorder that could not be considered secondary to the mood disorder itself. Four had sleep apnea (three obstructive, one central), two had periodic leg movements in sleep (PLMS), and one had a disorder of initiating or maintaining sleep with an atypical polysomnograph showing frequent alpha intrusions into delta sleep and increased spindling. The three treatment-resistant depressives with obstructive sleep apnea showed improvement of depression (mean Hamilton Depression scores decreased from 20.5 to 12.1) after 1 month of CPAP. Benzodiazepine treatment of the PLMS subjects did not affect depression. Though a small study, and lacking a comparison group, this study suggests that clinicians managing treatment-resistant depressed patients may want to consider the possibility that a primary sleep disorder may be contributing to the treatment-resistant condition. Fig. 5.2 provides guidelines for how to proceed with such a sleep disorder evaluation in treatment-resistant depressed patients.

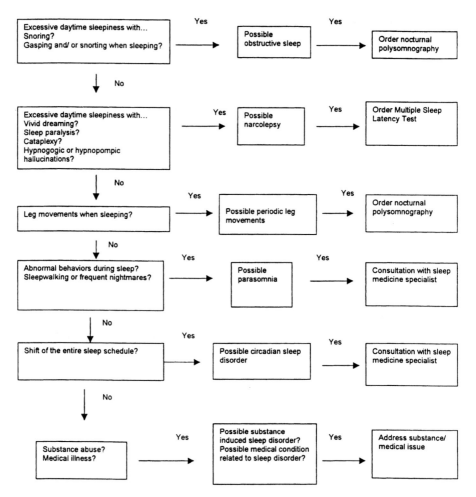

Fig. 5.2     Diagnostic algorithm for evaluating the possible contribution of primary sleep disorders to treatment-resistant mood states.

## Conclusions

To date, few investigators have devoted effort specific to sleep in treatment-resistant mood disorders, though that may be changing, as this chapter outlines. What work has been done shows promise for the understanding and treatment of these treatment-resistant conditions. Data from ECT, pharmacotherapy and psychotherapy studies suggest that some sleep EEG changes may be predictive of treatment-resistant depressions. Further work is need in this area, as is work on the potential predictive value of sleep changes for treatment-resistant manic states. In both manic and depressed states, patients appear to suffer a degree of sleep state misperception. During manic episodes, patients tend to underestimate and depressive patients tend to overestimate their insomnia. Thus, over-reliance on patient sleep reports could contribute to the misidentification of some patients as treatment-resistant. The application of sleep deprivation to treat treatment-resistant depressions and sleep induction to treat treatment-resistant manic states holds promise. Finally, the relative contribution of primary sleep disorders to treatment-resistant mood states is virtually unknown and warrants investigation. Certainly scientific study within the areas described in this chapter could enhance understanding of the pathophysiologic mechanisms contributing to treatment-resistant mood disorders. The knowledge thus garnered could lead to the development of other therapies to reduce the suffering and enhance the lives of those patients burdened with treatment-resistant mood disorders.

## REFERENCES

Amsterdam, J.D. & Hornig-Rohan, M. (1996). Treatment algorithms in treatment resistant depression. *Psychiatric Clinics of North America*, **19**, 371–85.

Anonymous (1997). Practice parameters for the indications for polysomnography and related procedures. Polysomnography Task Force, American Sleep Disorders Association Standards of Practice Committee. *Sleep*, **20**(6), 406–22.

Barbini, B., Bertelli, S., Colombo, C., & Smeraldi, E. (1996). Sleep loss, a possible factor in augmenting manic episode. *Psychiatry Research*, **65**, 121–5.

Benca, R., Obermeyer, W., Thisted, R., & Gillin, J.C. (1992). Sleep and psychiatric disorders, a meta analysis. *Archives of General Psychiatry*, **49**, 651–6.

Billiard, M., Dolenc, L., Aldaz, C., Ondze, B., & Besset, A. (1994). Hypersomnia associated with mood disorders: a new perspective. *Journal of Psychosomatic Research*, **38** (Suppl 1), 41–7.

Breslau, N., Roth, T., Rosenthal, L., & Andreski, P. (1996). Sleep disorders and psychiatric disorders: a longitudinal epidemiologic study of young adults. *Biological Psychiatry*, **39**(6), 411–18.

Buysse, D.J., Reynolds, C.F. 3rd, Kupfer, D.J. et al. (1994). Clinical diagnoses in 216 insomnia patients using the International Classification of Sleep Disorders (ICSD), DSM-IV and ICD-10 categories: a report from the APA/NIMH DSM-IV Field Trial. *Sleep*, **17**(7), 630–7.

Campbell, R.J. (1985). Miscellaneous organic therapies. In *Comprehensive Textbook of Psychiatry*, vol 2. 4th edn. ed. H.I. Kaplan & B.J. Sadock, pp. 1569–75. Baltimore, MD: Williams & Wilkins.

Chemelli, R.M., Willie, J.T., Sinton, C.M. et al. (1999). Narcolepsy in orexin knockout mice: molecular genetics of sleep regulation. *Cell*, **8**(4), 437–51.

Dessauer, M., Goetze, U., & Tölle, R. (1985). Periodic sleep deprivation in drug-refractory depression. *Neuropsychobiology*, **13**(3), 111–16.

Dew, M.A., Reynolds, C.F. 3rd, Houck, P.R. et al. (1997). Temporal profiles of the curse of depression during treatment. Predictors of pathways toward recovery in the elderly [see comments]. *Archives of General Psychiatry*, **54**(11), 1016–24.

Dolenc, L., Besset, A., & Billiard, M. (1996). Hypersomnia in association with dysthymia in comparison with idiopathic hypersomnia and normal controls. *Pflugers Archiv – European Journal of Physiology.* **431**(6 Suppl 2), R303–4.

Engelman, H.M., Martin, S.E., Deary, I.J., & Douglas, N.J. (1997). Effect of CPAP therapy on daytime function in patients with mild sleep apnea/hypopnea syndrome. *Thorax*, **52**(2), 114–19.

Finch, N., Altshuler, L.L., Szuba, M.P., & Mintz, J. (1994). Rapid resolution of first manias: sleep related? *Journal of Clinical Psychiatry*, **55**, 26–9.

Ford, D.E. & Kamerow, D.B. (1989). Epidemiologic study of sleep disturbances and psychiatric disorders: an opportunity for prevention? *Journal of American Medical Association*, **162**, 1479–84.

Gessa, G.L., Pani, L., Fadda, P., & Fratta, W. (1995). Sleep deprivation in the rat: an animal model of mania. *European Neuropsychopharmacology*, **5** Suppl. (-HD-), 89–93.

Gillin, J.C. (1983). The sleep therapies of depression. *Progress in Neuro-Psychopharmacology and Biological Psychiatry*, **7**(2–3), 351–64.

Gillin, J.C. (1987). Sleep reduction: factor in the genesis of mania? [letter]. *American Journal of Psychiatry*, **144**(9), 1248–9.

Gillin, J.C., Sitaram, N., Wehr, T. et al. (1984). Sleep and affective illness. In *Neurobiology of Sleep Disorders*, ed. R. Post & J. Ballenger, pp. 157–89. MD: Williams and Wilkins.

Goodwin, F.K. & Jamieson, K.R. (1990). Sleep and biological rhythms. In *Manic-Depressive Illness*, ed. F.K. Goodwin & K.R. Jamieson, pp. 541–75. Oxford University Press.

Grunhaus, L., Shipley, J., Eiser, A. et al. (1996). Polysomnographic studies in patients referred for ECT: pre-ECT studies. *Convulsive Therapy*, **12**(4), 224–31.

Grunhaus, L., Shipley, J., Eiser, A. et al. (1997). Sleep onset rapid eye movement after electroconvulsive therapy is more frequent in patients who respond less well to electroconvulsive therapy. *Biological Psychiatry*, **42**, 191–200.

Hamilton, M. (1960). A rating scale for depression. *Journal of Neurology, Neurosurgery and Psychiatry*, **23**, 56–62.

Hartman, E. (1968). A polygraphic study. *Archives of General Psychiatry*, **18**, 99–111.

Hudson, J., Lipinski, J., Frankenburg, F., Grochochinski, V., & Kupfer, D. (1988). Electroencephalographic sleep in mania. *Archives of General Psychiatry*, **45**, 568–75.

James, S.P., Potter, L., Berwish, N., & Amsterdam, J.D. (1991). Polysomnography in refractory depression. In *Advances in Neuropsychiatry and Psychopharmacology*, ed. J.D. Amsterdam. Vol 2: *Refractory Depression.* New York: Raven Press.

Janssen, P.A. (1988). The relevance of pharmacological studies to sleep research in psychiatry. *Pharmacopsychiatry*, **21**(1), 33–7.

Kaplan, R. (1992). Obstructive sleep apnea and depression – diagnostic and treatment implications. *Australian and New Zealand Journal of Psychiatry*, **26**(4), 586–91.

Kloss, J.D., Szuba, M.P., Ball, W.A., McManus, K.S., & Dinges, D.F. (2000). A blinded comparative trial of partial and total sleep deprivation during major depressive episodes. *Sleep*, **23**(Suppl. 1).

Koyama, T. & Yamashita, I. (1992). Biological markers of depression: WHO multi-center studies and future perspective. *Progress in Neuropsycholpharmacology and Biological Psychiatry*, **16**(6), 791–6.

Kupfer, D. (1995). Sleep research in depressive illness: clinical implications – a tasting menu. *Biological Psychiatry*, **38**, 391–403.

Kupfer, D. & Reynolds, C. (1992). Sleep and psychiatric disorders. *Archives of General Psychiatry*, **49**, 669–970.

Liebenluft, E., Albert, P.S., Rosenthal, N.E., & Wehr, T.A. (1996). Relationship between sleep and mood in patients with rapid-cycling bipolar disorder. *Psychiatry Research*, **63**(2–3), 161–8.

Lin, L., Faraco, J., Li, R. et al. (1999). The sleep disorder canine narcolepsy is caused by a mutation in the hypocretin (orexin) receptor 2 gene. *Cell*, **98**(3), 365–76.

Linkowski, P., Kerkhofs, M., Rielaert, C., & Mendlewicz, J. (1986). Sleep during mania in manic-depressive males. *European Archives of Psychiatry and Neurological Science*, **235**(6), 339–41.

Linkowski, P., Kerkhofs, M., Van Onderbergen, A. et al. (1994). The 24-hour profiles of cortisol, prolactin, and growth hormone secretion in mania. *Archives of General Psychiatry*, **51**(8), 616–24.

Malkoff-Schwartz, S., Frank, E., Anderson, B. et al. (1998). Stressful life events and social rhythm disruption in the onset of manic and depressive bipolar episodes: a preliminary investigation. *Archives of General Psychiatry*, **55**(8), 702–7.

Mefford, I.N., Foutz, A., Baker, T.L. et al. (1981). Regional distribution of biogenic amines in CNS of normal and narcoleptic canines. *Sleep Research*, **10**, 69.

Millman, R.P., Fogel, B.S., McNamara, M.E., & Carlisle, C.C. (1989). Depression as a manifestation of obstructive sleep apnea; reversal with nasal continuous positive airway pressure. *Journal of Clinical Psychiatry*, **50**(9), 348–51.

Monti, J.M., Alterwain, P., Estevez, F. et al. (1993). The effects of ritanserin on mood and sleep in abstinent alcoholic patients. [Randomized Controlled Trial] *Sleep*, **16**(7), 647–54.

Mosko, S., Zetin, M., Glen, S. et al. (1989). Self reported depressive symptomatolgy, mood ratings, and treatment outcome in sleep disorder patients. *Journal of Clinical Psychology*, **45**(1), 51–60.

Neylan, T. (1995). Treatment of sleep disturbances in depressed patients. *Journal of Clinical Psychiatry*, **56**, suppl 2, 56–61.

Nishino, S., Ripley, B., Overeem, S., Lammers, G.J., & Mignot, E. (2000). Hypocretin (orexin) deficiency in human narcolepsy [letter]. *Lancet*, **355**(9197), 39–40.

Nofzinger, E.A., Thase, M.E., Reynolds, C.F. 3rd et al. (1991). Hypersomnia in bipolar depression: a comparison with narcolepsy using the multiple sleep latency test. *American Journal of Psychiatry*, **148**(9), 1177–81.

Parrino, L., Spaggiari, M.C., Boselli, M., Di Giovanni, G., & Terzano, M.G. (1994). Clinical and polysomnographic effects of trazodone CR in chronic insomnia associated with dysthymia. *Psychopharmacology*, **116**(4), 389–95.

Pflüg, B. & Tölle, R. (1971). Disturbance of the 24-hour rhythm in endogenous depression and the treatment of endogenous depression by sleep deprivation. *International Pharmacopsychiatry*, **6**(3), 187–96.

Piccinin, B. & Ansseau, M. (1991). [Value of sleep and neuroendocrine tests as biological markers of depression in children and adolescents]. [French] *Encephale*, **17**(5), 457–66.

Post, R.M. (1992). Transduction of psychosocial stress into the neurobiology of recurrent affective disorder. *American Journal of Psychiatry*, **149**(8), 999–1010.

Ramos Platon, M.J. & Espinar Sierra, J. (1992). Changes in psychopathological symptoms in sleep apnea patients after treatment with nasal continuous positive airway pressure. *International Journal of Neuroscience*, **62**(3–4), 173–95.

Reynolds, C.D. 3rd, Christiansen, C.L., Taska, L.S., Coble, P.A. & Kupfer, D.J. (1983). Sleep in Narcolepsy and depression. Does it all look alike? *Journal of Nervous and Mental Disease*, **171**(5), 290–5.

Roth, B. & Nevsimalova, S. (1975). Depression in narcolepsy and hypersomnia. *Schweizer Archiv fur Neurologie, Neurochirurgie und Psychiatrie*, **116**(2), 291–300.

Roth, T. & Ancoli-Israel, S. (1999). Daytime consequences and correlates of insomnia in the United States: results of the 1991 National Sleep Foundation Survey II. *Sleep*, **22**(2), S354–8.

Schülte, R. (1966). Kombierte psycho- und pharmakotherapie bei melancholikern. In *Probleme Pharmakopsychiatrischer Kombinations und Langzeitbehandlungen*, ed. H. Kranz & N. Petrillowitsch, pp. 150–69. Basel, Switzerland: Karger.

Singh, N.A., Clements, K.M., & Fiatarone, M.A. (1997). A randomized controlled trial of the effect of exercise on sleep. *Sleep*, **20**(2), 95–101.

Strousse, T., Szuba, M.P., & Baxter, L.R. (1992). Response to sleep deprivation in three women with postpartum psychosis. *Journal of Clinical Psychiatry*, **53**, 204–6.

Szuba, M.P., Baxter, L.R., Fairbanks, L.A., Guze, B.H., & Bergman, K.S. (1991). Effects of partial sleep deprivation on the diurnal variation of mood and motor activity in major depression. *Biological Psychiatry*, **30**, 817–29.

Thase, M.E., Simons, A.D., & Reynolds, C.F. 3rd. (1996). Abnormal electroencephalographic sleep profiles in major depression: association with response to cognitive behavior therapy. *Archives of General Psychiatry*, **53**(2), 99–108.

Tiberge, M. (1995). (Poorly understood sleep disorders in depression). Review. Les pathologies meconnues du sommeil au cours de la depression. *Encephale*, **21** spec# 7, 29–33.

Wehr, T.A. (1987). Sleep reduction as a final common pathway in the genesis of mania. *American Journal of Psychiatry*, **144**, 201–4.

Wirz-Justice, A. & Van den Hoofdakker, R.H. (1999). Sleep deprivation in depression: what do we know, where do we go? *Biological Psychiatry*, **46**(4), 445–53.

Zammit, G.K., Weiner, J., Damato, N., Sillup, G., & McMillan, C.A. (1999). Quality of life in people with insomnia. *Sleep*, **22**(2), S379–85.

**6**

# Structural and functional brain imaging in treatment-resistant depression

Terence A. Ketter, Christopher J. Bench, Mark S. George,
Tim A. Kimbrell, and Robert M. Post

## Introduction

Mood disorders are a heterogeneous group of illnesses which vary in clinical features such as symptoms, severity, and longitudinal course. Emerging research suggests that clinical diversity reflects biologic heterogeneity, and this notion is supported by the fact that the effectiveness of treatments can vary markedly across patients. Methods to more effectively target therapeutics in treatment-resistant mood disorder patients are sorely needed. In this chapter we consider the insights that structural and functional brain imaging methods have offered into the neural substrates of affective processes as well as the current and possible future utility of these methods in the evaluation and management of patients with treatment-resistant mood disorders.

## The neuroanatomy of affective processes

### Neuroanatomic models

Neuroanatomic models of the substrates of affective processes were originally derived from non-human animal studies in addition to postmortem and in vivo studies of humans with brain trauma, neurologic, and psychiatric disorders. More recently, brain imaging studies of healthy volunteers and mood disorder patients have helped refine models of healthy and pathologic affective processes.

Midline cerebral structures have long been considered possible mediators of affective experiences. Over a century ago, Broca defined the great limbic lobe as a midline cortical limbus (border or ring) around the brainstem in mammals (Broca, 1878). In 1937 Papez proposed a corticothalamic mechanism of emotion in which the hypothalamus was the origin of emotional impulses, that were sent to mamillary body, thence to anterior thalamus, and then on to cingulate, which through cortical projections could add affective valence to various cerebral processes (Papez, 1937). In 1952 MacLean introduced the term limbic system to describe the cortex of the limbic lobe and closely related brainstem structures (Fig. 6.1) (MacLean, 1952; 1990; Mesulam, 1985). Yakolev and colleagues noted thalamolimbic connections in which clusters of adjacent nuclei in the anterior portion of the thalamus projected to components of the limbic system in a topographic fashion (Yakolev et al., 1966).

Alexander and colleagues (1986, 1990) described a series of basal ganglia–thalamocortical circuits, three of which involve anterior cerebral structures with particular relevance to psychiatric disorders. The limbic circuit involves anterior paralimbic structures, going from anterior cingulate and medial orbitofrontal cortices to ventral striatum (limbic striatum – nucleus accumbens and olfactory tubercle), to ventral pallidum, to medial dorsal nucleus of thalamus and back to anterior cingulate and medial orbitofrontal cortices. This circuit may serve as a positive feedback loop, while a side loop involving the subthalamic nucleus may allow it also to serve as a negative feedback loop. As noted below, functional imaging studies suggest that structures in this limbic circuit are involved in the mediation of emotional experience in healthy subjects and are functionally abnormal in mood disorders. The lateral orbitofrontal circuit (lateral orbitofrontal cortex to caudate, to globus pallidus, to substantia nigra, to medial dorsal nucleus of thalamus, and back to lateral orbitofrontal cortex) is implicated by imaging studies in the pathophysiology of obsessive compulsive disorder (McGuire et al., 1994). The dorsolateral prefrontal circuit is from dorsolateral prefrontal cortex to caudate, to globus pallidus, to substantia nigra, to medial dorsal nucleus of thalamus, and back to dorsolateral prefrontal cortex. Dysfunction of structures in this circuit may contribute to the clinical profiles of schizophrenia and mood disorders, in particular, certain aspects of psychomotor slowing (Dolan et al., 1993).

Recent evidence supports division of the limbic system into anterior and posterior components based on differences in cytoarchitecture, connections, and functions (Vogt et al., 1992; Devinsky et al., 1995). The anterior (amygdalocentric) limbic system includes the amygdala, septum, orbitofrontal, insular, and anterior cingulate cortices, and the ventral striatum, and appears related to affective, motivational and endocrine functions. In contrast, the posterior (hippocampo-centric) limbic system includes the hippocampus, posterior parietal, posterior parahippocampal, and posterior cingulate cortices, and the dorsal striatum, and may be more related to learning and memory (Devinsky et al., 1995; MacLean & Delgado, 1953; Mesulam, 1998). Thus, the last century has seen progressively more detailed models of the putative cerebral substrates of affective experience. The most recent studies implicate a distributed circuit involving prefrontal, anterior paralimbic, and related subcortical structures.

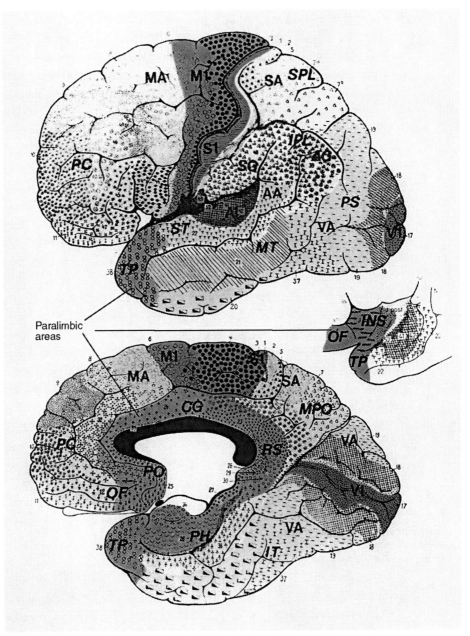

Fig. 6.1.    The limbic system. Lateral aspect of the left hemisphere (*top*) and the mesial aspect of the right hemisphere (*bottom*) showing paralimbic structures. Recent basic and clinical brain imaging research suggests that anterior paralimbic structures contribute to affective processes. (Adapted from Mesulam, 1985 with permission.)

### PET studies in healthy volunteers

Recent positron emission tomography (PET) studies in healthy volunteers have examined the functional anatomy of affective changes induced by physiologic or pharmacologic means. Thus, induction of transient emotions (sadness, happiness, anger and anxiety) by recalling affectively congruous events is associated with changes in anterior paralimbic function (George et al., 1995a,b,c,d; Kimbrell et al., 1999). Acute intravenous procaine yields diverse affective and psychosensory symptoms in concert with robust changes in global and anterior paralimbic cerebral blood flow (Ketter et al., 1996). Moreover, regional cerebral blood flow (rCBF) responses to procaine are related to various clinical responses. Figure 6.2 shows the anterior paralimbic activation pattern observed with induction of acute affective changes by procaine. This pattern is similar to that seen with self-induced emotions, and this concordance even extends to regional correlational relationships, as left amygdala activation correlates with the degree of negative affect (procaine-induced dysphoria and self-induced sadness) and deactivation with the intensity of positive affect (procaine-induced euphoria and self-induced happiness). These studies complement recent reports of the role of the amygdala in the recognition of facial emotion (Adolphs et al., 1994).

In the following sections, we review brain imaging studies in mood disorders, which in many cases demonstrate disruptions in anterior paralimbic structures and anterior basal ganglia–thalamocortical circuits. Many of these studies involved treatment-resistant patients or patients in tertiary care institutions and thus may be particularly indicative of the neurobiology of treatment-resistant mood disorders. As this chapter emphasizes recent studies, readers with particular interest in earlier studies may wish to refer to prior review articles (Dolan & Friston, 1989; Baxter, 1991; Sackeim & Prohovnik, 1993).

## Brain imaging in secondary mood disorders

### Primary vs. secondary mood disorders

A useful initial approach to the treatment-resistant mood disorder patient is to reassess the diagnosis, as diverse neurologic, general medical, or substance use disorders can cause psychiatric symptoms. In the past, such conditions were termed 'organic' on the basis of detectable abnormalities in macroscopic or microscopic cerebral tissue structure or blood biochemistry. Disorders in which abnormalities were not evident with such methods were considered 'functional.' With advances in medical technology, it is apparent that there are abnormalities in cerebral metabolism and biochemistry in a variety of 'functional' psychiatric disorders. Such conditions are now termed 'primary' disorders, suggesting primary disruptions of cerebral biochemical processes. Disorders caused by other

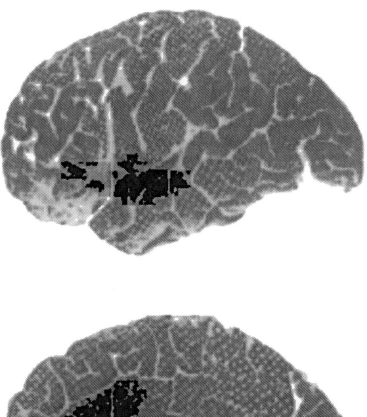

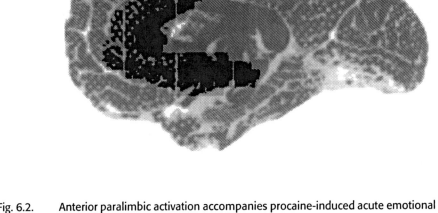

Fig. 6.2.     Anterior paralimbic activation accompanies procaine-induced acute emotional changes in healthy volunteers. Statistical parametric maps (SPMs) of significant ($P < 0.001$) increases in globally normalized cerebral blood flow rendered on the lateral aspect of the left hemisphere (*top*) and the mesial aspect of the right hemisphere (*bottom*), during acute intravenous procaine-induced emotional symptoms in 32 healthy volunteers. Note the concordance of this activation pattern with the anterior paralimbic structures in Fig. 6.1.

neurologic, general medical, or substance use problems are called 'secondary,' suggesting that the psychiatric symptoms are due to disruptions of cerebral biochemical processes caused by different primary problems. This nomenclature serves to emphasize similarities rather than differences between primary and secondary psychiatric disorders. This aids in conceptualizing similarities in pathophysiology and could help to destigmatize primary psychiatric disorders by emphasizing their physical basis in disrupted cerebral processes.

Thus, a useful initial approach to the treatment-resistant mood disorder patient is to reassess whether the disorder is primary or secondary. This yields the clear therapeutic distinction that, in secondary mood disorders, symptoms may be alleviated by treating the primary disease, and by implication reversing its cerebral metabolic sequelae. The primary vs. secondary distinction may be viewed as a continuum rather than as a simple dichotomy, with subclinical neurologic or general medical disorders increasing the liability to mood disorders. For example, as noted below, some patients with late life or late onset depressions have subtle brain changes suggestive of mild cerebrovascular insufficiency, which is not severe enough to merit a diagnosis of depression secondary to stroke. Also, some mood disorder patients have subtle changes in thyroid function, which are not sufficiently severe to merit a diagnosis of depression secondary to hypothyroidism. Preliminary data suggest that plasma thyroid stimulating hormone levels may correlate inversely with global and regional cerebral blood flow and metabolism in mood disorder patients (Marangell et al., 1997), so that varying degrees of thyroid dysfunction could yield varying degrees of disruption of cerebral metabolism and hence contribute to psychiatric symptoms.

The initial assessment of the treatment-resistant mood disorder patient for the existence of a secondary mood disorder includes a careful history and general physical and neurologic examinations. Secondary compared to primary mood disorders often have later onset ages and less family history of psychiatric illness, and are often treatment resistant. Laboratory studies of blood and urine can help evaluate the possibility of a variety of primary medical and substance use disorders. Specific neurologic investigations such as electroencephalography and structural brain imaging can exclude other primary medical disorders. These methods are generally well tolerated, and when used judiciously may provide substantial financial as well as human benefits, if they detect a reversible primary neurologic or general medical disorder which has yielded an otherwise treatment-resistant secondary mood disorder.

## Structural brain imaging in secondary mood disorders

Structural brain imaging using computerized tomography (CT) and magnetic resonance imaging (MRI) can be used to diagnose conditions associated with secondary mood disorders. In addition, structural imaging studies of patients with secondary mood disorders can offer new insights into the anatomy and pathophysiology of such disorders.

The high prevalence of mood disorders in patients with stroke, Huntington's disease, Parkinson's disease, traumatic brain injury, epilepsy, multiple sclerosis, and brain tumors has resulted in a provocative and at times controversial literature concerning the neuroanatomy of secondary mood disorders. Thus, the risk of depression may be greater after anterior compared to posterior and after left hemisphere compared to right hemisphere strokes, while the risk of mania may be greater after right hemisphere compared to left hemisphere strokes (Starkstein & Robinson, 1989; Stern & Bachmann, 1991). Basal ganglia strokes may also be associated with secondary depression (Mendez et al., 1989). The profound basal ganglia damage noted in Huntington's disease and Parkinson's disease and the high prevalence of mood symptoms in these disorders also provide support of a role for basal ganglia dysfunction in secondary mood disorders (Folstein & Folstein, 1983; Caine & Shoulson, 1983; Horn, 1974; Mindham, 1970). With traumatic brain injury, left dorsolateral prefrontal and/or left basal ganglia lesions may increase the risk of depression (Federoff et al., 1992), while right temporal basal polar lesions may increase the risk of mania (Jorge et al., 1993). The risk of secondary depression in patients with epilepsy may be greater with left than with right temporal lobe lesions (Altshuler et al., 1990). Temporal (Honer et al., 1987) and left frontal lobe (George et al., 1994) lesions may also increase the risk of depression secondary to multiple sclerosis, although a recent study failed to replicate these findings (Moller et al., 1994). Finally, frontal lobe brain tumors may be associated with secondary depression (Direkze et al., 1971; Kanakaratnam & Direkze, 1976).

## Functional brain imaging in secondary mood disorders

Functional brain imaging has much more limited clinical application in the diagnosis of conditions associated with secondary mood disorders, due to its expense and the less extensive data supporting its diagnostic utility. However, such studies offer important insights into the pathophysiology of secondary mood disorders, and provide intriguing evidence of similarities between these and primary mood disorders.

A substantial literature supports anterior cerebral hypoactivity in secondary depressions. Patients with depression secondary to diverse neurologic and medical (stroke (Mayberg et al., 1991b), epilepsy (Bromfield et al., 1992), Parkinson's (Mayberg et al., 1990; Ring et al., 1994) and Huntington's (Mayberg et al., 1992) diseases, and acquired immunodeficiency syndrome (Renshaw et al., 1992)), or other psychiatric (obsessive-compulsive (Baxter et al., 1989), bulimia (Andreason et al., 1992), and cocaine abuse (Volkow et al., 1991)) disorders have consistently had anterior cerebral (commonly prefrontal and anterior cingulate) hypoactivity compared to either healthy controls or euthymic controls matched for the primary illness. In addition, the degree of anterior cerebral hypoactivity has often correlated with the severity of rated depression. These findings are convergent with the observations in primary mood disorders described below. Hence, anterior cerebral hypoactivity may represent a common substrate of depressive symptoms independent of illness etiology.

There is a paucity of functional imaging studies in secondary mania. Starkstein and colleagues reported right temporal lobe hypometabolism in three patients with mania secondary to stroke (Starkstein et al., 1990). In summary, preliminary functional imaging findings in mania and depression secondary to stroke are in convergence with other clinical and structural imaging evidence that left-sided lesions may be associated with secondary depression and right-sided lesions with secondary mania. However, this evidence of lateralization in secondary mood disorders should be considered with caution in view of the limited data, as well as the apparent lack of robust lateralization in primary depression.

## Brain imaging in primary mood disorders

Many patients with treatment-resistant mood disorders are deemed to have a primary psychiatric disorder as there is no clinical or laboratory evidence of the mood problem being secondary to another neurologic, medical, or substance abuse process. In many cases this is supported by a family history of psychiatric problems, suggesting an inherited disorder of brain metabolism that manifests itself as a primary mood disorder. The evaluation of such treatment-resistant patients should include re-evaluation of the primary psychiatric diagnosis. Generally this is done by careful assessment of the patient's history with an emphasis on symptom profile, comorbidity, responses to treatments, and family history of psychiatric symptoms and treatment responses. Of particular interest, some patients appear to have a progressive course with mood episodes advancing from reactive to spontaneous, and increasing in frequency and severity to the point that the illness is autonomous, continuous, and treatment-resistant (Post, 1992). This suggests that some primary cerebral metabolic disruptions (presenting as primary psychiatric disorders) may be progressive in a fashion similar to degenerative neurologic disorders. Serial brain imaging studies may allow assessment of this theory.

Although brain imaging does not yet have a direct clinical application in the evaluation and management of primary mood disorders, research studies have advanced our understanding of the neuroanatomy and pathophysiology of mood disorders, and in some instances suggested mechanisms of treatment resistance. In addition, such studies have begun to explore ways to more effectively target existing treatments, and even provide the bases for the development of new treatments.

## Structural brain imaging in primary mood disorders

Structural brain imaging studies can diagnose conditions capable of causing secondary mood disorders and even detect differences between groups of patients with primary psychiatric disorders and healthy controls, but cannot diagnose primary mood disorders in individual patients. The challenge raised by the discovery of structural changes is to relate them to specific symptomatic, cognitive or physiological dysfunctions. Recent observations, consensus findings, and results of meta-analyses in this area, are reviewed below. Readers interested in details of individual structural imaging studies are referred to prior review articles (Sackeim & Prohovnik, 1993; Jeste et al., 1988; Nasrallah et al., 1989; Schlegel, 1991; Hauser, 1991).

### Subcortical hyperintensities

Subcortical hyperintensities (SCHs) are bright areas in periventricular white, deep white, or subcortical gray matter observed on $T_2$-weighted MRI images (Fig. 6.3, left). Both bipolar (Dupont et al., 1990, 1995; Swayze et al., 1990; Figiel et al., 1991b; Aylward et al., 1994) and elderly unipolar (Kanaya & Yonekawa, 1990; Krishnan et al., 1988, 1993; Brown et al., 1992; Coffey et al., 1988, 1989, 1990; Lesser et al., 1991) mood disorder patients have been reported to have increased SCHs compared to controls. SCHs may (Botteron et al., 1991; Miller et al., 1989) or may not (Swayze et al., 1990) also be increased in psychoses. These lesions vary with age, and may be related to a number of factors including hypertension, carotid arteriosclerosis, arteriolar hyalinization, and dilated perivascular spaces. Their exact significance in mood disorder patients and relationships to other variables, such as dexamethasone suppression status or post-dexamethasone cortisol levels (Rao et al., 1989; Deicken et al., 1991; Coffey et al., 1993b), remain to be determined.

Dupont and colleagues recently reported that younger bipolar patients had increased volumes of white matter SCHs compared to unipolar patients and healthy controls (Dupont et al., 1995). The distribution of SCHs appeared relatively frontal compared to controls, and total volume of SCHs was associated with increased cognitive impairment, increased rate of psychiatric illness in the family and onset after adolescence. Altshuler and colleagues reported increased periventricular SCHs in bipolar I but not bipolar II patients compared to healthy controls, and provided a meta-analysis of eight studies (including a total of 198 bipolar I

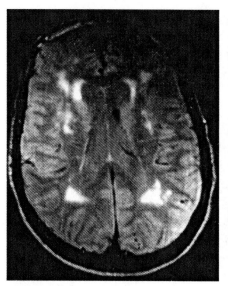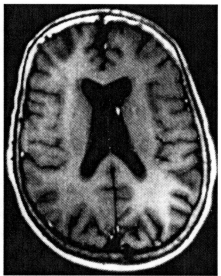

Fig. 6.3.     Subcortical hyperintensities and ventricular enlargement. *Left*: Intermediate
$(T_1–T_2)$-weighted spin-echo MRI showing multiple subcortical hyperintensities (SCHs) in
periventricular and deep white matter and in basal ganglia. *Right*: $T_1$-weighted spin-echo
MRI showing enlarged lateral ventricles. These findings are often seen in patients with
primary mood disorders. (Reproduced from Coffey, 1996 with permission.)

disorder patients and 307 healthy controls) which found a common odds ratio of
3.3 for the presence of any SCH in bipolar I patients vs. healthy controls (*P*
0.00001) (Altshuler et al., 1995).

Patients with late life depression appear to have an excess of SCHs (Kanaya &
Yonekawa, 1990; Krishnan et al., 1988, 1993; Brown et al., 1992; Coffey et al., 1988,
1989, 1990; Lesser et al., 1991) and some (Coffey et al., 1989; Lesser et al., 1991;
Figiel et al., 1991a; Salloway et al., 1996; Keshavan et al., 1996; Hickie et al., 1995;
O'Brien et al., 1996) but not all (Greenwald et al., 1996) studies suggest that SCHs
are more common where the first episode of depression is of late onset. However,
the interpretation of many of these studies is limited because only a minority
(O'Brien et al., 1996) control adequately for cardiovascular risk factors and age.
The mechanisms mediating the link between SCHs and depression remain uncertain as is their clinical significance, though one study suggests severity of white
matter SCHs may predict poorer responses to physical treatments (Hickie et al.,
1995).

### Ventricular enlargement

A recent meta-analysis has confirmed that older mood disorder patients have
ventricular enlargement (VE, Fig. 6.3, right) and sulcal prominence (Elkis et al.,

1995). Longitudinal studies suggest that the association between ventricular brain ratio (VBR) and cognitive impairment persists into clinical recovery from depression (Beats et al., 1996), suggesting that structural change relates to neuropsychologic impairment independent of depressed mood. VE may even increase with disease duration, perhaps in excess of the increase noted with normal aging (Vita et al., 1988; Woods et al., 1990). An initial report has raised the possibility that structural changes can also be seen in much younger patients (Steingard et al., 1996).

Reliable clinical correlates of VE remain elusive. There do not appear to be consistent relationships with severity of mood symptoms (Luchins et al., 1984; Schlegel et al., 1989a,b,c; Van den Bossche et al., 1991), polarity (Swayze et al., 1990; Elkis et al., 1995; Andreason et al., 1990; Dolan et al., 1985; Schlegel & Kretzschmar, 1987), psychotic symptoms (Schlegel et al., 1989b; Schlegel & Kretzschmar, 1987; Luchins & Meltzer, 1983; Targum et al., 1983; Dewan et al., 1988b; Nasrallah et al., 1984; Pearlson et al., 1984), cognitive dysfunction or gender (Elkis et al., 1995). Several studies have examined the relationship between VE and dexamethasone suppression status, pre- and postdexamethasone cortisol levels and urinary free cortisol, given the glucocorticoid cascade hypothesis which proposes that prolonged activation of the hypothalamic–pituitary–adrenal axis can produce permanent brain damage (O'Brien, 1997). However, most (Coffey et al., 1993b; Van den Bossche et al., 1991; Schlegel & Kretzschmar, 1987; Targum et al., 1983; Standish-Barry et al., 1985; Dewan et al., 1988a; Risch et al., 1992), but not all (Rao et al., 1989; Rothschild et al., 1989; Schlegel et al., 1989a,b,c; Kellner et al., 1983) studies have failed to detect a significant relationship.

### Other structural abnormalities

In contrast to the above, the literature concerning other structural changes in mood disorders is less extensive and consistent. There are conflicting data regarding third ventricular enlargement in mood disorders (Schlegel & Kretzschmar, 1987; Dewan et al., 1988b). Decreased frontal (Tanaka et al., 1982; Strakowski et al., 1993) (Coffey et al., 1993a; Kumar et al., 1996a,b), caudate (Krishnan et al., 1992), putamen (Husain et al., 1991), and brainstem and cerebellar vermis (Shah et al., 1992) areas or volumes in mood disorder patients compared to controls have been reported, but other studies have failed to replicate these findings (Aylward et al., 1994; Strakowski et al., 1993; Swayze et al., 1992; Yates et al., 1987; Raine et al., 1992). Patients with recurrent major depression may have hippocampal atrophy which is related to the duration of depression, consistent with the notion that chronic hypercortisolemia could yield progressive hippocampal degeneration (Sheline et al., 1996). Bipolar patients have been reported to have decreased temporal lobe areas (Hauser et al., 1989) (relative to cerebellum) and volumes (Altshuler et al., 1991). However, other groups failed to find altered temporal lobe areas (Johnstone et al., 1989) or volumes in bipolar disorder. Corpus callosum size has been reported decreased in bipolar (Hauser et al., 1989; Coffman et al., 1990) and unchanged (Lammers et al., 1991) or increased in the anterior and posterior quadrants (Wu et al., 1993) in unipolar patients. Pituitary enlargement has been reported in mood disorder patients (Krishnan et al., 1991), and may be related to the degree of adrenal escape from suppression by dexamethasone (Axelson et al., 1992).

## PET and SPECT studies in primary depression
### Brain mapping studies

PET and single photon emission computed tomography (SPECT) studies have demonstrated cerebral blood flow and metabolic abnormalities in primary depression. The majority of resting state or continuous performance task studies have noted decreased anterior cortical and paralimbic activity in depressed patients (Fig. 6.4: see footnote), which has often correlated with the severity of depression (Table 6.1). In the literature between 1984 and 1995, we found a total of 38 papers and abstracts comparing cerebral blood flow and metabolism in a total of 576 mood disorder patients with 590 healthy controls (references available upon request). Half (19) of these reports studied cerebral glucose metabolism as assessed by fluorine-18-deoxyglucose ($^{18}$FDG), while the other half studied cerebral blood flow by oxygen-15 water ($H_2{}^{15}O$), technetium-99m-hexamethyl-propylene-amineoxime ($^{99m}$Tc-HMPAO), technetium-99m-exametazime ($^{99m}$Tc-EMZ) and iodine-123-$N$-isopropyl-4-iodo-amphetamine ($^{123}$I-IMP), or other tracers. Studies found abnormal (decreased much more often than increased) cerebral activity in anterior cortical, paralimbic and subcortical structures (prefrontal > temporal > basal ganglia > anterior cingulate) in primary depression. Most studies did not report lateralized cerebral functional changes in primary depression.

In summary, resting state and continuous performance task studies in patients with depression have identified focal deficits in brain function. The relationship of these deficits to specific symptoms has been explored by a minority of studies (Bench et al., 1993). Such correlational analyses have suggested that the dorsolateral prefrontal cortex is an area of dysfunction common to depressed and schizophrenic patients who show the clinical feature of psychomotor slowing (Dolan et al., 1993).

'Activation' studies targeting specific brain regions, cognitive processes and neurotransmitter systems have also been applied to depressed patients. The results from recent cognitive and pharmacologic activation studies complement the previously described resting state and continuous performance task studies. Thus,

At the time of going to press a colour version of this figure was available for download from http://www.cambridge.org/9780521593410

**Table 6.1.** Negative correlations between Hamilton depression ratings and cerebral blood flow and metabolism in primary depression

| Study | Region | r | P |
|---|---|---|---|
| Baxter et al. (1989) | L DLPF/hemisphere | −0.49[a] | 0.0002 |
|  | R DLPF/hemisphere | −0.41 | 0.005 |
| O'Connell et al. (1989) | FL/cerebellum | −0.32[a] | 0.001 |
|  | TL/cerebellum | −0.45 | 0.001 |
| Schlegel et al. (1989a) | L TL | −0.44 | 0.05 |
| Kanaya & Yonekawa (1990) | Cerebrum/cerebellum | −0.58 | 0.01 |
| Kumar et al. (1991) | Cerebrum/cerebellum | −0.75 | 0.01 |
| Austin et al. (1992) | R FL/occipital | −0.37[a] | 0.05 |
| Cohen et al. (1992) | M PF | −0.95[a] | 0.02 |
| Drevets et al. (1992) | L PF/global | −0.62[a] | 0.05 |
| Yazici et al. (1992) | L PF/slice | −0.68[a] | 0.006 |
|  | M PF/slice | −0.58 | 0.02 |
| O'Connell et al. (1995) | FL/cerebellum | −0.34[a] | 0.01 |

L = left; R = right; M = mesial; FL = frontal lobe; TL = temporal lobe; PF = prefrontal; DLPF = dorsolateral prefrontal

[a] 7 studies with significant negative correlations between prefrontal activity and severity of depression.

depressed patients show blunted anterior paralimbic rCBF responses compared to healthy controls during facial emotion recognition (George et al., 1993), Stroop colour-word interference (George et al., 1995d), and transient sadness self-induction (George et al., 1995b) tasks, and following pharmacologic activation with acute intravenous procaine (Ketter et al., 1993), and acute oral amphetamine (Trivedi et al., 1995). Mann et al. (1996) used $^{18}$FDG PET to assess the functional effects of DL-fenfluramine challenge on regional glucose metabolism in untreated depressed patients in comparison with healthy controls. Whereas control subjects showed activations in the left prefrontal and temporo-parietal cortex, areas implicated in resting state studies in depression, no such activations were seen in the depressed patients, suggesting a blunted serotonergic responsivity in depression.

The few studies reporting increased anterior cerebral activity in primary depression tended to include patients with affective illness subtypes with unique phenomenologic, pathophysiologic and treatment response characteristics. Increased cerebral activity compared to controls has been reported in familial pure depressive disorder (Drevets et al., 1992), bipolar II patients with summer seasonal affective disorder (Goyer et al., 1992), bipolar I depression (Ketter et al., 1994), antidepressant responders to sleep deprivation (Ebert et al., 1991; Wu et al., 1992), responders to carbamazepine (Ketter et al., 1999), and prior non-responders to a wide variety of antidepressants (Hornig et al., 1997). The brain regions with increased activity in these subtypes tended to be the same (prefrontal and anterior paralimbic) areas in which decreases were noted in the majority of studies. These findings suggest that in these subtypes, different or opposing biochemical disruptions may occur in structures which are involved in the mediation of emotional experience.

This is further supported by differential clinical responses in some of these subtypes. For example, patients with anterior limbic hyperactivity (compared to those without this marker) may be more likely to have antidepressant responses to sleep deprivation or carbamazepine, interventions which appear to decrease cerebral activity. Many responders to either of these interventions have bipolar illness. Preliminary evidence suggests that bipolar I depression may be more likely to be associated with hypermetabolism, bipolar II depression with intermediate heterogeneous metabolic patterns, and unipolar depression with hypometabolism (Fig. 6.5: see footnote) (Ketter et al., 1994).

Reports comparing euthymic and depressed patients, matched for medication status, have generally found that with euthymia there is attenuation (or resolution) of abnormalities observed in depression (Drevets et al., 1992; Kimbrell et al., 1996; Bench et al., 1995; Post et al., 1987; Amsterdam et al., 1995). Residual abnormalities in medication-free euthymic patients have been proposed to represent possible trait markers of depressive illnesses (Drevets et al., 1992), but the clinical relevance of these changes needs to be further clarified. For example, elderly depressed patients may have decreases in global and regional CBF which persist during remission, as well as diminished CBF responses during hypercapnea challenge which could reflect decreased vasodilatory reserve, and are consistent with the notion that progressive mild cerebrovascular insufficiency may underlie some cases of late life depression (Sackeim, 1996). If true, this would offer a mechanism for the high prevalence of treatment refractoriness in late life depression, and suggest that particular caution ought to be taken with such patients to avoid causing iatrogenic hypotension with tricyclic antidepressants or monoamine oxidase inhibitors, as this could exacerbate this putative cerebrovascular insufficiency.

Treatment responders, compared with their own depressed, pretreatment baseline often show attenuation (or resolution) of pretreatment cerebral functional abnormalities in response to various therapies, including medication (Baxter et al., 1989; Kanaya & Yonekawa, 1990; Ketter et al., 1999), light (Cohen et al., 1992), sleep deprivation (Ebert et al., 1991; Wu et al., 1992), and (non-convulsive) transcranial magnetic stimulation (Pascual-Leone & Pallardó, 1996; George et al., 1995c). In contrast, successful electroconvulsive therapy appears to further exacerbate decreased anterior cerebral activity (Nobler et al., 1994; Schmidt et al., 1996). Also, recent data suggest that chronic but not acute paroxetine decreases prefron-

At the time of going to press a colour version of this figure was available for download from http://www.cambridge.org/9780521593410

tal and anterior paralimbic metabolism (Kennedy et al., 1996), while venlafaxine therapy decreases prefrontal and paralimbic CBF in responders but not non-responders (Little et al., 1997).

Comparisons of baseline (pretreatment) cerebral function in patients who later respond or fail to respond to therapy suggest possible baseline markers of treatment responses; these may offer important insights into the heterogeneity of mood disorders, and perhaps even be used someday to more effectively target treatments in treatment-resistant illness. Thus, anterior limbic hyperactivity may be a baseline marker for patients who attain antidepressant responses to sleep deprivation (Ebert et al., 1991; Wu et al., 1992). In addition, preliminary data suggest that baseline temporal hypermetabolism and frontal hypometabolism may be markers for patients who are more likely to respond to carbamazepine and nimodipine, respectively (Ketter et al., 1999). Finally, in never hospitalized outpatients with mild to moderate depression, responders to bupropion or venlafaxine appear to have the classic pattern of baseline prefrontal and paralimbic hypometabolism which was not observed in non-responders (Little et al., 1996).

## Receptor Imaging Studies

PET and SPECT studies of specific neurotransmitter systems combining medication challenges with $^{18}FDG$ and $H_2{}^{15}O$, or using more biochemically specific radiotracers have noted altered serotonergic (Mann et al., 1996; Agren et al., 1993; D'haenen et al., 1992), dopaminergic (Agren et al., 1993; Pearlson et al., 1995; Ebert et al., 1994; Suhara et al., 1992), and opiatergic (Mayberg et al., 1991b) function in mood disorder patients compared to controls. However, this literature is much less extensive than that for cerebral blood flow and metabolism, primarily due to the lack of good radioligands for serotonergic and noradrenergic receptors, and most of these findings require replication.

## PET and SPECT studies in primary mania

The few cerebral blood flow and metabolism studies in primary mania have had variable and at times conflicting findings. Global cerebral metabolism in medication-free hypomanic or euthymic bipolar patients may not differ from healthy controls but may be increased compared to bipolar patients in depressed or mixed states (Schwartz et al., 1987). Kishimoto and colleagues noted widespread increases in $^{11}C$-glucose uptake in three medication-free manic patients compared to controls, and in contrast to widespread decreases in nine unipolar depressed patients (Kishimoto et al., 1987). O'Connell and colleagues reported that 11 manic patients had increased (globally normalized) temporal lobe CBF compared to controls, in a fashion similar to patients with schizophrenia (O'Connell et al., 1989, 1995) and atypical psychosis (O'Connell et al., 1989). Also, decreased normalized frontal and basal ganglia CBF was noted in both mania and schizo-phrenia patients compared to controls (O'Connell et al., 1995). Moreover, across mixed subjects (schizophrenia, mania, and controls), mania ratings had positive correlations with caudate ($r = 0.25$, $n = 100$, $P < 0.01$) (O'Connell et al., 1989) and right temporal ($r = 0.41$, $n = 48$, $P < 0.01$) CBF (O'Connell et al., 1995). In contrast, Migliorelli and colleagues found that five medication-free manic patients had decreased right temporal basal cortical CBF (normalized to cerebellum) compared to controls as well as (right less than left) temporal basal and (basal less than dorsal) right temporal CBF asymmetries (Migliorelli et al., 1993). Their group found a trend towards a negative correlation ($r = -0.86$, $n = 5$, $P = 0.06$) between mania ratings and right basotemporal CBF. In a recent xenon SPECT study, no global differences were found between 11 manic and 11 depressed (seven unipolar, four bipolar) patients and 11 controls, but both patient groups had relative hypofrontality compared to controls (Rubin et al., 1995).

## MRS studies in primary mood disorders

Magnetic resonance spectroscopy (MRS) uses modified structural MRI scanners to study resonance spectra of compounds containing paramagnetic (odd atomic number) elements. An emerging MRS literature is beginning to suggest biochemi-cally specific abnormalities in mood disorder patients, and allow assessment of brain concentrations of lithium and fluorinated medications.

Proton ($^1$H) MRS allows determination of lactate, glutamate, aspartate, gamma-aminobutyric acid, creatine, choline and N-acetylaspartate (Fig. 6.6). Choline is of particular interest as it is a precursor of acetylcholine and involved in second messenger cascades. Unipolar depressed patients have been observed to have increased basal ganglia choline, which was decreased with nefazodone ther-apy (Charles et al., 1994). Increased basal ganglia choline has also been reported in bipolar patients on lithium (Sharma et al., 1992). Kato et al. also noted increased basal ganglia choline in euthymic bipolar patients, with no differences between patients on, compared to off, lithium (Kato et al., 1996). Rapid cycling compared to non-rapid cycling bipolar patients tended to have lower basal ganglia choline (Demopulos et al., 1996). Brain choline uptake appears to decrease markedly with age (Cohen et al., 1995), and the development of cerebral choline depletion has been proposed as a possible mechanism of the deteriorating course seen in some patients with bipolar disorders (Renshaw et al., 1996). Preliminary evidence suggests that the addition of choline bitartrate may yield improvement in treat-ment-resistant rapid cycling bipolar patients on lithium (Stoll et al., 1996). Thus, brain imaging studies of patients with treatment-resistant mood disorders may aid not only in understanding mechanisms of, but also in devising treatments for, treatment-resistant affective illness.

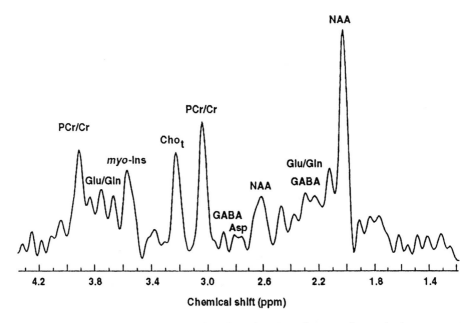

Fig. 6.6. Typical normal proton ($^1$H) MRS of left dorsolateral prefrontal cortex. The cerebral proton metabolites are assigned as follows: PCr/Cr = phosphocreatine plus creatine, Glu = glutamate, Gln = glutamine, *myo*-Ins = *myo*-inositol, Cho$_t$ = choline containing compounds, GABA = gamma-aminobutyric acid, Asp = aspartate, NAA = *N*-acetylaspartate. (Reproduced from Stanley et al., 1995 with permission.)

Lithium ($^7$Li) MRS studies, primarily in bipolar patients, have fairly consistently reported brain lithium concentrations to be about one half of serum lithium levels. Across nine studies the mean brain/serum lithium ratio was 0.54 (standard deviation 0.11, range 0.40 to 0.77). Brain lithium concentrations may correlate better with serum ($r = 0.66$) than with red blood cell ($r = 0.33$) lithium levels (Kato et al., 1993), suggesting that red blood cell lithium levels may be less relevant than plasma levels. Moreover, improvement in manic symptoms correlated with brain lithium ($r = 0.64$, Fig. 6.7) and brain/serum lithium ratio ($r = 0.60$), but not serum lithium or lithium dose/weight (Kato et al., 1994). Preliminary evidence suggests that brain lithium concentrations may need to be at least 0.2 mM (Kato et al., 1994; Gyulai et al., 1991) for adequate therapeutic effects. This raises the possibility that some patients could be resistant to lithium due to insufficient transport of this ion into the central nervous system.

Phosphorous ($^{31}$P) MRS allows determination of high energy phosphates, intracellular pH and free magnesium, and some phospholipids, including phosphomonoesters (PMEs – putative cell membrane 'building blocks') and phosphodiesters (PDEs – putative cell membrane 'breakdown products'). $^{31}$P MRS

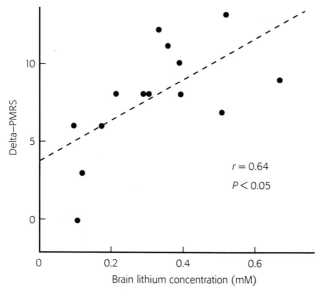

Fig. 6.7.     Cerebral lithium concentrations correlate with antimanic responses. Brain lithium levels assessed by lithium ($^7$Li) MRS. The correlation coefficient is 0.64 ($P < 0.05$). The regression line is shown as a dotted line. (Reproduced from Kato et al., 1994 with permission.)

studies of medicated and unmedicated euthymic bipolar patients have found decreased frontal and temporal PMEs and increased PDEs, while manic or depressed bipolar patients had increased PMEs (Deicken et al., 1995a,b; Kato et al., 1993). Despite lithium's inhibitory effect on the inositol phosphatase pathway, lithium therapy failed to alter PMEs (which include an inositol phosphate component) in schizophrenia and schizoaffective patients (Keshaven et al., 1992). Decreased left prefrontal phosphocreatine was noted in bipolar depression, with the degree of decrease correlated with the severity of depression, while decreased right prefrontal phosphocreatine was observed in euthymic and manic bipolar patients (Kato et al., 1995).

## Conclusions

### Current clinical and clinical research applications

Brain imaging methods have already had substantial impact on neuropsychiatry (Table 6.2). Structural brain imaging is currently used clinically in the diagnosis and management of a number of conditions associated with secondary mood disorders. Judiciously applied, this modality may allow improved management of patients with mood disorders which are treatment-resistant by virtue of their being secondary to a reversible neurologic or medical disorder. Functional brain

**Table 6.2.** Clinical and clinical research applications of brain imaging

| Methods | Clinical applications | Clinical research applications |
|---|---|---|
| CT / MRI | Detect neurologic and general medical disorders associated with secondary mood disorders | Assess structural abnormalities in primary and secondary mood disorders |
| PET / SPECT / functional MRI (Cerebral blood flow and metabolism) | Not currently used in psychiatry. Limited use in neurology (e.g. dementia diagnosis, epileptic foci lateralization) | Assess neuroanatomy of functional abnormalities in primary and secondary mood disorders, effects of therapies, and baseline markers of treatment response |
| PET / SPECT (Specific radiotracers) MRS | Not currently used | Assess biochemical abnormalities in primary and secondary mood disorders, effects of therapies, and baseline markers of treatment response |

imaging is not currently routinely applied in clinical psychiatry, due to expense, invasiveness, lack of general availability, and still emerging knowledge of its clinical significance with respect to diagnosis and treatment. However, this modality has seen limited clinical applications in neurology, such as in the diagnosis of dementia and in the determination of lateralization of seizure foci prior to epilepsy surgery. Functional brain imaging studies of cerebral blood flow and metabolism have confirmed the importance of prefrontal and anterior paralimbic structures in mood disorders, and have suggested subtype heterogeneity and the possibility that different topographies at baseline may be related to treatment responses.

## Future directions

Technologic refinements to enhance spatial and temporal resolution, decrease or eliminate exposure to ionizing radiation (such as functional MRI, MRS, and more sensitive PET and SPECT scanners), increase biochemical specificity (such as MRS and new PET and SPECT radiotracers), and increase availability and decrease expense (such as using generally available scanners and avoiding the need for on-site cyclotrons) should allow further advances in our knowledge of the neuroanatomic and biochemical substrates of mood disorders. Will some patients with otherwise treatment-resistant unipolar or bipolar illness be discovered to have the atypical pattern of temporal hypermetabolism and be treated with agents such as carbamazepine, which could normalize this dysfunction, while others are found to have remediable deficits in brain choline levels or in transport of lithium into the central nervous system? It remains of great promise, but it is yet to be seen whether methodologic and research advances will ultimately yield more widespread clinical applications of functional brain imaging methods to facilitate diagnosis and treatment in psychiatry. If this does occur, patients with treatment treatment-resistant mood disorders will be a crucial target population.

## REFERENCES

Adolphs, R., Tranel, D., Damasio, H. et al. (1994). Impaired recognition of emotion in facial expressions following bilateral damage to the human amygdala. *Nature*, 372(6507), 669–72.

Agren, H., Reibring, L., Hartvig, P. et al. (1993). Monoamine metabolism in human prefrontal cortex and basal ganglia. PET studies using [$\beta$-$^{11}$C]L-5-hydroxytryptophan and [$\beta$-$^{11}$C]L-DOPA in healthy volunteers and patients with unipolar major depression. *Depression*, 1(2), 71–81.

Alexander, G.E., DeLong, M.R., & Strick, P.L. (1986). Parallel organization of functionally segregated circuits linking basal ganglia and cortex. *Annual Review of Neuroscience*, 9, 357–81.

Alexander, G.E., Crutcher, M.D., & DeLong, M.R. (1990). Basal ganglia-thalamocortical circuits: parallel substrates for motor, oculomotor, prefrontal and limbic functions. *Progress in Brain Research*, 85, 119–46.

Altshuler, L.L., Devinsky, O., Post, R.M. et al. (1990). Depression, anxiety, and temporal lobe epilepsy. Laterality of focus and symptoms. *Archives of Neurology*, 47(3), 284–8.

Altshuler, L.L., Conrad, A., Hauser, P. et al. (1991). Reduction of temporal lobe volume in bipolar disorder: a preliminary report of magnetic resonance imaging [letter]. *Archives of General Psychiatry*, 48(5), 482–3.

Altshuler, L.L., Curran, J.G., Hauser, P. et al. (1995). T$_2$ hyperintensities in bipolar disorder: magnetic resonance imaging comparison and literature meta-analysis. *American Journal of Psychiatry*, 152(8), 1139–44.

Amsterdam, J.D., Mozley, P.D., & Hornig-Rohan, M. (1995). $^{123}$I-iofetamine (IMP) SPECT brain imaging in depressed patients: normalization of temporal lobe asymmetry during clinical recovery. *Depression*, 6(3), 273–3.

Andreasen, N.C., Swayze, V.W. 2nd, Flaum, M. et al. (1990). Ventricular abnormalities in affective disorder: clinical and demographic correlates. *American Journal of Psychiatry*, 147(7), 893–900.

Andreason, P.J., Altemus, M., Zametkin, A.J. et al. (1992). Regional cerebral glucose metabolism in bulimia nervosa. *American Journal of Psychiatry*, 149(11), 1506–13.

Austin, M.P., Dougall, N., Ross, M. et al. (1992). Single photon emission tomography with $^{99m}$Tc-exametazime in major depression and the pattern of brain activity underlying the psychotic/neurotic continuum. *Journal of Affective Disorders*, 26(1), 31–43.

Axelson, D.A., Doraiswamy, P.M., Boyko, O.B. et al. (1992). In vivo assessment of pituitary volume with magnetic resonance imaging and systematic stereology: relationship to dexamethasone suppression test results in patients. *Psychiatry Research*, **44**(1), 63–70.

Aylward, E.H., Roberts-Twille, J.V., Barta, P.E. et al. (1994). Basal ganglia volumes and white matter hyperintensities in patients with bipolar disorder. *American Journal of Psychiatry*, **151**(5), 687–93.

Baxter, L.R, Jr. (1991). PET studies of cerebral function in major depression and obsessive-compulsive disorder. The emerging prefrontal consensus. *Annals of Clinical Psychiatry*, **3**, 103–9.

Baxter, L.R. Jr., Schwartz, J.M., Phelps, M.E. et al. (1989). Reduction of prefrontal cortex glucose metabolism common to three types of depression. *Archives of General Psychiatry*, **46**(3), 243–50.

Beats, B.C., Sahakian, B.J., & Levy, R. (1996). Cognitive performance in tests sensitive to frontal lobe dysfunction in the elderly depressed. *Psychological Medicine*, **26**, 591–603.

Bench, C.J., Friston, K.J., Brown, R.G. et al. (1992). The anatomy of melancholia – focal abnormalities of cerebral blood flow in major depression. *Psychological Medicine*, **22**(3), 607–15.

Bench, C.J., Friston, K.J, Brown, R.G. et al. (1993). Regional cerebral blood flow in depression measured by positron emission tomography: the relationship with clinical dimensions. *Psychological Medicine*, **23**(3), 579–90.

Bench, C.J., Frackowiak, R.S., & Dolan, R.J. (1995). Changes in regional cerebral blood flow on recovery from depression. *Psychological Medicine*, **25**(2), 247–61.

Botteron, K.N., Figiel, G.S., & Zorumski, C.F. (1991). Electroconvulsive therapy in patients with late-onset psychosis and structural brain changes. *Journal of Geriatric Psychiatry and Neurology*, **4**(1), 44–7.

Broca, P. (1878). Anatomie comparée des circonvolutions cérébrales: le grand lobe limbique et la scissure limbique dans la série des mammifères. [Anatomic considerations of cerebral convolutions: the great limbic lobe and limbic sulci in a series of mammals]. *Reviews of Anthropology*, **1**(Ser. 2), 385–498.

Bromfield, E.B., Altshuler, L., Leiderman, D.B. et al. (1992). Cerebral metabolism and depression in patients with complex partial seizures. *Archives of Neurology*, **49**(6), 617–23.

Brown, F.W., Lewine, R.J., Hudgins, P.A. et al. (1992). White matter hyperintensity signals in psychiatric and nonpsychiatric subjects. *American Journal of Psychiatry*, **149**(5), 620–5.

Caine, E.D. & Shoulson, I. (1983). Psychiatric syndromes in Huntington's disease. *American Journal of Psychiatry*, **140**(6), 728–33.

Charles, H.C., Lazeyras, F., Krishnan, K.R. et al. (1994). Brain choline in depression: in vivo detection of potential pharmacodynamic effects of antidepressant therapy using hydrogen localized spectroscopy. *Progress in Neuropsychopharmacological Biology and Psychiatry*, **18**(7), 1121–7.

Coffey, C.E. (1996). Brain morphology in primary mood disorders: implications for electroconvulsive therapy. *Psychiatric Annals*, **26**(11), 713–16.

Coffey, C.E., Figiel, G.S., Djang, W.T. et al. (1988). Leukoencephalopathy in elderly depressed patients referred for ECT. *Biological Psychiatry*, **24**(2), 143–61.

Coffey, C.E., Figiel, G.S., Djang W.T. et al. (1989). White matter hyperintensity on magnetic resonance imaging: clinical and neuroanatomic correlates in the depressed elderly. *Journal of Neuropsychiatry and Clinical Neuroscience*, 1(2), 135–44.

Coffey, C.E., Figiel, G.S., Djang, W.T. et al. (1990). Subcortical hyperintensity on magnetic resonance imaging: a comparison of normal and depressed elderly subjects. *American Journal of Psychiatry*, **147**(2), 187–9.

Coffey, C.E., Wilkinson, W.E., Weiner, R.D. et al. (1993a). Quantitative cerebral anatomy in depression. A controlled magnetic resonance imaging study. *Archives of General Psychiatry*, **50**(1), 7–16.

Coffey, C.E., Wilkinson, W.E., Weiner, R.D. et al. (1993b). The dexamethasone suppression test and quantitative cerebral anatomy in depression. *Biological Psychiatry*, **33**(6), 442–9.

Coffman, J.A., Bornstein, R.A., Olson, S.C. et al. (1990). Cognitive impairment and cerebral structure by MRI in bipolar disorder. *Biological Psychiatry*, **27**(11), 1188–96.

Cohen, R.M., Gross, M., Nordahl, T.E. et al. (1992). Preliminary data on the metabolic brain pattern of patients with winter seasonal affective disorder. *Archives of General Psychiatry*, **49**(7), 545–52.

Cohen, B.M., Renshaw, P.F., Stoll, A.L. et al. (1995). Decreased brain choline uptake in older adults. An in vivo proton magnetic resonance spectroscopy study. *Journal of the American Medical Association*, **274**(11), 902–7.

Deicken, R.F., Reus, V.I., Manfredi, L. et al. (1991). MRI deep white matter hyperintensity in a psychiatric population. *Biological Psychiatry*, **29**(9), 918–22.

Deicken, R.F., Fein, G., Weiner, M.W. (1995a). Abnormal frontal lobe phosphorous metabolism in bipolar disorder. *American Journal of Psychiatry*, **152**(6), 915–18.

Deicken, R.F., Weiner, M.W., & Fein, G. (1995b). Decreased temporal lobe phosphomonoesters in bipolar disorder. *Journal of Affective Disorders*, **33**(3), 195–9.

Demopulos, C.D., Renshaw, P.F., Sachs, G.S. et al. (1996). Rapid cycling tended to be associated with low choline in the basal ganglia. 149th Annual Meeting of the American Psychiatric Association, New York, May 4–9, Abstract NR2, p. 74.

Devinsky, O., Morrell, M.J., & Vogt, B.A. (1995). Contributions of anterior cingulate cortex to behaviour. *Brain*, **118**(1), 279–306.

Dewan, M.J., Haldipur, C.V., Boucher, M. et al. (1988a). Is CT ventriculomegaly related to hypercortisolemia? *Acta Psychiatrica Scandinavica*, **77**(2), 230–1.

Dewan, M.J., Haldipur, C.V., Lane, E.E. et al. (1988b). Bipolar affective disorder. I. Comprehensive quantitative computed tomography. *Acta Psychiatrica Scandinavica*, **77**(6), 670–6.

D'haenen, H., Bossuyt, A., Mertens, J. et al. (1992). SPECT imaging of serotonin$_2$ receptors in depression. *Psychiatry Research*, **45**(4), 227–37.

Direkze, M., Bayliss, S.G., & Cutting, J.C. (1971). Primary tumours of the frontal lobe. *British Journal of Clinical Practice*, **25**(5), 207–13.

Dolan, R.J. & Friston, K.J. (1989). Positron emission tomography in psychiatric and neuropsychiatric disorders. *Seminars in Neurology*, **9**(4), 330–7.

Dolan, R.J., Calloway, S.P., & Mann, A.H. (1985). Cerebral ventricular size in depressed subjects. *Psychological Medicine*, **15**(4), 873–8.

Dolan, R.J., Bench, C.J., Liddle, P.F. et al. (1993). Dorsolateral prefrontal cortex dysfunction in the major psychoses; symptom or disease specificity? *Journal of Neurology, Neurosurgery and Psychiatry*, **56**(12), 1290–4.

Drevets, W.C., Videen, T.O., Price, J.L. et al. (1992). A functional anatomical study of unipolar depression. *Journal of Neuroscience*, **12**(9), 3628–41.

Dupont, R.M., Jernigan, T.L., Butters, N. et al. (1990). Subcortical abnormalities detected in bipolar affective disorder using magnetic resonance imaging. Clinical and neuropsychological significance. *Archives of General Psychiatry*, **47**(1), 55–9.

Dupont, R.M., Jernigan, T.L., Heindel, W. et al. (1995). Magnetic resonance imaging and mood disorders. Localization of white matter and other subcortical abnormalities. *Archives of General Psychiatry*, **52**(9), 747–55.

Ebert, D., Feistel. H., & Barocka, A. (1991). Effects of sleep deprivation on the limbic system and the frontal lobes in affective disorders: a study with Tc-99m-HMPAO SPECT. *Psychiatry Research*, **40**(4), 247–51.

Ebert, D., Feistel, H., Kaschka, W. et al. (1994). Single photon emission computerized tomography assessment of cerebral dopamine $D_2$ receptor blockade in depression before and after sleep deprivation – preliminary results. *Biological Psychiatry*, **35**(11), 880–5.

Elkis, H., Friedman, L., Wise, A. et al. (1995). Meta-analyses of studies of ventricular enlargement and cortical sulcal prominence in mood disorders. Comparisons with controls or patients with schizophrenia. *Archives of General Psychiatry*, **52**(9), 735–46.

Federoff, J.P., Starkstein, S.E., Forrester, A.W. et al. (1992). Depression in patients with acute traumatic brain injury. *American Journal of Psychiatry*, **149**(7), 918–23.

Figiel, G.S., Krishnan, K.R., Doraiswamy, P.M. et al. (1991a). Subcortical hyperintensities on brain magnetic resonance imaging: a comparison between late age onset and early onset elderly depressed subjects. *Neurobiology of Aging*, **12**(3), 245–7.

Figiel, G.S., Krishnan, K.R., Rao, V.P. et al. (1991b). Subcortical hyperintensities on brain magnetic resonance imaging: a comparison of normal and bipolar subjects. *Journal of Neuropsychiatry and Clinical Neuroscience*, **3**(1), 18–22.

Folstein, S.E. & Folstein, M.F. (1983). Psychiatric features of Huntington's disease: recent approaches and findings. *Psychiatric Development*, **1**(2), 193–205.

George, M.S., Ketter, T.A., Gill, D. et al. (1993). Blunted CBF with emotion recognition in depression. 146th Annual Meeting of the American Psychiatric Association, San Francisco, May 22–27, Abstract NR114.

George, M.S., Kellner, C.H., Bernstein, H. et al. (1994). A magnetic resonance imaging investigation into mood disorders in multiple sclerosis. *Journal of Nervous and Mental Diseases*, **182**(7), 410–12.

George, M.S., Ketter, T.A., Parekh, P.I. et al. (1995a). Brain activity during transient sadness and happiness in healthy women. *American Journal of Psychiatry*, **152**(3), 341–51.

George, M.S., Kimbrell, T., Parekh, P.I. et al. (1995b). Actively depressed subjects have difficulty inducing, and blunted limbic rCBF during, transient sadness. 148th Annual Meeting of the American Psychiatric Association, Miami, May 20–25, 1995. Abstract NR167. pp. 99–100.

George, M.S., Wassermann, E.M., Williams, W.A. et al. (1995c). Daily repetitive transcranial magnetic stimulation (rTMS) improves mood in depression. *Neuroreport*, **6**(14), 1853–6.

George, M.S., Ketter, T.A., Parekh, P.I. et al. (1995d). Blunted left cingulate activation in mood disorder subjects during a response interference task (the Stroop). *Journal of Neuropsychiatry and Clinical Neuroscience*, **9**(1), 55–63.

Goyer, P.F., Schulz, P.M., Semple, W.E. et al. (1992). Cerebral glucose metabolism in patients with summer seasonal affective disorder. *Neuropsychopharmacology*, **7**(3), 233–40.

Greenwald, B.S., Kramer-Ginsberg, E., Krishnan, R.R. et al. (1996). MRI signal hyperintensities in geriatric depression. *American Journal of Psychiatry*, **153**(9), 1212–15.

Gyulai, L., Wicklund, S.W., Greenstein, R. et al. (1991). Measurement of tissue lithium concentration by lithium magnetic resonance spectroscopy in patients with bipolar disorder. *Biological Psychiatry*, **29**(12), 1161–70.

Harvey, I., Persaud, R., Ron, M.A. et al. (1994). Volumetric MRI measurements in bipolars compared with schizophrenics and healthy controls. *Psychological Medicine*, **24**(3), 689–99.

Hauser, P. (1991). Magnetic resonance imaging in primary affective disorder. In *Brain Imaging in Affective Disorders*, ed. P. Hauser, pp. 25–53. Washington: American Psychiatric Press, Inc.

Hauser, P., Altshuler, L.L., Berrettini, W. et al. (1989). Temporal lobe measurement in primary affective disorder by magnetic resonance imaging. *Journal of Neuropsychiatry and Clinical Neuroscience*, **1**(2), 128–34.

Hauser, P., Dauphinais, I.D., Berrettini, W. et al. (1989). Corpus callosum dimensions measured by magnetic resonance imaging in bipolar affective disorder and schizophrenia. *Biological Psychiatry*, **26**(7), 659–68.

Hickie, I., Scott, E., Mitchell, P. et al. (1995). Subcortical hyperintensities on magnetic resonance imaging: clinical correlates and prognostic significance in patients with severe depression. *Biological Psychiatry*, **37**(3), 151–60.

Honer, W.G., Hurwitz, T., Li, D.K. et al. (1987). Temporal lobe involvement in multiple sclerosis patients with psychiatric disorders. *Archives of Neurology*, **44**(2), 187–90.

Horn, S. (1974). Some psychological factors in Parkinsonism. *Journal of Neurology, Neurosurgery and Psychiatry*, **37**(1), 27–31.

Hornig, M., Mozley, P.D., & Amsterdam, J.D. (1997). HMPAO SPECT brain imaging in treatment-resistant depression. *Progress in Neuropsychopharmacological Biology and Psychiatry*, **21**(7), 1097–114.

Husain, M.M., McDonald, W.M., Doraiswamy, P.M. et al. (1991). A magnetic resonance imaging study of putamen nuclei in major depression. *Psychiatry Research*, **40**(2), 95–9.

Jeste, D.V., Lohr, J.B., & Goodwin, F.K. (1988). Neuroanatomical studies of major affective disorders. A review and suggestions for further research. *British Journal of Psychiatry*, **153**, 444–59.

Johnstone, E.C., Owens, D.G., Crow, T.J. et al. (1989). Temporal lobe structure as determined by nuclear magnetic resonance in schizophrenia and bipolar affective disorder. *Journal of Neurology, Neurosurgery and Psychiatry*, **52**(6), 736–41.

Jorge, R.E., Robinson, R.G., Starkstein, S.E. et al. (1993). Secondary mania following traumatic brain injury. *American Journal of Psychiatry*, **150**(6), 916–21.

Kanakaratnam, G. & Direkze, M. (1976). Aspects of primary tumours of the frontal lobe. *British Journal of Clinical Practice*, **30**(11–12), 220–1.

Kanaya, T. & Yonekawa, M. (1990). Regional cerebral blood flow in depression. *Japanese Journal of Psychiatry and Neurology*, **44**(3), 571–6.

Kato, T., Shioiri, T., Inubushi, T. et al. (1993). Brain lithium concentrations measured with lithium-7 magnetic resonance spectroscopy in patients with affective disorders: relationship to erythrocyte and serum concentrations. *Biological Psychiatry*, **33**(3), 147–52.

Kato, T., Takahashi, S., Shioiri, T. et al. (1993). Alterations in brain phosphorous metabolism in bipolar disorder detected by in vivo $^{31}$P and $^7$Li magnetic resonance spectroscopy. *Journal of Affective Disorders*, **27**(1), 53–9.

Kato, T., Inubushi, T., & Takahashi, S. (1994). Relationship of lithium concentrations in the brain measured by lithium-7 magnetic resonance spectroscopy to treatment response in mania. *Journal of Clinical Psychopharmacology*, **14**(5), 330–5.

Kato, T., Shioiri, T., Murashita, J. et al. (1995). Lateralized abnormality of high energy phosphate metabolism in the frontal lobes of patients with bipolar disorder detected by phase-encoded $^{31}$P-MRS. *Psychological Medicine*, **25**(3), 557–66.

Kato, T., Hamakawa, H., Shioiri, T. et al. (1996). Choline-containing compounds detected by proton magnetic resonance spectroscopy in the basal ganglia in bipolar disorder. *Journal of Psychiatry and Neuroscience*, **21**(4), 248–54.

Kellner, C.H., Rubinow, D.R., Gold, P.W. et al. (1983). Relationship of cortisol hypersecretion to brain CT scan alterations in depressed patients. *Psychiatry Research*, **8**(3), 191–7.

Kennedy, S.H., Vaccarino, F.J., Houle, S. et al. (1996). Effects of acute and chronic paroxetine on regional brain metabolism in depression. 149th Annual Meeting of the American Psychiatric Association, New York, May 4–9. Abstract NR657, p. 250.

Keshavan, M.S., Pettegrew, J.W., & Panchalingam, K.S. (1992). Membrane phospholipids and lithium response in schizophrenia: a $^{31}$P-MRS study. Abstract VIII.B.1. *Schizophrenia Research*, **6**, 134.

Keshavan, M.S., Mulsant, B.H., Sweet, R.A. et al. (1996). MRI changes in schizophrenia in late life: a preliminary controlled study. *Psychiatry Research*, **60**(2–3), 117–23.

Ketter, T.A., Andreason, P.J., George, M.S. et al. (1993). Blunted CBF response to procaine in mood disorders. 146th Annual Meeting of the American Psychiatric Association, San Francisco, May 22–27. Abstract NR297.

Ketter, T.A., George, M.S., Andreason, P.J. et al. (1994). rCMRglu in unipolar versus bipolar depression. 147th Annual Meeting of the American Psychiatric Association, Philadelphia, May 21–26. Abstract NR444.

Ketter, T.A., Andreason, P.J., George, M.S. et al. (1996). Anterior paralimbic mediation of procaine-induced emotional and psychosensory experiences. *Archives of General Psychiatry*, **53**(1), 59–69.

Ketter, T.A., Kimbrell, T.A., George, M.S. et al. (1999). Baseline cerebral hypermetabolism associated with carbamazepine response, and hypometabolism with nimodipine response in mood disorders. *Biological Psychiatry*, **46**(10), 1364–74.

Kimbrell, T., Ketter, T.A., George, M.S. et al. (1996). Anterior paralimbic hypometabolism in patients with unipolar depression in remission. 149th Annual Meeting of the American Psychiatric Association, New York, May 4–9. Abstract NR462, p. 196.

Kimbrell, T.A., George, M.S., Parekh, P.I. et al. (1999). Regional brain activity during transient self-induced anxiety and anger in healthy adults. *Biological Psychiatry*, **46**(4), 454–65.

Kishimoto, H., Takazu, O., Ohno, S. et al. (1987). $^{11}$C-glucose metabolism in manic and depressed patients. *Psychiatry Research*, **22**(1), 81–8.

Krishnan, K.R., Goli, V., Ellinwood, E.H. et al. (1988). Leukoencephalopathy in patients diagnosed as major depressive. *Biological Psychiatry*, **23**(5), 519–22.

Krishnan, K.R., Doraiswamy, P.M., Lurie, S.N. et al. (1991). Pituitary size in depression. *Journal of Endocrinology and Metabolism*, **72**(2), 256–9.

Krishnan, K.R., McDonald, W.M., Escalona, P.R. et al. (1992). Magnetic resonance imaging of the caudate nuclei in depression. Preliminary observations. *Archives of General Psychiatry*, **49**(7), 553–7.

Krishnan, K.R., McDonald, W.M., Doraiswamy, P.M. et al. (1993). Neuroanatomical substrates of depression in the elderly. *European Archives of Psychiatry and Clinical Neuroscience*, **243**(1), 41–6.

Kumar, A., Mozley, D., Dunham, C. et al. (1991). Semiquantitative I-123 IMP SPECT studies in late onset depression before and after treatment. *International Journal of Geriatric Psychiatry*, **6**, 775–7.

Kumar, A., Miller, D.S., Cowell, P. et al. (1996a). Focal anatomic substrates in late-life depression. 149th Annual Meeting of the American Psychiatric Association, New York, May 4–9. Abstract NR435, p. 188.

Kumar, A., Miller, D.S., Schweizer, E.E. et al. (1996b). Focal neuroanatomic correlates of minor depression. 149th Annual Meeting of the American Psychiatric Association, New York, May 4–9. Abstract NR655, p. 249.

Lammers, C.S., Doraiswamy, P.M., Husain, M.M. et al. (1991). MRI of corpus callosum and septum pellucidum in depression [letter]. *Biological Psychiatry*, **29**(3), 300–1.

Lesser, I.M., Miller, B.L., Boone, K.B. et al. (1991). Brain injury and cognitive function in late-onset psychotic depression. *Journal of Neuropsychiatry and Clinical Neuroscience*, **3**, 33–40.

Little, J.T., Ketter, T.A., Kimbrell, T.A. et al. (1996). Venlafaxine or bupropion responders but not nonresponders show baseline prefrontal and paralimbic hypometabolism compared with controls. *Psychopharmacology Bulletin*, **32**(4), 629–35.

Little, J.T., Ketter, T.A., Kimbrell, T.A. et al. (1997). Anterior paralimbic blood flow decreased after venlafaxine response. 52nd Annual Meeting of the Society of Biological Psychiatry, San Diego, May 14–18. Abstract 270. *Biological Psychiatry*, **41**(Suppl. 7S), 79S–80S.

Luchins, D.J. & Meltzer, H.Y. (1983). Ventricular size and psychosis in affective disorder. *Biological Psychiatry*, **18**, 1197–8.

Luchins, D.J., Lewine, R.R., & Meltzer, H.Y. (1984). Lateral ventricular size, psychopathology, and medication response in the psychoses. *Biological Psychiatry*, **19**(1), 29–44.

McGuire, P.K., Bench, C.J., Frith, C.D. et al. (1994). Functional anatomy of obsessive-compulsive phenomena. *British Journal of Psychiatry*, **164**(4), 459–68.

MacLean, P.D. (1952). Some psychiatric implications of physiological studies on the frontotemporal portion of limbic system (visceral brain). *Electroencephalography and Clinical Neurophysiology*, **4**, 407–18.

MacLean, P.D. (1990). *The Triune Brain in Evolution. Role in Paleocerebral Functions*. New York: Plenum Press.

MacLean, P. & Delgado, J.M.R. (1953). Electrical and chemical stimulation of frontopolar portion of limbic system in the waking animal. *Electroencephalogical and Clinical Neuro-*

*physiology*, **5**, 91–100.

Mann, J.J., Malone, K.M., Diehl, D.J. et al. (1996). Demonstration in vivo of reduced serotonin responsivity in the brain of untreated depressed patients. *American Journal of Psychiatry*, **153**(2), 174–82.

Marangell, L.B., Ketter, T.A., George, M.S. et al. (1997). Inverse relationship of peripheral thyrotropin-stimulating hormone levels to brain activity in mood disorders. *American Journal of Psychiatry*, **154**(2), 224–30.

Mayberg, H.S., Starkstein, S.E., Sadzot, B. et al. (1990). Selective hypometabolism in the inferior frontal lobe in depressed patients with Parkinson's disease. *Annals of Neurology*, **28**(1), 57–64.

Mayberg, H.S., Dannals, R.F., Ross, C.A. et al. (1991a). Mu opiate receptor binding is increased in depressed patients measured by PET and C-11-carfentanil. 30th Annual Meeting of the American College of Neuropsychopharmacology, San Juan, Puerto Rico, December 9–13. Abstract. p. 61.

Mayberg, H.S., Starkstein, S.E., Morris, P.L. et al. (1991b). Remote cortical hypometabolism following focal basal ganglia injury: relationship to secondary changes in mood. Abstract 540S. *Neurology*, **41**(Suppl. 1), 266.

Mayberg, H.S., Starkstein, S.E., Peyser, C.E. et al. (1992). Paralimbic frontal lobe hypometabolism in depression associated with Huntington's disease. *Neurology*, **42**(9), 1791–7.

Mendez, M.F., Adams, N.L., & Lewandowski, K.S. (1989). Neurobehavioral changes associated with caudate lesions. *Neurology*, **39**, 349–54.

Mesulam, M.M. (1985). Patterns in behavioral neuroanatomy: association areas, the limbic system, and hemispheric specialization. In *Principles of Behavioral Neurology*, ed. M.M. Mesulam, pp. 1–70. Philadelphia: F.A. Davis Company.

Mesulam, M.M. (1998). Neural substrates of behavior: the effects of brain lesions upon mental state. In *The New Harvard Guide to Psychiatry*, ed. A.M. Nicholi, pp. 91–128. Cambridge, MA: Harvard University Press.

Migliorelli, R., Starkstein, S.E., Teson, A. et al. (1993). SPECT findings in patients with primary mania. *Journal of Neuropsychiatry and Clinical Neuroscience*, **5**(4), 379–83.

Miller, B.L., Lesser, I.M., Boone, K. et al. (1989). Brain white-matter lesions and psychosis. *British Journal of Psychiatry*, **155**, 73–8.

Mindham, R.H. (1970). Psychiatric symptoms in Parkinsonism. *Journal of Neurology, Neurosurgery and Psychiatry*, **33**(2), 188–91.

Moller, A., Wiedemann, G., Rohde, U. et al. (1994). Correlates of cognitive impairment and depressive mood disorder in multiple sclerosis. *Acta Psychiatrica Scandinavica*, **89**(2), 117–21.

Nasrallah, H.A., McCalley-Whitters, M., & Pfohl, B. (1984). Clinical significance of large cerebral ventricles in manic males. *Psychiatry Research*, **13**(2), 151–6.

Nasrallah, H.A., Coffman, J.A., & Olson, S.C. (1989). Structural brain-imaging findings in affective disorders: an overview. *Journal of Neuropsychiatry and Clinical Neuroscience*, **1**(1), 21–6.

Nobler, M.S., Sackeim, H.A., Prohovnik, I. et al. (1994). Regional cerebral blood flow in mood disorders, III. Treatment and clinical response. *Archives of General Psychiatry*, **51**(11), 884–97.

O'Brien, J.T. (1997). The 'glucocorticoid cascade' hypothesis in man. *British Journal of Psychiatry*, **170**, 199–201.

O'Brien, J., Desmond, P., Ames, D. et al. (1996). A magnetic resonance imaging study of white matter lesions in depression and Alzheimer's disease. *British Journal of Psychiatry*, **168**(4), 477–85.

O'Connell, R.A., Van Heertum, R.L., Billick, S.B. et al. (1989). Single photon emission computed tomography (SPECT) with [123I]IMP in the differential diagnosis of psychiatric disorders. *Journal of Neuropsychiatry and Clinical Neuroscience*, **1**(2), 145–53.

O'Connell, R.A., Van Heertum, R.L., Luck, D. et al. (1995). Single-photon emission computed tomography of the brain in acute mania and schizophrenia. *Journal of Neuroimaging*, **5**(2), 101–4.

Papez, J.W. (1937). A proposed mechanism of emotion. *Archives of Neurological Psychiatry*, **38**, 725–43.

Pascual-Leone, A. & Pallardó, F. (1996). Beneficial effects of repetitive transcranial magnetic stimulation (rTMS) in depression are associated with normalization of prefrontal hypometabolism. 8th Congress of the Association of European Psychiatrists, London, July 7–12. Abstract. *European Psychiatry*, **11**(Suppl. 4), 354s.

Pearlson, G.D., Garbacz, D.J., Tompkins, R.H. et al. (1984). Clinical correlates of lateral ventricular enlargement in bipolar affective disorder. *American Journal of Psychiatry*, **141**(2), 253–6.

Pearlson, G.D., Wong, D.F., Tune, L.E. et al. (1995). In vivo $D_2$ dopamine receptor density in psychotic and nonpsychotic patients with bipolar disorder. *Archives of General Psychiatry*, **52**(6), 471–7.

Post, R.M. (1992). The transduction of psychosocial stress into the neurobiology of recurrent affective illness. *American Journal of Psychiatry*, **149**, 999–1010.

Post, R.M., DeLisi, L.E., Holcomb, H.H. et al. (1987). Glucose utilization in the temporal cortex of affectively ill patients: positron emission tomography. *Biological Psychiatry*, **22**(5), 545–53.

Raine, A., Lencz, T., Reynolds, G. et al. (1992). An evaluation of structural and functional prefrontal deficits in schizophrenia: MRI and neuropsychological measures. *Psychiatry Research*, **45**, 123–37.

Rao, V.P., Krishnan, K.R., Goli, V. et al. (1989). Neuroanatomical changes and hypothalamo–pituitary–adrenal axis abnormalities. *Biological Psychiatry*, **26**(7), 729–32.

Renshaw, P.F., Johnson, K.A., Worth, J.L. et al. (1992). New onset depression in patients with AIDS dementia complex (ADC) is associated with frontal lobe perfusion defects on HMPAO-SPECT scan. 31st Annual Meeting of the American College of Neuropsychopharmacology, San Juan, Puerto Rico, December 14–18. Abstract, p. 94.

Renshaw, P.F., Stoll, A.L., Sachs, G.S. et al. (1996). A choline deficit hypothesis for the progression of bipolar disorder with age. 35th Annual Meeting of the American College of Neuropsychopharmacology, San Juan, Puerto Rico, December 9–13. Abstract, p. 85.

Ring, H.A., Bench, C.J., Trimble, M.R. et al. (1994). Depression in Parkinson's disease. A positron emission study. *British Journal of Psychiatry*, **165**(3), 333–9.

Risch, S.C., Lewine, R.J., Kalin, N.H. et al. (1992). Limbic–hypothalamic–pituitary–adrenal axis activity and ventricular-to-brain ratio studies in affective illness and schizophrenia. *Neuropsychopharmacology*, **6**(2), 95–100.

Rothschild, A.J., Benes, F., Hebben, N. et al. (1989). Relationships between brain CT scan findings and cortisol in psychotic and nonpsychotic depressed patients. *Biological Psychiatry*, 26(6), 565–75.

Rubin, E., Sackeim, H.A., Prohovnik, I. et al. (1995). Regional cerebral blood flow in mood disorders: IV. Comparison of mania and depression. *Psychiatry Research*, 61(1), 1–10.

Sackeim, H.A. (1996). Physiological perturbations in late-life depression: implications for neuronal circuitry and effects of treatment. 35th Annual Meeting of the American College of Neuropsychopharmacology, San Juan, Puerto Rico, December 9–13. Abstract, p. 73.

Sackeim, H.A. & Prohovnik, I. (1993). Brain imaging studies of depressive disorders. In *The Biology of Depressive Disorders*, ed. J.J. Mann & D.J. Kupfer, pp. 205–58. New York: Plenum.

Salloway, S., Malloy, P., Kohn, R. et al. (1996). MRI and neuropsychological differences in early- and late-life-onset geriatric depression. *Neurology*, 46(6), 1567–74.

Schlegel, S. (1991). Computed tomography in affective disorders. In *Brain Imaging in Affective Disorders*, ed. P. Hauser, pp. 1–24. Washington, DC: American Psychiatric Press.

Schlegel, S. & Kretzschmar, K. (1987). Computed tomography in affective disorders. Part I: ventricular and sulcal measurements. *Biological Psychiatry*, 22(1), 4–14.

Schlegel, S., Aldenhoff, J.B., Eissner, D. et al. (1989a). Regional cerebral blood flow in depression: associations with psychopathology. *Journal of Affective Disorders*, 17(3), 211–18.

Schlegel, S., Frommberger, U., & Buller, R. (1989b). Computerized tomography (CT) in affective disorders: relationship with psychopathology. *Psychiatry Research*, 29(3), 271–2.

Schlegel, S., von Bardeleben, U., Wiedemann, K. et al. (1989c). Computerized brain tomography measures compared with spontaneous and suppressed plasma cortisol levels in major depression. *Psychoneuroendocrinology*, 14(3), 209–16.

Schmidt, M.E., Henry, M., Matochik, J.A. et al. (1996). The effects of ECT on cerebral glucose metabolism. 149th Annual Meeting of the American Psychiatric Association, New York, May 4–9. Abstract NR474, p. 199.

Schwartz, J.M., Baxter, L.R. Jr, Mazziotta, J.C. et al. (1987). The differential diagnosis of depression. Relevance of positron emission tomography studies of cerebral glucose metabolism to the bipolar–unipolar dichotomy. *Journal of the American Medical Association*, 258(10), 1368–74.

Shah, S.A., Doraiswamy, P.M., Husain, M.M. et al. (1992). Posterior fossa abnormalities in major depression: a controlled magnetic resonance imaging study. *Acta Psychiatrica Scandinavica*, 85(6), 474–9.

Sharma, R., Venkatasubramanian, P.N., Barany, M. et al. (1992). Proton magnetic resonance spectroscopy of the brain in schizophrenic and affective patients. *Schizophrenia Research*, 8(1), 43–9.

Sheline, Y.I., Wang, P.W., Gado, M.H. et al. (1996). Hippocampal atrophy in recurrent major depression. *Proceedings of the National Academy of Sciences, USA*, 93(9), 3908–13.

Standish-Barry, H.M., Hale, A.S., Honig, A. et al. (1985). Ventricular size, the dexamethasone suppression test and outcome of severe endogenous depression following psychosurgery. *Acta Psychiatrica Scandinavica*, 72(2), 166–71.

Stanley, J.A., Drost, D.J., Williamson, P.C. et al. (1995). In vivo proton MRS study of glutamate and schizophrenia. In *NMR Spectroscopy in Psychiatric Brain Disorders*, ed. H.A. Nasrallah & J.W. Pettegrew, pp. 21–44. Washington: American Psychiatric Press, Inc.

Starkstein, S.E. & Robinson, R.G. (1989). Affective disorders and cerebrovascular disease. *British Journal of Psychiatry*, **154**, 170–82.

Starkstein, S.E. & Mayberg, H.S., Berthier, M.L. et al. (1990). Mania after brain injury: neuroradiological and metabolic findings. *Annals of Neurology*, **27**(6), 652–9.

Steingard, R.J., Renshaw, P.F., Yurgelun-Todd, D. et al. (1996). Structural abnormalities in brain magnetic resonance images of depressed children. *Journal of American Academy of Child and Adolescent Psychiatry*, **35**(3), 307–11.

Stern, R.A. & Bachmann, D.L. (1991). Depressive symptoms following stroke. *American Journal of Psychiatry*, **148**, 351–6.

Stoll, A.L., Sachs, G.S., Cohen, B.M. et al. (1996). Choline in the treatment of rapid-cycling bipolar disorder: clinical and neurochemical findings in lithium-treated patients. *Biological Psychiatry*, **40**(5), 382–8.

Strakowski, S.M., Wilson, D.R., Tohen, M. et al. (1993). Structural brain abnormalities in first-episode mania. *Biological Psychiatry*, **33**(8–9), 602–9.

Suhara, T., Nakayama, K., Inoue, O. et al. (1992). $D_1$ dopamine receptor binding in mood disorders measured by positron emission tomography. *Psychopharmacology*, **106**(1), 14–18.

Swayze, V.W. 2nd, Andreasen, N.C., Alliger, R.J. et al. (1990). Structural brain abnormalities in bipolar affective disorder. Ventricular enlargement and focal signal hyperintensities. *Archives of General Psychiatry*, **47**(11), 1054–9.

Swayze, V.W. 2nd, Andreasen, N.C., Alliger R.J. et al. (1992). Subcortical and temporal structures in affective disorder and schizophrenia: a magnetic resonance imaging study. *Biological Psychiatry*, **31**(3), 221–40.

Tanaka, Y., Hazama, H., Fukuhara, T. et al. (1982). Computerized tomography of the brain in manic-depressive patients – a controlled study. *Folia Psychiatrica Neurologica Japan*, **36**, 137–43.

Targum, S.D., Rosen, L.N., DeLisi, L.E. et al. (1983). Cerebral ventricular size in major depressive disorder: association with delusional symptoms. *Biological Psychiatry*, **18**(3), 329–36.

Trivedi, M.H., Blackburn, T., Lewis, S. et al. (1995). Effects of amphetamine in major depressive disorder using functional MRI. 50th Annual Meeting of the Society of Biological Psychiatry, Miami, May 17–20, 1995. Abstract 228. *Biological Psychiatry*, **37**(9), 657.

Van den Bossche, B., Maes, M., Brussaard, C. et al. (1991). Computed tomography of the brain in unipolar depression. *Journal of Affective Disorders*, **21**(1), 67–74.

Vita, A., Sacchetti, E., & Cazzullo, C.L. (1988). A CT follow-up study of cerebral ventricular size in schizophrenia and major affective disorder. *Schizophrenia Research*, **1**, 165–6.

Vogt, B.A., Finch, D.M., & Olson, C.R. (1992). Functional heterogeneity in cingulate cortex: the anterior executive and posterior evaluative regions. *Cerebral Cortex*, **2**(6), 435–43.

Volkow, N.D., Fowler, J.S., Hitzemann, R. et al. (1991). Abnormal dopamine brain activity in cocaine abusers. 30th Annual Meeting of the American College of Neuropsychopharmacology, San Juan, Puerto Rico, December 9–13. Abstract, p. 30.

Woods, B.T., Yurgelun-Todd, D., Benes, F.M. et al. (1990). Progressive ventricular enlargement in schizophrenia: comparison to bipolar affective disorder and correlation with clinical course. *Biological Psychiatry*, **27**(3), 341–52.

Wu, J.C., Gillin, J.C., Buchsbaum, M.S. et al. (1992). Effect of sleep deprivation on brain metabolism of depressed patients. *American Journal of Psychiatry*, **149**(4), 538–43.

Wu, J.C., Buchsbaum, M.S., Johnson, J.C. et al. (1993). Magnetic resonance and positron emission tomography imaging of the corpus callosum: size, shape and metabolic rate in unipolar depression. *Journal of Affective Disorders*, **28**(1), 15–25.

Yakolev, P.I., Locke, S., & Angevine, J.B. Jr (1966). The limbus of the cerebral hemisphere, limbic nuclei of the thalamus, and the cingulum bundle. In *The Thalamus*, ed. D.P. Purpura & M.D. Yahr, pp. 77–97. New York: Columbia University Press.

Yates, W.R., Jacoby, C.G., & Andreasen, N.C. (1987). Cerebellar atrophy in schizophrenia and affective disorder. *American Journal of Psychiatry*, **144**(4), 465–7.

Yazici, K.M., Kapucu, O., Erbas, B. et al. (1992). Assessment of changes in regional cerebral blood flow in patients with major depression using the $^{99m}$Tc-HMPAO single photon emission tomography method. *European Journal of Nuclear Medicine*, **19**(12), 1038–43.

# 7

# Immunologic factors in treatment-resistant depression

Anna Sluzewska, Janusz Rybakowski, Mady Hornig,
and Jay D. Amsterdam

## Introduction

Nearly 30% of depressed patients fail to achieve an adequate response to psycho-pharmacological treatment and at least 60% fail to achieve complete remission from their major depressive episode (MDE). Thus, the majority of depressed patients suffer from some degree of treatment-resistant depression (TRD) (Fawcett, 1994; O'Reardon & Amsterdam, 1999). Despite advances in psychopharmacological treatment, the mortality and morbidity of this disorder make depression a major public health problem in most countries.

The biological basis of TRD is still unclear. However, several lines of research have suggested the possibility of alterations in central stress-induced neuroendocrine and immunoendocrine compensatory mechanisms. These appear to result in a variety of hormonal and immunologic 'markers' in TRD. The study of these indices may enhance our understanding of why some patients do not respond to apparently adequate antidepressant treatment, and may help identify which therapies might be successful for particular patients. Both clinical and experimental studies indicate that the susceptibility to MDE reflects an interplay between environmental and genetic factors.

The immune system may be viewed as a sensory organ that recognizes physical and emotional stress, and relays this information to the central nervous system (CNS) and endocrine system via immunoendocrine protein messengers or cytokines. There is compelling experimental evidence of an intimate interaction between the CNS, endocrine and immune system, and putative links between these systems have been recognized. The dysregulations in the central stress response in patients with MDE could potentially reflect a generalized stress adaptation response that has escaped its normal counter-regulatory restraint mechanisms (Chrousos & Gold, 1992). In this model, the central stress mechanism has become excessively activated, continually responding to many distinct circadian, neurosensory, blood-borne and limbic–hypothalamic signals. These signals include cytokines produced by immune-mediated inflammatory reactions such as tumor necrosis factor (TNF) α, interleukin-1 (IL-1) and interleukin-6 (IL-6) (Chrousos & Gold, 1992). Local activation of immunological and immune-accessory cells ensues, and cytokines, lipid-bound mediators of inflammation, and neuropeptides are generated (Paul & Seder, 1994). It is, therefore, not surprising that some patients with MDE report the onset of their depressive symptoms occurred after a protracted viral infection (Amsterdam et al., 1998); nor is it surprising that some antidepressant medications possess antiviral activity (Amsterdam, et al., 1998), or that antiinfective agents possess antidepressant activity (Amsterdam et al., 1994).

Central stress-induced events are generally clinically silent and handled effectively by the autonomic nervous system and immunoendocrine system. However, in a vulnerable host these stress-induced responses cause a more severe inflammatory with further activation of the central stress system, resulting in the onset of systemic affective symptoms and signs. Among the many mediators of the stress-induced inflammatory response, inflammatory cytokines, TNF α, IL-1α and β, and IL-6 are responsible for most of the hypothalamic–pituitary–adrenal (HPA) axis stimulation that is associated with immune/inflammatory reactions, with hypercortisolism being one of the most consistent findings in depression (Carroll et al., 1976; Amsterdam et al., 1989; Nemeroff, 1996). Substantial evidence from clinical studies indicates that the hypercortisolemia associated with major depression is due to hypersecretion of corticotropin-releasing hormone (CRH) (Holsboer et al., 1984; Amsterdam et al., 1989). Findings further suggest involvement of HPA axis hyperactivity in the pathogenesis of TRD (Amsterdam et al., 1994). Christiansen et al. (1989) found poor response to antidepressant treatment in MDE patients with high spontaneous cortisol levels. Others (McLeod, 1972; Amsterdam et al., 1983) observed poor response to tricyclic antidepressants in patients demonstrating excessive cortisol secretion after dexamethasone suppression (DST). Moreover, the findings of Murphy et al. (1991) and Amsterdam et al. (1994) suggest that steroid suppressive treatment may be useful in some TRD patients with persistent HPA axis abnormalities.

## Acute phase response (APR) in MDE

The status of the immune system in MDE has been extensively studied since the 1980s. There is increasing evidence that acute episodes of MDE may be accompanied by an activation of the immune system which results in the release of immune factors called an acute phase response (APR) (Maes et al., 1992b). The APR is one means by which the organism responds and adapts to a disturbance of its homeostasis through the influence of factors such as infection, tissue injury, neoplastic growth, or immunological disorders (Heinrich et al., 1990). In the addition to the systemic reaction of the immune, endocrine and metabolic axes, compensatory behavioral changes are also seen (Kushner & Mackiewicz, 1993). These behaviors are expressed as 'sickness' and characterized by psychomotor retardation, sleep disturbances, anorexia, anergy, and lethargy (Kent et al., 1992).

Several studies have found that some individuals with MDE can demonstrate alterations in plasma levels of several positive acute phase proteins (APPs) including haptoglobin (HP) (Maes et al., 1992a), α-1-acid glycoprotein (AGP) (Nemeroff et al., 1990; Kehoe et al., 1992; Joyce et al., 1992; Sluzewska & Rybakowski, 1993), α-1 antichymotrypsin (ACT) (Joyce et al., 1992; Sluzewska et al., 1995b), C-reactive protein (CRP) (Sluzewska & Rybakowski, 1993), and transferrin and albumin (Maes et al., 1992a; Song & Leonard, 1993). However, not all studies have demonstrated these findings (Hornig-Rohan et al., 1998; Hornig et al., 1999).

In particular (AGP) had been implicated in the patho-physiology of MDE as a result of its being an endogenous inhibitor of serotonin (5HT) reuptake and of $^3$H-imipramine binding sites (Abraham et al., 1987). AGP also functions as an important binding protein for plasma-bound antidepressants (Kremer et al., 1988), and as an inhibitor of platelet aggregation (Costello et al., 1979).

Specific alterations in the glycosylation of AGP can occur in many patho-physiological states (Turner, 1992). These alternations in AGP glycosylation are due to variations in the structure of the oligosaccharides present at a given molecular site and have been referred to as 'microheterogeneity.' Shifts in glyco-forms can accompany changes in serum concentrations of AGP, but are independent of AGP synthesis rate. Different glycoforms of serum AGP have varied immunoregulatory effects. Con-A unreactive variants show significant (50–75%) inhibition of thymocyte proliferation (Pos et al., 1990), and are also more effective in inducing release of IL-1 inhibitor (Durand, 1989). Furthermore, these AGP glycoform variants are also involved in chemotaxis and oxidative metabolism and decrease neutrophils (Vasson et al., 1994). Changes in serum concentration of AGP result primarily from the effects of inflammatory cytokines and humoral factors on its hepatic biosynthesis (Kushner & Mackiewicz, 1993). Changes in the proportions of AGP glycoforms originate in the liver following modifications in glycosylation mechanisms which are mediated by cytokines (IL-6, IL-1, TNF and interferon) and by glucocorticoids (Van Dijk et al., 1994).

We have observed several altered patterns of AGP microheterogeneity in 75% of patients with MDE (Sluzewska et al., 1996a). Type I alterations in AGP micro-heterogeneity in MDE are similar to those seen in acute inflammatory states. They consist of elevated AGP levels, high values of AGP-RC, and reactivity to Con-A. Such patterns were observed in one-third of MDE patients. Patients having a type I pattern had longer episode duration and were treatment-resistant to pharmacotherapy.

The pattern of type II changes in AGP glycosylation which include elevated levels of AGP, low levels of AGP-RC and no reactivity to Con-A, are similar to those seen in chronic inflammatory states. This pattern was generally observed in patients with shorter duration of MDE who did not have TRD.

## Acute phase proteins (APP) and TRD

We have studied three separate positive APPs in 201 patients with MDE. Patients were recruited from the Departments of Psychiatry in Bydgoszcz ($n=60$), Poznan ($n=81$) and Philadelphia ($n=60$). All patients met DSM-III-R criteria for MDE: 175 had recurrent unipolar MDE and 26 had bipolar MDE (Sluzewska et al., 1996a). Elevated levels of APPs were observed in 75% of patients. A micro-heterogeneity pattern showing type I glycosylation of AGP and ACT indicated the presence of a variant with high Con A reactivity and high AGP-RC and ACT-RC values in one-third of MDE patients. This pattern of glycosylation is generally observed in patients with burns, rheumatoid arthritis and lupus erythematosus (Pawłowski et al., 1989; Breborowicz & Mackiewicz, 1989). MDE patients with this glycosylation patterns demonstrated more severe stage 2 or 3 TRD (see Thase & Rush, 1995). These patients also demonstrated the longest illness duration ($12.6 \pm 5$ years) and episode duration ($11.6 \pm 5.3$ months). In contrast, non-TRD patients demonstrated a type II glycosylation pattern with significantly lower concentrations of CRP and low levels of Con-A reactivity, AGP-RC and ACT-RC. A similar pattern of APP glycosylation has also been observed in patients with chronic inflammation, hepatic cirrhosis and rheumatoid arthritis (Turner, 1992).

## Cytokines and TRD

In addition to the immune-inflammatory markers described above, there have been several studies examining the role of pro-inflammatory cytokin IL-6, soluble IL-6 receptor (sIL-6R), soluble IL-2 receptor (sIL-2R) and soluble transferrin receptor (sTfR) in MDE patients with and without TRD. Elevated concentrations of IL-6, sIL-6R, sIL-2R and sTfR have been reported during an acute MDE (Maes et al., 1995a; Sluzewska et al., 1995a, 1996b) and in patients remitted from MDE (Maes et al., 1995). Interaction of sIL-6R with IL-6 has the effect of intensifying its bioactivity (Bock et al., 1992). The product term sIL-6R × IL-6 may be computed in clinical studies as an index of the potentiation effect of plasma sIL-6R on IL-6. We observed a value of sIL-6R × IL-6 three times higher in MDE patients compared to healthy controls (Sluzewska et al., 1996b). In addition, we also found markedly elevated levels of IL-6, sIL-6R and sIL-6R × IL-6 in TRD vs. non-TRD patients (Sluzewska et al., 1995b). Moreover, a significant association was observed in TRD patients between the levels of AGP, ACT and IL-6 (Sluzewska et al., 1995b).

Shifts in plasma concentrations of cytokines, their soluble receptors, and of glucocorticoids during MDE may be involved in the regulation of AGP and ACT glycosylation. It appears that IL-6 may influence glycosylation of APPs (Van Dijk et al., 1994), while glucocorticoids may modulate the effects of cytokines on APP glycosylation. Van Dijk & Mackiewicz (1993) found that the magnitude and type of glycosylation were dependent on the composition and plasma level of interacting cytokines, and that these effects could be modulated by increased levels of glucocorticoids. Finally, Pos et al. (1988) demonstrated that elevated levels of glucocorticoids could result in a type I glycosylation pattern of AGP. An increased frequency of type I glycosylation pattern and elevated glucocorticoid appear to characterize patients with TRD (Amsterdam et al., 1994; Sluzewska et al. 1996a).

## Cytokines and HPA axis in TRD

Many studies have demonstrated an excessive hypothalamic–pituitary axis (HPA) activity in TRD (Christiansen et al., 1989; McLeod, 1972; Amsterdam et al., 1983, 1994). We administered the dexamethasone suppression test (DST) to 60 MDE inpatients and observed significantly higher levels of AGP in the DST cortisol non-suppressors (Sluzewska et al., 1995b). Thirty-eight percent of these patients had TRD. Morning plasma cortisol and AGP levels were significantly correlated and suggested an influence of glucocorticoids on AGP synthesis (Sluzewska & Rybakowski, 1993). We also observed a positive correlation between morning cortisol levels and concentration of IL-6, AGP and ACT in TRD patients (Sluzewska et al., 1996d). This observation supports studies by Navarra et al. (1991) and Tominga et al. (1991) who reported that IL-6 stimulates HPA axis activity by increasing production of corticotropin-releasing hormone (CRH), corticotropin (ACTH) and cortisol. These findings suggest that the alterations in the concentration and microheterogeneity pattern of AGP and ACT seen in patients TRD could be linked to both HPA axis disturbances and increased production of cytokines such as IL-6 and sIL-6R. Patients resistant to antidepressant therapy are more likely to demonstrate these abnormalities.

## Electrophoretic protein fraction in TRD

The acute phase response (APR) seen in MDE (Nemeroff et al., 1990; Maes et al. (1992a,b) is often accompanied by reduced levels of total serum protein (TSP) and changes in electrophoretically separated serum protein fractions. Several investigators have observed lower levels of serum albumin in MDE patients compared to normal controls (Joyce et al., 1992; Song et al., 1994; Maes et al., 1991, 1995b). This observation is supported by animal experiments using the olfactory bulbectomized rat model of depression. Song and Leonard (1994b) found lower levels of serum albumin and $\gamma$-globulin fractions. Acute phase proteins (APPs) migrate electrophoretically between albumin and $\gamma$-globulin fractions. APPs such as AGP, ACT, CRP migrate in $\alpha_1$ zone, while haptoglobin (Hp) and Cp migrate in the $\alpha_2$ zone. Fibrinogen and C3 migrate in $\beta$ zone, and immunoglobulins migrate in the $\gamma$ zone (Ritzmann & Daniels, 1976). This may partly explain why during the acute phase response (APR) there are alterations in TSP and in electrophoretically seperated protein fractions (Putnam 1984a,b).

Only a few studies have examined serum protein fractions in MDE. Song et al. (1994) reported increased levels of $\alpha_1$ and $\alpha_2$-globulin fractions. Similarly, Maes et al. (1995b) found increased levels of $\alpha_2$ and $\gamma$-globulin. More recently, Van Hunsel et al. (1996) reported lower levels of TSP, albumin, $\beta$- and $\gamma$-globulin in 37 MDE patients (of whom 29 had TRD). Additionally, the percentages of $\alpha_1$- and $\alpha_2$-globulin fractions were significantly higher in MDE and TRD patients compared to controls, while $\alpha_2$-globulin was lower in TRD vs. non-TRD patients.

We have also observed decreased levels of TSP and albumin, and elevated levels of $\alpha_1$, $\alpha_2$ and $\gamma$-globulin in 49 MDE patients compared to controls (Sluzewska et al., 1996d). Even higher percentages of $\alpha_1$ and $\gamma$-globulin were seen in 25 TRD patients compared to controls. Moreover, a positive correlations between $\alpha_1$-globulin and AGP, and between ACT and cortisol was observed, as well as a negative correlation between albumin and $\alpha_1$-, $\alpha_2$-, $\beta$-, $\gamma$-globulin and cortisol in TRD patients (Sluzewska et al., 1996d). There was a positive correlation between IL-6 and $\alpha_1$-globulin, and a negative correlation between IL-6 and albumin.

The finding of increased proportion of $\alpha_1$-, $\alpha_2$- and $\gamma$-globulin fractions, together with lower TSP and albumin levels, suggests the presence of elevated APPs migrating in the $\alpha_1$- and $\alpha_2$-immunoglobulins in the $\gamma$ electrophoretical zone. These observations support the hypothesis that MDE and, in particular, TRD is accompanied by an APR.

## Antibodies against serotonin (5HT) and gangliosides in TRD

The presence of antinuclear, antiphospholipid, anti-5HT and antihistone antibodies have been reported in MDE (Villemain, et al., 1988; Irwin et al., 1990; Maes et al., 1991; Schott et al., 1992). Some autoimmune disorders have been related to the induction of antihormone and antireceptor antibodies (Cohen, 1984). We observed antibodies against 5HT and gangliosides in patients with MDE (Sluzewska et al., 1996d). Antibodies against gangliosides have been shown to be cross-reactive with a portion of the 5HT receptor (Fishman, 1988). Antibody reactivity of IgG or IgM to 5HT (55%) or to gangliosides (50%) was observed in MDE patients. In most, the presence of antibodies to 5HT was associated with the presence of antibodies to gangliosides, of which 73% had TRD. Moreover, patients with antibodies to both 5HT and gangliosides also had higher levels of CRP, AGP and ACT, and had pattern of microheterogeneity characterized by higher AGP-RC (type I glycosylation), IL-6, and decreased levels of 5HT in comparison to normal controls (Sluzewska et al., 1996c).

As one of several proinflammatory cytokines, IL-6 may play a role in stimulating production of antibodies (Cavallo et al., 1994). Antinuclear and antiphospholipid antibodies have also been described in MDE (Maes et al., 1991). In addition, decreased levels of serum 5HT have been observed in TRD patients (Sluzewska et al., 1996c). The frequent co-occurrence of anti-5HT antibodies with anti-ganglioside antibodies, together with the observation that gangliosides are a component of some 5HT receptors (Fishman, 1988), suggests the possibility that ganglioside antibodies may also be directed against the 5HT receptor. The presence of APPs might further suggest that 5HT system disregulation may be related to the APR and to autoimmune pathogenesis in some MDE patients. The induction of anti-5HT and antiganglioside antibodies has been found to occur with viral infections and in response to stress and the production of cytokines such as IL-6 (Balkwill & Burke, 1989; Balkwill, 1993).

## Antibodies against viral agents

The role of the acute phase reaction (APR) in the pathogenesis of TRD is unclear. In animal experiments, the chronic stress model of depression is associated with signs of an APR, including elevated levels of AGP and Hp (Sluzewska et al., 1994a, 1996e). Various forms of psychological stress may induce the secretion of IL-6 in rodents (LeMay et al., 1990; Zhou et al., 1993), and it is possible that the central stress response of MDE could be related to and APR with increased IL-6 and other APPs in humans, especially those with TRD. In studies of transgenic mice overexpressing IL-6 in the CNS, there is evidence suggesting that IL-6 could be a potent pathogenic agent in neurodegenerative diseases and neuropsychiatric disease (Campbell & Chiang, 1995). Some investigators have hypothesized that, in humans, a viral-induced APR could occur in individuals genetically vulnerable to develop MDE. Several viral agents have been proposed as likely candidates including Herpes simplex virus (HSV) (Amsterdam et al., 1986, 1998), Epstein–Barr virus (Amsterdam et al., 1986) and Borna Disease (BD) virus (Amsterdam et al., 1985). Studies linking human affective disorders to specific viral agents have produced intriguing results (Kurstak 1987, 1991). For example, antibodies against HSV have been reported in some, but not all, studies of MDE patients (see

Amsterdam & Hernz, 1993). Similarly, an association between MDE and BD virus antibodies has been reported (Amsterdam et al., 1985; Fu et al., 1993). Persistent BD virus infection in experimental animals has been found to induce neuro-behavioral and cognitive changes suggestive of human bipolar disorder (see Amsterdam et al., 1985; Gosztonyi & Ludwig, 1995). This intriguing psychoneurovirologic model of MDE suggests that a multiplicity of factors (e.g. genetic, environmental, immunologic and endocrinologic) may contribute to the immune dysregulation seen in TRD.

## Clinical applications

### Lithium augmentation

Lithium carbonate has consistently been shown to potentiate the therapeutic effect of antidepressant drugs in TRD (de Montigny et al., 1981; Rybakowski & Mat-kowski, 1992; de Montigny, 1994; Katona et al., 1995). However, reliable pre-dictors of clinical outcome have been lacking. Lithium potentiation of antide-pressant activity has been linked to its effect on 5HT functions in TRD (see de Montigny, 1994).

In clinical studies of the effect of lithium on APPs in MDE, we have found that lithium may exert a 'normalizing' influence on the levels and microheterogeneity of APPs (Sluzewska et al., 1994b). This effect might be related to cytokine shifts induced by lithium therapy. In this regard, during short-term treatment with lithium, we observed a reduction of IL-6 levels and in sIL-6R $\times$ IL-6 (Sluzewska et al., 1995c). Moreover, lithium augmentation of an antidepressant drug in TRD produced a significant decrease in plasma levels of CRP, AGP, and in the glycosylation values of AGP and ACT. Seventy-five percent of these TRD patients exhibited a beneficial response to lithium potentiation after a 4-week trial. In contrast, non-responders to lithium potentiation differed in their immunological indices prior to lithium, with non-responders having higher values of reactivity coefficients (indicating an inflammatory immune pattern) (Sluzewska et al., 1997c).

These observations suggest that alterations in serum levels of APPs may have 'psychotropic' consequences. AGP is an endogenous inhibitor of platelet 5HT reuptake (Abraham et al., 1987) and may also functions as a binding protein of many antidepressants (Kremer et al., 1988). Thus, a reduction in AGP might stimulate 5HT transport and/or increase the amount of free, unbound antide-pressant drug crossing into the CNS. Our study indicates the presence of a difference in the pattern of APPs prior to lithium augmentation between respon-ders and non-responders in TRD. After 4 weeks of lithium therapy, non-respon-ders maintain higher values of AGP-RC and less of a reduction in AGP levels compared to the TRD responders. We have postulated that that altered APP microheterogeneity in TRD non-responders to lithium potentiation may be due to elevations of glucocorticoids in TRD. In this context, glucocorticoids can modulate cytokine production, thus altering the rate of synthesis and glycosylation of APPs. This suggests that some TRD patients with an immune disturbance may be candidates for treatment that modulate glucocorticoid levels (Amsterdam et al., 1994).

## Steroid suppression and acute phase proteins (APP)

In one chronic stress model of depression in rats which produces increased glucocorticoids, elevated levels of Hp and AGP were observed (Willner et al., 1992). After chronic treatment with ketoconazole (an inhibitor of glucocorticoid synthesis), Hp and AGP levels were reduced (Sluzewska et al., 1994a, 1996e). Studies of steroid suppression in patients with TRD have suggested that a reduction in steroid synthesis may have antidepressant effects (Amsterdam et al., 1994). Murphy et al. (1991) reported a robust efficacy of steroid suppression therapy with ketoconazole in 80% of TRD patients.

Similarly, Amsterdam et al. (1994) reported an overall response rate of 70% and a remission rate of 50% to ketoconazole therapy in six highly treatment-resistant, hypercortisolic, TRD patients. We have subsequently undertaken a preliminary study of serum APP levels in hypercorticolemic TRD patients who have received antidepressant ketoconazole therapy. Preliminary results have shown a decreased level of AGP, ACT and Hp following adjunctive ketoconazole therapy in several highly TRD patients (Sluzewska et al., unpublished data). The complex interrelationship within the psycho-neuro-immuno-endorine system, and its modulation by genetic and environmental (e.g. infectious) factors, suggests both a model for understanding the pathophysiology of TRD and potential mechanisms for the treatment of TRD.

## Conclusions

There is considerable evidence that MDE in general, and TRD in particular, may be accompanied by an immune-inflammatory response, as demonstrated by: (i) an acute phase response (APR); (ii) an increased production of cytokines such as IL-6; and, (iii) activation of lymphocytes (T cells). The role of such immune activation in the pathophysiology of MDE and TRD remains to be determined. Clinical strategies that modulate immune function might be explored in TRD, including treatment with steroid antagonists, protein blockers amd antibodies to IL-6 or sIL-1R. In this context, patients receiving anti-IL-6 antibody as a therapeutic adjuvant for TRD should show striking reductions in serum APP levels

(Klein et al., 1991). Recent antidepressant drug trials in MDE with several CNS peptide blockers that alter immunoendocrine function have been undertaken, and these studies suggest that the immunoendocrine laboratory findings since the 1980s will be the clinical treatment of the near future.

## Acknowledgments

This work was supported by grants KBN 502-3-326, 501-1-020 from Karol Marcinkowski University of Medical Sciences in Poznan, Poland, and by the Jack Warsaw Fund of the Depression Research Unit, University of Pennsylvania School of Medicine, Philadelphia, PA.

## REFERENCES

Abraham, K.I., Ieni, J.R., & Meyerson, L.R. (1987). Purification and properties of human plasma endogenous modulator for platelet tricyclic binding /serotonine transport complex. *Biochemica Biophysica Acta*, **923**, 8–21.

American Psychiatric Association (1994). *Diagnostic and Statistical Manual of Mental Disorders*. 4th edn. Washington, DC: American Psychiatric Association.

Amsterdam, J.D. & Hernz, W.H. (1993). Serum antibodies to herpes simplex virus types I and II in depressed patients and healthy controls. *Biological Psychiatry*, **34**, 417–20.

Amsterdam, J.D., Winokur, A., Bryant, S., Larkin, J., & Rickels, K. (1983). The dexamethasone suppression test as a predictor of antidepressant response. *American Journal of Psychiatry*, **80**, 43–5.

Amsterdam, J.D., Winokur, A., Dyson, W. et al. (1985). Borna disease virus: a possible etiologic factor in human affective disorders. *Archives of General Psychiatry*, **42**, 1093–6.

Amsterdam, J.D., Henle, W., Winokur, A., Wolwowitz, O., Pickar, D., & Paul, S.M. (1986). Serum antibodies to Epstein–Barr virus in patients with major depressive disorder. *American Journal of Psychiatry*, **143**, 1593–6.

Amsterdam, J.D., Maislin, G., Winokur, A., Phillips, J., Berwish, N., & Gold, P. (1989). The assessment of abnormalities in hormonal responsiveness at multiple levels of the hypothalamic–pituitary–adrenocortical axis in depressive illness. *Psychoneuroendocrinology*, **14**, 43–62.

Amsterdam, J.D., Rosenzweig, M., & Mozley, P.D. (1994). Assessment of adrenocortical activity in refractory depression: steroid suppression with ketoconazole. In *Refractory Depression: Current Strategies and Future Directions*, ed. W.A. Nolen, J. Zohar, S.P. Roose, & J.D. Amsterdam. Chichester, UK: John Wiley.

Amsterdam, J.D., Garcia-Espana, F., & Rybakowski, J. (1998). Rates of flu-like infections in patients with affective illness. *Journal of Affective Disorders*, **47**, 177–82.

Balkwill, F. (1993). Cytokines in health and disease. *Immunology Today*, **14**, 149–50.

Balkwill, F.R. & Burke, F. (1989). The cytokine network. *Immunology Today*, **10**, 299–303.

Bock, G.R., Marsh, J., & Widdows, K. (1992). In *Polyfunctional Cytokines: IL-6 and LIF. Ciba Foundation Symposium* 167. Chichester, UK: John Wiley.

Breborowicz, J. & Mackiewicz, A. (1989). Affinity electrophoresis for diagnosis of cancer and inflammatory conditions. *Electrophoresis*, **10**, 568–73.

Campbell, I.L. & Chiang, Ch-Sh. (1995). Cytokine involvement in central nervous system disease: Implications from transgenic mice. In *Stress; Basic Mechanisms and Clinical Implications. Annals NY Academy of Sciences*, **771**, 301–12.

Carroll, B.J., Curtis, G.C., Davies, B.M., Mendels, J., & Sugerman, A.A. (1976). Urinary free cortisol excretion in depression. *Psychological Medicine*, **6**, 43–50.

Cavallo, MG., Pozzilli, P., & Thorpe, R. (1994). Cytokines and autoimmunity. *Clinical and Experimental Immunology*, **96**, 1–7.

Christiansen, P., Lolk, A., & Gram, L.F. (1989). Cortisol and treatment of depression: predictive value of spontaneous and suppressed cortisol levels and course of spontaneous plasma cortisol. *Psychopharmacology*, **97**, 471–5.

Chrousos, G.P. & Gold, P.W. (1992) The concepts of stress and stress system disorders: overview of physical and behavioral homeostasis. *Journal of the American Medical Association*, **268**, 200.

Cohen, I.R. (1984). Autoimmunity: physiologic and pernicious. *Advances in Internal Medicine*, **29**, 147–65.

Costello, M., Field, B.A., & Gewurz, H. (1979). Inhibition of platelet aggregation by native and disialised alpha-1-acid glycoprotein. *Nature*, **281**, 677–81.

de Montigny, C. (1994). Lithium addition in refractory depression. In *Refractory Depression: Current Strategies and Future Directions*, ed. W. A. Nolen, J. Zohar, S. P. Roose, & J.D. Amsterdam, pp. 47–57. New York: Wiley.

de Montigny, C., Grunberg, F., Mayer, A., & Deschenes, J.P. (1981). Lithium induces rapid relief of depression in tricyclic antidepressant drug nonresponders. *British Journal of Psychiatry*, **138**, 252–6.

Durand, G. (1989). Glycan variations of human alpha-1-acid glycoprotein modulate the biology of macrophages. *Progress in Clinical Biological Research*, **300**, 247–52.

Fawcett, J. (1994). Progress in treatment-resistant and treatment-refractory depression: we still have a long way to go. *Psychiatric Annals*, **24**, 214–16.

Fishman, P.H. (1988). Gangliosides as cell surface receptors and transducers of biological signals. In *New Trends in Ganglioside Research: Neurochemical and Neuroregenerative Aspects*, ed. R.W. Ledeen, E.L. Hogan, G. Tettamanti, A.J. Yates, & R.R. Yu, pp. 183–217. Padova: Liviana Press.

Fu, Z.F., Amsterdam, J.D., Kao, M., Shankar, V., Koprowski, H., & Dietzschold, B. (1993). Detection of Borna disease virus-specific antibodies from patients with affective disorders by western immunoblot technique. *Journal of Affective Disorders*, **27**, 61–8.

Gosztonyi, G. & Ludwig, H. (1995). Borna disease – neuropathology and pathogenesis. In *Borna Disease. Current Topics in Microbiology and Immunology*, ed. H. Koprowski & W.I. Lipkin, Vol. 190, pp. 39–73.

Heinrich, P.C., Castell, J.V., & Andus, T. (1990). Review article: interleukin-6 and the acute phase response. *Biochemical Journal*, **265**, 621–36.

Holsboer, F., Girken, A., Stalia, G.K., & Muller, O.A. (1984). Blunted corticotropin and normal cortisol response to human corticotropin-releasing factor in depression. *New England Journal of Medicine*, **311**, 1127.

Hornig, M., Amsterdam, J., Camoun, A., & Goodman, D. (1999). Auto-antibodies in affective disorders. *Journal of Affective Disorders*, **55**, 29–37.

Hornig-Rohan, M., Goodman, D., Camoun, A., & Amsterdam, J. (1998). Positive and negative acute phase proteins in affective subtypes. *Journal of Affective Disorders*, **49**, 9–18.

Irwin, M., Patterson, T., Smith, T.L. et al. (1990). Reduction of immune function in life stress and depression. *Biological Psychiatry*, **27**, 22–30.

Joyce, P.R., Hawes, C.R., & Mulder, R.T. (1992). Elevated levels of acute phase plasma proteins in major depression. *Biological Psychiatry*, **32**, 1035–41.

Katona, C.L.E., Abou-Saleh, M.T., & Harrison, D.A. (1995). Placebo-controlled trial of lithium augmentation of fluoxetine and lofepramine. *British Journal of Psychiatry*, **166**, 80–6.

Kehoe, W., Kwentus, J., Sheffel, W., & Harralson, A. (1992). Increased alpha-1-acid glyco-protein in depression lowers free fraction of imipramine. *Biological Psychiatry*, **29**, 489–93.

Kent, S., Bluthe, R.M., Kelly, K.W., & Dantzer, R. (1992). Sickness behavior as a new target for drug development. *Trends in Pharmacological Sciences*, **13**, 24–8.

Klein, R., Richter, C., & Berg, P.A. (1991). Antibodies against central nervous system tissue (anti-CNS) detected by ELISA and western blotting: marker antibodies for neuropsychiatric manifestations in connective tissue diseases. *Autoimmunity*, **10**, 133–44.

Kremer, J.M.H., Wilting, J., & Janssen, L.H.M. (1988). Drug binding to human alpha-1-acid glycoprotein in health and disease. *Pharmacology Review*, **40**, 1–47.

Kurstak, E. (ed.) (1987). *Viruses, Immunity, and Mental Diseases.* New York: Plenum.

Kurstak, E. (ed.) (1991). *Psychiatry and Biological Factors.* New York: Plenum.

Kushner, I. & Mackiewicz, A. (1993). The acute phase response: an overview. In *Acute Phase Proteins. Molecular Biology, Biochemistry and Clinical Applications*, ed. A. Mackiewicz, I. Kushner, & H. Baumann, pp. 3–19. Boca Raton, FL: CRP Press.

Le May, L.G., Vander, A.J., & Kluger, M.J. (1990). The effect of psychological stress on plasma interleukin-6 activity in rats. *Physiology and Behavior*, **47**, 957–61.

McLeod, W.R. (1972). Poor response to antidepressants and dexamethasone nonsuppression. In *Depressive Illness: Some Research Studies*, ed. B. Davis, B.J. Carroll, & R.M. Mowbray, pp. 202–6. Springfield, IL: Thomas.

Maes, M., Bosmans, E., Suy, E., Vandervorst, C., Dejonckheere, C., & Raus, J. (1991). Antiphospholipid, antinuclear, Epstein–Barr and cytomegalovirus antibodies and soluble interleukin-2 receptor in depressive patients. *Journal of Affective Diseases*, **21**, 133–40.

Maes, M., Scharpe, S., Van Grootel, L. et al. (1992a). Higher alpha-1-antitrypsin, haptoglobin, cerurlplasmin and lower retinol protein plasma levels during depression. Further evidence for the existence of an inflammatory process during that illness. *Journal of Affective Diseases*, **24**, 183–92.

Maes, M., Scharpe, S., Bosmans, E. et al. (1992b). Disturbances in acute phase proteins during melancholia: additional evidence for presence of inflammatory process during that illness. *Progress in Neuropsychopharmacological and Biological Psychiatry*, **16**, 501–15.

Maes, M., Meltzer, H.Y., & Bosmans, E. (1995a). Increase plasma levels of interleukin-6, soluble interleukin-2 and transferrin receptors in major depression. *Journal of Affective Disorders*, **34**, 301–9.

Maes, M., Wautwers, A., Neels, H. et al. (1995b). Total serum protein and serum protein fractions in depression: relationships to depressive symptoms and glucocorticoid activity. *Journal of Affective Disorders*, **34**, 61–9.

Murphy, B.E.P., Dhar, V., Ghadirian, A.M., Chouinard, G., & Keller, R. (1991). Response to steroid suppression in major depression resistant to antidepressant therapy. *Journal Clinic of Psychopharmacology*, **2**, 121–5.

Navarra, P., Tsagarakis, S., Faria, M.S., Rees, L.H., Besser, G.M., & Grossman, A.B. (1991). Interleukin-1 and interleukin-6 stimulate the release of corticotropin-releasing hormone from rat hypothalamus in vitro via the elicosanoid cyclooxygenase pathway. *Endocrinology*, **128**, 37–44.

Nemeroff, C.B. (1996). The corticotropin-releasing factor (CRF) hypothesis of depression: new findings and new directions. *Molecular Psychiatry*, **4**, 336–42.

Nemeroff, C.B., Krisnam, R.R., Blazer, D.G., Knight, D.L., Benjamin, D. & Meyerson, I.R. (1990). Elevated plasma concentration of alpha-1-acid glycoprotein, a putative endogenous inhibitor of tritiated imipramine binding site in depressed patients. *Archives of General Psychiatry*, **47**, 337–40.

O'Reardon, J. & Amsterdam, J. (1999). Mechanisms and management of treatment-resistant affective disorders. In *Pharmacotherapy of Mood and Cognition*, ed. S. Montgomery & U. Halbreich. Washington, DC: American Psychiatric Press. 295ff.

Paul, W.E. & Seder, R.A. (1994). Lymphocyte responses and cytokines. *Cell*, **76**, 241–51.

Pawłowski, P., Mackiewicz, S., & Mackiewicz, A. (1989). Microheterogeneity of alpha-1-acid glycoprotein in detection of intercurrent infection in rheumatoid arthritis. *Arthritis and Rheumatology*, **32**, 347–51.

Pos, O., Van Dijk, W., Ladiges, N., Sala, M., Van Tiel, D., & Boers, W. (1988). Glycosylation of four acute-phase glycoproteins secreted by rat liver cells in vivo and in vitro. Effects of inflammation and dexamethasone. *European Journal of Cell Biology*, **46**, 121–8.

Pos, O., Van der Stelt, M.E., & Wolbik, G.J. (1990). Changes in the serum concentration and glycosylation of human alpha-1-acid glycoprotein and alpha-1-protease inhibitor in severely burned patients: relation to interleukine-6 levels. *Clinical and Experimental Immunology*, **82**, 579–82.

Putnam, F.W. (1984a). Progress in plasma proteins. In *The Plasma Proteins: Structure, Function and Genetic Control*. 2nd edn, pp. 2–44. Orlando: Academic Press.

Putnam, F.W. (1984b). Alpha, beta, gamma, omega – the structure of plasma proteins. In *The Plasma Proteins: Structure, Function and Genetic Control*. 2nd edn, pp. 46–166. Orlando, FL: Academic Press.

Ritzmann, S.E. & Daniels, J.C. (1976). Serum protein electrophoresis and total serum proteins. In *Serum Protein Abnormalities: Diagnostic and Clinical Aspects*, pp. 3–25. Boston, MA: Little, Brown and Company.

Rybakowski, J.K. & Matkowski, K. (1992). Adding lithium to antidepressant therapy: factors related to therapeutic potentiation. *European Neuropsychopharmacology*, **2**, 161–5.

Schott, K., Batra, A., Klein, R., Bartels, M., Koch, W., & Berg, P.A. (1992). Antibodies against serotonin and gangliosides in schizophrenia and major depressive disorder. *European Psychiatry*, 7, 209–12.

Sluzewska, A. & Rybakowski, J.K. (1993). Cortisol levels and immunological indices in depression. *Neuropsychopharmacology*, 9, 107S.

Sluzewska, A., Nowakowska, E., Gryska, K., & Mackiewicz, A. (1994a). Haptoglobin levels in chronic mild stress model of depression in rats before and after treatment. *European Neuropsychopharmacology*, 4(3), 302.

Sluzewska, A., Rybakowski, J.K., Sobieska, M., & Wiktorowicz, K. (1994b). The effect of lithium, carbamazepine and fluoxetine on alpha-1-acid glycoprotein and alpha-1-antichymotrypsin in depressed patients. *Neuropsychopharmacology*, 10, 202.

Sluzewska, A., Wiktorowicz, K., Mackiewicz, S., & Rybakowski, J.K. (1994c). The effect of short-term treatment with lithium and carbamazepine on some immunological indices in depressed patients. *Lithium*, 5, 41–6.

Sluzewska, A., Rybakowski, J.K., Laciak, M., Mackiewicz, A., Sobieska, M., & Wiktorowicz, K. (1995a). Interleukin-6 levels in depressed patients before and after treatment with fluoxetine. *Annals of New York Academy of Science*, 762, 474–7.

Sluzewska, A., Rybakowski, J.K., Sobieska, M., Bosmans, E., Pollet, H., & Wiktorowicz, K. (1995b). Increased levels of alpha-1-acid glycoprotein and interleukin-6 in refractory depression. *Depression*, 3, 170–5.

Sluzewska, A., Rybakowski, J.K., Bosmans, E., Maes, M., Berhmans, R., & Pollet, H. (1995c). The effects of treatment with lithium and carbamazepine on some interleukins and their receptors in depressed patients. *Pharmacological Research*, 3, 366.

Sluzewska, A., Rybakowski, J.K., Sobieska, M., & Wiktorowicz, K. (1996a). Concentration and microheterogeneity glycophorms of alpha-1-acid glycoprotein in major depression. *Journal of Affective Disorders*, 39, 149–55.

Sluzewska, A., Rybakowski, J., Bosmans, E. et al. (1996b). Indicators of immune activation in major depression. *Psychiatry Research*, 63(3), 161–7.

Sluzewska, A., Samborski, W., Sobieska, M., & Klein, R. (1996c). Clinical relevance of antibodies against serotonin and gangliosides and acute phase proteins in major depression. *European Neuropsychopharmacology*, 6(4), S4–75.

Sluzewska, A., Gryska, K., & Mackiewicz, A. (1996d). Acute phase proteins in chronic mild stress model of depression. *Behavioural Pharmacology*, 7(1), 105–6.

Sluzewska, A., Rybakowski, J.K., Sobieska, M., & Amsterdam, J.D. (1996e). Changes in concentration and microheterogeneity of two acute phase proteins in major depression. *Glycoconjugate Journal*, 13, 891–2.

Sluzewska, A., Samborski, W., Sobieska, M., Klein, R., Bosmans, E., & Rybakowski, J.K. (1997a). Serum antibodies in relation to immune activation in major depression. *Human Psychopharmacology*, 12, 453–8.

Sluzewska, A., Rybakowski, J.K., & Sobieska, M. (1997b). Total serum protein and serum protein fractions in major depression and treatment resistant depression. *Biological Psychiatry*, 42(1S), 114.

Sluzewska, A., Sobieska, M., & Rybakowski, J.K. (1997c). Changes in acute-phase proteins during lithium potentiation of antidepressants in refractory depression. *Neuropsychobiology*, **35**, 123–7.

Song, C. & Leonard, B.L. (1993). Changes in plasma proteins in depressed patients and rodent model of depression. *Neuropsychopharmacology*, **9**, 106S.

Song, C. & Leonard, B.E. (1994). An acute phase protein response in the olfactory bulbectomised rat: effect of sertraline treatment. *Medical Science Research*, **22**, 313–14.

Song C., Dinan, T., & Leonard, B.E. (1994). Changes in immunoglobulins, compliment component and acute phase proteins levels in depressed patients and normal controls. *Journal of Affective Disorders*, **30**, 283–8.

Thase, M.E. & Rush A.J. (1995). Treatment-resistant depression. In *Psychopharmacology: The Fourth Generation of Progress*, ed. F.E. Bloom & D.J. Kupfer, pp. 1081–98. New York: Raven Press.

Tominga, T., Fukata, J., & Naito, Y. (1991). Prostaglandin-dependent in vitro stimulation of adrenocortical steroidogenesis by interleukins. *Endocrinology*, **128**, 526–31.

Turner, G.A. (1992). N-glycosylation of serum proteins in disease and its investigation using lectins. *Clinica et Chemica Acta*, **208**, 149–71.

Van Dijk, W. & Mackiewicz, A. (1993). Control of glycosylation alterations of acute phase proteins. In *Acute Phase Glycoproteins: Molecular Biology, Biochemistry and Applications*, ed. A. Mackiewicz, I. Kushner, & H. Bauman, pp. 559–80. Boca Raton, FL: CRC Press.

Van Dijk, W., Turner, G.A., & Mackiewicz, A. (1994). Changes in glycosylation of acute phase proteins in health and disease: occurrence, regulation and function. *Glycosylation and Disease*, **1**, 5–14.

Van Hunsel, F., Wauters, A., Vandoolaeghe, E., Neels, H., Demedts, P., & Maes, M. (1996). Lower total serum protein, albumin, beta- and gamma-globulin in major and treatment resistant depression: effects of antidepressant treatment. *Psychiatry Research*, **65**, 159–69.

Vasson, M.P., Roche-Arvellier, M., Coudrec, R., Baguet, J.C., & Raichvarg, D. (1994). Effects of alpha-1-acid glycoprotein on human polynuclear neutrophils: influence of glycan microheterogeneity. *Clinica Chemica Acta*, **224**, 65–71.

Villemain, F., Magnin, H., Feuillet-Fieux, M.N., Zarifian, E., Loo, H., & Bach, J.H. (1988). Anti-histone antibodies in schizophrenia and affective disorders. *Psychiatry Research*, **24**, 53–60.

Willner, P., Muscat, R., & Papp, M. (1992). Chronic mild stress-induced anhedonia: a realistic animal model of depression. *Neuroscience Biobehavior Review*, **16**, 525–34.

Zhou, D., Kusnecov, A.W., Shurin, M.R., DePaoli, M., & Rabin, B.S. (1993). Exposure to physical and psychological stressor elevates plasma interleukin-6: relationships to the activation of hypothalamic–pituitary–adrenal axis. *Endocrinology*, **133**, 2523–30.

# Part III

## Treatment approaches

# 8

# Selective serotonin reuptake inhibitors and serotonin–norepinephrine reuptake inhibitors in treatment-resistant depression

William Boyer and Richard Bunt

## Introduction

The selective serotonin reuptake inhibitors (SSRIs) represent one of the biggest advances in antidepressant pharmacotherapy in recent years, arguably the most important development since the accidental discovery of the antidepressant activity of a chlorpromazine analogue called imipramine. However the SSRIs' advantages lie primarily in an improved side effect profile and greatly improved safety in overdose; not efficacy. A newer class of antidepressants, the selective serotonin and norepinephrine reuptake inhibitors (SNRIs) holds the potential for increased efficacy plus a benign side effect profile.

This chapter will consider the use of SSRIs and SNRIs in resistant depression. We will consider two main situations: (i) the patient who has had no previous treatment with one of these medications, and (ii) the patient who does not respond to one of these treatments. This will naturally lead to a consideration of some general principles of managing the non-responder.

## Patients who have not been treated with an SSRI or SNRI

It has become uncommon to encounter a treatment-resistant patient who has not had a trial of at least one SSRI. The relative rarity of these patients makes it unlikely that many studies of SSRI-naïve treatment-resistant patients will be conducted or published. Nevertheless it is worthwhile to briefly review the limited literature on SSRI monotherapy in treatment-resistant depression.

### Efficacy of SSRI monotherapy

An open label study by Amsterdam and colleagues (1994) demonstrated fluoxetine's efficacy in resistant major depression. The authors defined complete response conservatively, as a greater than 50% reduction in HDRS and final score less than 7. Fifty-six percent of the 41 treatment-resistant patients responded.

**Table 8.1.** SSRIs in antidepressant (non-SSRI) non-responders

| Authors/Year | SSRI | $n$ | Pct responders |
|---|---|---|---|
| Amsterdam et al. (1994) | fluoxetine | 41 | 56.0% |
| Beasley et al. (1990) | fluoxetine | 53 | 51.8% |
| Simpson and DePaulo (1991) | fluoxetine | 16 | 62.5% |
| White et al. (1990) | fluvoxamine | 11 | 81.8% |
| Delgado et al. (1988) | fluvoxamine | 28 | 28.6% |
| Gagiano et al. (1988) | paroxetine | 28 | 64.3% |
| Peselow et al. (1989) | paroxetine | 10 | 50.0% |
| Thase et al. (1995) | sertraline | 27 | 63.0% |
| | | | Average 54.3% |

Table 8.1 summarizes this and other studies of SSRIs in antidepressant non-responders. These trials varied in important design aspects, including the degree and definition of treatment resistance. Response rates ranged from a low of 28.6% up to 81.8%, with fluvoxamine accounting for both extremes. Perhaps the most reasonable interpretation of these disparate results is that the SSRIs have shown at least modest efficacy in patients who failed to respond to other antidepressants.

## SNRI monotherapy

The situation concerning SNRI monotherapy is different than the SSRIs. Currently, there is only one of this class, venlafaxine, approved for marketing in the United States. Venlafaxine, like the SSRIs, has minimal direct effects on the neuronal receptors responsible for typical TCA side effects (e.g. acetylcholine and histamine). It therefore shares the quality of a relatively benign side effect profile with the SSRIs. However, venlafaxine's safety in overdose is relatively less well established and it must be given at least twice a day. Furthermore, most patients given venlafaxine require dosage titration, while this is not true for the SSRIs.

Available data suggest that venlafaxine might enjoy two important characteristics: more rapid speed of onset and enhanced antidepressant efficacy. A number of studies support the apparent rapidity of onset of antidepressant activity (Benkert et al., 1994; Derivan et al., 1995; Rickels et al., 1995). However, this claim has been made before for other antidepressants (Barranco et al., 1979; Fabre, 1985) and later abandoned. A major stumbling problem in establishing speed of onset is the lack of agreement over 'onset.' Speed of onset may also be related to speed of dosage titration, therefore the quicker one reaches a higher dose the quicker one sees onset. This in turn is linked to side effects, since patients are more likely to tolerate rapid titration of a medication with few side effects.

**Venlafaxine in resistant depression**

Two major studies of venlafaxine in well-defined resistant depression have been reported. De Montigny and colleagues reported a response rate of 70% in a series of 90 patients who had failed at least one antidepressant trial (average = 3.2 trials) (De Montigny et al., 1995). In contrast, Nierenberg and associates reported a response rate of only 32.9% (Hamilton Depression scale) to 40% (on the Clinical Global Impressions scale) among 82 patients who had failed to respond to at least three separate antidepressant trials (Nierenberg et al., 1994b). The difference in results may be due to different criteria for treatment resistance.

The efficacy of venlafaxine compared to SSRIs is also relevant for this discussion. Two major studies have been performed. Fluoxetine served as the comparison drug in both cases. In the first, 68 inpatients with major depression were randomized to fluoxetine (40 mg/day) or venlafaxine (200 mg/day) for 7 weeks (Clerc et al., 1994). Venlafaxine was significantly superior in reducing depressive symptoms. Fewer venlafaxine-treated patients dropped out of the trial due to side effects.

The second study was a 6-week placebo-controlled, randomized comparison of venlafaxine and fluoxetine in 314 outpatients with major depression (Dierick et al., 1996). A clinical response, defined as at least a 50% decrease from the baseline HAM-D score, was attained in 72% of patients on venlafaxine and 60% of patients on fluoxetine ($P = 0.023$). Among patients who increased their dose at 2 weeks, venlafaxine was significantly ($P < 0.05$) superior from week 3 onward. These four studies therefore suggest that venlafaxine may be useful for patients who have failed to respond to an antidepressant of a different class, including SSRIs.

Whether and to what extant venlafaxine's characteristics are shared by other SNRIs is unclear. Milnacipran is an SNRI available in some countries. In comparative trials, milnacipran, at 100 mg/day, was significantly more effective than placebo (60% responders vs. 46%); SSRIs (65% vs. 52%), and similar to the TCAs, even in more severe endogenous or melancholic patients (Briley, 1996). Duloxetine is an investigational SNRI which has been studied in depression. However, it currently appears that initial licensing approval will be sought for urologic rather than psychiatric indications.

## Managing the patient who fails to respond to an SSRI or SNRI

A patient who fails to respond to an SSRI or SNRI will become a much more common clinical problem than the patient who has not yet had a trial of one of these medications. A large number of possible treatment strategies are already available. However, before trying to sort through them, it is worthwhile to go through a formal or informal 'checklist' of possible causes for non-response.

**Is this non-response or intolerance?**

The difference between non-response and intolerance due to side effects has clinically significant implications. A patient who does not respond to an adequate trial of an antidepressant should usually next be treated with an antidepressant from a different class. A patient who is intolerant of a medication cannot (and should not) have an 'adequate' trial of that agent. It is less important to exclude drugs from the same class if there is an alternative less likely to produce these side effect(s). A common example is the patient who cannot tolerate a tertiary amine TCA (e.g. amitriptyline or imipramine) because of anticholinergic side effects, but responds well to a secondary amine compound (e.g. desipramine or nortriptyline).

Patients often present some combination of non-response and intolerance. Occasionally, it is impossible to determine whether certain symptoms represent side effects or depression. An example is the anhedonia and anergia occasionally seen with SSRIs, especially in higher than average doses. Some general guidelines can be offered. If the patient appears intolerant of even a small dose or a very short duration of treatment, a same-class alternative with a presumably better side effect profile might be considered. However, if the patient has taken a regular dose for at least 2 to 3 weeks with absolutely no subjective or objective improvement then it may be wisest to regard this as non-response and select the next medication from a different class.

**How severe is the depression and is it worse, the same or somewhat better?**

This question is also clinically relevant. Those who are somewhat better are the most likely to respond to 'more of the same;' meaning a longer trial and/or higher dosage of the antidepressant. Mild depressions are often chronic, and chronicity often indicates a need for prolonged antidepressant trials.

Patients who are worse or those with stable but severe depression deserve the most aggressive treatment, such as adjunctive and/or combination therapies. Patients who are initially moderately or severely depressed and make modest improvements risk losing their gains if the antidepressant is changed. Patients with mild to moderate depression who are neither significantly better or worse may usually be managed with sequential trials of single antidepressants.

**Is the diagnosis correct?**

It is axiomatic that depressed patients require appropriate medical screening and evaluation prior to starting antidepressant treatment. This is especially true for patients who have had no previous affective episodes. The screening may be helpful for diagnosis and management of organic conditions associated with affective disorders (e.g. cardiovascular problems) as well as those which contribute to, or even cause, the disturbance.

One of the most common psychiatric findings in patients referred for treatment-resistant depression is a bipolar-spectrum disorder. The concept of a bipolar spectrum holds that the condition may present with signs and symptoms ranging from the classical bipolar I disturbance to very mild or highly atypical bipolar II and rapid or even ultra-rapid cycling. Patients with more atypical presentations are often (mis)diagnosed as having a personality disorder because their profound and rapid mood shifts are seen as characterological 'lability' rather than a mood swing.

Some features can help with the distinction. A family history of bipolar disorder is very strong evidence in favor or bipolar disorder in the patient. Bipolar spectrum patients also often have a characteristically different attitude about their mood swings than those with Axis II disorders. The latter typically see their moodiness as part of who they are. They persistently minimize the significance of, and externalize blame for, their emotional behavior. Patients with a bipolar diathesis are more likely to have some objectivity and psychological 'distance' concerning their mood swings and are puzzled about the profoundly different ways they see the world at times. Occasionally, it is impossible to distinguish between mood swings and mood lability. In this case the patient is then usually better served by diagnosis and treatment for the more treatable disorder, the affective one.

## Treatment options for non-responders

There is no lack of treatment options for the depressed patient unresponsive to medication. A dozen or more have been described. The problem lies in the very profusion of options: how to choose between them, when and how to combine them, and what order in which to employ them.

One way to simplify and categorize the options is 'wait,' 'change,' 'augment,' or 'combine.' 'Waiting' means to have the patient continue the same treatment longer, perhaps at a different (usually higher) dose. 'Switching' means changing from one antidepressant to another. 'Augmentation' is the use of an antidepressant plus medication not considered to be an antidepressant by itself. 'Combination' is the simultaneous use of more than one antidepressant, usually of different classes.

### Waiting (longer trials)

There continues to be debate in the literature as to what is a 'long-enough' trial for an antidepressant. Recommendations range from four to eight and even twelve weeks. Some of this disagreement seems due to imprecise definitions. Although a clinically meaningful response may require more than 4 weeks, some improvement is typically seen before then. Most clinicians would suspect that a patient whose depression suddenly resolves over the course of one or even a few days is having a placebo response.

Another source of confusion is that investigators usually pose the research question as whether and to what extent early improvement correlates with later response. The more important clinical question is how well does lack of early improvement predict non-response? This is more relevant because the question of whether and how long to continue an antidepressant arises from patients who do not improve, not those who show an early response.

Boyer and Feighner investigated this issue by pooling data from several similar antidepressant studies conducted at the Feighner Research Institute (Boyer & Feighner, 1994). Patients who failed to show at least 20% improvement at some point in the first 4 weeks had only a 4% chance of a meaningful response at 6 weeks. Similar results were obtained using two different definitions of improvement.

Early, partial improvement can be difficult to gauge, especially in patients with ongoing life stresses. These patients may continue to report symptoms such as anxiety-related insomnia, anhedonia, tension headaches and gastrointestinal disturbances for weeks or months if the stresses continue. In this situation we have found that improvement in a sense of being able to cope or not feeling as overwhelmed is a favorable prognostic indicator.

## Changing antidepressants

It is axiomatic among many psychopharmacologists that when changing antidepressants one should select the next one from a different chemical class. The theory is that since the depression did not respond to one type of physiological 'attack,' another avenue is more likely to be effective. There is surprisingly little systematic data to either support or refute this theory, however. Most of what support there is comes from studies which showed good response rates to monoamine oxidase inhibitors among patients who failed a tricyclic antidepressant (Nolen et al., 1988; Quitkin et al., 1990; Thase et al., 1992a,b). Whether the same principle applies to the newer antidepressant classes is uncertain.

Three studies of changing from one SSRI to another have been published or presented (Joffe et al., 1996; Thase et al., 1995; Zarate et al., 1996). Globally defined response rates in these papers ranged between 42 and 68%, with an average of 56% ($n = 148$). We were able to locate only two studies which described patients switched to a TCA after failing an SSRI (Peselow et al., 1989; Thase et al., 1995). In these a virtually identical percentage (54%) of SSRI non-responders responded to the TCA ($n = 65$). There is currently no data on SSRI non-responders crossed over to an SNRI. However, comparative SSRI–SNRI studies suggest that the latter may be a worthwhile option for SSRI non-responders (Clerc et al., 1994; Dierick et al., 1996).

In the absence of clear scientific data, it remains a clinical judgement whether to prescribe a second SSRI for a patient who fails an initial trial with of one. As previously mentioned, it is important to try to tease apart non-response from side effects, since 'pure' non-response argues more heavily for changing antidepressant class. It is doubtful that three or more consecutive trials of different SSRIs is often justified unless there is a very clear reason to prefer this class of medication (e.g. proven efficacy in treating another of the patient's diagnoses, such as obsessive-compulsive disorder or low toxicity in overdose).

## Antidepressant augmentation
### Lithium

Most published data concerning lithium augmentation of SSRIs concerns fluoxetine. Ontiveros and coworkers conducted an open trial comparing lithium augmentation of fluoxetine and desipramine (Ontiveros et al., 1991). The 60 patients had failed to respond to 6 weeks of therapy with either 150–300 mg/day of desipramine or 20–80 mg/day of fluoxetine. Exclusion criteria included most other Axis I or Axis II disorders, as well as patients with significant intercurrent major life events. Both groups achieved an approximate 60% response rate. Results were not significantly related to the dosage, or blood level of lithium.

Katona and colleagues published a placebo-controlled, prospective study of 62 patients. Their patients had failed to respond to either fluoxetine or lofepramine which, like desipramine, is a relatively noradrenergic antidepressant (Kopala & Honer, 1994). Lithium augmentation was significantly superior to placebo overall. The magnitude of superiority increased when only patients with 'therapeutic' blood levels of lithium were considered. Other, uncontrolled reports suggest that lithium augmentation may be useful for paroxetine and sertraline non-responders (Camprubi & Puri, 1995; Dinan, 1993; Hawley et al., 1994).

It is clear from the available data that typical 'therapeutic' blood levels of lithium are not always required for successful lithium augmentation (Dinan, 1993). However, there is also strong suggestive evidence that success is more likely with therapeutic levels (Stein & Bernardt, 1993). Important unanswered questions include whether once daily administration is as effective as divided doses (which should lead to better compliance), how long to continue lithium augmentation and if, when, and how to discontinue (Hardy et al., 1997). Although some have suggested that lithium augmentation is effective only in depressed patients with a bipolar-spectrum disorder, the balance of data does not support this contention.

Lithium augmentation may be the most dangerous of the augmentation strategies to be discussed here. Adverse effects may include signs and symptoms of lithium toxicity and/or serotonergic over-activity, which is referred to as he 'serotonin syndrome.' The more severe side effects appear to occur most frequently in the elderly, a population which is also more likely to tolerate lithium monotherapy poorly (Austin et al., 1990; Flint & Rifat, 1994).

## Thyroid

Thyroid augmentation has not been systematically studied with either SSRIs or SNRIs. Published experience includes only case reports and small case series (Crowe et al., 1990; Gupta et al., 1991; Joffe, 1992). Thyroid hormone has exhibited efficacy as an adjunctive agent in several controlled TCA studies. For example, in a 1993 study of 50 unipolar depressed patients by Joffe et al. (1993), triiodothyronine (T3) and lithium augmentation were equally effective.

Another study by Joffe and Singer (1990) had previously shown that triiodothyronine (T3) was significantly more effective adjunct than thyroxine (T4) in treating TCA non-responders. It should be noted that peripheral and CNS T3 levels are not necessarily proportionately linked and in fact have been said to vary conversely due to complex feedback mechanisms. Normal results on thyroid screening tests does not preclude a positive response (Schwarcz et al., 1984).

Thyroid augmentation appears, on average, to be better tolerated than lithium. The acute side effect of most concern is induction or worsening of cardiac dysrhythmias or heart failure due to thyroid's tendency to accelerate the heart rate. Cardiology consultation should be considered prior to starting patients with cardiac pathology on thyroid augmentation. As with lithium augmentation, the best length of time to continue thyroid and the best way to discontinue it are unknown.

## Buspirone

Buspirone has been used with some success both to augment SSRIs in treatment of depression and also as treatment for SSRI-induced sexual dysfunction. Bakish presented case histories of three depressed patients with 'obsessional traits, marked anxiety, and a history of eating disorders' (Bakish, 1992). The patients had previously been treated with various agents including phenelzine, clomipramine, desipramine, imipramine, alprazolam, clonazepam, ECT, fluoxetine and trazodone. Buspirone was added to the patients' regimens at low dosages and titrated up to 30 mg per day split into two or three doses. All three of the patients reportedly achieved complete remission of their depressive symptoms and none suffered any significant adverse effects.

An open study was conducted by Joffe and coworkers to assess the efficacy of buspirone augmentation of SSRIs (Joffe & Schuller, 1993). The authors reported their experience with 25 patients whose depression had failed to respond to multiple trials including: desipramine, phenelzine, tranylcypromine, lithium alone, and several TCAs. Each patient had had to two three such trials. The patients were started on either fluoxetine or fluvoxamine which was titrated according to side-effect tolerance and continued for a minimum of 5 weeks. Finally, buspirone 10 mg twice a day was added and increased over the first week to a maximum of 50 mg/day. No changes in SSRI dosages were made during this phase of treatment. Twelve of the 16 fluoxetine patients and five of the nine fluvoxamine patients experienced moderate to complete improvement. Of the 17 responders, 13 had a sustained response at 3 months' follow-up. The remaining four patients were either lost to follow-up or changed their therapy 'for reasons other than antidepressant efficacy' (Joffe & Schuller, 1993).

### Pindolol

The beta-blocker pindolol is another adjunct which has produced a rapid response in very limited trials. Two of these reported response rates of 6/8 and 13/19 at a dosage of 2.5 mg three times a day (Artigas et al., 1994; Blier & Bergeron, 1995).

The rationale for this combination is that pindolol, by blocking 5HT1a auto-receptors, may prevent a compensatory (but detrimental) down-regulation of serotonergic function provoked by the increased synaptic serotonin activity associated with SSRIs. It is possible that pindolol and buspirone act by similar mechanisms, even though buspirone is an agonist at the 5HT1a receptor. The key point is that buspirone is a relatively weak agonist compared to the endogenous ligand (Eison, 1990). If there is a high level of initial activity at the receptor, its net effect would be antagonistic, like pindolol.

Pindolol is subject to the cautions and contra-indications of other beta blockers. These include aggravation of asthma and masking of hypoglycemic symptoms. A serious behavioral 'toxicity' of both buspirone and pindolol is the worsening of irritability in some SSRI-treated patients (Blier & Bergeron, 1995; Norden, 1995).

### Stimulants

Stoll and colleagues reported rapid response to methylphenidate augmentation of SSRIs at dosages of 5–20 mg three times a day. These response were sustained at follow-up, which ranged from 2–10 months. The five patients described had had a variety of prior antidepressant trials. Several had been on SSRIs for extended periods (Stoll et al., 1996).

Metz and Shader (1991) reported four cases in which depressed patients were treatment-resistant to TCAs. Three of these patients obtained either partial responses to fluoxetine or relapsed while on fluoxetine. They improved when pemoline 9.375 to 18.75 mg a day was added. These responses lasted between 9 and 23 months. There are also reports of successful augmentation of fluoxetine with dextroamphetamine, pergolide and bromocriptine (Linet, 1989).

We have found stimulants to be especially helpful in treating residual fatigue and anergia after an otherwise successful antidepressant trial. They have also been used successfully to counteract medication-associated sexual dysfunction. Significant side effects, including dependence and abuse, are uncommon.

## Antidepressant combinations

One of the most common antidepressant combinations with SSRIs or SNRIs is the adjunctive use of a sedating antidepressant to treat insomnia. Trazodone is frequently used for this purpose. In one of the earliest such reports Nierenberg and colleagues (1992) described improvement in sleep and depression in three of eight patients when trazodone was added to their regimen. These patients had not responded to fluoxetine alone. These results were largely replicated in a subsequent placebo-controlled trial (Nierenberg et al., 1994a).

Other sedating antidepressants are sometimes used in combination with an SSRI or SNRI. These include amitriptyline, doxepin and trimipramine. Mianserin, where available, is also used. Mianserin's relatively new cousin, mirtazapine, is also likely to be used for this purpose.

Although the concomitant use of a sedating antidepressant usually helps insomnia, the antidepressant efficacy of this combination has not been well studied. More attention has focused on the combination of a relatively noradrenergic TCA such as desipramine with an SSRI (Eisen, 1989). An initial observation that this combination promoted down-regulation of beta-adrenergic receptors (which is thought to be related to antidepressant activity) faster than either drug alone (Baron et al., 1988) also prompted speculation that combined neurotransmitter reuptake blockade may produce faster antidepressant effects (Horgan, 1993). These hypotheses may also be related to the clinical characteristics of SNRIs.

Whether and to what extent the addition of desipramine to an SSRI confers additional antidepressant benefit is unclear. In an early open trial low-dose desipramine plus fluoxetine was effective in 13 of 20 outpatients who failed to respond to fluoxetine alone (Weilburg et al., 1991). However, a subsequent rigorously controlled study reported essentially negative results. This study included only patients who had failed separate 6-week trials of both desipramine and fluoxetine. Six of these patients were treated with fluoxetine plus desipramine and five remained on desipramine plus placebo. Only one patient in each group responded (Miller et al., 1995). This study suggests that the combination of fluocetine and desipramine has no value over either antidepressant by itself. However, patients who have failed to respond to two consecutive antidepressants in a study (and probably more prior to the study) are a relatively treatment-resistant group. Therefore, the study's sample size ($n = 11$) was probably not large enough.

Another important moderating variable may be the type of non-response, i.e. complete or partial. Fava and collaborators reported that desipramine augmentation was more effective than either fluoxetine dose increase or lithium augmentation among complete non-responders to at least eight weeks of fluoxetine monotherapy (Fava et al., 1994). Partial fluoxetine responders did best with fluoxetine dosage increase.

The concomitant use of bupropion plus an SSRI has received even less attention. Boyer and Feighner presented their experience with this combination in a series of 23 patients who were treated with both fluoxetine and bupropion. Each patient had had a significant but partial initial response to either fluoxetine (20–60 mg/day) or bupropion (150–450 mg/day), which did not improve with continued treatment. Fluoxetine or bupropion was continued at the most effective dose while the second treatment was added. Eight patients (35%) had a moderate or marked response to the combination and six (26%) a minimal response. Nine patients (39%) had combination therapy discontinued because of side effects. The side effects were the same type as those seen with either drug alone, such as anxiety, agitation, headaches, and insomnia. No seizures or other serious side effects were seen (Boyer & Feighner, 1993).

Marshall and colleagues (1995) reported the successful use of sertraline plus bupropion with four treatment-resistant depressed patients who had failed to respond to sertraline alone. Bupropion has also been successfully employed as an adjunct or alternative to an SSRI for patients with significant sexual dysfunction (Labbate & Pollack, 1994; Walker et al., 1993). Its mechanism of action in this regard may involve dopamine uptake inhibition.

*Pharmacokinetic considerations in combined antidepressant therapy*
The concomitant use of a heterocyclic antidepressant and an SSRI requires consideration of possible drug–drug interactions (Preskorn et al., 1990). A thorough discussion of this issue is beyond the scope of this chapter. However the most important clinical consequence of the interaction is that SSRIs, by saturating hepatic metabolic pathways, may slow the metabolism of the heterocyclic enough to cause very high blood levels to develop (Preskorn et al., 1994). The clinician should therefore be aware that relatively low doses of the heterocyclic may produce significant therapeutic and side effects and that this interaction may not be immediately apparent. Initial doses should therefore be relatively low and combined with conservative upward dose titration.

Venlafaxine is less prone to significantly inhibit the hepatic enzymes affected by

SSRIs (Otton et al., 1994). Therefore, it is theoretically less likely to cause the same type and severity of adverse drug–drug interactions. However, this has not been studied to the same degree as with SSRIs, so caution is still advisable.

## Other considerations in managing non-response

### Concurrent symptoms and choice of antidepressant

Antidepressants are often helpful in syndromes other than depression. Examples include obsessive-compulsive disorder (OCD), panic disorder, and bulimia. If a patient has symptoms of another antidepressant-responsive syndrome, it is tempting to choose an antidepressant which is known to be helpful for the other disorder as well. Unfortunately, there is little evidence that antidepressants selected this way will be more (or less) effective against the core depressive syndrome. There is, in fact, evidence that improvement in one of these other disorders may occur independently of depression (Capstick, 1975). Similarly, there is no evidence that depressed patients with insomnia or agitation have a superior antidepressant response to sedating antidepressants or that 'activating' medications work better for patients with hypersomnolence or psychomotor retardation (Filteau et al., 1992, 1993).

The syndrome of atypical depression is a notable exception. This has been shown to be more responsive to the monoamine oxidase inhibitor (MAOI) phenelzine than to tricyclic antidepressants. The symptoms of atypical depression which are helpful in making this distinction are hypersomnolence, hyperphagia, hypersensitivity to interpersonal rejection and a subjective sense of 'leaden' paralysis when depressed. The presence of any of these symptoms tends to predict a superior response to phenelzine, and presumably other MAOIs (McGrath et al., 1992).

### Suicide risk

Although all patients with affective disorders are in some danger of suicide, some patients are at especially high risk (Appleby, 1992). One of the strongest risk factors is a history of one or more suicide attempts. Others include lack of social support, poor health, living alone, male gender and substance abuse (Appleby, 1992).

A significant risk of suicide should be considered in antidepressant treatment choice. Tricyclic antidepressants are known to be highly toxic in overdose. Considerable experience suggests that the risk with SSRIs and trazodone is considerably lower (de Jonghe & Swinkels, 1992). Human data with other antidepressants and psychotropics is more limited, but lithium, non-reversible MAOIs (i.e. tranylcypromine and phenelzine) and probably thyroid augmentation, are likely to be

toxic in overdose. Pindolol, a beta-blocker which shows promise for antidepressant augmentation, would also be serious if taken in overdose. Case reports suggest
that overdoses with venlafaxine, bupropion, nefazodone and mirtazapine are
relatively well tolerated (Hoes & Zeijpveld, 1996; Montgomery, 1995; Robinson et
al., 1996; Rudolph & Derivan, 1996; Spiller et al., 1994). Buspirone, which has also
been used for augmentation, also appears to be relatively safe in overdose
(Schweizer & Riskels, 1991).

## Optimizing concurrent therapies

It is not unusual for depressed patients to be under treatment for other illnesses. It
is good practice to review these medications with a goal of, if possible, maximizing
their positive impact on the mood disorder. For example, patients taking thyroid
replacement are typically treated with liothyronine (T4). However there is experimental evidence that triiodothyronine (T3) may be more beneficial as an antidepressant adjunct (Ballantine et al., 1987; Cooke et al., 1992; Joffe & Singer, 1990).

Antihypertensives are sometimes suspected of causing or contributing to depression. Their liability in this regard differs between classes. Pindolol is a beta
blocker which potently inhibits the (primarily) presynaptic 5HT1a receptor.
Angiotensin converting enzyme (ACE) inhibitors have been noted to have antidepressant effects and are even suspected of inducing mania in isolated cases (Cohen
& Zubenko, 1988). In some situations it may be possible, with consultation, to
change the patient's antihypertensive regimen to one of these agents.

## Efficacy of the treatment options for treatment-resistant depression

Depending on the definition, there are a dozen or more possible treatments for
antidepressant non-response. It is therefore safe to predict that there will never be
an 'ideal' randomized, comparative study of all of these options. Lacking this, one
must pursue the data which is available. One approach is to survey practitioners as
to what they find useful. This is somewhat circular, since practitioners are likely to
do what they have learned. However, it is reasonable to suppose that a clearly
ineffective intervention would not enjoy wide acceptance for very long, and that a
clearly superior treatment is likely to be more widespread and long-lived.

Chaimowitz and colleagues (1991) surveyed Canadian psychiatrists concerning
their preferred order of pharmacological treatments for Major Depression. This
study was conducted before the widespread acceptance of SSRIs as first-line
treatment. Almost equal portions of respondents preferred trying an antidepressant of the same class (TCA), a different class (MAOI) or lithium augmentation.
Similar portions of respondents chose lithium augmentation or change to a
different class of antidepressant as second-line treatments in a later survey of

**Table 8.2.** Antidepressant augmentation[a] vs. change of antidepressants[b]

| Advantages | Allows continuing trial of current antidepressant – especially useful if |
|---|---|
| | 1. *there has not yet been an adequate trial* |
| | 2. *the risk of not achieving an equivalent response with another antidepressant is considered unacceptable (e.g. the patient has failed multiple other antidepressants but responded partially to current treatment)* |
| | Well-documented efficacy in resistant depression – *lithium* |
| | May be combined – *lithium and thyroid may help different patient populations* |
| Disadvantages | Multiple dosing required – *likely to cause compliance problems*[b] |
| | Dangerous in overdose – *lithium, thyroid, pindolol*[c] |
| | Relatively low therapeutic index – *lithium, thyroid, pindolol*[c] |
| | Potential interactions between the antidepressant and augmenting agent |
| | Lack of guidelines for length of therapy |

[a] lithium, thyroid hormone, buspirone, pindolol.
[b] venlafaxine, nefazodone, bupropion and MAOIs also usually require divided dosing.
[c] also applies to TCAs and first-generation MAOIs (i.e. phenelzine, tranylcupromine).

psychiatrists in the northeastern US (Nierenberg, 1991). Thyroid augmentation was not widely endorsed in either survey.

We have recently conducted a meta-analysis of published or presented data concerning the efficacy of the several treatment options for resistant depression (Boyer, 2000). The two highest effect sizes were associated with dosage increase and switch to an MAOI. The efficacy of MAOIs in treatment-resistant depression was not limited to patients with an 'atypical' symptom picture.

There was no significant difference in efficacy (effect sizes) between lithium and thyroid augmentation. Both were significantly superior to placebo. Data concerning augmentation with buspirone or pindolol were much more scarce, but suggested at least equal efficacy to lithium or thyroid augmentation.

One may generalize that, with the exception of MAOIs, there is no reason from an efficacy standpoint to choose between augmentation strategies and changing antidepressants. Other reasons for and against these categories should be examined. The advantages and disadvantages of antidepressant augmentation compared to change of antidepressants are summarized in Table 8.2.

The importance of these factors will vary from one patient to the next. However, in most cases change of antidepressant is preferable. There are two important exceptions. One is the patient who has had a definite, but partial response to the current antidepressant. A change of antidepressant in this situation entails the risk of partial or even complete relapse. If the initial depression was moderate to severe this danger may shift the risk/benefit evaluation in favor of augmentation. An-

**Table 8.3.** Patient and symptom characteristics

| Patient | Clinical considerations |
|---|---|
| Compliance risk | Simple regimen, fewest medications given fewest times a day. Usually means change antidepressant rather than augment |
| Advanced age | Most likely to have adverse effects with lithium augmentation |
| Suicide risk | Avoid TCAs, MAOIs, lithium, thyroid |
| Any atypical symptoms | |
| 1. hypersomnolence | |
| 2. hyperphagia | Predicts better response to MAOIs than TCAs |
| 3. rejection sensitivity | |
| 4. 'leaden' paralysis | |

other exception is the patient whose depression is worsening. In this condition augmentation allows the current antidepressant to be continued (i.e. allows a longer trial) while one or more other therapies may be added. It should be stressed that as depression worsens, ECT becomes an increasingly important alternative and that some medications (e.g. lithium) may be less attractive options because they must be withdrawn prior to ECT.

## Summary and discussion

In this chapter we have discussed evidence concerning the efficacy of SSRIs and SNRIs in resistant depression. Following this we examined the variety of options available for managing non-responders to these medications. We have avoided presenting formal treatment algorithms for two reasons. First, such algorithms have been presented elsewhere (Nelson et al., 1996) and to do so here would be unnecessarily redundant. Secondly, we have presented a moderately large number of considerations in treatment choice. The most practical way to present and use all of these factors would be a computer program. To include all of them in a two-dimensional diagram would lead to an illegible, and unusable, mess.

These treatment considerations can, however, be summarized in a general way. (Tables 8.3 and 8.4). These tables can be reviewed in the treatment decision-making process.

We have presented the data and recommendations in this chapter as aids to the clinical decision-making process. Ultimately, the 'best' decision in any particular context will remain one arrived at by careful consideration of the evidence, collaboration with the patient, and the 'art' which is the practice of medicine.

**Table 8.4.** Treatment principles and example interventions for antidepressant non-responders

| And now is | Depression was initially<br>Mild to moderate severity | Moderate to severe |
|---|---|---|
| Partially improved | *Conservative*<br>• Longer trial<br>• Increase dose | *Moderately conservative*<br>• Increase dose<br>• Augmentation<br>• Change antidepressant |
| No change | *Moderately conservative*<br>• Change antidepressant<br>• Longer trial | *Moderately aggressive*<br>• Change antidepressant<br>• Add augmentation soon after change |
| Worse | *Moderately aggressive*<br>• Change antidepressant<br>• Add augmentation soon after change | *Aggressive*<br>• Augmentation<br>• Add an antidepressant at time of, or soon after augmentation<br>• ECT |

## REFERENCES

Amsterdam, J.D., Maislin, G., & Potter, L. (1994). Fluoxetine efficacy in treatment resistant depression. *Progress in NeuroPsychopharmacology and Biological Psychiatry*, **18**, 243–61.

Appleby, L. (1992). Suicide in psychiatric patients: risk and prevention. *British Journal of Psychiatry*, **161**, 749–58.

Artigas, F., Perez, V., & Alvarez, E. (1994). Pindolol induces a rapid improvement of depressed patients treated with serotonin reuptake inhibitors. *Archives of General Psychiatry*, **51**, 248–51.

Austin, L.S., Arana, G.W. & Melvin, J.A. (1990). Toxicity resulting from lithium augmentation of antidepressant treatment in elderly patients. *Journal of Clinical Psychiatry*, **51**, 344–5.

Bakish, D. (1992). Fluoxetine potentiation by buspirone: three case histories. *Canadian Journal of Psychiatry*, **36**, 749–50.

Ballantine, H.T., Bouckoms, A.J., Thomas, E.K., & Giriunas, I.E. (1987). Treatment of psychiatric illness by stereotactic cingulotomy. *Biological Psychiatry*, **22**, 807–19.

Baron, B.M., Ogden, A.M., Siegel, B.W., Stegeman, J., Ursillo, R.C., & Dudley, M.W. (1988). Rapid down regulation of beta-adrenoceptors by co-administration of desipramine and fluoxetine. *European Journal of Pharmacology*, **154**, 125–34.

Barranco, S.F., Thrash, M.L., Hackett, E., Frey, J., Ward, J., & Norris, E. (1979). Early onset of response to doxepin treatment. *Journal of Clinical Psychiatry*, **40**, 265–9.

Beasley, C.M. Jr, Sayler, M.E., Cunningham, G.E., Weiss, A.M., & Masica, D.N. (1990). Fluoxetine in tricyclic refractory major depressive disorder. *Journal of Affective Disorders*, **20**, 193–200.

Benkert, O., Hackett, D., Realini, R., White, C., & Wilde, J.D. (1994). A randomised, double blind, comparison of a rapidly escalating dose of venlafaxine and imipramine in inpatients with major depression and melancholia. Presented at the XIX CINP meeting, Washington, DC.

Blier, P. & Bergeron, R. (1995). Effectiveness of pindolol with selected antidepressant drugs in the treatment of major depression. *Journal of Clinical Psychopharmacology*, 15, 217–22.

Boyer, W. (2000). A quantitative review of treatments for antidepressant non-responders. In submission.

Boyer, W.F. & Feighner, J.P. (1993). The combined use of fluoxetine and bupropion. Presented at the American Psychiatric Association Annual Meeting, San Francisco CA.

Boyer, W.F. & Feighner, J.P. (1994). Clinical significance of early non-response in depressed patients. *Depression*, 2, 32–5.

Briley, M. (1996). Milnacipran: a Na and 5-HT reuptake inhibitor. X World Congress of Psychiatry, Madrid, August.

Camprubi, M.E. & Puri, B.K. (1995). The treatment of refractory depression using paroxetine with lithium augmentation. *Progress in NeuroPsychopharmacology and Biological Psychiatry*, 19, 515–17.

Capstick, N. (1975). Depressive reactions in the course of clomipramine therapy used in the treatment of obsessional conditions. *Scottish Medical Journal*, 20(1 Suppl.), 45–8.

Chaimowitz, G.A., Links, P.S., Padgett, R.W., & Carr, A.C. (1991). Treatment-resistant depression: a survey of practice habits of Canadian psychiatrists. *Canadian Journal of Psychiatry*, 36, 353–6.

Clerc, G.E., Ruimy, P., & Verdeau-Pailles, J. (1994). A double-blind comparison of venlafaxine and fluoxetine in patients hospitalized for major depression and melancholia. *International Clinical Psychopharmacology*, 9, 139–43.

Cohen, B.M., & Zubenko, G.S. (1988). Captopril in the treatment of recurrent major depression. *Journal of Clinical Psychopharmacology*, 8, 143–4.

Cooke, R.G., Joffe, R.T., & Levitt, A.J. (1992). T3 augmentation of antidepressant treatment in T4-replaced thyroid patients. *Journal of Clinical Psychiatry*, 53, 16–18.

Crowe, D., Collins, J.P.. & Rosse, R.B. (1990). Thyroid hormone supplementation of fluoxetine treatment. *Journal of Clinical Psychopharmacology*, 10, 150–1.

de Jonghe, F. & Swinkels, J.A. (1992). The safety of anti-depressants. *Drugs*, 43(Suppl. 2), 40–6.

Delgado, P.L., Price, L.H., Charney, D.S., & Heninger, G.R. (1988). Efficacy of fluvoxamine in treatment-refractory depression. *Journal of Affective Disorders*, 15, 55–60.

de Montigny, C., Debonnel, G., Bergeron, R., & Blier, P. (1995). Venlafaxine in treatment-resistant depression: an open-label multicenter study. Presented at the American College of Neuropsychopharmacology annual meeting, San Juan, Puerto Rico.

Derivan, A., Entsuah, A.R., & Kikta, D. (1995). Venlafaxine: Measuring the onset of antidepressant action. *Psychopharmacology Bulletin*, 31, 439–47.

Dierick, M., Ravizza, L., Realini, R., & Martin, A. (1996). A double-blind comparison of venlafaxine and fluoxetine for treatment of major depression in outpatients. *Progress in NeuroPsychopharmacology and Biological Psychiatry*, 20, 57–71.

Dinan, T.G. (1993). Lithium augmentation in sertraline-resistant depression: a preliminary dose-response study. *Acta Psychiatrica Scandinavica,* **88**, 300–1.

Eisen, A. (1989). Fluoxetine and desipramine: a strategy for augmenting antidepressant response. *Pharmacopsychiatry,* **22**, 272–3.

Eison, M.S. (1990). Azapirones: Clinical uses of serotonin partial agonists. *Drug Therapy,* Suppl. (August), 1–7.

Fabre, L.F. (1985). Treatment of depression in outpatients: a controlled comparison of the onset of action of amoxapine and maprotiline. *Journal of Clinical Psychiatry,* **46**, 521–4.

Fava, M., Rosenbaum, J.F., McGrath, P.J., Stewart, J.W., Amsterdam, J.D., & Quitkin, F.M. (1994). Lithium and tricyclic augmentation of fluoxetine treatment for resistant major depression: a double-blind, controlled study. *American Journal of Psychiatry,* **151**, 1372–4.

Filteau, M.J., Lapierre, Y.D., Bakish, D., & Blanchard, B. (1992). Clinical profiles of antidepressants: a meta-analysis on 400 patients. Presented at the American Psychiatric Association Annual Meeting, Washington, DC.

Filteau, M.J., Baruch, P., Bakish, D., Blanchard, A., Pourcher, E., & Lapierre, Y.D. (1993). Specific Serotonin Reuptake Inhibitors and Agitated Depression. Presented at the American Psychiatric Association Annual Meeting. San Francisco, CA.

Flint, A.J. & Rifat, S.L. (1994). A prospective study of lithium augmentation in antidepressant-resistant geriatric depression. *Journal of Clinical Psychopharmacology,* **14**, 353–6.

Gagiano, C.A., Mueller, P.G.M., Fourie, J., & LeRoux, J.F. (1989). The therapeutic efficacy of paroxetine: (a) an open study in patients with major depression not responding to antidepressants; (b) a double-blind comparison with amitriptyline in depressed outpatients. *Acta Psychiatrica Scandinavica,* **80**(Suppl. 350), 130–1.

Gupta, S., Masand, P., & Tanquary, J.F. (1991). Thyroid supplementation of fluoxetine in the treatment of major depression. *British Journal of Psychiatry,* **159**, 866–7.

Hardy, B.G., Shulman, K.I., & Zucchero, C. (1997). Gradual discontinuation of lithium augmentation in elderly patients with unipolar depression. *Journal of Clinical Psychopharmacology,* **17**, 22–6.

Hawley, C.J., Roberts, A.G., & Walker, M.H. (1994). Tolerability of combined treatment with lithium and paroxetine: 19 cases treated under open conditions. *Journal of Psychopharmacology,* **8**, 266–7.

Hoes, M.J. & Zeijpveld, J.H. (1996). First report of mirtazapine overdose. *International Clinical Psychopharmacology,* **11**, 147.

Horgan, D. (1993). Combined fluoxetine and desipramine in resistant depression. *Autralia and New Zealand Journal of Psychiatry,* **27**, 166, 168.

Joffe, R.T. (1992). Triiodothyronine potentiation of fluoxetine in depressed patients. *Canadian Journal of Psychiatry,* **37**, 48–50.

Joffe, R.T. & Schuller, D.R. (1993). An open study of buspirone augmentation of serotonin reuptake inhibitors in refractory depression. *Journal of Clinical Psychiatry,* **54**, 269–71.

Joffe, R.T. & Singer, W. (1990). A comparison of triiodothyronine and thyroxine in the potentiation of tricyclic antidepressants. *Psychological Research,* **32**, 241–51.

Joffe, R.T., Singer, W., Levitt, A.J., & MacDonald, C. (1993). A placebo-controlled comparison of lithium and triiodothyronine augmentation of tricyclic antidepressants in unipolar refractory depression. *Archives of General Psychiatry,* **50**, 387–93.

Joffe, R.T., Levitt, A.J., Sokolov, S.T.H., & Young, L.T. (1996). Response to an open trial of a second SSRI in major depression. *Journal of Clinical Psychiatry*, **57**, 114–15.

Kopala, L. & Honer, W.G. (1994). Risperidone, serotonergic mechanisms, and obsessive-compulsive symptoms in schizophrenia. *American Journal of Psychiatry*, **151**, 1714–15.

Labbate, L.A. & Pollack, M.H. (1994). Treatment of fluoxetine-induced sexual dysfunction with bupropion: a case resport. *Annals of Clinical Psychiatry*, **6**, 13–15.

Linet, L.S. (1989). Treatment of a refractory depression with a combination of fluoxetine and D-amphetamine. *American Journal of Psychiatry*, **146**, 803–4.

Marshall, R.D., Johannet, C.M., Collins, P.Y., Smith, H., Kahn, D.A., & Douglas, C.J. (1995). Bupropion and sertraline combination treatment in refractory depression. *Journal of Psychopharmacology*, **9**, 284–6.

McGrath, P.J., Stewart, J.W., Harrison, W.M. et al. (1992). Predictive value of symptoms of atypical depression for differential drug treatment outcome. *Journal of Clinical Psychopharmacology*, **12**, 197–202.

Metz, A. & Shader, R.I. (1991). Combination of fluoxetine with pemoline in the treatment of major depressive disorder. *International Clinical Psychopharmacology*, **6**, 93–6.

Miller, H.L., Delgado, P.L., Salomon, R.M., Berman, R.M., & Charney, D.S. (1995). Combined desipramine and fluoxetine treatment in refractory depression. Presented at the American Psychiatric Association Annual Meeting, Miami, FL.

Montgomery, S.A. (1995). Safety of mirtazapine: a review. *International Clinical Psychopharmacology*, **10**, Suppl. 4, 3745.

Nelson, J.C., Docherty, J.P., Kasper, S., Nierenberg, A., & Ward, G. (1996). Algorithms for the treatment of subtypes of unipolar major depression. *Psychopharmacology Bulletin*, **31**, 475–82.

Nierenberg, A.A. (1991). Treatment choice after one antidepressant fails: a survey of northeastern psychiatrists. *Journal of Clinical Psychiatry*, **52**, 383–5.

Nierenberg, A.A., Adler, L.A., Peselow, E., Zornberg, G., & Rosenthal, M. (1994a). Trazodone for antidepressant-associated insomnia. *American Journal of Psychiatry*, **151**, 1069–72.

Nierenberg, A.A., Cole, J.O., & Glass, L. (1992). Possible trazodone potentiation of fluoxetine: a case series. *Journal of Clinical Psychiatry*, **53**, 83–5.

Nierenberg, A.A., Feighner, J.P., Rudolph, R., Cole, J.O., & Sullivan, J. (1994b). Venlafaxine for treatment-resistant unipolar depression. *Journal of Clinical Psychopharmacology*, **14**, 419–23.

Nolen, W.A., van-de-Putte, J.J., Dijken, W.A. et al. (1988). Treatment strategy in depression. II. MAO inhibitors in depression resistant to cyclic antidepressants: two controlled crossover studies with tranylcypromine versus L-5-hydroxytryptophan and nomifensine. *Acta Psychiatrica Scandinavica*, **78**, 676–83.

Norden, M.J. (1995). Buspirone treatment of sexual dysfunction associated with selective serotonin reuptake inhibitors. *Depression*, **2**, 109–12.

Ontiveros, A., Fontaine, R., & Elie, R. (1991). Refractory depression: the addition of lithium to fluoxetine or desipramine. *Acta Psychiatrica Scandinavica*, **83**, 188–92.

Otton, S.V., Ball, S.E., Inaba, T., & Sellers, E.M. (1994). Interaction of Venlafaxine, a new antidepressant, with CYP2D6 in human liver microsomes. Presented at the XIX CINP meeting, Washington, DC.

Peselow, E.D., Filippi, A.M., Goodnick, P., Barouche, F., & Rieve, R.R. (1989). The short- and long-term efficacy of paroxetine hcl: B. Data from a double-blind crossover study and from a year-long term trial vs. imipramine and placebo. *Psychopharmacology Bulletin*, **25**, 272–6.

Preskorn, S.H., Alderman, J., Chung, M., Harrison, W., Messign, M., & Harris, S. (1994). Pharmacokinetics of desipramine coadministered with sertraline or fluoxetine. *Journal of Clinical Psychopharmacology*, **14**, 90–8.

Preskorn, S.H., Beber, J.H., Faul, J.C., & Hirschfield, R.M.A. (1990). Serious adverse effects of combining fluoxetine and tricyclic antidepressants. *American Journal of Psychiatry*, **147**, 532.

Quitkin, F.M., McGrath, P.J., Stewart, J.W. et al. (1990). Atypical depression, panic attacks, and response to imipramine and phenelzine. A replication. *Archives of General Psychiatry*, **47**, 935–41.

Rickels, K., Derivan, A., Entsuah, R., Miska, S., & Rudolph, R. (1995). Rapid onset of antidepressant activity with venlafaxine treatment. *Depression*, **3**, 146–53.

Robinson, D.S., Roberts, D.L., Smith, J.M. et al. (1996). The safety profile of nefazodone. *Journal of Clinical Psychiatry*, **57** Suppl. 2, 31–8.

Rudolph, R.L. & Derivan, A.T. (1996). The safety and tolerability of venlafaxine hydrochloride: analysis of clinical trials database. *Journal of Clinical Psychopharmacology*, **16** Suppl. 2, 54–61.

Schwarcz, G., Halaris, A., Baxter, L., Escobar, J., Thompson, M., & Young, M. (1984). Normal thyroid function in desipramine nonresponders converted to responders by the addition of L-triiodothyronine. *American Journal of Psychiatry*, **141**, 1614–16.

Schweizer, E. & Riskels, K. (1991). Serotonergic antidepressants: a review of their clinical efficacy. In *5HT1a Agonists, 5-HT3 Antagonists and Benzodiazepines: Their Comparative Behavioral Pharmacology*, ed. R.J. Rodgers & S.J. Cooper, pp. 366–76. Chichester: John Wiley.

Simpson, S.G. & DePaulo, J.R. (1991). Fluoxetine treatment of bipolar II depression. *Journal of Clinical Psychopharmacology*, **11**, 52–4.

Spiller, H.A., Ramoska, E.A., Krenzelok, E.P., Sheen, S.R., Borys, D.J., Villalobos, D. et al. (1994). Bupropion overdose: a 3-year multi-center retrospective analysis. *American Journal of Emerging Medicine*, **12**, 43–5.

Stein, G. & Bernardt, M. (1993). Lithium augmentation therapy in tricyclic-resistant depression: a controlled trial using lithium in low and normal doses. *British Journal of Psychiatry*, **162**, 634–40.

Stoll, A.L., Pillay, S.S., Diamond, L., Workum, S.B., & Cole, J.O. (1996). Methylphenidate augmentation of serotonin selective reuptake inhibitors: a case series. *Journal of Clinical Psychiatry*, **57**, 72–6.

Thase, M.B., Blomgren, S.L., Birkett, M.A., Apter, J.T., & Tepner, R. (1997). Fluoxetine treatment of patients with major depressive disorder who failed initial treatment with sertraline. *Journal of Clinical Psychiatry*, **58**, 16–21.

Thase, M.E., Frank, E., Mallinger, A.G., Hamer, T., & Kupfer, D.J. (1992a). Treatment of imipramine-resistant recurrent depression, III: Efficacy of monoamine oxidase inhibitors. *Journal of Clinical Psychiatry*, **53**, 5–11.

Thase, M.E., Mallinger, A.G., McKnight, D., & Himmelhoch, J.M. (1992b). Treatment of imipramine-resistant recurrent depression. IV: A double-blind crossover study of tranylcypromine for anergic bipolar depression. *American Journal of Psychiatry*, **149**, 195–8.

Thase, M.E., Keller, M.D., Gelenberg, A., Hirschfield, S., & Schatzberg, A. (1995). Double-blind crossover antidepressant study: sertraline vs. imipramine. Presented at the New Clinical Drug Evaluation Unit Conference.

Walker, P.W., Cole, J.O., Gardner, E.A. et al. (1993). Improvement in fluoxetine-associated sexual dysfunction in patients switched to bupropion. *Journal of Clinical Psychiatry*, **54**, 459–65.

Weilburg, J.B., Rosenbaum, J.F., Meltzer-Brody, S., & Shushtari, J. (1991). Tricyclic augmentation of fluoxetine. *Annals of Clinical Psychiatry*, **3**, 209–13.

White, K., Wykoff, W., Tynes, L.L., Schneider, L., & Zemansky, M. (1990). Fluvoxamine in the treatment of tricyclic-resistant depression. *Psychiatric Journal of the University of Ottawa*, **15**, 156–8.

Zarate, Jr C.A., Kando, J.C., Tohen, M., Weiss, M.K., & Cole, J.O. (1996). Does intolerance or lack of response with fluoxetine predict the same will happen with sertraline? *Journal of Clinical Psychiatry*, **57**, 67–71.

# 9

# Conventional and second generation monoamine oxidase inhibitors in treatment-resistant depression

David Bakish and Cynthia L. Hooper

## Introduction

The treatment of patients with treatment-resistant depressive illness can be frustrating to clinicians as, by definition, conventional antidepressant treatments have failed. This, despite having effective treatment-resistant depression therapies such as tricyclic antidepressants (TCAs), monoamine oxidase inhibitors (MAOIs), reversible inhibitors of monoamine oxidase A (RIMAs); dopamine reuptake inhibitors, specific serotonin reuptake inhibitors (SSRIs), 5-HT$_2$ antagonists, serotonin–noradrenaline reuptake inhibitors (SNRIs), and electroconvulsive treatment (ECT). This chapter will examine the efficacy of conventional and second generation monoamine oxidase inhibitors in treatment-resistant depression.

Both classical monoamine oxidase inhibitors and reversible inhibitors of monoamine oxidase A have been underutilized in the treatment of treatment-resistant depression. There are several potential reasons for this including the food and drug interactions found in classical monoamine oxidase inhibitor treatment (Blackwell et al., 1967) and early negative research findings including the Medical Research Council study of 1965, where the monoamine oxidase inhibitor phenelzine was found to be less effective than imipramine or electroconvulsive therapy (Medical Research Council, 1965). The conclusion was that MAOIs are 'drugs of narrow therapeutic utility and have not emerged as drug of choice in the treatment of any type of depressive illness' (Simpson & Cabot, 1974, p. 155).

Further research has now shown that both the specific and non-specific types of monoamine oxidase inhibitors have therapeutic utility and are starting to become more widely used in the treatment of treatment-resistant depression (Martin et al., 1994).

## Classical monoamine oxidase inhibitors (Fig. 9.1)

The three classical monoamine oxidase inhibitors used at present are phenelzine, tranylcypromine, and isocarboxazid. Iproniazid was the first of the classical

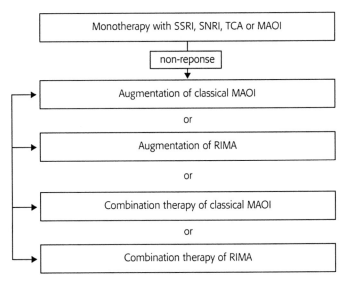

Fig. 9.1.     Treatment of treatment-resistant depression with monoamine oxidase inhibitors.

monoamine oxidase inhibitors, discovered by accident in 1957 through investigations of the side effects of tuberculosis treatment. It was found that as many as 75% of patients with depressive illness improved as much or more with iproniazid as with ECT (Kline, 1958). In England, West and Dally (1959) conducted clinical trials with iproniazid and found that it was of particular value in treating patients with 'atypical' depressive illness, characterized by self-reproach, p.m. diurnal variation, phobias, hysterical conversion symptoms, tremor, and personality disorder. They found that iproniazid was less effective in the typical endogenous depressive illness. However, soon after the publication of their trials, there were reports of fatal hepatitis caused by the administration of iproniazid, and it was pulled from the market.

More negative research results occurred in the early 1960s when phenelzine was found not to be statistically effective either alone (Harris & Robin, 1960) or when compared to imipramine or electroconvulsive therapy (Greenblatt et al., 1964). However, phenelzine had been used to treat severe inpatient endogenous depression, which, it is now clear, is not the ideal patient group for MAOIs. Sargant and Dally (1962) discovered through clinical experience that monoamine oxidase inhibitors seem to have a beneficial effect in depressed patients with phobic and anxiety symptoms. Patients with self-reproach, no early morning awakening, phobias, depressed mood which is better in the morning, and what was called 'inadequate personalities' appeared to do better on MAOIs.

Blackwell (1963; Blackwell et al., 1967) found that there was a potential tyramine interaction between monoamine oxidase inhibitors and certain foods.

There are also differences between the MAOIs in terms of safety and efficacy. Iproniazid is the most dangerous, but also the most powerful, while the safest of the monoamine oxidase inhibitors is isocarboxazid, which is also the weakest (Tyrer, 1982). The compound in the middle of the therapeutic and toxic range is phenelzine, which has emerged as the preferred choice of all the MAOIs, providing a balance between safety and efficacy. Tranylcypromine is different as it is not a hydrazine like the other MAOIs. It is also different in that clinical response occurs within 3 weeks of the start of treatment, it possibly has amphetamine-like action, and it possesses greater energizing properties, which may make it useful in the treatment of resistant depression (Shawcross & Tyrer, 1987).

With the knowledge about interactions and MAOIs, in addition to the studies showing poor efficacy in certain types of depression, the use of monoamine oxidase inhibitors decreased markedly. They were used only for very specific patient cases and were not studied in any great detail. MAOIs were so under-utilized that Garfinkel et al. (1979) showed that only 7% of psychiatry residents in Canada received supervision in the use of MAOIs.

It has been shown that dose is likely the best predictor of response (Young et al., 1986). Phenelzine doses of 30 mg per day were no more effective than placebo, but a dose of 60 mg per day was statistically superior (Ravaris et al., 1976). Robinson et al. (1973) stated that an adequate trial of phenelzine appears to require a dose of 1 mg per kilogram of body weight per day. The guideline doses for isocarboxazid and tranylcypromine are not as clear. For tranylcypromine, doses of 30 mg/day to 60 mg/day may be adequate, but higher doses of 60 to 90 mg/day are often required. In resistant depression higher doses of up to 200 mg may be necessary (Martin et al., 1994).

Maximal platelet MAO inhibition occurs within 2 to 4 weeks of starting treatment (Robinson et al., 1978). Therefore, it is important to realize that maximum effect may not be reached until 6 weeks of treatment (Tyrer, 1976). It has also been reported that there may be continued improvement with phenelzine up to 4 months after initiating the trial (Hamilton, 1982). It is thus also important in the treatment of depression, and especially treatment-resistant depression, to take into account: (i) the dose of the MAOI, and (ii) the length of time that the patient has been treated at an adequate dose.

McGrath et al. (1987) treated patients in a crossover design with high doses of phenelzine (maximum 90 mg), imipramine (maximum 300 mg) or placebo and found that of the non-responders, only 4 of 14 patients responded to a tricyclic crossover vs. 17 of 26 patients who responded to a MAOI crossover. This difference was statistically significant and there seemed to be a preferential re-sponse in resistant patients with atypical depression symptoms to the use of phenelzine. Nolen et al. (1988) subsequently showed that not only patients with atypical depressive symptoms but also patients with major depression and melancholia responded to MAOIs, in particular tranylcypromine.

Because of the risk of interaction with tyramine and their adverse side effects, classical MAOIs are usually recommended as a second or third step after unsuccessful treatment with a standard tricyclic antidepressant, SSRI, other new generation drug, or lithium augmentation (Nolen & Haffmans, 1989).

## Selective monoamine oxidase A inhibitors

The new reversible and selective monoamine oxidase A inhibitors (RIMAs) such as moclobemide, brofaromine and toloxatone have fewer adverse effects and, because MAO-B is still available for tyramine degradation, no diet restrictions. These drugs have an ease of use and safety profile which is much improved compared to the classical MAOIs (Amrein et al., 1989; Möller et al., 1991). Moclobemide and brofaromine inhibit monoamine oxidase A by 80% within 30 minutes of administration and the enzyme activity recovers almost completely within 24 hours. Thus, both of these drugs are short acting and when stopped, the antidepressant effect disappears in 3 to 8 days. (Bieck & Antonin, 1989). The safety of these drugs is much greater than classical non-reversible, non-selective monoamine oxidase inhibitors. Moclobemide is the most thoroughly investigated of these compounds and has been shown, in multiple clinical trials, to be an effective antidepressant in doses of 300–600 mg per day. It is comparable in antidepressant effectiveness to tranylcypromine (Rossel & Moll, 1990); isocarboxazid (Larsen et al., 1991); tricyclic antidepressants such as amitriptyline (Bakish et al., 1992; Newburn et al., 1990; Norman et al., 1985), imipramine (Baumhackl et al., 1989), clomipramine (Guelfi et al., 1992) and desipramine (Stefanis et al., 1984); as well as the newer SSRIs such as fluvoxamine (Bougerol et al., 1992).

There are few studies with moclobemide in resistant depressed patients. Nolen et al. (1994) switched patients with resistant depression in remission (mean treatment year of 4.3 years) receiving tranylcypromine to moclobemide. The dose of moclobemide varied from 450 to 900 mg per day and patients were followed for 2 months. Sixteen of the 28 patients showed deterioration and were put back on tranylcypromine, nine because of relapse.

Brofaromine trials have shown it to be as effective as tranylcypromine or imipramine (Möller et al., 1991). Chouinard et al. (1994) demonstrated in a multinational placebo-controlled trial with brofaromine and placebo that, when the sleep items were taken out of the Hamilton Rating Depression scale, brofaromine was significantly better than placebo. In resistant major depressive patients, brofaromine was found to be as efficacious as tranylcypromine (Nolen et al., 1993; Volz et al., 1994). Brofaromine appeared to be an effective, easy-to-use

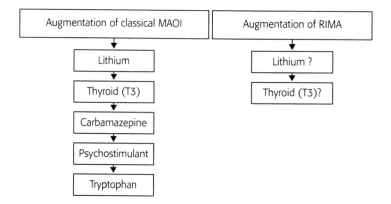

Fig. 9.2.    Suggestions for augmentation therapies with classical MAOIs or RIMAs.

antidepressant. However, because of its adverse effect on sleep, it has not been developed further as an antidepressant.

## Potentiation strategies (Fig. 9.2)

### Lithium carbonate

Lithium carbonate is an effective potentiator of tricyclic antidepressants. It prevents recurrent affective episode in bipolar patients possibly by augmenting neuronal postsynaptic serotonin receptor sensitivity. Lithium has been combined with MAOIs with good efficacy (de Montigny et al., 1983; Nelson & Byck 1982; Blier et al., 1984; Price et al., 1985). It is important to ensure that patients on both lithium and classical MAOIs are monitored closely, completing lithium levels regularly to monitor for toxicity. At present, there are no comparative studies evaluating the safety and efficacy of lithium potentiation of RIMAs.

### Other mood stabilizers

Carbamazepine is the best studied of the anticonvulsants in both unipolar and bipolar affective disorders. The use of classical MAOIs with carbamazepine should be done carefully as early studies have shown that MAOIs increase the carbamazepine drug level (Wright et al., 1982; Valsalan & Cooper, 1982). Recently Ketter et al. (1995) combined phenelzine with carbamazepine in treatment resistant patients and found that four out of ten patients improved. There are no reports of trials combining RIMAs and other mood stabilizers.

### Thyroid hormone

There have been no controlled studies examining the combination of MAOIs or RIMAs with T3 or T4, although there is good evidence for the usefulness of thyroid augmentation of tricyclic antidepressants (Earle, 1970; Prange et al., 1969).

### Psychostimulants

Case studies have reported treatment response in treatment-resistant patients when using a classical MAOI combined with a psychostimulant (Fawcett et al., 1991; Feighner et al., 1985). However, these case studies also found that severe adverse reactions can occur. Therefore, psychostimulants should be used in combination with classical MAOIs only for the most treatment-resistant patients and under very close observation. There are no reported studies on the use of psychostimulants and RIMAs in the treatment of treatment-resistant depressive illness.

### Tryptophan

There are placebo-controlled trials which have found tryptophan superior to placebo in augmenting phenelzine, tranylcypromine and nialimide (Coppen et al., 1963; Glassman & Platman, 1969; Gutierrez & Alino, 1971). However, one must be careful with this combination as there have also been reports of serotonin syndrome, characterized by fever, hyperactivity, sedation, hypertension, and myoclonus (Insel et al., 1982; Pope et al., 1985). An excellent review by Young (1991) stated quite clearly that potentiation of MAOI by tryptophan implies, but does not prove, that it should be effective in treatment-resistant patients. There have been no published studies of tryptophan used to augment RIMAs.

## Combination treatment with other antidepressants (Fig. 9.3)

Classical MAOIs have been combined with other antidepressants since their earliest days of use. RIMAs offer a relatively safer option which can benefit the treatment-resistant patient.

### Tricyclic antidepressants

Tricyclic antidepressants have been used in combination with MAOIs since the early 1960s and are, in general, safe and effective if the MAOI is added to the tricyclic or if both medications are started simultaneously (Pandy et al., 1991). Berlanga and Ortega-Soto (1995) showed that a group of resistant depressed patients did well on a combination of amitriptyline and isocarboxazid. In an open study by Sethna (1974), 12 treatment-resistant patients were noted to be improved on a combination of phenelzine and amitriptyline. The use of amitriptyline along with phenelzine seems to be one of the safest combinations (Davidson et al., 1978). However, the combination of MAOIs with clomipramine or imipramine is much

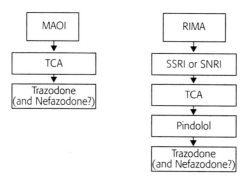

Fig. 9.3.    Suggestions for combination therapy with classical MAOIs or RIMAs.

more risky especially when clomipramine is added to tranylcypromine (Ananth & Luchins, 1977). There is a possibility of serious adverse events such as agitation, hyperthermia, delirium, and death (White & Simpson, 1984; Oefele et al., 1986). It is recommended that clomipramine be used in combination with MAOIs only in extreme circumstances and with close supervision.

The reversible inhibitors of MAO-A, in particular, moclobemide, are able to be combined safely with amitriptyline if the RIMA is added to a therapeutic dose of amitriptyline. Moclobemide in combination with clomipramine or citalopram (an SSRI available in Canada and the United Kingdom); however, has been shown to have a significant hazard of serotonin syndrome (Norman & Burroughs, 1995; Neuvonen et al., 1993).

### Specific serotonin reuptake inhibitors

The use of specific serotonin reuptake inhibitors in combination with classical MAOIs is not recommended. Virtually all patients develop some degree of serotonin syndrome, and some have died (Feighner et al., 1990). It is particularly dangerous to use fluoxetine, which has an active metabolite with an extremely long half-life, with phenelzine, which is a non-competitive, non-selective MAOI. The combination could lead to a serotonin syndrome which would continue for many days upon stopping the combination (Sternbach, 1988).

Research on the combination of moclobemide with SSRIs has demonstrated efficacy and safety in treatment-resistant patients, if the precaution is taken to either start low doses of both agents together or to add moclobemide at lower than normal doses to lower than normal doses of SSRIs (Ebert et al., 1995; Joffe & Bakish, 1994; Bakish et al., 1995).

### Serotonin and noradrenergic reuptake inhibitors – Venlafaxine

The development of a serotonin and noradrenergic reuptake inhibitor (SNRI) venlafaxine led to its use in combination with classical MAOIs. The results were poor and led to a patient developing serotonin syndrome when he was rapidly switched from a non-reversible classical MAOI phenelzine to venlafaxine (Heisler et al., 1996; Klysner et al., 1995). There have yet been no reports of any adverse reaction of venlafaxine with RIMAs.

### SSRI and 5-HT2 antagonists – trazodone and nefazodone

Nefazodone is an antidepressant which is a mild serotonin and noradrenergic reuptake inhibitor but primarily a 5-HT2 antagonist with enhanced 5-HT1A neurotransmission (Taylor et al., 1995). There have been no reports of any untoward reactions with the combination of nefazodone and a classical MAOI or a RIMA. In addition, trazodone, a chemical cousin of nefazodone, has been used clinically for years to treat the insomnia which is often a side effect of classical MAOI treatment (Nierenberg & Keck, 1989). Trazodone has also been used safely in combination with SSRIs such as fluvoxamine, sertraline, paroxetine and fluoxetine and with moclobemide (Bakish et al., 1995), suggesting nefazodone might be safely and efficaciously combined with moclobemide.

### Other medications

Buspirone, marketed as an anxiolytic but thought to have antidepressant effects, has led to adverse interactions with classical MAOIs in which patients' blood pressure ratings increased significantly after a 5 mg dose of buspirone was added to the treatment regimen (Gelenberg, 1990). There are no reports on combining RIMAs with buspirone.

There is some suggestion that bupropion can be combined with tranylcypromine with efficacious effect in resistant depression (Abbuzzahab, 1994).

Tranylcypromine was combined with mianserin, a tricyclic compound used in the United Kingdom, and resulted in many depressed patients responding markedly within the first week and a majority of patients responding by 2 weeks (Graham, 1988; Nierenberg & Keck, 1989). They were not treatment-resistant patients, but the study demonstrated that the combination was relatively safe.

Thornton et al. (1996) gave patients with treatment-resistant depressive illness combinations of moclobemide, venlafaxine, nefazodone, trazodone, fluoxetine, paroxetine, sertraline, fluvoxamine and/or lithium carbonate. Several patients experienced a reduction in symptoms, although it was often transitory. The combinations were all well tolerated. It is important to note that, in all cases, the doses of the medications were less than standard doses.

## Clinical applications

The first-line treatment for treatment-resistant depression should be a specific serotonin reuptake inhibitor (SSRI) such as fluoxetine, paroxetine, sertraline, and fluvoxamine, or a serotonin and norepinephrine reuptake inhibitor (SNRI) such as venlafaxine. If, after an adequate trial, symptoms remain, combination treatment with a reversible inhibitor of monoamine oxidase A (RIMA – moclobemide, brofaromine) should be considered. We recommend the use of moclobemide over standard MAOIs as there are no dietary restrictions, reduced risk of interactions, and a reduced risk of serotonin syndrome. In all cases, lower than standard doses of SSRIs and SNRIs should be combined with lower than standard doses of moclobemide. In particular, a starting dose of 75 mg/day of moclobemide can be added to fluoxetine 10 mg/day, paroxetine 10 mg/day, sertraline 15 mg/day, fluvoxamine 50 mg/day or venlafaxine 75 mg/day. If symptoms remain, moclobemide can be increased up to 300 mg/day. If insomnia develops as a side effect of the combination, trazodone 25–75 mg/day can be added to aid sleep. In our clinic we have also found that combining moclobemide to low dose nefazodone (75 mg/day) can be helpful in treatment-resistant cases, particularly in patients with phobic and avoidance symptoms. It is important to remember that these combination strategies should be used in extreme cases only, should always use lower than standard dosages, and require careful monitoring of the patient for signs of serotonin syndrome.

The second-line treatment strategy should be the combination of a tricyclic antidepressant and moclobemide. We recommend using amitriptyline 150 mg/day with moclobemide 75 mg bid up to 300 mg bid. Do not use clomipramine in combination with moclobemide as the combination can result in the serotonin syndrome.

Finally, there have been a number of studies recently examining the combination of pindolol, a $\beta$-adrenergic antagonist and pre-synaptic 5-HT$_{1A}$ antagonist, with SSRIs (Blier & Bergeron, 1996; Bakish et al., 1997). Blier and Bergeron (1995) in one study included two patients taking moclobemide for drug-resistant depression. They added pindolol 2.5 mg tid to moclobemide 300 mg tid. One patient stopped the pindolol augmentation after 3 days of treatment because of increased irritability, but the other patient experienced a drop of 15 points on the Hamiliton Depression Scale after 1 week of treatment. This is certainly an exciting new area of research and may contribute greatly to the treatment of patients with treatment-resistant depression.

The use of monoamine oxidase inhibitors in the treatment of depressive illness has a long history. Research has provided us with guidelines for using MAOIs in particular cases (atypical depression, anxiety symptoms), and has led to the development of reversible and specific inhibitors of MAO-A. The particular advantage of MAOIs in treatment-resistant depressive illness is in combination treatment, where the RIMA moclobemide can be combined safely and effectively with SSRIs, SNRIs, TCAs and possibly pindolol.

## REFERENCES

Abbuzzahab, F.S. Sr. (1994). Combination therapy: monoamine oxidase inhibitors and bupropion HCI, *Neuropsychopharmacology*, **10**(3S)2, 74S.

Amrein, R., Allen, S.R., Guentert, T.W. et al. (1989). The pharmacology of reversible monoamine oxidase inhibitors. *British Journal of Psychiatry*, **155**(6), 66–71.

Ananth, F. & Luchins, D. (1977). A review of combined tricyclic and MAOI therapy. *Comprehensive Psychiatry*, **18**, 221–30.

Bakish, D., Bradwejn, J., Nair, N., McClure, J., Remick, R., & Bulger, L. (1992). A comparison of moclobemide, amitriptyline and placebo in depression: a Canadian multicentre study. *Psychopharmacology*, **106**, S98–S101.

Bakish, D., Hooper, C.L., West, D.L., Miller, C., Blanchard, A., & Bashir, F. (1995). Moclobemide and specific serotonin reuptake inhibitor combination treatment of resistant anxiety and depressive disorders. *Human Psychopharmacology*, **10**(2), 105–9.

Bakish, D., Hooper, C.L., Thornton, M.D., Wiens, A., Miller, C.A., & Thibaudeau, C.A. (1997). Rapid onset: an open study of the treatment of major depressive disorder with nefazodone and pindolol combination therapy. *International Clinical Psychopharmacology*, **12**(2), 91–7.

Baumhackl, U., Biziere, K., Fischbach, R. et al. (1989). Efficacy and tolerability of moclobemide compared with imipramine in depressive disorder (DSM III): an Australian double-blind, multicentre study. *British Journal of Psychiatry*, **155**(6), 78–83.

Berlanga, C. & Ortega-Soto, H.A. (1995). A 3-year follow-up of a group of treatment-resistant depressed patients with a MAOI/tricyclic combination. *Journal of Affective Disorder*, **34**(3), 187–92.

Bieck, P.R. & Antonin, K.H. (1989). Tyramine potentiation during treatment with MAO inhibitors: brofaromine and moclobemide vs irreversible inhibitors. *Journal of Neural Transmission*, **28**, 21–31.

Blackwell, B. (1963). Hypertensive cases due to monoamine oxidase inhibitors. *Lancet*, **ii**, 849–51.

Blackwell, B., Marley, E., Price, J., & Taylor, D. (1967). Hypotensive interactions between monoamine oxidase inhibitors and foodstuffs. *British Journal of Psychiatry*, **113**, 349–65.

Blier, P. & Bergeron, R. (1995). Effectiveness of pindolol with selected antidepressant drugs in the treatment of major depression. *Journal of Clinical Psychopharmacology*, **15**(3), 217–22.

Blier, P., de Montigny, C., & Azzaro, A.J. (1984). Modification of serotonergic and noradrenergic neurotransmission by long term administration of monoamine oxidase inhibitors. *Society of NeuroScience*, Abstract, **10**, 6.

Bougerol, T., Uchida, C., Gachoud, J.P. et al. (1992). Efficacy and tolerability of moclobemide as compared to fluvoxamine in depressive disorder (DSM III): a French/Swiss double-blind trial. *Psychopharmacology (Berl.)*, **106**(Suppl.), 102–8.

Chouinard, G., Saxena, B.M., Nair, N.P.V. et al. (1994). A Canadian multicentre, placebo-controlled study of a fixed dose of brofaromine, a reversible selective MAO-A inhibitor, in the treatment of major depression. *Journal of Affective Disorders*, **32**, 105–14.

Coppen, A., Shaw, D.M., & Farrell, J.P. (1963). Potentiation of the antidepressive effect of a monoamine oxidase inhibitor by tryptophan. *Lancet*, **1**, 79–81.

Davidson, J., McLeod, M.N., Law-Yone, B. et al. (1978). Comparison of electroconvulsive therapy and combined phenelzine–amitriptyline in refractory depression. *Archives of General Psychiatry*, **35**, 639–42.

de Montigny, C., Cournoyer, G., Morisette, R., Langlois, R., & Caille, G. (1983). Lithium carbonate addition in tricyclic antidepressant-resistant unipolar depression. *Archives of General Psychiatry*, **40**, 1327–34.

Earle, B.V. (1970). Thyroid hormone and tricyclic antidepressants in resistant depressions. *American Journal of Psychiatry*, **126**, 1667–9.

Ebert, D., Albert, R., May, A., Stosiek, I., & Kaschka, W. (1995). Combined SSRI–RIMA treatment in refractory depression. Safety data and efficacy. *Psychopharmacology*, **119**(3), 342–4.

Fawcett, J., Kravitz, H.M., Zajecka, J.M. et al. (1991). CNS stimulant potentiation of monoamine oxidase inhibitors in treatment-refractory depression. *Journal of Clinical Psychopharmacology*, **11**, 127–32.

Feighner, J.P., Herbstein, J., & Damlouji, N. (1985). Combined MAOI, TCA and direct stimulant therapy of treatment-resistant depression. *Journal of Clinical Psychiatry*, **46**, 206–9.

Feighner, J.P., Boyer, W.F., Tyler, D.L., & Neborsky, R.J. (1990). Adverse consequences of fluoxetine–MAOI combination therapy. *Journal of Clinical Psychiatry*, **51**(6), 222–5.

Garfinkel, P.E., Cameron, P., & Kingstone, E. (1979). Psychopharmacology education in psychiatry. *Canadian Journal of Psychiatry*, **24**, 644–51.

Gelenberg, A.J. (1990). Buspirone–MAOI interaction. *Biological Therapy and Psychiatry*, **13**(9), 36.

Glassman, A.H. & Platman, S.R. (1969). Potentiation of a monoamine oxidase inhibitor by tryptophan. *Journal of Psychiatric Research*, **7**, 83–8.

Graham, P.M. (1988). Combined mianserin and tranylcypromine (letter to the editor). *British Journal of Psychiatry*, **153**, 415–16.

Greenblatt, M., Grosser, G.H., & Wechsler, H. (1964). Differential response of hospitalized depressed patients to somatic therapy. *American Journal of Psychiatry*, **120**, 935–43.

Guelfi, J.D., Payan, C., Fermanian, J. et al. (1992). Moclobemide versus clomipramine in endogenous depression: a double-blind randomized clinical trial. *British Journal of Psychiatry*, **160**, 519–24.

Gutierrez, J.L.A. & Alino, J.J.L. (1971). Tryptophan and an MAOI (Nialimide) in the treatment of depression, *International Pharmacopsychiatry*, **6**, 92–7.

Hamilton, M. (1982). The effect of treatment on the melancholias (depressions). *British Journal of Psychiatry*, **140**, 223–30.

Harris, J.A. & Robin, A.A. (1960). A controlled trial of phenelzine in depressive reactions. *Journal of Mental Science*, **106**, 1432–7.

Heisler, M.A., Guibry, J.R., & Arnecke, B. (1996). Serotonin syndrome induced by administration of venlafaxine and phenelzine (letter to the editor). *Annals of Pharmacotherapy*, **30**, 84.

Insel, T.R., Roy, B.F., & Cohen, R.M. (1982). Possible development of the serotonin syndrome in man. *American Journal of Psychiatry*, **139**, 954–5.

Joffe, R.T. & Bakish, D. (1994). Combined SSRI-moclobemide treatment of psychiatric illness. *Journal of Clinical Psychiatry*, **55**, 24–5.

Ketter, T.A., Post, R.M., Parekh, P.I., & Worthington, K. (1995). Addition of monoamine oxidase inhibitors to carbamazepine. Preliminary evidence of safety and antidepressant efficacy in treatment-resistant depression. *Journal of Clinical Psychiatry*, **56**(10), 471–5.

Kline, N.S. (1958). Clinical experience with iproniazid (Marsilid). *Journal of Clinical Experimental Psychopathology*, **19** (Suppl. 1), 72–8.

Klysner, R., Larsen, J.K., Sorensen, P., Hyllested, M., & Pedersen, B.D. (1995). Toxic interaction of venlafaxine and isocarboxacide (letter). *Lancet*, **346**(8985), 1298–9.

Larsen, J.K., Gjerris, A., Holme, P. et al. (1991). Moclobemide in depression: a randomized, multicentre trial against isocarboxazid and clomipramine emphasizing atypical depression. *Acta Psychiatrica Scandinavica*, **84**(55), 564–70.

McGrath, P.J., Stewart, J.W., Harrison, W., & Quitkin, F.M. (1987). Treatment of refractory depression with a monoamine oxidase inhibitor antidepressant. *Psychopharmacology Bulletin*, **23**, 169–72.

Martin, L., Bakish, D., & Joffe, R. (1994). MAOI treatment of depression. In *Clinical Advances in Monoamine Oxidase Inhibitor Therapies*, ed. S.H. Kennedy. Washington, DC: American Psychiatric Press Inc.

Medical Research Council (1965). Clinical Trials Subcommittee. Clinical trial on the treatment of depressive illness. *British Medical Journal*, **2**, 881–6.

Möller, H.J., Wendt, G., & Waldmeier, P. (1991). Brofaromine – a selective, reversible and short-acting MAO-A inhibitor: review of the pharmacological and clinical findings. *Pharmacopsychiatry*, **24**, 50–4.

Nelson, J.C. & Byck, R. (1982). Rapid response to lithium in phenelzine non-responders. *British Journal of Psychiatry*, **141**, 85–6.

Neuvonen, P.J., Pohjola-Sintonen, S., Tacke, U., & Vuori, E. (1993). Five fatal cases of serotonin syndrome after moclobemide-citalopram or moclobemide-clomipramine overdoses (letter to the editor). *Lancet*, **342**, 1419.

Newburn, G.M., Fraser, A.R., Menkes, D.B. et al. (1990). A double blind trial of moclobemide versus amitriptyline in the treatment of depressive disorders. *Australia and New Zealand Journal of Psychiatry*, **24**, 475–9.

Nierenberg, A.A. & Keck, P.E. Jr (1989). Management of monamine oxidase inhibitor associated insomnia with trazodone. *Journal of Clinical Psychopharmacology*, **9**, 42–5.

Nolen, W.A. & Haffmans, P.M.J. (1989). The treatment of resistant depression. *International Journal of Clinical Psychopharmacology*, **4**, 217–28.

Nolen, W.A., Van de Putte, J.J., Dijken, W.A. et al. (1988). Treatment strategy in depression. *Acta Psychiatrica Scandinavica*, **78**, 676–83.

Nolen, W.A., Hoencamp, E., Haffmans, P.M.J., & Bouvy, P.F. (1992). Classical and seclective monoamine oxidase inhibitors in refractory major depression. In *Refractory Depression Current Strategies and Future Directions*, ed. W.A. Nolen, J. Zohar, S.P. Roose, & J.D. Amsterdam, pp. 59–68. Chichester, UK: John Wiley.

Nolen, W.A., Haffmans, P.M.J., Bouvy, P.F., & Duivenvoorden, H.J. (1993). Monoamine oxidase inhibtors in resistant major depression: a double-blind comparison of brofaromine and tranylcypromine in patients resistant to tricylic antidepressants. *Journal of Affective Disorders*, **28**, 189–97.

Nolen, W.A., Hoencamp, E., Hallmans, P.M.J. et al. (1994). Classical and selective monoamine oxidase inhibitors in refractory major depression. In *Refractory Depression: Current Strategies and Future Directions*, ed. W.A. Nolen, J. Zohar, S.P. Roose, & J.D. Amsterdam, pp. 59–68. Chichester, UK: John Wiley.

Norman, T.R. & Burroughs, G.D. (1995). A risk-benefit assessment of moclobemide in the treatment of depressive disorders. *Drug Safety*, **12**(1), 46–54.

Norman, T.R., Aims, D., Burroughs, G.D. et al. (1985). A controlled study of a specific MAO A reversible inhibitor (RO 11–1163) and amitriptyline in depressive illness. *Journal of Affective Disorders*, **8**, 29–35.

Oefele, K.V., Grohmann, R., & Rüther, E. (1986). Adverse drug reactions in combined tricyclic and monoamine oxidase inhibitor therapy. *Pharmacopsychiatry*, **19**, 243–4.

Pandy, A.C., Calarco, M.N., & Grunhaus, L.J. (1991). Combined monoamine oxidase inhibitor TCA treatment in refractory depression. In *Refractory Depression*, ed. J. Amsterdam, pp. 115–21. New York: Raven Press.

Pare, C.N.B. (1963). Potentiation of MAOI by tryptophan. *Lancet*, **2**, 527–8.

Pope, H.G., Jonas, J.M., Hudson, J.I. et al. (1985). Toxic reactions to combination of monoamine oxidase inhibitors and tryptophan. *American Journal of Psychiatry*, **142**, 491–2.

Prange, A.J. Jr, Wilson, I.C., Rabon, A.M., & Lipton, M.A. (1969). Enhancement of imipramine antidepressant activity by thyroid hormone. *American Journal of Psychiatry*, **126**, 457–69.

Price, L.H., Charney, D.S., & Heninger, G.R. (1985). Efficacy of lithium-tranylcypromine treatment in refractory depression. *American Journal of Psychiatry*, **142**, 619–23.

Ravaris, C.L., Nies, A., Robinson, D.S., Ives, J.O., Lamborn, K.R., & Korson, L. (1976). A multiple dose, controlled study of phenelzine in depressive-anxiety states. *Archives of General Psychiatry*, **33**, 347–50.

Robinson, D.S., Nies, A., & Ravaris, C.L. (1973). Clinical pharmacology of phenelzine. *Archives of General Psychiatry*, **37**, 629–35.

Robinson, D.S., Nies, A., Ravaris, C.L., Ives, J.O., & Bartlett, D. (1978). Clinical pharmacology of phenelzine. *Archives in General Psychiatry*, **35**(5), 629–35.

Rossel, L. & Moll, E. (1990). Moclobemide versus tranylcypromine in the treatment of depression. *Acta Psychiatrica Scandinavica*, **360**, 61–2.

Sargant, W. & Dally, P. (1962). Treatment of anxiety states by antidepressant drugs. *British Medical Journal*, **1**, 6–9.

Sethna, E.R. (1974). A case of refractory cases of depressive illness and their response to combined antidepressant treatment. *British Journal of Psychiatry*, **124**, 265–72.

Shawcross, C. & Tyrer, P. (1987). The place of monoamine oxidase inhibitors in the treatment of resistant depression. In *Treating Resistant Depression*, ed. J. Zohar & R.H. Belmaker, pp. 113–30. New York: PMA Publishing Corp.

Simpson, L. & Cabot, B. (1974). Monoamine oxidase inhibitors. In *Drug Treatment of Mental Disorders*, ed. L. Simpson. New York: Raven Press, p. 155.

Stefanis, C.N., Alevizos, B., & Papadimitriou, G. (1984). Moclobemide (RO 11–1163) versus desipramine: a double-blind study in depressive patients. In *Monoamine Oxidase and Disease: Prospects for Therapy with Reversible Inhibitors*, ed. K.F. Tipton, P. Dostert, & M. Strolin Benedetti, pp. 377–92. London: Academic Press.

Sternbach, H. (1988). Danger of monoamine oxidase inhibitor therapy after fluoxetine withdrawal. *Lancet*, **ii**(8615), 850–1.

Taylor, D.P., Carter, R.B., Eison, A.S. et al. (1995). Pharmacology and neurochemistry of nefazodone, a novel antidepressant drug. *Journal of Clinical Psychiatry*, **56**(6), 3–11.

Thornton, M., Bakish, D., & Hooper, C.L. (1996). Examples of combination therapy in treatment-resistant mood disorders. Poster presented at the *19th Annual Meeting of the Canadian College of Neuropsychopharmacology (CCNP)*, June 2–5. Toronto, ON, Canada.

Tyrer, P.J. (1976). Toward rational treatment with monoamine oxidase inhibitors. *British Journal of Psychiatry*, **128**, 354–60.

Tyrer, P.J. (1982). Monoamine oxidase inhibitors and amine precursors. In *Drugs in Psychiatric Practice*, ed. P.J. Tyrer, pp. 249–79, London: Butterworths.

Valsalan, V.C. & Cooper, G.L. (1982). Carbamazepine intoxication caused by interaction with isoniazid. *British Medical Journal*, **285**, 261–2.

Volz, H.P., Faltus, F., Magyar, I., & Moller, H.J. (1994). Brofaromine in treatment-resistant depressed patients – a comparative trial versus tranylcypromine. *Journal of Affective Disorders*, **30**(3), 209–17.

West, E.D. & Dally, P.J. (1959). Effects of iproniazid in depressive syndromes. *British Medical Journal*, **1**, 1491–4.

White, K. & Simpson, G. (1984). The combined use of MAOIs and tricyclics. *Journal of Clinical Psychiatry*, **45**(7, sect 2), 67–9.

Wright, J.M., Stokes, E.F., & Sweeney, V.P. (1982). Isoniazid-induced carbamazepine toxicity and vice versa. *Medical Intelligence*, **307**, 1325–7.

Young, S.N. (1991). Use of tryptophan in combination with other antidepressant treatments. *Journal of Psychiatry and Neuroscience*, **16**(5), 241–6.

Young, W.P., Laws, E.R., Sharbrough, F.W. et al. (1986). Human monoamine oxidase: lack of brain and platelet correlation. *Archives of General Psychiatry*, **43**, 604–9.

# 10

# Drug combination strategies

Lawrence H. Price, Linda L. Carpenter, and Steven A. Rasmussen

## Introduction

Notwithstanding their extraordinary popularity, the new classes of antidepressants introduced during the past decade have not solved the problem of refractory depression. If anything, challenges to the clinician have grown more daunting: more patients are receiving antidepressants, their expectations are higher, third-party payors are now actively involved in monitoring treatment cost and efficiency, and the proliferation of treatment options has made choices among those options more complicated. Moreover, for all of their advantages in terms of safety, tolerability, and efficacy across a range of non-affective disorders, the new agents are not substantially more effective as antidepressants than the older tricyclics and monoamine oxidase inhibitors (MAOIs) (Montgomery, 1995).

Three basic operational strategies have emerged in the pharmacologic management of refractory depression (Table 10.1): (i) optimization of the current drug regimen; (ii) substitution of the current drug with a different drug; and (iii) combination of two or more drugs, one of which may be the current drug. This chapter will review and evaluate various combination approaches through a consideration of the following factors: mechanism of action, evidence of efficacy (including study designs and patient samples), specificity and predictors of response, safety (including common adverse effects and potential major toxicity), and clinical use (including dosage and special requirements). Before turning to this, however, a brief discussion of the terminology of refractory depression and all three management strategies will place the role of combination approaches in proper clinical perspective.

### Refractory depression: basic concepts

Numerous formal definitions of refractory depression have been proposed (Nierenberg, 1990; Thase & Rush, 1995; Fava & Davidson, 1996). Some authorities have distinguished between refractoriness and treatment resistance, using the latter term to indicate failure to respond to an initial drug trial, with refractoriness reserved for non-response to multiple trials. Efforts have been made to quantify

**Table 10.1.** Basic strategies in the pharmacological treatment of refractory depression

1. Optimization – change in the current drug regimen to maximize its efficacy
2. Substitution – discontinuation of the current drug and initiation of another drug
3. Combination – simultaneous use of two or more different drugs acting on the core symptoms of affective illness

**Table 10.2.** 'Refractoriness': Operational definitions used by clinicians

After some duration of treatment with an appropriate agent given in some dosage,

1. the patient is insufficiently improved or worse, or
2. the patient (or family) believes s/he is insufficiently improved or worse, or
3. the patient's physical health is endangered by adverse effects, or
4. the patient is unable to tolerate adverse effects

and it is believed that this situation is unlikely to change significantly for the better within a tolerable period of time.

refractoriness (Grunhaus & Remen, 1993), although empirical justification for these systems is still limited. A theoretically important distinction has been drawn between resistance/refractoriness and intolerance, which refers to an inability to tolerate a drug dosage within the usual therapeutic range due to the development of adverse effects. However useful such refinements might be from a research perspective, they fail to capture the clinical reality of the practitioner confronted with a patient who is still depressed despite the practitioner's ministrations. For this reason, we define refractoriness in the broad but easily operationalized and clinically relevant terms delineated in Table 10.2. It must be emphasized that any discussion of refractoriness in a given patient should prompt a thorough reconsideration of the diagnosis of depression (Depression Guide Panel, 1993a).

The nature of clinical improvement in depression, the obverse of refractoriness, also deserves consideration. The term improvement itself is generally taken to mean any clinically significant amelioration of symptoms. In recent years, a distinction has been made between response and remission. The former usually connotes symptomatic improvement of a substantial magnitude, whereas the latter refers to a state in which symptoms have been rendered minimal or eliminated. Response may be defined in terms of a change from the pretreatment baseline (e.g. a 50% improvement) or the attainment of some cutoff score on a rating scale of depressive symptoms (e.g. less than 10 on the 17-item Hamilton Depression Rating Scale (HDRS). Remission, however, usually indicates a minimal level of symptoms (e.g. less than 7 on the HDRS) rather than a degree of improvement. However these terms are operationally defined, they are useful in underscoring the notion that improvement exists as a graded spectrum of clinical states.

Related to the issue of refractoriness is the concept of tachyphylaxis. This refers to the loss of an initial response to treatment despite maintenance of the drug at the initially effective dosage. Tachyphylaxis usually occurs after several months of treatment, and anecdotally appears to be more common with selective serotonin reuptake inhibitors (SSRIs) and MAOIs than with tricyclics.

## Management of refractory depression: basic strategies

### Optimization

This most conservative strategy involves changing the parameters of the current drug regimen in order to enhance its efficacy. By definition, optimization always entails the use of a primary antidepressant, i.e. an agent that can be used as an independent treatment for depression. At a preliminary level, optimization includes selection of the current drug: one class of agents might be preferred in a particular patient on the basis of greater efficacy for that patient's depressive subtype, e.g. an MAOI for atypical depression (McGrath et al., 1992), greater efficacy for comorbid conditions, e.g. an SSRI for comorbid obsessive compulsive disorder (Goodman et al., 1990), or better tolerability, e.g. a norepineprine-selective tricyclic in a patient with a history of serotonin syndrome (Sternbach, 1991). More typically, though, optimization involves ensuring an adequate duration of treatment, e.g., 4–6 weeks (Quitkin et al., 1996) or longer (Greenhouse et al., 1987) or an adequate dosage. Dosage adjustment of tricyclics can be guided by steady-state drug plasma levels (Preskorn & Burke, 1993), while MAOI dosing can be facilitated by measurement of platelet MAO activity (Davidson et al., 1978). Even with the SSRIs and newer heterocyclics, for which plasma levels have not yet been shown to predict clinical response, enhanced efficacy can result from dosage alterations (Montgomery, 1995).

### Substitution

Stopping the current agent and trying another is the most frequently employed approach when optimization fails. The conventional wisdom has been that substitution is most effective when a different class of agents is used (Thase & Rush, 1995; Price, 1990; Amsterdam & Hornig-Rohan, 1996). Evidence seems to support this when substituting MAOIs (McGrath et al., 1993) or SSRIs (Amsterdam et al., 1994) for tricyclics, or tricyclics for SSRIs (Peselow et al., 1989). The implicit assumption here is that the greater the difference in the mechanism of action between the two agents, the more likely the new agent will be effective. However, recent studies suggest that substituting a different SSRI for a previously ineffective (Joffe et al., 1996a) or untolerated (Brown & Harrison, 1992) SSRI may also be successful. This may indicate that the differences in the chemical structures of the SSRIs are functionally important enough to override the similarities in their mechanism of action.

**Table 10.3.** Combination approaches to the treatment of refractory depression

1. Augmentation – the simultaneous use of two or more agents to increase efficacy (i.e. the amount of improvement) over what might be obtained with any one of the agents used
2. Acceleration – the simultaneous use of two or more agents to hasten the onset of therapeutic effects
3. Stabilization – simultaneous use of two or more agents to prevent the occurrence of mania or hypomania

The major advantage of substitution over combination approaches is that of simplicity: using a single agent minimizes the sources of adverse effects, eliminates the possibility of adverse interactions between agents, and facilitates identification of the specifically effective components of the treatment regimen. Conversely, the major disadvantage of this approach is the loss of time: any further benefit that might have occurred with continuation of the initial agent is lost, time must be taken to taper the initial agent, time might be required for a washout between agents (especially if MAOIs are being used), and another 6 weeks of treatment with the new agent might be required to obtain a response. Moreover, even with such highly effective second-line treatments as electroconvulsive therapy (ECT), a history of refractoriness diminishes the chances of response (Prudic et al., 1996).

## Combination

Combination involves the simultaneous use of multiple drugs acting on the core symptoms of affective illness. This definition excludes the use of adjunctive agents to manage secondary symptoms (e.g. benzodiazepines for anxiety) or drug adverse effects (e.g. cyproheptadine for SSRI-induced dysorgasmia). Combination approaches have had a checkered career in psychopharmacology, reaching a nadir with the 'polypharmacy' of the 1970s. At that time, it was commonplace for multiple agents with similar chemical structures and mechanisms of action to be used together, often with little regard to diagnostic distinctions or optimization of any one agent. This therapeutic flailing-about was succeeded by an era of intensive monotherapy, which often saw the use of heroic doses of single agents. The past decade has witnessed a renewed interest in combination approaches, now guided by both a better appreciation of the importance (and limits) of optimization and a better understanding of the role of antidepressant neuropharmacology. We now distinguish between three combination strategies on the basis of treatment objective: augmentation, acceleration, and stabilization (Table 10.3). Previous efforts to define combination approaches in terms of mechanism of action, while theoretically stimulating, have been of limited practical use (Price, 1990).

Augmentation refers to the simultaneous use of multiple agents to increase efficacy (i.e. the amount of improvement) over what might be obtained with any one of the agents used. In practice, this often involves the addition of a new agent to a previously ineffective ongoing primary antidepressant. The simultaneous initiation of multiple drugs from the start of treatment, however, would be included in this definition if the objective were to enhance efficacy.

Acceleration refers to the simultaneous use of multiple drugs to hasten the onset of therapeutic effects. The delayed latency of onset of antidepressants, long considered a major limitation of these agents, has again become a focus of attention in the current managed care environment. Acceleration almost always involves the simultaneous initiation of drugs from the start of treatment.

Stabilization refers to the simultaneous use of multiple drugs to prevent the occurrence of mania or hypomania. Obviously, this approach is relevant only to patients in the bipolar spectrum, and a detailed discussion is beyond the scope of this chapter (cf. Sachs, 1996). Delineation of this strategy is important, however, because of the frequency with which mood-stabilizing, or thymoleptic, agents are used in patients with refractory depression. Often, this use is for antimanic prophylaxis, but some of these agents (e.g. lithium) are used extensively for purposes of augmentation, in both bipolar and unipolar illness. Thymoleptics used for stabilization are clearly not adjunctive, since they meet our criterion of 'acting on the core symptoms of affective illness' and generally constitute a key element of the treatment regimen in such cases.

What distinguishes this organizational scheme from others is the emphasis on treatment objective, rather than presumed mechanism of action or sequence of initiation of agents. Importantly, this terminology more accurately reflects the common usage of the term 'augmentation' in clinical practice. It should be underscored that these combination strategies are not mutually exclusive: it is conceivable that a drug-free refractory bipolar depressed patient might be started on lithium in addition to a primary antidepressant in order to increase the antidepressant's efficacy (augmentation), hasten its onset (acceleration), and prevent it from precipitating mania (stabilization). Evaluation of the benefits of lithium in this context, however, requires attention to three different outcome measures. These distinctions are important clinically, and critical in the design and interpretation of research studies.

## Combination agents

### Lithium

Lithium augmentation was first popularized by de Montigny et al. (1981), who reported dramatic improvement in an uncontrolled series of 8 inpatients with refractory unipolar depression within 48 hours after lithium was added to their ongoing tricyclic regimens. This report was seminal for three reasons: (i) it triggered a flowering of research on the efficacy and parameters of lithium augmentation; (ii) it helped legitimize combination treatment in refractory depression; and (iii) it convincingly established the relevance of preclinical neuropharmacology to the development of novel clinical treatment approaches. On the basis of findings in laboratory animals, de Montigny et al. (1981) hypothesized that lithium's ability to increase presynaptic serotonin (5-hydroxytryptamine [5-HT]) function (Price et al., 1990a) would interact with postsynaptic 5-HT receptors sensitized by long-term tricyclic treatment (de Montigny & Aghajanian, 1978), resulting in enhanced clinical efficacy.

Support for this receptor sensitization hypothesis of lithium augmentation has been mixed. Lithium added to desipramine in rats has been shown to be more effective than either drug alone in enhancing $5\text{-HT}_{1A}$ receptor-mediated effects on adenylate cyclase and $5\text{-HT}_2$ receptor-mediated effects on inositol phosphate (Newman et al., 1990). Clinical studies in depressed patients have also suggested that 5-HT function is increased after long-term, but not short-term, treatment with tricyclics (Price et al., 1989a), as well as by short-term lithium treatment (Price et al., 1989b). Perhaps most relevant, 5-HT function in refractory depressed patients is enhanced by lithium augmentation of primary antidepressants (Cowen et al., 1989; McCance-Katz et al., 1992).

On the other hand, the degree of enhancement of 5-HT function in depressed patients following lithium augmentation does not correlate with the magnitude of clinical improvement (Cowen et al., 1989; McCance-Katz et al., 1992). Moreover, clinical augmentation effects have not been observed with fenfluramine, a presynaptic 5-HT releaser (Price et al., 1990b). Among alternative mechanisms proposed to account for lithium augmentation, Yoshida et al. (1989) suggested the involvement of pharmacokinetic effects of lithium on tricyclic metabolism in the brain. Wolf et al. (1989) hypothesized that lithium might enhance the presynaptic 5-HT uptake blockade of monoamine uptake-inhibiting antidepressants. Mørk et al. (1990) found that the combination of lithium and imipramine was more effective than either drug alone in reducing $\beta$-adrenoceptor-stimulated adenylate cyclase activity in rat cortex, which is relevant because of the hypothesis that down-regulation of $\beta$-adrenoceptor number and function is a major mechanism of antidepressant action (Sulser et al., 1978). Finally, the possibility remains that lithium exerts antidepressant effects of its own that are entirely independent of the primary antidepressants with which it is given (Price, 1989).

Evidence for the clinical efficacy of lithium augmentation is strong. Seven of the 10 placebo-controlled trials in refractory patients (total $n = 226$) have reported positive findings, for a cumulative response rate of 46% (Table 10.4). Findings from the ten largest $(n \geqslant 15)$ open-label studies of lithium augmentation are remarkably similar, with a cumulative response rate of 56% in 354 refractory

**Table 10.4.** Placebo-controlled trials of lithium augmentation in refractory depression

| Study | n | Response rate (%) | Outcome |
|---|---|---|---|
| *Double-blind parallel groups* | | | |
| Heninger et al. (1983) | 15 | 63 | + |
| Cournoyer et al. (1984) | 12 | 50 | + |
| Kantor et al. (1986) | 7 | 25 | − |
| Zusky et al. (1988) | 16 | 38 | − |
| Stein and Bernadt (1993) | 24 | 14 | + |
| Schöpf et al. (1989) | 27 | 50 | + |
| Browne et al. (1990) | 17 | 27 | − |
| Joffe et al. (1993) | 33 | 53 | + |
| Katona et al. (1995) | 60 | 52 | + |
| *Blind placebo-substitution study* | | | |
| Kramlinger and Post (1989) | 15 | 53 | + |
| Cumulative: | 226 | 46 | + |

**Table 10.5.** Large open-label trials ($n \geqslant 15$) of lithium augmentation in refractory depression

| Study | n | Response rate (%) |
|---|---|---|
| Nelson and Mazure (1986) | 21 | 52 |
| Price et al. (1986) | 84 | 57 |
| Dinan and Barry (1989) | 15 | 73 |
| Thase et al. (1989) | 20 | 65 |
| van Marwijk et al. (1990) | 51 | 65 |
| Cowen et al. (1991) | 23 | 44 |
| Zimmer et al. (1991) | 15 | 67 |
| Ontiveros et al. (1991) | 60 | 42 |
| Rybakowski and Matkowski (1992) | 51 | 55 |
| Strober et al. (1992) | 24 | 42 |
| Cumulative: | 364 | 56 |

patients (Table 10.5). Of the negative controlled studies, two evaluated patients after only 48 hours of lithium (Kantor et al., 1986; Browne et al., 1990), while the third used lithium doses that were too low to be effective (Zusky et al., 1988).

Although the successful use of lithium augmentation has been described across diagnostic subtypes of depression, some variability in response has been reported. Price et al. (1986) observed marked improvement in 57% of non-psychotic melancholic patients vs. 25% of non-melancholics. Some investigators have re-ported higher response rates in bipolar than unipolar depressed patients (Nelson

& Mazure, 1986; Rybakowski & Matkowski, 1992), but others have detected no difference (Price et al., 1986; Schöpf et al., 1989). Other variables, such as number of previous antidepressant trials, family history, age, gender, and dexamethasone non-suppression, have not been correlated with outcome (Price et al., 1986; Schöpf et al., 1989; Rybakowski & Matkowski 1992). At present, the best predictor of response is a serum lithium level $> 0.5$ meq/l (Stein & Bernadt, 1993; Katona et al., 1995).

None of the larger studies of lithium augmentation has identified unique safety or tolerability problems with this combination. Early concerns about potentially toxic interactions between lithium and the SSRIs have generally not been supported (Bauer et al., 1996). Probably the most common adverse effects are tremor and myoclonic jerks. It is true, however, that lithium has a distinctly narrow therapeutic index, a high propensity for 'nuisance' adverse effects, and a potential for major toxicity.

The usual dose of lithium for augmentation is 900 mg/day, adjusted to achieve serum levels of 0.5–1.0 mmol/l. Efficacy has been reported with all major classes of primary antidepressants, including tricyclics, SSRIs, and MAOIs; trazodone may be less effective (Price et al., 1986), but the literature on the non-tricyclic heterocyclics is generally limited. The latency of response has been reported to vary from 48 hours (de Montigny et al., 1981, 1983; Cournoyer et al., 1984) to 6 weeks (Thase et al., 1989), but most studies suggest that a 3–4 week trial is appropriate. Special requirements include standard screening laboratory tests for lithium (Price & Heninger, 1994) and periodic serum lithium levels (especially at the end of the first week to ensure an adequate level).

Lithium acceleration has also been examined in several controlled trials, but results have been inconsistent. The earliest study found lithium + tricyclic slightly superior to placebo + tricyclic only at week 4 in 45 depressed patients treated at nine hospitals (Lingjaerde et al., 1974). In a secondary analysis at the only site enrolling more than a few patients ($n = 13$), lithium + tricyclic was superior to placebo + tricyclic at weeks 1, 2, and 4, with no difference at week 6. Shortly thereafter, Nick et al. (1976) detected no differences after 2 weeks in 30 patients randomized to lithium + clomipramine or placebo + clomipramine, but clomipramine doses were low (mean, $80 \pm 20$ mg/day). More recently, Ebert et al. (1995) found lithium + tricyclic superior to placebo + tricyclic in 40 non-refractory bipolar melancholic inpatients after 5 weeks, with no difference at weeks 1 and 2, while Cappiello et al. (1998) found lithium + desipramine superior to placebo + desipramine in 29 largely refractory patients at weeks 1 and 2 of a 4-week trial. However, concurrent lithium conferred no advantage over placebo + tricyclic in two recent Israeli studies of non-refractory depressed inpatients ($n = 22$) (Shahal et al., 1996) and outpatients ($n = 31$) (Bloch et al., 1994).

In sum, lithium augmentation is supported by a strong empirical foundation and appears as safe and well tolerated as lithium monotherapy. Probably the major impediment to its use is patient acceptance, since many patients are apprehensive about possible side effects or fear that taking lithium implies that they have a severe 'mental illness.' The data on lithium acceleration are still too ambiguous to justify its routine use.

## Triiodothyronine (T₃)

Interest in the antidepressant properties of $T_3$ dates back to the late 1950s (Flach et al., 1958; Feldmesser-Reiss, 1958), with numerous studies since that time examining the role of thyroid function in the pathogenesis of refractory (Howland, 1993) and non-refractory (Prange et al., 1987) depression. Early investigators speculated that $T_3$ acted by correcting subclinical hypothyroidism, with subsequent refinements of this focusing on the interaction of $T_3$ with catecholamines and unspecified adrenergic receptors (Whybrow & Prange, 1981). More recent work has suggested that the effects of $T_3$ are mediated via $\beta$-adrenoceptors (Howland, 1993), which have been implicated in antidepressant action, as noted above (Sulser et al., 1978). The major competing theory argues that exogenous $T_3$ corrects a relative hyperthyroid state in the central nervous system (CNS) by suppressing thyroxine ($T_4$) synthesis in the thyroid gland (Joffe & Singer, 1990; Joffe & Sokolov, 1994). Unlike $T_3$, $T_4$ readily crosses the blood–brain barrier into the CNS, where it is converted to $T_3$, so suppression of peripheral $T_4$ levels by exogenous $T_3$ paradoxically decreases $T_3$ in the CNS. Supporting this theory is evidence that $T_4$ levels tend to decline in depressed patients who respond to antidepressants (Duval et al., 1996) or cognitive/behavioral therapy (Joffe et al., 1996b).

Evidence for the efficacy of $T_3$ augmentation is limited. On the basis of a meta-analysis including eight comparative trials in mostly refractory patients (total $n = 292$) and a cumulative response rate of 57% (Table 10.6), Aronson et al. (1996) recently concluded that $T_3$ augmentation 'may be ... effective' (p. 842). Although the meta-analysis was statistically significant, only four studies (total $n = 95$) utilized randomized, double-blind designs with a placebo or comparator control (Joffe & Singer, 1990; Gitlin et al., 1987; Steiner et al., 1978; Joffe et al. 1993), and two of these studies (total $n = 71$) were from the same research group; meta-analysis of this subset of four studies was not significant.

Successful use of $T_3$ augmentation has been described in both unipolar and bipolar patients, but no diagnostic specificity has been reported. Some studies have suggested that a positive clinical response to $T_3$ is predicted by subclinical hypothyroidism, as reflected in lower thyroid hormone levels or exaggerated thyrotropin responses to thyrotropin-releasing hormone (Targum et al., 1984;

**Table 10.6.** Comparative trials of T$_3$ augmentation in refractory depression

| Study | $n$ | Response rate (%) | Outcome |
|---|---|---|---|
| Banki (1975) | 96 | 75 | + |
| Banki (1977) | 49 | 67 | + |
| Steiner et al. (1978) | 8 | 75 | − |
| Goodwin et al. (1982) | 12 | 33 | + |
| Gitlin et al. (1987) | 16 | 0 | − |
| Thase et al. (1989) | 40 | 25 | − |
| Joffe & Singer (1990) | 38 | 53 | + |
| Joffe et al. (1993) | 33 | 59 | + |
| Cumulative: | 292 | 57 | + |

Baruch et al., 1985; Nakamura & Nomura, 1992). However, other investigators have failed to replicate this (Gitlin et al., 1987, Schwarcz et al., 1984).

T$_3$ augmentation is extremely well tolerated, with only rare complaints of tremor or activation. Caution is indicated in patients with cardiovascular disease, and chronic elevation of thyroid function may promote osteoporosis, which would be of special concern in depressed women (Michaelson et al., 1996); however, clinically significant effects on thyroid function are uncommon. The usual dose of T$_3$ is 25–50 mcg/day, and a 3–4 week trial would be considered adequate to evaluate efficacy. Special requirements include baseline and periodic thyroid function tests and thyrotropin levels.

Interestingly, placebo-controlled trials of T$_3$ acceleration preceded the more recent augmentation studies. These trials, conducted in non-refractory euthyroid depressed patients, generally suggested a hastening of the onset of tricyclic antidepressant effects by T$_3$, especially in women (Prange et al., 1969; Coppen et al., 1972; Wheatley 1972; Wilson et al., 1979). The increased importance of rapidity of onset in the current health-care climate warrants a modern replication of these early findings.

While the efficacy of T$_3$ augmentation is not established, this approach remains popular with some clinicians because of its tolerability, safety, ease of use, and patient acceptance. However, it should be noted that the systematic efficacy data on T$_3$ augmentation and acceleration derive entirely from studies with tricyclics; the published experience with other primary antidepressants is limited to case reports.

### SSRI + heterocyclic

Shortly after the introduction of fluoxetine in the US, Weilburg et al. (1989) reported that addition of this SSRI to the ongoing heterocyclic (mostly tricyclic)

regimens of 30 refractory depressed outpatients resulted in an 87% response rate. Similar findings were reported by Eisen (1989). A simplistic understanding of this might be that greater therapeutic effects result from potently inhibiting uptake of the two biogenic amines most clearly implicated in the pathogenesis of depression, 5-HT by fluoxetine and norepinephrine (NE) by the heterocyclic. This rationale has been used in the promotion of the novel heterocyclic venlafaxine, which inhibits uptake of both amines. A more sophisticated explanation has been suggested by Baron et al. (1988), who reported that concurrent administration of fluoxetine and the selective NE uptake inhibitor desipramine resulted in a more rapid and profound decrease in cortical $\beta$-adrenoceptor binding and function in rats than did either drug alone. These findings would predict both augmentation and acceleration effects. However, the observed changes in $\beta$-adrenoceptors could result simply from the elevation of brain and blood desipramine levels due to inhibition of its metabolism by fluoxetine (Goodnough & Baker, 1994).

Evidence for the efficacy of SSRI + heterocyclic combinations is limited to open-label studies. Using historical controls for comparison, Nelson et al. (1991) found evidence of both acceleration and augmentation in 14 mostly non-refractory depressed inpatients given fluoxetine and desipramine from the start of treatment. A strength of this study was careful attention to pharmacokinetic factors, so that changes in drug blood levels could be excluded as an explanation of the findings. Seth et al. (1992) described eight highly refractory patients who responded to SSRI + nortriptyline combination treatment, while Zajecka et al. (1995) reported a 48% response rate to heterocyclic augmentation in 25 depressed patients with varying degrees of refractoriness to fluoxetine. However, in a double-blind, comparator-controlled study, Fava et al. (1994) found no evidence of efficacy for adding low-dose (25–50 mg) desipramine to ongoing fluoxetine in refractory patients.

A disadvantage of SSRI + heterocyclic combination treatment is that the adverse effects of either or both agents can be enhanced, primarily due to the tendency of these drugs to inhibit each other's metabolism and consequently increase blood levels (Taylor, 1995). Sertraline may be slightly less problematic than other SSRIs in this regard, but caution is still warranted. Most published reports have utilized fluoxetine or sertraline as the SSRI and desipramine, nortriptyline, or amoxapine as the heterocyclic, although anecdotal reports have involved most agents in both classes. There has been particular interest in bupropion because of its dopamine (DA) uptake-inhibiting properties (Bodkin et al., 1997), but clinicians should bear in mind the increased risk of seizures with higher blood levels of this agent. All sequences of drug initiation (SSRI first, heterocyclic first, or both started simultaneously) have been reported to be effective. Dosing will depend on which sequence is used, but should take into account the likelihood of pharmacokinetic interactions: when adding to an ongoing regimen or initiating both drugs simultaneously, SSRIs should be started at the low end of the therapeutic dose range, while heterocyclics should be started at one-third of the lowest therapeutic dose and titrated up to achieve therapeutic blood levels. Special requirements include heterocyclic plasma level monitoring, which is useful to establish the safety as well as the adequacy of dosing. A 4-week trial would be considered adequate to evaluate efficacy.

The current vogue for this approach reflects the popularity of the SSRIs rather than the efficacy or safety database. In many cases, SSRI + heterocyclic treatment seems to represent a compromise between substitution and combination: in the light of positive anecdotal and published reports, it seems reasonable to the clinician to simply continue the preceding agent rather than start all over. The fallacy in this is that many patients who appear to respond in these circumstances are responding to the new agent, rather than to the combination. As a result, patients may end up continuing on agents which are actually contributing little beyond the potential for toxic pharmacokinetic interactions. Only well-designed controlled trials can clarify this issue.

## Buspirone

Buspirone is an azapirone derivative which acts as an agonist at the 5-HT$_{1A}$ receptor (Eison & Temple, 1986). Although this agent is marketed as an anxiolytic, other 5-HT$_{1A}$ agonists (e.g. gepirone, ipsapirone, flesinoxan) have generated considerable interest as potential antidepressants. It was in this regard that buspirone augmentation was initially tried by Jacobsen (1991), who reported full or partial responses in an open series of seven of eight refractory and eight of nine tachyphylactic depressed patients. Based on electrophysiologic studies in laboratory animals, Blier and de Montigny (1994) have suggested that stimulation of postsynaptic 5-HT$_{1A}$ receptors constitutes a major mechanism of antidepressant action. However, an alternative mechanism for buspirone's effects in this context has also been proposed, involving the ability of its active metabolite, 1-(-2-pyrimidinyl)-piperazine (1-PP), to block $\alpha_2$ adrenoceptors (Howland, 1995).

Further evidence of buspirone's efficacy as an augmenting agent is limited to open-label studies. Joffe and Schuller (1993) reported marked responses in 17/25 refractory patients, while Bakish (1991) described three additional cases. The dose range of buspirone in these studies has been 20–50 mg/day, with an average of 30 mg/day, and 3-week trials have been considered adequate. Most reports have involved SSRIs, although efficacy has been described with tricyclics. Hypertensive episodes have infrequently been reported when buspirone is added to an MAOI. Buspirone is otherwise very safe and usually well tolerated, with occasional complaints of nausea or paradoxically increased nervousness. The favorable adverse effect profile of buspirone has been a major source of its popularity in augmentation, but efficacy data are still limited.

## Stimulants

Placebo-controlled studies do not support the use of these agents as primary antidepressants (Satel & Nelson, 1989). Despite this, their use in refractory depression, both alone and in combination approaches, has been the subject of numerous case reports. The generally accepted mechanism of action has invoked the ability of stimulants to release biogenic amines (particularly the catecholamines NE and DA, but also the indoleamine 5-HT), which might enhance the net effects of the aminergic uptake inhibition characteristic of most primary antidepressants. However, it has also been suggested that stimulants could act by inhibiting the metabolism of primary antidepressants, and thereby increasing their blood levels.

Ayd and Zohar (1987) identified five uncontrolled studies totalling 67 patients in which stimulants had been used to augment ineffective primary treatment in refractory depression. In a subsequent report, Fawcett et al. (1991) observed a response rate of 78% in 32 patients. Importantly, these investigators and some others (Feighner et al., 1985) have indicated that response is sustained over extended periods, in contrast to the tachyphylaxis observed with stimulants when used alone.

The most common adverse effects of stimulants in this context are anxiety, motor activation, and insomnia, but the precipitation or exacerbation of psychosis or mania may also occur. Possible elevations in blood pressure and heart rate require regular monitoring, but other significant cardiovascular effects are unlikely in healthy individuals. Abuse and dependence are rare in this population in the absence of predisposing comorbid conditions.

Dextroamphetamine and methylphenidate have been most frequently used, generally in doses of 5–30 mg/day, starting at low doses given early in the day and titrating upward. Pemoline has also been employed, although recent reports of acute hepatic failure with this agent now necessitate monitoring of liver function tests during its use. A 2–3-week trial is probably adequate to evaluate efficacy. Non-response to one stimulant does not preclude response to another. Most reports describe stimulant augmentation of tricyclics; use with MAOIs requires lower initial doses and slower upward titration because of the theortical risk of severe hypertensive reaction, although orthostatic hypotension occurs more frequently.

The absence of controlled trials supporting efficacy, plus an unfavorable side-effects profile, relegate the stimulants to selective use only. However, most experts acknowledge at least occasional dramatic benefits with stimulant augmentation, and recent ancedotal reports have claimed utility in reversing the tachyphylaxis sometimes associated with SSRIs.

## Neuroleptics

In the mid-1970s, investigators noted that patients with delusional depression responded poorly to tricyclic monotherapy, even when blood levels were monitored to ensure optimization (Glassman et al., 1975). This led to trials of neuroleptic plus tricyclic in such patients, with Nelson and Bowers (1978) reporting a 92% response rate in an open-label study primarily utilizing perphenazine and imipramine. The rationale for this combination relates directly to the antipsychotic properties of the neuroleptics, now believed to be mediated through their ability block DA $D_2$ receptors.

Numerous subsequent uncontrolled studies have replicated the original finding of Nelson and Bowers (1978), albeit with lower response rates in the 65–80% range, roughly comparable to the efficacy of ECT in this population (Parker et al., 1992). In the only controlled study ($n = 58$ psychotic depressed inpatients), Spiker et al. (1985) observed response rates of 19% for perphenazine alone, 41% for amitriptyline alone, and 78% for the combination.

Neuroleptic augmentation is unique in the specificity of its indication for a particular subtype of depression. Some other patients may benefit from neuroleptic augmentation, particularly those with near-psychotic rumination or marked psychomotor agitation (Nelson, 1987). The risk/benefit ratio in refractory patients lacking such features generally does not favor this approach. One open-label study has suggested that thioridazine may accelerate the antidepressant response to desipramine in non-refractory, non-psychotic depressed patients, perhaps by blocking presynaptic $\alpha_2$-adrenoceptors rather than through effects on the DA system (Bennett et al., 1984).

The major drawback of neuroleptic augmentation is the long-term risk of tardive dyskinesia, to which mood disorder patients seem especially vulnerable. More acute problems include extrapyramidal symptoms, anticholinergic side effects, and orthostatic hypotension, the latter two particularly troublesome when tricyclics are involved. Pharmacokinetic interactions are known to result in increased blood levels of both neuroleptics and tricyclics when these agents are used together.

Any of the conventional neuroleptics may be used for augmentation, with drug selection contingent upon consideration of adverse effects (more extrapyramidal symptoms with high-potency drugs, more cardiovascular and anticholinergic effects with low-potency agents). Evidence suggests that neuroleptic should be given for a conventionally adequate duration and at doses in the antipsychotic range (Nelson et al., 1986), although some patients may respond at lower doses.

Most published reports have involved tricyclics, but MAOIs and SSRIs (Roths-child et al., 1993) have also been successfully used. Some authorities have suggested that the benefits of neuroleptic plus tricyclic treatment may be obtained more conveniently by monotherapy with amoxapine, a tricyclic with $D_2$ antagonist properties (Anton & Burch, 1990). A disadvantage of this agent, however, is that its use precludes the independent titration of antipsychotic and antidepressant doses.

There is little published experience yet with the newer neuroleptics (e.g. risperidone, olanzapine, sertindole), but their superior side-effect profile relative to conventional neuroleptics may prove to be a major advantage in combination treatment. Preliminary findings have been reported from a controlled comparison of fluoxetine, olanzapine, and the combination of both drugs in patients with treatment-resistant depression (Shelton et al., 1998). Olanzapine plus fluoxetine showed greater efficacy than either monotherapy, with no increase in significant adverse effects. Also intriguing is a report from Ostroff and Nelson (1999), in which eight of eight SSRI-resistant patients responded to augmentation with low ($\leqslant 1$ mg/day) doses of risperidone. Confirmation of these preliminary observations could dramatically broaden the indications for atypical neuroleptics in refractory depression. A more cautious approach is warranted with the older atypical neuroleptic clozapine, which should be reserved only for highly resistant cases because of its plethora of minor side effects (hypersalivation, sedation) and major toxicities (decreased seizure threshold, agranulocytosis).

### 5-HT$_{1A}$ antagonists

Interest in these agents stems from electrophysiological studies of antidepressants in laboratory animals, which have indicated that long-term treatment with SSRIs and MAOIs causes desensitization of presynaptic 5-HT$_{1A}$ autoreceptors. Since these autoreceptors are inhibitory, the net result of this effect is enhanced 5-HT neurotransmission (Blier & de Montigny, 1994). The same effect can be induced more rapidly by administering the SSRI in conjunction with a 5-HT$_{1A}$ antagonist (Hjorth & Sharp, 1993). Since selective 5-HT$_{1A}$ antagonists are not generally available, studies to date have used $\beta$-adrenergic blockers, some of which also block the presynaptic 5-HT$_{1A}$ receptor.

Based on these findings, Artigas et al. (1994) tried to hasten the therapeutic onset of paroxetine by combining it with the $\beta$-adrenergic/5-HT$_{1A}$ antagonist pindolol. Five of seven depressed patients responded within 1 week in this open-label acceleration trial, while six of eight SSRI-resistant patients responded to augmentation with pindolol. The sucessful use of pindolol to accelerate response to SSRIs, especially paroxetine, has now been replicated in both open and controlled trials (Blier & Bergeron, 1998; Bordet et al., 1998). However, Berman et al. (1999) recently found no beneficial effects of pindolol acceleration of fluoxetine in a double-blind, placebo-controlled study of 86 depressed patients, and other investigators have questioned the robustness of the effect (McAskill et al., 1998). An earlier placebo-controlled study by Tang et al. (1990) found no benefit from propranolol in 16 depressed patients treated with desipramine.

Two placebo-controlled studies have failed to demonstrate efficacy for pindolol added to ongoing SSRI treatment in clearly refractory depressed patients (Moreno et al., 1997; Perez et al., 1999).

No major adverse effects have been reported with this strategy. Some patients have experienced increased irritability, and decreases in heart rate and blood pressure are routinely observed. The usual contraindications to $\beta$ blockers should be observed, such as bronchospastic disease, diabetes, congestive heart failure, and cardiac conduction abnormalities. Theoretically, this approach should work with any $\beta$ blocker possessing significant affinity for the 5-HT$_{1A}$ receptor and with any SSRI or MAOI. Thus far, however, positive reports have generally used pindolol 2.5 mg t.i.d. as the $\beta$ blocker and paroxetine as the SSRI, with efficacy evident by 3–4 weeks; negative findings have been reported with fluoxetine and sertraline. Despite the elegant theoretical rationale, the contradictory clinical studies suggest that this approach currently be considered experimental.

## Other agents

Numerous other combination strategies have been described or proposed. For various reasons, they should not be considered first-line approaches at this time.

### Mirtazapine

A novel antidepressant which blocks $\alpha_2$-adrenoceptors and 5-HT$_2$ receptors, this was recently found effective in 55% of 20 refractory depressed patients following open-label augmentation of another primary antidepressant (Carpenter et al., 1999); placebo-controlled trials are present under way.

### DA D$_2$ receptor agonists

These have been reported to have some antidepressant properties when used alone. Positive augmentation effects have been described for pergolide (Bouckoms & Mangini, 1993) and bromocriptine (Inoue et al., 1996). Anecdotal reports suggest these agents may have a role in the treatment of SSRI tachyphylaxis.

### $\alpha_2$ adrenoceptor antagonists

$\alpha_2$ adrenoceptor antagonists (e.g. yohimbine, idazoxan) have shown accelerant properties in animal studies; these findings have not been replicated in depressed patients treated with tricyclics (Charney et al., 1986), but augmentation studies with SSRIs have suggested some promise (Cappiello et al., 1995). $\alpha_2$ adrenoceptor blockade has been invoked as a major mechanism of action of the newly released antidepressant mirtazapine (de Montigny et al., 1995).

### Thyroxine (T$_4$)

This was recently reported by Bauer and colleagues (1998) to be safe and effective as an augmenting agent in refractory depression when given in supraphysiological doses of 300–600 mcg/d. These intriguing findings, which are contrary to predictions based on the theory of Joffe and Sokolov (1994) mentioned above, have not yet been replicated.

### Inositol

Inositol is an isomer of glucose that serves as a key precursor in the phosphatidylinositol pathway. This pathway plays a major role as a second-messenger system in the brain. Both open (Levine et al., 1993) and placebo-controlled (Levine et al., 1995) studies have documented modest but significant effects of inositol monotherapy in the treatment of depressed patients, most of whom were refractory. Studies of inositol as an augmenting agent are currently in progress.

### Novel anticonvulsants

Novel anticonvulsants (e.g. lamotrigine, gabapentin, topiramate) are currently under investigation with respect to their mood-stabilizing properties. Antidepressant augmenting efficacy for these drugs has not yet been established, although there have been positive open-label reports (Yasmin et al. in press).

### 5-HT precursors

5-HT precursors (i.e. tryptophan, 5-hydroxytryptohan) were the subject of numerous controlled trials in the 1970s, which generally suggested that these compounds might have modest antidepressant properties (Byerley & Risch, 1985). Several methodologically sophisticated studies in the 1960s and 1970s demonstrated acceleration effects of tryptophan in non-refractory patients concurrently receiving MAOIs or the potent but non-selective tricyclic SRI clomipramine (SSRIs were not yet available) (e.g. Glassman & Platman, 1969; Walinder et al., 1976). Efficacy with other tricyclics, or as an augmentation agent in refractory patients, is less clear. Significant neuromotor side effects ('serotonin syndrome') have occasionally occurred when tryptophan has been combined with an SSRI (Sternbach 1991). Unfortunately, tryptophan was implicated in the pathogenesis of the eosinophilia–myalgia syndrome, probably reflecting a contaminant arising during synthesis (Kamb et al., 1992). As a result, tryptophan has been banned from clinical use in the US, although it is still available in Canada and other countries.

## Sleep deprivation

This has shown transient antidepressant effects in numerous studies, with some evidence that it may have value as an augmenting agent (Dessauer et al., 1985), but it is not practical for long-term treatment.

## Captopril

An angiotensin II-converting enzyme inhibitor approved for use as an antihypertensive, this was reported to be of benefit in augmenting primary antidepressants in a very preliminary open study of nine treatment-resistant patients (Vuckovic et al., 1991).

## Estrogen

This has long been of interest with respect to possible antidepressant properties, probably reflecting its unequivocal benefits in the treatment of menopausal symptoms. The limited controlled data do not support claims of efficacy in treatment-resistant depression (Oppenheim et al., 1987), but the recent introduction of selective estrogen receptor modulators (SERMs; e.g. raloxifene) should stimulate new work in this area.

## MAOI + tricyclic combination

This treatment has been found effective in several studies (Razani et al., 1983), and appears to be safe in the hands of clinicians highly experienced with these drugs. However, because of concerns about the risk of potentially lethal interaction effects, as well as the increased availability of safer alternatives, this approach is now rarely used.

Some drugs that have previously been proposed for use in treating refractory depression no longer merit consideration. Reserpine was shown in early studies to rapidly augment tricyclics when given in large parenteral doses, but more recent controlled trials failed to replicate these findings (Amsterdam & Berwish, 1987; Price et al., 1987). Fenfluramine has been hypothesized to act as an augmenting agent similar to lithium on the basis of its ability to potently release and block reuptake of 5-HT. However, the racemic mixture of D,L-fenfluramine showed no efficacy (Price et al., 1990b), and the stereoisomer D-fenfluramine has been withdrawn from the market due to its induction of valvular heart disease (Connolly et al., 1997).

**Table 10.7.** Factors affecting choice of treatment

(i) Efficacy – how well the agent treats the condition for which it is given

(ii) Specificity – how well specific clinical or neurobiological features predict preferential response to the agent

(iii) Safety – how frequent and serious are the complications associated with use of the agent

(iv) Convenience – how easy it is for the physician to initiate and maintain treatment with the agent

(v) Patient acceptance –

       (a) common ('nuisance') adverse effects

       (b) convenience (for the patient)

       (c) cost

(vi) 'Other' factors –

       (a) the 'new drug' effect

       (b) 'press'

## Clinical applications

There are numerous options available to the clinician for managing treatment-resistant depression. Choosing among these alternatives can be daunting, but simple drug choice algorithms run the risk of minimizing the importance of individualized treatment for each patient. We believe that a more useful approach combines the systematic assessment of the patient's clinical state (Depression Guide Panel 1993b) with a systematic consideration of the risks and benefits associated with each treatment option.

Table 10.7 summarizes key factors affecting the choice of a specific treatment. It must be emphasized that the weight assigned to each factor will vary according to the clinical circumstances. Thus, in a severely depressed patient, efficacy may be of paramount importance, so that an agent with strongly supportive efficacy data (e.g. lithium) will be optimal. In a psychotic patient, specificity would be of greatest concern, leading to the selection of a neuroleptic. Safety is, of course, always a major factor, but even more so in patients with pre-existing medical conditions which put them at special risk. Convenience to the physician should be a secondary consideration, particularly in refractory illness, but patient acceptance is not, as it is a key determinant of whether the chosen treatment will be successful. Finally, both physicians and patients may be influenced by the 'new drug' effect, the enthusiasm associated with a newly released drug or a newly described combination. Moreover, the publicity, or 'press,' generated by an agent, whether positive or negative, can often affect choice in ways that are far more profound than most physicians would care to acknowledge.

Whatever options are selected, a crucial ingredient in the successful management of refractory depression is persistence. Although short-term studies underscore the high degree of morbidity associated with refractory depression (Nierenberg et al., 1990), longer-term follow-up confirms the Kraepelinian perspective that depression tends to be a remitting illness (Stoudemire et al., 1993; Mueller et al., 1996). These findings constitute a strong argument against therapeutic nihilism in the treatment of refractory patients.

## Acknowledgments

This work was supported in part by a Stanley Foundations Research Award to Dr Price and a NARSAD Young Investigator Award to Dr Carpenter.

## REFERENCES

Amsterdam, J.D. & Berwish, N. (1987). Treatment of refractory depression with combination reserpine and tricyclic antidepressant therapy. *Journal of Clinical Psychopharmacology*, 7, 238–42.

Amsterdam, J.D. & Hornig-Rohan, M. (1996). In *Treatment Algorithms in Treatment-Resistant Depression*, ed. M. Hornig-Rohan & J.D. Amsterdam, pp. 371–86. Philadelphia: W.B. Saunders Co.

Amsterdam, J.D., Maislin, G., & Potter, L. (1994). Fluoxetine efficacy in treatment resistant depression. *Progress in Neuro-Psychopharmacology and Biological Psychiatry*, 18, 243–61.

Anton, R.F. & Burch, E.A. (1990). Amoxapine versus amitriptyline combined with perphenazine in the treatment of psychotic depression. *American Journal of Psychiatry*, 147, 1203–8.

Aronson, R., Offman, H., Joffe, R.T., & Naylor, C.D. (1996). Triiodothyronine augmentation in the treatment of refractory depression. *Archives of General Psychiatry*, 53, 842–8.

Artigas, F., Perez, V., & Alvarez, E. (1994). Pindolol induces a rapid improvement of depressed patients treated with serotonin reuptake inhibitors. *Archives of General Psychiatry*, 51, 248–51.

Ayd, F.J. Jr & Zohar, J. (1987). Psychostimulant (amphetamine or methylphenidate) therapy for chronic and treatment-resistant depression. In *Treating Resistant Depression*, ed. J. Zohar & R.H. Belmaker, pp. 343–55. New York: PMA Publishing.

Bakish, D. (1991). Fluoxetine potentiation by buspirone: three case histories. *Canadian Journal of Psychiatry*, 36, 749–50.

Banki, C. (1975). The use of triiodothyronine in the treatment of depression [in Hungarian]. Orv Hetil. 116, 2543–6.

Banki, C.M. (1977). Cerebrospinal fluid amine metabolites after combined amitriptyline-triiodothyronine treatment of depressed women. *European Journal of Pharmacology*, 11, 311–15.

Baron, B.M., Ogden, A.M., Siegel, B.W., Stegeman, J., Ursillo, R.C., & Dudley, M.W. (1988). Rapid down regulation of $\beta$-adrenoceptors by co-administration of desipramine and fluoxetine. *European Journal of Pharmacology*, **154**, 125–34.

Baruch, P., Jouvent, R., & Widlocher, D. (1985). Increased TSH response to TRH in refractory depressed women. *American Journal of Psychiatry*, **142**, 145–6.

Bauer, M., Linden, M., Schaaf, B., & Weber, H.J. (1996). Adverse events and tolerability of the combination of fluoxetine/lithium compared with fluoxetine. *Journal of Clinical Psychopharmacology*, **16**, 130–4.

Bauer, M., Hellweg, R., Graf, K., & Baumgartner, A. (1998). Treatment of refractory depression with high-dose thyroxine. *Neuropsychopharmcology*, **18**, 444–55.

Bennett, J.A., Hirschowitz, J., Zemlan, F., Thurman, D.N., & Garver, D.L. (1984). Combined thioridazine and desipramine: early antidepressant response. *Psychopharmacology*, **82**, 263–5.

Berman, R.M., Anand, A., Cappiello, A. et al. (1999). The use of pindolol with fluoxetine in the treatment of major depression: final results from a double-blind, placebo-controlled trial. *Biological Psychiatry*, **45**, 1170–7.

Blier, P. & Bergeron, R. (1998). The use of pindolol to potentiate antidepressant medication. *Journal of Clinical Psychiatry*, **59**, 16–23.

Blier, P. & de Montigny, C. (1994). Current advances and trends in the treatment of depression. *Trends in Pharmacological Science*, **15**, 220–6.

Bloch, M., Schwartzman, Y., Bonne, O., & Lerer, B. (1994). Concurrent treatment of major depression with desipramine and lithium: a double-blind, placebo-controlled clinical study. Presented at the 9th ECNP Congress, Jerusalem, Israel.

Bodkin, J.A., Lasser, R.A., Wines, J.D., Gardner, D.M., & Baldessarini, R.J. (1997). Combining serotonin reuptake inhibitors and bupropion in partial responders to antidepressant monotherapy. *Journal of Clinical Psychiatry*, **58**, 137–45.

Bordet, R., Thomas, P., & Dupuis, B. (1998). Effect of pindolol on onset of action of paroxetine in the treatment of major depression: intermediate analysis of a double-blind, placebo-controlled trial. Reseau de Recherche et d'Experimentation Psychopharmacologique. *American Journal of Psychiatry*, **155**, 1346–51.

Bouckoms, A. & Mangini, L. (1993). Pergolide: an antidepressant adjuvant for mood disorders? *Psychopharmacological Bulletin*, **29**, 207–11.

Brown, W.A. & Harrison, W. (1992). Are patients who are intolerant to one SSRI intolerant to another? *Psychopharmacological Bulletin*, **28**, 253–6.

Browne, M., Lapierre, Y.D., Hrdina, P.D., & Horn, E. (1990). Lithium as an adjunct in the treatment of major depression. *International Clinical Psychopharmacology*, **5**, 103–10.

Byerley, W.F. & Risch, S.C. (1985). Depression and serotonin metabolism: rationale for neurotransmitter precursor treatment. *Journal of Clinical Psychopharmacology*, **5**, 191–206.

Cappiello, A., McDougle, C.J., Malison, R.T., Heninger, G.R., & Price, L.H. (1995). Yohimbine augmentation of fluvoxamine in refractory: a single-blind study. *Biological Psychiatry*, **38**, 765–7.

Cappiello, A., McDougle, C.J., Delgado, P.L. et al. (1998). Lithium + desipramine vs. desipramine alone in the treatment of major depression: a preliminary study. *International Clinical Psychopharmacology*, **13**, 191–8.

Carpenter, L., Jocic, Z., Hall, J., Rasmussen, S., & Price, L. (1999). Mirtazapine augmentation in the treatment of refractory depression. *Journal of Clinical Psychiatry*, **60**, 45–9.

Charney, D.S., Price, L.H., & Heninger, G.R. (1986). Desipramine-yohimbine combination treatment of refractory depression: implications for the beta-adrenergic receptor hypothesis of antidepressant action. *Archives of General Psychiatry*, **43**, 1155–61.

Connolly, H., Crary, J., McGoon, M. et al. (1997). Valvular heart disease associated with fenfluramine-phentermine. *New England Journal of Medicine*, **337**, 581–8.

Coppen, A., Whybrow, P.C., Noguera, R., Maggs, R., & Prange, A.J. Jr (1972). The comparative antidepressant value of L-tryptophan and imipramine with and without attempted potentiation by liothyronine. *Archives of General Psychiatry*, **26**, 234–41.

Cournoyer, G., de Montigny, C., Ouellette, J. et al. (1984). Lithium addition in tricyclic-resistant unipolar depression: a placebo-controlled study. Abstracts, 14th Coll International Neuropsychopharmacology Congress 179.

Cowen, P.J., McCance, S.L., Cohen, P.R., & Juiler, D.L. (1989). Lithium increases 5-HT-mediated neuroendocrine responses in tricyclic resistant depression. *Psychopharmacology*, **99**, 230–2.

Cowen, P.J., McCance, S.L., Ware, C.J., Cohen, P.R., Chalmers, J.S., & Juler, D.L. (1991). Lithium in tricyclic-resistant depression. Correlation of increased brain 5-HT function with clinical outcome. *British Journal of Psychiatry*, **159**, 341–6.

Davidson, J., McCleod, M., & Blum, M. (1978). Acetylation phenotype, platelet monoamine oxidase inhibition, and effectiveness of phenelzine in depression. *American Journal of Psychiatry*, **135**, 467–9.

de Montigny, C. & Aghajanian, G.K. (1978). Tricyclic antidepressants: long-term treatment increases responsivity of rat forebrain neurons to serotonin. *Science*, **202**, 1303–6.

de Montigny, C., Grunberg, F., Mayar, A., & Deschenes, J.P. (1981). Lithium induces rapid relief of depression in tricyclic antidepressant drug non-responders. *British Journal of Psychiatry*, **138**, 252–6.

de Montigny, C., Cournoyer, G., Morrissette, R., Langlois, R., & Caillé, G. (1983). Lithium carbonate addition in tricyclic antidepressant-resistant unipolar depression: correlations with the neurobiologic actions of tricyclic antidepressant drugs and lithium ion on the serotonin system. *Archives of General Psychiatry*, **40**, 1327–34.

de Montigny, C., Haddjeri, N., Mongeau, R., & Blier, P. (1995). The effects of mirtazapine on the interactions between central noradrenergic and serotonergic systems. *CNS Drugs*, **4** Suppl. 17.

Depression Guide Panel (1993a). Depression in primary care: Vol. 1. Detection and diagnosis. Clinical Practice Guideline, Number 5. Rockville, MD, US Dept. of Health and Human Services, Public Health Services, Report # 93–0550.

Depression Guide Panel (1993b). Depression in primary care: Vol. 2. Treatment of major depression. Clinical Practice Guideline, Number 5. Rockville, MD, US Dept. of Health and Human Services, Public Health Services, Report # 93–0551.

Dessauer, M., Goetze, U., & Tolle, R. (1985). Periodic sleep deprivation in drug-refractory depression. *Neuropsychobiology*, **13**, 111–16.

Dinan, T.G. & Barry, S. (1989). A comparison of electroconvulsive therapy with a combined lithium and tricyclic combination among tricyclic nonresponders. *Acta Psychiatrica Scandinavica*, **80**, 97–100.

Duval, F., Mokrani, M-C., Crocq, M-A. et al. (1996). Effect of antidepressant medication on morning and evening thyroid function tests during a major depressive episode. *Archives of General Psychiatry*, **53**, 833–40.

Ebert, D., Jaspert, A., Murata, H., & Kaschka, W.P. (1995). Initial lithium augmentation improves the antidepressant effects of standard TCA treatment in non-resistant depressed patients. *Psychopharmacology*, **118**, 223–5.

Eisen, A. (1989). Fluoxetine and desipramine: a strategy for augmenting anti-depressant response. *Pharmacopsychiatry*, **22**, 272–3.

Eison, A.S. & Temple, D.S. (1986). Buspirone: review of its pharmacology and current perspectives on its mechanism of action. *American Journal of Medicine*, **80**(Suppl. 3B), 1–9.

Fava, M., Rosenbaum, J.F., McGrath, P.J., Stewart, J.W., Amsterdam, J.D. & Quitkin, F.M. (1994). Lithium and tricyclic augmentation of fluoxetine treatment for resistant major depression: a double-blind, controlled study. *American Journal of Psychiatry*, **151**, 1372–4.

Fava, M. & Davidson, K.G. (1996). Definition and epidemiology of treatment-resistant depression. In *Treatment Algorithms in Treatment-resistant Depression*, ed. M. Hornig-Rohan & J.D. Amsterdam, pp. 179–200. Philadelphia: W.B. Saunders Co.

Fawcett, J., Kravitz, H.M., Zajecka, J.M., & Schaff, M.R. (1991). CNS stimulant potentiation of monoamine oxidase inhibitors in treatment-refractory depression. *Journal of Clinical Psychopharmacology*, **11**, 127–32.

Feighner, J.P., Herbstein, J., & Damlouji, N. (1985). Combined MAOI, TCA, and direct stimulant therapy of treatment-resistant depression. *Journal of Clinical Psychiatry*, **46**, 206–9.

Feldmesser-Reiss, E.E. (1958). The application of triiodothyronine in the treatment of mental disorders. *Journal of Nervous and Mental Diseases*, **127**, 540–5.

Flach, F.F., Celian, C.I., & Rawson, R.W. (1958). Treatment of psychiatric disorders with triiodothyronine. *American Journal of Psychiatry*, **114**, 841–2.

Gitlin, M.J., Weiner, H., Fairbanks, L., Hershman, J.M., & Friedfeld, N. (1987). Failure of T3 to potentiate tricyclic antidepressant response. *Journal of Affective Diseases*, **13**, 267–72.

Glassman, A.H. & Platman, S.R. (1969). Potentiation of a monoamine oxidase inhibitor by tryptophan. *Journal of Psychiatric Research*, **7**, 83–8.

Glassman, A.H., Kantor, S.J., & Shostak, M. (1975). Depression, delusions, and drug response. *American Journal of Psychiatry*, **132**, 716–19.

Goodman, W.K., Price, L.H., Delgado, P.L. et al. (1990). Specificity of serotonin reuptake inhibitors in the treatment of obsessive compulsive disorder: comparison of fluvoxamine and desipramine. *Archives of General Psychiatry*, **47**, 577–85.

Goodnough, D.B. & Baker, G.B. (1994). 5-Hydroxytryptamine$_2$ and $\beta$-adrenergic receptor regulation in rat brain following chronic treatment with desipramine and fluoxetine alone and in combination. *Journal of Neurochemistry*, **62**, 2262–8.

Goodwin, F.K., Prange, A.J., Jr, Post, R.M., Muscettola, G., & Lipton, M.A. (1982). Potentiation of antidepressant effects by L-triiodothyronine in tricyclic nonresponders. *American Journal of Psychiatry*, **139**, 34–8.

Greenhouse, J.B., Kupfer, D.J., Frank, E., Jarrett, D.B., & Rezman, K.A. (1987). Analysis of time to stabilization in the treatment of depression: biological and clinical correlates. *Journal of Affective Disorders*, **13**, 259–66.

Grunhaus, L. & Remen, A. (1993). Assessment of treatment-resistant major depression: The Michigan Adequacy of Treatment Scale. *Journal of Clinical Psychopharmacology*, **13**, 221–3.

Heninger, G.R., Charney, D.S., & Sternberg, D.E. (1983). Lithium carbonate augmentation of antidepressant treatment: an effective prescription for treatment-refractory depression. *Archives of General Psychiatry*, **40**, 1335–42.

Hjorth, S. & Sharp, T. (1993). 5-HT1A autoreceptor blockade potentiates the ability of the 5-HT reuptake inhibitor citalopram to increase nerve terminal output of 5-HT in vivo: a microdialysis study. *Journal of Neurochemistry*, **60**, 776–9.

Howland, R.H. (1993). Thyroid dysfunction in refractory depression: implications for pathophysiology and treatment. *Journal of Clinical Psychiatry*, **54**, 47–54.

Howland, R.H. (1995). Biochemical effects of antidepressant augmentation. *Archives of General Psychiatry*, **52**, 156.

Inoue, T., Tsuchiya, K., Miura, J. et al. (1996). Bromocriptine treatment of tricyclic and heterocyclic antidepressant-resistant depression. *Biological Psychiatry*, **40**, 151–3.

Jacobsen, F.M. (1991). Possible augmentation of antidepressant response by buspirone. *Journal of Clinical Psychiatry*, **52**, 217–20.

Joffe, R.T. & Schuller, D.R. (1993). An open study of buspirone augmentation of serotonin reuptake inhibitors in refractory depression. *Journal of Clinical Psychiatry*, **54**, 269–71.

Joffe, R.T. & Singer, W. (1990). A comparison of triiodothyronine and thyroxine in the potentiation of tricyclic antidepressants. *Psychiatry Research*, **32**, 241–51.

Joffe, R.T. & Sokolov, S.T.H. (1994). Thyroid hormones, the brain, and affective disorders. *Critical Reviews in Neurobiology*, **8**, 45–63.

Joffe, R.T., Singer, W., Levitt, A.J., & MacDonald, C. (1993). A placebo-controlled comparison of lithium and triiodothyronine augmentation of tricyclic antidepressants in unipolar refractory depression. *Archives of General Psychiatry*, **50**, 387–93.

Joffe, R.T., Levitt, A.J., Sokolov, S.T.H., & Young, L.T. (1996a). Response to an open trial of a second SSRI in major depression. *Journal of Clinical Psychiatry*, **57**, 114–15.

Joffe, R.T., Segal, Z., & Singer, W. (1996b). Change in thyroid hormone levels following response to cognitive therapy for major depression. *American Journal of Psychiatry*, **153**, 411–13.

Kamb, M.L., Murphy, J.J., Lones, J.L. et al. (1992). Eosinophilia-myalgia syndrome in L-tryptophan-exposed patients. *Journal of the American Medical Association*, **267**, 77–82.

Kantor, D., McNevin, S., Leichner, P., Harper, D., & Krenn, M. (1986). The benefit of lithium carbonate adjunct in refractory depression – fact or fiction? *Canadian Journal of Psychiatry*, **31**, 416–18.

Katona, C.L.E., Abou-Saleh, T., Harrison, D.A. et al. (1995). Placebo-controlled trial of lithium augmentation of fluoxetine and lofepramine. *British Journal of Psychiatry*, **166**, 80–6.

Kramlinger, K.G. & Post, R.M. (1989). The addition of lithium to carbamazepine: antidepressant efficacy in treatment-resistant depression. *Archives of General Psychiatry*, **46**, 794–800.

Levine, J., Gonsalves, M., Babur, I. et al. (1993). Inositol 6 gm daily may be effective in depression but not in schizophrenia. *Human Psychopharmacology*, **8**, 49–53.

Levine, J., Barak, Y., Gonzalves, M. et al. (1995). Double-blind, controlled trial of inositol treatment of depression. *American Journal of Psychiatry*, **152**, 792–4.

Lingjaerde, O., Edlund, A.H., Gormsen, C.A. et al. (1974). The effect of lithium carbonate in combination with tricyclic antidepressants in endogenous depression: a double-blind multi-center trial. *Acta Psychiatrica Scandinavica*, **50**, 233–42.

McAskill, R., Mir, S., & Taylor, D. (1998). Pindolol augmentation of antidepressant therapy. *British Journal of Psychiatry*, **173**, 203–8.

McCance-Katz, E.F., Price, L.H., Charney, D.S., & Heninger, G.R. (1992). Serotonergic function during lithium augmentation of refractory depression. *Psychopharmacology*, **108**, 93–7.

McGrath, P.J. Stewart, J.W., Harrison, W.M. et al. (1992). Predictive value of symptoms of atypical depression for differential drug treatment outcome. *Journal of Clinical Psychopharmacology*, **12**, 197–202.

McGrath, P.J., Stewart, J.W., Nunes, E.V. et al. (1993). A double-blind crossover trial of imipramine and phenelzine for outpatients with treatment-refractory depression. *American Journal of Psychiatry*, **250**, 118–23.

Michaelson, D., Stratakis, C., Hill, L. et al. (1996). Bone mineral density in women with depression. *New England Journal of Medicine*, **335**, 1176–81.

Montgomery, S.A. (1995). Selective serotonin reuptake inhibitors in the acute treatment of depression. In *Psychopharmacology: The Fourth Generation of Progress*, ed. F.E. Bloom & D.J. Kupfer, pp. 1043–51. New York: Raven Press.

Moreno, F.A., Gelenberg, A.J., Bachar, K., & Delgado, P.D. (1997). Pindolol augmentation of treatment-resistant depressed patients. *Journal of Clinical Psychiatry*, **58**, 437–9.

Mørk, A., Klysner, R., & Geisler, A. (1990). Effects of treatment with a lithium-imipramine combination on components of adenylate cyclase in the cerebral cortex of the rat. *Neuropharmacology*, **29**, 261–7.

Mueller, T., Keller, M.B., Leon, A.C. et al. (1996). Recovery after 5 years of unremitting major depressive disorder. *Archives of General Psychiatry*, **53**, 794–9.

Nakamura, T. & Nomura, J. (1992). Comparison of thyroid function between responders and nonresponders to thyroid hormone supplementation in depression. *Japanese Journal of Psychiatry and Neurology*, **46**, 905–9.

Nelson, J.C. (1987). The use of antipsychotic drugs in the treatment of depression. In *Treating Resistant Depression*, ed. J. Zohar & R.H. Belmaker, pp. 131–45. New York: PMA Publishing.

Nelson, J.C. & Bowers, M.B. (1978). Delusional unipolar depression. *Archives of General Psychiatry*, **35**, 1321–8.

Nelson, J.C. & Mazure, C.M. (1986). Lithium augmentation in psychotic depression refractory to combined drug treatment. *American Journal of Psychiatry*, **143**, 363–6.

Nelson, J.C., Price, L.H., & Jatlow, P. (1986). Neuroleptic dose and desipramine concentrations during combined treatment of unipolar delusional depression. *American Journal of Psychiatry*, **143**, 1151–4.

Nelson, J.C., Mazure, C.M., Bowers, M.B., Jr & Jatlow, P.I. (1991). A preliminary, open study of the combination of fluoxetine and desipramine for rapid treatment of major depression. *Archives of General Psychiatry*, **48**, 303–7.

Newman, M.E., Drummer, D., & Lerer, B. (1990). Single and combined effects of desimipramine and lithium on serotonergic receptor number and second messenger function in rat brain. *Journal of Pharmacological Experimental Therapy*, **252**, 826–31.

Nick, J., Luaute, J.P., Des Lauriers, A., Moinet, A., & Monfort, J. (1976). L'association clomipramine-lithium essai controle. *Encephale*, **2**, 5–16.

Nierenberg, A.A. (1990). Methodological problems in treatment-resistant depression research. *Psychopharmacology Bulletin*, **26**, 461–4.

Nierenberg, A.A., Price, L.H., Charney, D.S., & Heninger, G.R. (1990). After lithium augmentation: a retrospective follow-up of patients with antidepressant-refractory depression. *Journal of Affective Diseases*, **18**, 167–75.

Ontiveros, A., Fontaine, R., & Elie, R. (1991). Refractory depression: the addition of lithium to fluoxetine or desipramine. *Acta Psychiatrica Scandinavia*, **83**, 188–92.

Oppenheim, G., Zohar, J., Shapiro, B., & Belmaker, R.H. (1987). The role of estrogen in treating resistant depression. In *Treating Resistant Depression*, ed. J. Zohar & R.H. Belmaker, pp. 357–65. New York: PMA Publishing.

Ostroff, R.B. & Nelson, J.C. (1999). Risperidone augmentation of selective serotoinin reuptake inhibitors in major depression. *Journal of Clinical Psychiatry*, **60**, 256–9.

Parker, G., Roy, K., Hadzi-Pavlovic, D., & Pedic, F. (1992). Psychotic (delusional) depression: a meta-analysis of physical treatments. *Journal of Affective Diseases*, **24**, 17–24.

Perez, V., Soler, J., Puigdemont, D. et al. (1999). A double-blind, randomized, placebo-controlled trial of pindolol augmentation in depressive patients resistant to serotonin reuptake inhibitors. *Archives of General Psychiatry*, **56**, 375–9.

Peselow, E.D., Filippi, A.M., Goodnick, P., Barouche, F., & Fieve, R.R. (1989). The short-and long-term efficacy of paroxetine HCl: B. Data from a double-blind crossover study and from a year-long trial vs. imipramine and placebo. *Psychopharmacology, Bulletin*, **25**, 272–6.

Prange, A.J., Wilson, I.C., Rabon, A.M., & Lipton, A.M. (1969). Enhancement of imipramine antidepressant effect by thyroid hormone. *American Journal of Psychiatry*, **126**, 457–69.

Prange, A.J., Garbutt, J.C., & Loosen, P.T. (1987). The hypothalamic–pituitary–thyroid axis in affective disorders. In *Psychopharmacology: The Third Generation of Progress*, ed. H.Y. Meltzer, pp. 629–36. New York, Raven Press.

Preskorn, S. & Burke, M. (1993). Therapeutic drug monitoring: principles and practice. *Psychiatric Clinins of North America*, **16**, 611–45.

Price, L.H. (1989). Lithium augmentation of tricyclic antidepressants. In *Treatment of Tricyclic Resistant Depression*, ed. I. Extein, pp. 49–79. Washington, DC: American Psychiatric Press.

Price, L.H. (1990). Pharmacological strategies in refractory depression. In *American Psychiatric Press Annual Review of Psychiatry*, ed. A. Tasman, S.M. Goldfinger, & C.A. Kaufmann, pp. 116–31. Vol. 9. Washington, DC: American Psychiatric Press.

Price, L.H. & Heninger, G.R. (1994). Lithium in the treatment of mood disorders. *New England Journal of Medicines*, **331**, 591–8.

Price, L.H., Charney, D.S., & Heninger, G.R. (1986). Variability of response to lithium augmentation in refractory depression. *American Journal of Psychiatry*, **143**, 1387–92.

Price, L.H., Charney, D.S., & Heninger, G.R. (1987). Reserpine augmentation of desipramine in refractory depression: clinical and neurobiological effects. *Psychopharmacology*, **92**, 431–7.

Price, L.H., Charney, D.S., Delgado, P.L., Anderson, G.M., & Heninger, G.R. (1989a). Effects of desipramine and fluvoxamine treatment on the prolactin response to tryptophan: serotonergic function and the mechanism of antidepressant action. *Archives of General Psychiatry*, **46**, 625–31.

Price, L.H., Charney, D.S., Delgado, P.L., Anderson, G.M., & Heninger, G.R. (1989b). Lithium treatment and serotonergic function: neuroendocrine, behavioral, and physiologic responses to intravenous L-tryptophan in affective disorder patients. *Archives of General Psychiatry*, **46**, 13–19.

Price, L.H., Charney, D.S., Delgado, P.L., & Heninger, G.R. (1990a). Lithium and serotonin function: Implications for the serotonin hypothesis of depression. *Psychopharmacology*, **100**, 3–12.

Price, L.H., Charney, D.S., Delgado, P.L., & Heninger, G.R. (1990b). Fenfluramine augmentation in tricyclic-refractory depression. *Journal of Clinical Psychopharmacology*, **10**, 312–17.

Prudic, J., Haskett, R.F., Mulsant, B. et al. (1996). Resistance to antidepressant medications and short-term clinical response to ECT. *American Journal of Psychiatry*, **153**, 985–92.

Quitkin, F., McGrath, P.J., Stewart, J.W. et al. (1996). Chronological milestones to guide drug change. *Archives of General Psychiatry*, **53**, 785–92.

Razani, J., White, K.L., White, J. et al.(1983). The safety and efficacy of combined amitriptyline and tranylcypromine treatment: a controlled trial. *Archives of General Psychiatry*, **40**, 557–661.

Rothschild, A.J., Samson, J.A., Bessette, M.P., & Carter-Campbell, J.T. (1993). Efficacy of the combination of fluoxetine and perphenazine in the treatment of psychotic depression. *Journal of Clinical Psychiatry*, **54**, 338–42.

Rybakowski, J. & Matkowski, K. (1992). Adding lithium to antidepressant therapy: factors related to therapeutic potentiation. *European Neuropsychopharmacology*, **2**, 161–5.

Sachs, G.S. (1996). Treatment-resistant bipolar depression. In *Treatment Algorithms in Treatment-resistant Depression*, ed. M. Hornig-Rohan & J.D. Amsterdam, pp. 371–86. Philadelphia, W.B. Saunders Co.

Satel, S.L. & Nelson, J.C. (1989). Stimulants in the treatment of depression: a critical overview. *Journal of Clinical Psychiatry*, **50**, 241–9.

Schöpf, J., Baumann, P., Lemarchand, T., & Rey, M. (1989). Treatment of endogenous depressions resistant to tricyclic antidepressants or related drugs by lithium addition. Results of a placebo-controlled double-blind study. *Pharmacopsychiatry*, **22**, 183–7.

Schwarcz, G., Halaris, A., Baxter, L., Escobar, J., Thompson, M., & Young, M. (1984). Normal thyroid function in desipramine nonresponders converted to responders by the addition of L-triiodothyronine. *American Journal of Psychiatry*, **141**, 1614–16.

Seth, R., Jennings, A.L., Bindman, J., Phillips, J., & Bergmann, K. (1992). Combination treatment with noradrenalin and serotonin reuptake inhibitors in resistant depression. *British Journal of Psychiatry*, **161**, 562–5.

Shahal, B., Piel, E., Mecz, L., Kremer, I., & Klein, E. (1996). Lack of advantage for imipramine combined with lithium versus imipramine alone in the treatment of major depression – a double-blind controlled study. *Biological Psychiatry*, **40**, 1181–3.

Shelton, R., Tollefson, G., Tohen, M. et al. (1998). The study of olanzapine plus fluoxetine in treatment-resistant major depressive disorder without psychotic features. Poster presented at the 30th Annual New Clinical Drug Evaluation Unit Mtg., Boca Raton, FL.

Spiker, D.G., Weiss, J.C., Dealy, R.S. et al. (1985). The pharmacological treatment of delusional depression. *American Journal of Psychiatry*, **142**, 430–6.

Stein, G. & Bernadt, M. (1993). Lithium augmentation therapy in tricyclic-resistant depression. A controlled trial using lithium in low and normal doses. *British Journal of Psychiatry*, **162**, 634–40.

Steiner, M., Radwan, M., Elizur, A., Blum, I., Atsmon, A., & Davidson, S. (1978). Failure of L-triiodothyronine to potentiate tricyclic antidepressant response. *Current Therapy Research*, **23**, 655–9.

Sternbach, H. (1991). The serotonin syndrome. *American Journal of Psychiatry*, **148**, 705–13.

Stoudemire, A., Hill, C.D., Morris, R., & Lewison, B.J. (1993). Long-term outcome of treatment-resistant depression in older adults. *American Journal of Psychiatry*, **150**, 1539–40.

Strober, M., Freeman, R., Rigali, J., Schmidt, S., & Diamond, R. (1992). The pharmacotherapy of depressive illness in adolescence: II. Effects of lithium augmentation in nonresponders to imipramine. *Journal of the American Academy of Child and Adolescent Psychiatry*, **31**, 16–20.

Sulser, F., Vetulani, J., & Mobley, P.L. (1978). Mode of action of antidepressant drugs. *Biochemical Pharmacology*, **27**, 257–61.

Tang, S.W., Remington, G., Persad, E., & Rosenblat, R. (1990). Coadministration of a beta-adrenergic antagonist and a tricyclic antidepressant: a pilot study. *Psychiatry Research*, **33**, 101–6.

Targum, S.D., Greenberg, R.D., Harmon, R.L., Kessler, K., Salerian, A.J. & Fram, D.H. (1984). Thyroid hormone and the TSH stimulation test in refractory depression. *Journal of Clinical Psychiatry*, **45**, 345–6.

Taylor, D. (1995). Selective serotonin reuptake inhibitors and tricyclic antidepressants in combination. Interactions and therapeutic uses. *British Journal of Psychiatry*, **167**, 575–80.

Thase, M.E. & Rush, A.J. (1995). Treatment-resistant depression. In *Psychopharmacology: The Fourth Generation of Progress*, ed. F.E. Bloom & D.J. Kupfer, pp. 1081–97. New York: Raven Press.

Thase, M.E., Kupfer, D.J., Frank, E., & Jarrett, D.B. (1989). Treatment of imipramine-resistant recurrent depression: II. An open clinical trial of lithium augmentation. *Journal of Clinical Psychiatry*, **50**, 413–17.

van Marwijk, H.W., Bekker, F.M., Nolen, W.A., Jansen, P.A., van Nieuwkerk, J.F. & Hop, W.C. (1990). Lithium augmentation in geriatric depression. *Journal of Affective Disorders*, **20**, 217–23.

Vuckovic, A., Cohen, B.M., & Zubenko, G.S. (1991). The use of captopril in treatment-resistant depression: an open trial. *Journal of Clinical Psychopharmacology*, **11**, 395–6.

Walinder, J., Skott, A., Carlsson, A., Nagy, A., & Bjorn-Erik, R. (1976). Potentiation of the antidepressant action of clomipramine by tryptophan. *Archives of General Psychiatry*, **33**, 1384–9.

Weilburg, J.B., Rosenbaum, J.F., Biederman, J., Sachs, G.S., Pollack, M.H. & Kelly, K. (1989). Fluoxetine added to non-MAOI antidepressants converts nonresponders to responders: a preliminary report. *Journal of Clinical Psychiatry*, **50**, 447–9.

Wheatley, D. (1972). Potentiation of amitryptyline by thyroid hormone. *Archives of General Psychiatry*, **26**, 229–33.

Whybrow, P.C. & Prange, A. (1981). A hypothesis of thyroid-catecholamine-receptor interaction. *Archives of General Psychiatry*, **38**, 106–13.

Wilson, I.C., Prange, A.J. Jr, McClane, T.K., Rabon, A.M., & Lipton, M.A. (1979). Thyroid-hormone enhancement of imipramine in non-retarded depressions. *New England Journal of Medicine*, **282**, 1063–7.

Wolf, M.A., Louis, J-C., & Vincendon, G. (1989). Antidepressant effect of lithium: a neurochemical study on neuronal uptake of norepinephrine and serotonin. *Progress in Neuro-Psychopharmacology and Biological Psychiatry*, **12**, 765–73.

Yasmin, S., Carpenter, L.L., Leon, Z., Siniscalchi, J.M., & Price, L.H. (in press). Adjunctive gabapentin in treatment-resistant depression: a retrospective chart review. *Journal of Affective Disorders*.

Yoshida, T., Suzuki, S., Sugita, S., Kobayashi, A., & Nakazawa, K. (1989). Effects of lithium on alterations of pharmacokinetics of imipramine and on the related changes of monoamines in rat brain. *European Journal of Pharmacology*, **173**, 143–9.

Zajecka, M., Jeffriess, H., & Fawcett, J. (1995). The efficacy of fluoxetine combined with a heterocyclic antidepressant in treatment-resistant depression: a retrospective analysis. *Journal of Clinical Psychiatry*, **56**, 338–43.

Zimmer, B., Rosen, J., Thornton, J.E., Perel, J.M., & Reynolds, C.F. III (1991). Adjunctive lithium carbonatee in nortriptyline-resistant elderly depressed patients. *Journal of Clinical Psychopharmacology*, **11**, 254–6.

Zusky, P.M., Biederman, J., Rosenbaum, J.F. et al. (1988). Adjunct low dose lithium carbonate in treatment-resistant depression: A placebo-controlled study. *Journal of Clinical Psychopharmacology*, **8**, 120–4.

# 11

# Electroconvulsive therapy in medication-resistant depression

Max Fink

## Introduction

Electroconvulsive therapy (ECT) is an effective treatment for major depressive disorders. It is usually reserved for patients who are so ill as to require hospital care. In direct comparisons between ECT and either tricyclic antidepressant drugs (TCA) or monoamine oxidase inhibitors (MAOI), ECT is more effective than either. (We lack information as to the relative efficacy of SSRI and ECT as such studies have not been done.)

The antidepressant efficacy of ECT is well established even in patients who have failed prior adequate courses of TCA and MAOI (Abrams, 1997; Avery & Lubrano, 1979; Fink 1979, 1999; Kantor & Glassman, 1977). In patients with delusional depression, TCA alone are approximately 35% effective while ECT elicits a robust response evaluated as 80% effective, equal to that reported for the combination of high doses of TCA and neuroleptic drugs (Kroessler et al., 1985; Parker et al., 1992). Despite its efficacy, and even superiority, in relieving severe depressive disorders, ECT is infrequently used. In modern guidelines and algorithms, it is almost always considered a treatment of last resort, if it is considered at all.

Many pundits have remarked that, were its merits available in capsule form, ECT would occupy a central role in treating major depressive disorders. Many reasons are given for the discrepancy between the experimental data and its present usage, and of these, three seem the most cogent.

ECT is a technical science that requires special facilities and special skills. Additional training and qualification is required of the psychiatrist. Unfortunately, training in ECT is rarely a feature of medical school experience and is unavailable in most psychiatric residency training programs (Lehrmann, 2000). Each treatment is complex, requiring the coordination of an anesthesiologist, a trained nurse, and the psychiatrist (APA, 1990). ECT requires more effort and greater experience than writing a prescription. Such an impediment would be hardly decisive if financial incentives and social pressures were encouraging, but they are not. The difficulties of coronary artery bypass surgery, tissue transplants, renal dialysis, and other highly technical procedures have not deterred almost every general hospital in the nation from developing these facilities. Very low reimbursement rates for ECT further discourage its use.

The hostility of the public and the profession is a more cogent reason for the professional disinterest. A negative attitude to ECT dominates present clinical psychiatric practice. It is codified in inadequate professional training and the scarcity of trained professionals, in public arguments in the press as to its safety, in negative images in film and television, and in legislative caveats and proscriptions. Few psychiatric leaders are grounded in ECT, and while many acknowledge an experience with the treatment, that experience is usually limited to their residency training. Public antipathy limits its use so that only the most established academic medical centers and a few private facilities in the United States provide ECT for their patients (Fink, 1993c, 1999; Hartmann, 1996). The negative attitudes to ECT are also encouraged by the massive advertising, extensive subvention of research, and direct financial payments by the pharmaceutical industry to lecturers and researchers in support of their products. None of the research granting agencies, public or private, and none of the national associations considers electroshock in their award, teaching, or research programs. It is nigh impossible for electroshock to obtain a public forum or its researchers to obtain support for their studies (Fink, 1999).

A more valid objection is that the benefits of the treatment 'do not last', that relapse is frequent. Renewed interest in ECT in the 1970s occurred at a time when public and professional opposition developed to all somatic treatments. It was the time of the California law that interdicted the use of electroshock and lobotomy in any individuals in the state. Although the law was finally modified, its chilling effect remains obvious in the scattered availability and use of ECT in the state. A similar sequence has developed in Texas where the legislature in 1994 interdicted the use of ECT in persons under 16 years of age. A review of the experience since 1995 finds the use of ECT limited to a few hospitals in the state and underutilization among populations of the non-white mentally ill (Reid et al., 1998). Electroshock, lobotomy, and psychotropic drugs were proscribed in many states and in many institutions (Endler & Persad, 1988; Fink, 1993c, 1999; Hartmann, 1996). Objections to the use of psychotropic medications dissolved rapidly when their efficacy and ease of use was recognized. The restrictions in leucotomy persist so that its use is limited to patients being treated in experimental protocols. While the restrictions and negative attitudes to electroshock also persist, ECT has sustained a national presence. But practitioners were intimidated and they prescribed minimal courses of ECT as they bargained to use the treatment. Short treatment courses, a failure to fix the benefits with continuation ECT, and dependence on inadequate continuation medication treatments (often the same medications which had failed before) encouraged early relapse. We have answered this objection by introducing continuation treatment with ECT. Patients now receive an index course of 6–10 ECT, followed by weekly and then bi-weekly treatments for up to six months (Monroe, 1991; Petrides et al., 1994; Fink, 1999). This practice is facilitated by our acceptance of outpatient (ambulatory) ECT as a feature in most ECT programs (Fink et al., 1996). Such practice assures prolonged successful results.

I have often defended the proposition that a severely depressed patient, especially one ill enough to warrant hospital care, should not be labeled pharmacotherapy resistant and treated interminably with medications without a trial of electroconvulsive therapy (see Fink 1987, 1989, 1993a,b, 1999). In this essay, I consider the questions:

(i) What is a reasonable role for ECT in the treatment of depressive mood disorders?
(ii) How many medication trials are reasonable before a change to ECT is considered?
(iii) Which psychopathological predictors urge consideration of ECT?
(iv) What changes in ECT practice encourage its freer use?
(v) How can ECT be reasonably integrated in treatment algorithms for severe depression?

## Defining medication resistance

When medicine is the first option in treating depression, how long should a trial continue before another tack is taken? For how many courses should a patient be treated before 'medication-resistant depression' is defined and ECT considered? I am aware of two suggested guidelines for such a determination. One is a sophisticated algorithm proposed by Sackeim and his associates in their studies of ECT (Sackeim et al., 1990); and a second is a model I derived from the evaluations of the efficacy of clozapine as a neuroleptic agent (Fink, 1993b).

Sackeim and his coworkers consider the type of medicine, the dosage, duration of the trial, and degree of compliance in developing a scale of adequacy of a medication trial in patients referred for ECT. In assessing the adequacy of a treatment course with a typical tricyclic antidepressant (i.e. imipramine, amitriptyline), medicine used for less than four weeks or with dosages less than 200 mg/day are deemed inadequate, while more than 200 mg/day for longer than 4 weeks are deemed adequate. After a successful course of ECT, the patients who had inadequate pre-ECT medicine trials often did well with continuation medication, usually because dosages were now set at adequate levels. But those who had failed adequate trials of medicines relapsed quickly (Sackeim et al., 1990; Prudic et al., 1990).

My definition of an adequate medication trial derives from studies of clozapine in schizophrenic patients. Because clozapine has the acknowledged risks of both agranulocytosis and induced seizures, experimentalists decided that a failed response to two trials with neuroleptic drugs of different classes, each for a minimum 4 weeks, was prerequisite to exposure to clozapine (Kane, 1989; Lieberman et al., 1989). I suggest that we define a failed trial of antidepressant medicines as the lack of response to a four week course of an SSRI and then a TCA (or a TCA followed by an SSRI) in doses of at least 200 mg/day for the TCA (and an equivalent of 40 mg/day of fluoxetine for the SSRI). In depressed patients with evidence of a bipolar illness, a trial of lithium therapy or an anticonvulsant medicine may replace the experience with an antidepressant medicine.

When depression is still debilitating after two adequate medication trials, ECT is the proper treatment. Only after an adequate ECT trial has failed, and such failure is remarkably infrequent, is it reasonable to use experimental augmentation and combination strategies or the latest marketed 'me, too' antidepressant medicines.

Other authors have come to the same opinion. In a special volume dedicated to treatment-resistant depression, Reus (1996) notes:

'ECT is as, or more, effective than any pharmacologic treatment for severe depression and should be considered in any identified treatment-resistant case. Its limited use reflects misconceptions about long-term effects and lack of training in its usage.' (p. 206).

Nelsen and Dunner (1995), in assessing their experience with therapy-resistant depression, note:

'... our TRD population reflects patients referred to a tertiary-care center ... [who] have been extensively treated and were characterized by chronic depression.'

They continue:

'... electroconvulsive therapy is underused in our particular sample. This is in spite of the fact that our patient population had chronic depression, had not responded to a number of treatments, and that over 25% of this population had made suicide attempts. Earlier and more frequent application of ECT may be an advantage to populations of patients who are referred for treatment-resistant depression.' (p. 48).

Medication resistance and persistent depression is encouraged by modern research practice. Experimentalists accept rating scale scores as outcome efficacy criteria. Item rating scales only partially reflect the quality of life of the individual and many who are evaluated as 'improved' are still ill and incapacitated. When patients begin a treatment trial with Hamilton Depression Rating Scale [HAM-D] scores of 24–30 (examples of severe depression), the accepted goal of a 50% reduction in the HAM-D leaves patients with scores of 12 to 18. They are still ill and unable to work, despite a 50% relief of symptoms. It is a poor trial that evaluates such persistent signs and symptoms in the HAMD as 'success'. On the other hand, ECT studies routinely accept 'single digit' (<9) and at least a 60% reduction in HAM-D scores as the minimal acceptable outcome criteria. Such relief is routinely achieved (Abrams, 1997; Fink, 1999).

# Depression subtypes

## Delusional depression

Psychosis, melancholia, agitated and catatonic motor behavior, and stupor predict a good outcome with ECT. Of these, the presence of delusions is the most useful. In the extended and careful ECT and sham-ECT studies undertaken by British authors between 1978 and 1981, the presence of delusions identified the patients with the best response (Palmer, 1981).

Delusional depression is a malignant depressive mood disorder. It responds poorly to standard antidepressant medicines when these are used alone (Kroessler, 1985; Parker et al., 1991, 1995; Coryell, 1996; Rothschild, 1996). In 1964, deCarolis and his associates reported the superior efficacy of ECT over adequate courses of imipramine (a minimum of 25 days at doses above 250 mg/day) in patients hospitalized for severe depressive mood disorders. The bulk of the poor results were in delusional depressed patients. Kantor and Glassman (1977) next reported that depressed patients who failed TCA trials even with careful medication dosing and blood level monitoring were characterized by the presence of delusions. Such patients responded well to courses of ECT. This finding has been repeatedly confirmed (Abrams, 1997).

Before a depressed patient is labeled 'medication resistant,' the presence of delusions must be carefully assessed. A delusional mood disorder warrants intensive therapy, either with the combination of a neuroleptic and a TCA, both in high doses, or a course of ECT. In the recommendations for the use of TCA and neuroleptic combined, much is made of the need for effective doses, usually described as equivalent to 32 to 64 mg perphenazine and 250 to 300 mg amitriptyline each day for a minimum of four weeks (Spiker et al., 1985). That such a necessary prescribed course of therapy is often overlooked is seen in the report by Mulsant et al. (1997) that the pretreatment medication trials were considered adequate in only 2 of 52 patients referred for ECT as medication resistant. The report is all the more astonishing, considering that the report comes from three of the premier academic treatment centers of the nation.

Many authors assume that an SSRI may substitute for a TCA in combination drug treatment. Such assumption is premature. We lack experimental data to warrant this substitution and such use may well encourage medication resistance.

Given the malignancy of delusional depression, its resistance and early relapse with high doses and extended courses of TCA with neuroleptics and even with ECT, the substitution of an SSRI or an atypical antidepressant is unjustified.

### Depression in adolescents

The recognition of a major depressive mood disorder in an adolescent is difficult, and few studies find medications effective. The same may be said for the role of ECT, although recent reviews culling case material report a surprising efficacy for it (Moise & Petrides, 1996; Rey & Walter, 1997; Walter & Rey, 1997). At a meeting of experts in adolescent depressive mood disorders in 1994, the participants recognized the paucity of experimental data to define the incidence of such disorders, their proper recognition, and their optimal treatment. They reviewed the available case material and their clinical experience, and concluded that, if an adolescent has the history and cross-sectional behavior sufficient to warrant a diagnosis of depressive mood disorder in an adult, the same diagnosis should be made and the same treatments considered. It is prudent to consider ECT in adolescents under the same conditions as ECT would be considered in adults.

What of therapy resistance in depressed adolescents? Considering the widespread belief that the primary cause of adolescent disorders is in family strife, maternal attitudes, and psychological turmoil and not in their biology, many adolescents suffer interminable and unsuccessful trials of special education, psychotherapy, group psychotherapy, and family counseling before they are considered therapy-resistant and medicines recommended. They are also disadvantaged that low and inadequate doses of popular and fashionable medicines are recommended. The practicing psychiatrist treating patients in this age group should recognize that suicide among adolescents is a severe risk, that psychosis is difficult to define, and that a smoke-screen of hallucinogenic and illicit drug use often clouds the diagnosis and treatment. When medication trials fail, it is prudent to reflect on the recent case literature of the efficacy and safety of ECT and consider its use (Fink, 1999).

### Depression in the elderly

Depressive mood disorders are frequent in the elderly. Bodily changes, loss of memory, loss of friends and family, social and sensory isolation, and retirement from work encourage depression. Such a mood disorder is accompanied by physical weakness, loss of initiative, appetite, and weight, insomnia, and decreased interest in sex. Systemic disabilities encourage questions whether relief will ever come, and whether the body that is left will sustain prior pleasures and interest (Meyers, 1995). Suicidal thoughts arise.

They also suffer disorders of thought. Their inability to work leads to the belief that they are worthless or penniless, or that governmental authorities are investigating their failure to pay taxes. Reduced interest in sex lead to thoughts that their spouse, or that they, are unfaithful. Such abnormal thoughts indicate a more severe depression, a condition for which antidepressant drug treatment alone is rarely successful. The addition of a neuroleptic drug to an antidepressant drug trial may be more successful.

The elderly are often sensitive to low doses of the medications given to treat depression and their systemic disorders. They develop side effects that compel their discontinuation. Since the elderly tolerate ECT well, it behoves practitioners to consider ECT earlier than later in their management.

## Suicidality

Suicidality, an ever-present risk in treating the severely ill, is an indication for ECT. Patients who are so driven to self-harm that their caretakers must provide 24-hour individual protection are of such high risk that the most rapidly effective treatment for this condition is compelled. Suicidality does not encourage proper random assignment experimental trials, so the best data are case analyses or retrospective studies of patients treated by various means. The efficacy of ECT and its speed of action is well documented (Avery & Winokur, 1978). Once a patient is defined as severely depressed with an active drive to self-harm, the security of delivering an adequate course of therapy and doing so rapidly compels the use of ECT.

## Borderline personality disorder and dysthymia

As best as I can tell, few therapies successfully alleviate these lifelong conditions. When character pathology leads to repeated episodes of wrist and face cutting and other acute episodes of self-harm, patients are seen as suicidal. When trials of medicines fail, ECT is considered. The evidence for the efficacy of ECT in such conditions is anecdotal and weak. While the immediate drive to suicide may be relieved by ECT, it usually recurs with severity as soon as the realities of family, housing, and work are discussed, and even more so when the patient returns to the community.

## Progress in ECT efficacy

ECT practice has changed and it is less riskful than described in all but the most recent texts. An adequate treatment and an adequate course of ECT are now better defined and readily achieved. The advantages of continuation ECT, the role of augmentation medications, and precise guidelines for electrode placements and energy dosing also contribute to treatment success (Abrams, 1997; Fink, 1994b, 1999; Fink et al., 1996).

## Electrode placement

For two decades electrotherapists were convinced that treatments through unilateral electrode placements were as effective as treatments through bilateral bitemporal electrode placements (Abrams, 1997). In a classical experiment, Sackeim and his associates (1993) reported an interaction between electrode placements and energy dosing that affected efficacy. Patients treated with unilateral electrode placements and threshold energies exhibited improvement in less than one-third of cases. When energies were increased to 2.5 times the threshold, improvement rates were higher, but not as high as either threshold or suprathreshold energies through bitemporal placement. Even in the most experienced hands, unilateral electrode placement requires special attention to electrical energy dosing to achieve a satisfactory outcome. Two new reports argue that energies in unilateral ECT must be set to at least five times the measured seizure threshold to achieve efficacy that is evaluated as equal to that of bilateral ECT. The full impact of such high energies are not fully assessed but the report by McCall (2000) shows a disturbing increase in cognitive effects with increasing energies above seizure threshold in unilateral ECT, an increase that has a steeper slope than the increase in efficacy. Furthermore, modern ECT devices are limited in their maximum output, and do not allow such energies to be delivered to patients with high initial seizure thresholds, a feature of many persons over the age of 50 (McCall, 2000; Sackeim et al., 2000).

Lately, some authors have examined the impact of bifrontal electrode placement on the efficacy and side effects of ECT (Bailine et al., 2000). The efficacy of bifrontal ECT is seen as the same as bitemporal ECT and the cognitive effects are less, when the energies are estimated by the half-age algorithm (Petrides & Fink, 1996). The assessment of this placement has assumed a high priority, and if the replications confirm the initial reports, both unilateral and bitemporal electrode placements will be replaced. For the present, however, bitemporal electrode placement is the preferred treatment practice.

## Adequate treatment

For decades, little attention was paid to the quality of each treatment. As we defined the relative merits of different electrode placements, the quality of the seizure became of interest. Seizure duration was one index of treatment adequacy (Fink & Johnson, 1982). But once energy dosing was seen as essential to unilateral electrode placement, attention was paid to EEG patterns and EEG endpoints to assure the most effective treatment. EEG criteria are now part of the definition of adequacy of treatment (Fink, 1994b, 1999; Kellner & Fink, 1996).

## Adequate course

Prescribing a fixed number of treatments leads to undertreatment. Short courses encourage early relapse, even with continuation medication. Present practice recommends a course of ECT of at least 4 months. The initial treatments are generally given in a hospital setting, the later treatments in ambulatory settings (Fink et al., 1996).

## Continuation ECT

For many patients, a course of ECT was predetermined as a fixed number of treatments, without correction for clinical progress. To sustain the antidepressant effect, patients were then prescribed medicines as continuation treatments. Unfortunately, the patients had often failed these same medications before their referral for ECT. Relapse rates were high. In the past decade, however, ECT treatment courses have been extended as continuation treatments in ambulatory ECT (Fink et al., 1996). The present recommendation is that the ECT course should extend for at least 4 months after the index course of ECT, a period close to that of a 6-month medication trial.

## Medications

Greater consideration is now given to the concurrent use of medications to augment the efficacy of treatments (Kellner, 1993; Fink, 1994a, 1999). In treating patients with psychosis, the action of neuroleptic drugs is augmented by ECT. The concurrent use of chlorpromazine, fluphenazine, thiothixene, and clozapine with ECT is documented, and present practice recommends such combined use (Fink, 1998).

Many therapists discontinue TCA, MAOI, and SSRI medications during the course of ECT as there are no studies supporting a favorable interaction. Also, these compounds are associated with cardiovascular effects that may increase risk, especially in the elderly and the systemically ill.

Lithium augmentation presents the hazard of an acute delirium when serum lithium levels are high. When lithium is continued during the course of ECT, dosing is generally reduced on the day before treatment to assure lower serum levels on the morning of treatment.

Anticonvulsants and benzodiazepines reduce the quality and efficacy of seizures. They are usually discontinued. If patients require anticonvulsants for a concurrent seizure disorder, treatment is continued with special attention to the quality of each treatment.

## Algorithms

It is now fashionable to develop clinical practice guidelines for the treatment of systemic disorders. These are of particular interest to managed care insurers, who

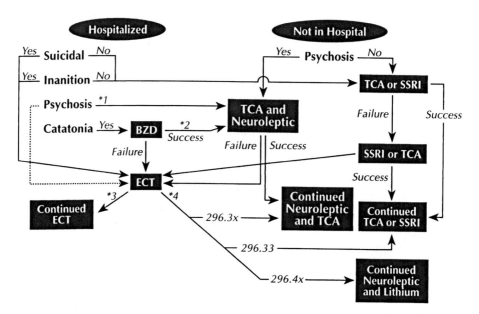

Fig. 11.1.  Major depressive disorder (× 296.3), bipolar disorder, depressed mood (× 296.4)
*1 Psychosis – ECT may be a primary treatment.
*2 Resolution of catatonia allows treatment for underlying condition.
*3 Prior adequate medication trial warrants continued ECT.
*4 Prior inadequate medication trial warrants continued medication.

seek rules under which the insured can be treated at minimal cost. One glaring omission is the severity of illness as a criterion for an algorithm. These are usually written as if all depressed patients are of the same degree of dysfunction. But, what may be a credible approach for a person complaining of feelings of inadequacy and depression, but is able to work, may not be credible if the disorder is associated with melancholia or suicidality that requires hospital protection. One defense of algorithm writers in recommending newer medications and ignoring established combined medication treatments or ECT is that their recommendations are designed for outpatients in offices and clinics. In such presentations, ECT is almost always either ignored or cited as the 'last resort' treatment option. Examples are widespread in clinical articles, in psychopharmacology texts, and in guidelines for practice developed by expert committees. (APA, 1993, 1994; Klein, 1994; De Battista & Schatzberg, 1994; Janicak et al., 1995; Preskorn et al., 1995; Amsterdam & Hornig-Rohan, 1996; Frances et al., 1996; Rush et al., 1998). The *Clinical Practice Guidelines* section on *Depression in Primary Care*, vol. 2 is an exception. These authors note that: 'Electroconvulsive therapy is a first-line treatment option only for patients with more severe or psychotic forms of major depressive disorder, those who have failed to respond to other therapies, those with medical conditions precluding the use of medications, and those with an essential need for rapid response.' (*USPHS AHCPR* Publication 93-0551, 1993, p. 41).

If ECT is cited, it is as an intervention after all else has been tried and failed. The 'all else' usually includes multiple medication trials, headed by the most recently introduced and often incompletely tested medicine, augmentation strategies based on little experience, and experimental combinations of new and old medications. In recent updates of a 1993 psychopharmacology text, priority of treatment is assigned to fluoxetine, paroxetine, sertraline, nefazadone, and venlafaxine (see Preskorn et al., 1995; Janicak et al., 1995). The authors infer their preferences from the open, clinical, ambulatory patient trials that, at best, show no difference from a comparison TCA. In another new supplement, these same authors recommend the use of risperidone and clozapine for manic disorders, despite the absence of supportive data. Similar algorithms with the same disinterest in ECT are prepared by expert committees (see Hales & Yudofsky, 1996; APA, 1993, 1994).

What is a reasonable algorithm for the role of ECT in treating depressive disorders? The principal decision nodes should consider severity of illness (need for in-hospital care), suicidality, presence of delusions, inanition, stupor, or catatonia, and then the adequacy of one or two established medication trials. New medicines proclaimed as equal in efficacy to existing standards but with lesser side effects are introduced to the market with increasing rapidity. None have been well tested in severely ill patients or compared to ECT at the time of introduction. Their recommendation for use early in the treatment algorithms is based wholly on the faith of the creators, many of whom are the same investigators who have done the premarket clinical trials and who continue as consultants and lecturers with industry support. Much of what we know about new medicines comes from postmarketing surveillance, and it generally requires many years before the proper role of a new medicine is established in clinical practice. At this time, none of the medicines introduced in the 1980s or the 1990s has been tested for efficacy against ECT. A decision tree for hospitalized patients that recognizes the superior and rapid efficacy of ECT is presented in Fig. 11.1. Unfortunately, such a decision tree can only be considered where a well trained and active ECT staff and facility is available.

A second algorithm is provided for the special needs of treating depression in the elderly (Fig. 11.2).

## Conclusions

Electroshock is an effective treatment for many mental disorders. It is safe. Its demonstrated efficacy in patients who have not responded to medications argues

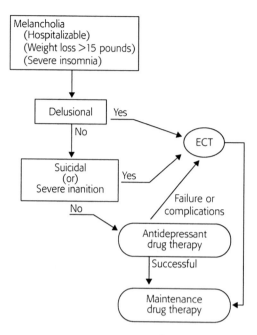

Fig. 11.2.    Severe depression in the elderly.

that ECT is more effective than our present variety of medicines. It has a specific role in treating the severely depressed, especially those defined as medication resistant. We should question the clinical and ethical justification of the widespread use of untested medications and combinations before a trial of ECT is considered in the severely depressed. (We should deplore any mental hospital that offers to treat mentally ill patients without an active, well staffed, and well equipped ECT facility.)

The use of ECT, however, is limited by its complexity and the need for trained personnel and well equipped facilities. ECT is favored in academic medical centers, where treatments are prescribed by the most sophisticated of our nation's medical practitioners.

Writing guidelines, algorithms, and diagrammatic flow charts is a popular occupation today. The role of ECT is generally ignored, first as the result of inexperience and ignorance, but also because the availability of ECT in mental hospitals is spotty. A greater acceptance of ECT as an effective and safe treatment and its reasonable consideration before less effective treatments are tried will do much to relieve the burdens of therapy resistance of the severe mentally ill – for themselves, for their families, and for society.

## Acknowledgment

Aided in part, by grants from the Scion Natural Science Association, Inc., St James, New York 11780.

## REFERENCES

Abrams, R. (1997). *Electroconvulsive Therapy*. 3rd edn. New York: Oxford University Press, 231 pp.

American Psychiatric Association (1990). *The Practice of Electroconvulsive Therapy: Recommendations for Treatment, Training and Privileging*. Washington, DC: APA Press.

American Psychiatric Association (1993). Practice guidelines for major depressive disorder in adults. *American Journal of Psychiatry*, **150**, 4 (Suppl.) pp. 1–26.

American Psychiatric Association (1994). Practice guidelines for the treatment of patients with bipolar disorder. *American Journal of Psychiatry*, **151**, 12 (Suppl. pp. 1–36).

Amsterdam, J.D. & Hornig-Rohan, M. (1996). Treatment algorithms in treatment-resistant depression. *Psychiatric Clinics of North America*, **19**, 371–86.

Anderson, I.M. & Tomenson, B.M. (1994). The efficacy of selective serotonin re-uptake inhibitors in depression: a meta-analysis of studies against tricyclic antidepressants. *Journal of Psychopharmacology*, **8**, 238–49.

Avery, D. & Lubrano, A. (1979). Depression treated with imipramine and ECT: the deCarolis study reconsidered. *American Journal of Psychiatry*, **136**, 559–62.

Avery, D. & Winokur, G. (1978). Suicide, attempted suicide, and relapse rates in depression. *Archives of General Psychiatry*, **35**, 749–53.

Bailine, S.H., Rifkin, A., Kayne, E. et al. (2000). Comparison of bifrontal and bitemporal ECT for major depression. *American Journal of Psychiatry*, **157**, 121–3.

Coryell, W. (1996). Psychotic depression. *Journal of Clinical Psychiatry*, **57** (Suppl 3), 27–31.

Davis, J.M., Ayd, F.J., & Preskorn, S.H. (1995). Advances in the pharmacotherapy of bipolar disorder. Update to *Principles and Practice of Pharmacotherapy*, vol. 1(3), pp. 1–20. Baltimore, MD: Williams & Wilkins.

De Battista, C. & Schatzberg, A.F. (1994). An algorithm for the treatment of major depression and its subtypes. *Psychiatric Annals*, **24**, 341–7.

Endler, N.S. & Persad, E. (1988). *Electroconvulsive Therapy. The Myths and the Realities*. Toronto: Hans Huber. 173 pp.

Fink, M. (1979). *Convulsive Therapy: Theory and Practice*. New York: Raven Press. 306 pp.

Fink, M. (1987). ECT: a last resort treatment for resistant depression? In *Treating Resistant Depression*, ed. J. Zohar & R. Belmaker, vol. 9, pp. 163–73. New York: PMA Publishing Co.

Fink, M. (1989). Electroconvulsive therapy: the forgotten option in the treatment of therapy-resistant depression. In *Treatment of Tricyclic Resistant Depression*, ed. I. Extein, pp. 135–50. Washington, DC: APA Press.

Fink, M. (1993a). A trial of ECT is essential before a diagnosis of refractory depression is made. In *Refractory Depression. Advances in Neuropsychiatry and Psychopharmacology*, ed. J.D. Amsterdam, vol. 2, pp. 87–92. New York: Raven Press.

Fink, M. (1993b). Who should get ECT? In *The Clinical Science of Electroconvulsive Therapy*, ed. C.E. Coffey, pp. 3–16. Washington, DC: APA Press.

Fink, M. (1993c). Impact of the anti-psychiatry movement on the revival of ECT in the U.S. *Psychiatric Clinics of North America*, **14**(4), 793–801.

Fink, M. (1994a). Combining electroconvulsive therapy and drugs: a review of safety and efficacy. *CNS Drugs*, **1**, 370–6.

Fink, M. (1994b). Optimizing ECT. *L'Encephale*, **20**, 297–302.

Fink, M. (1998). ECT and clozapine in schizophrenia. *Journal of Electroconvulsive Therapy*, **14**, 223–6.

Fink, M. (1999). *Electroshock: Restoring the Mind*. New York: Oxford University Press, 157 pp.

Fink, M. & Johnson, L. (1982). Monitoring duration of ECT seizures: 'Cuff' and EEG methods compared. *Archives of General Psychiatry*, **39**, 1189–91.

Fink, M. & Sackeim, H.A. (1996). Convulsive therapy for schizophrenia? *Schizophrenia Bulletin*, **22**, 27–39.

Fink, M. & Taylor, M.A. (1991). Catatonia: a separate category for DSM-IV? *Integrative Psychiatry*, **7**, 2–10.

Fink, M., Abrams, R., Bailine, S., & Jaffe, R. (1996). Ambulatory electroconvulsive therapy: report of a task-force of the Association for Convulsive Therapy. *Convulsive Therapy*, **12**, 41–55.

Frances, A., Docherty, J.P., & Kahn, D.A. (1996). Treatment of bipolar disorder. Expert consensus guideline series. *Journal of Clinical Psychiatry*, **57**, Suppl. 12A, 1–88.

Hales, R.E. & Yudofsky, S.C. (1996). *Practical Clinical Strategies in Treating Depression and Anxiety Disorders in a Managed Care Environment*, pp. 1–61. Washington DC: American Psychiatric Association.

Hartmann, E. (1996). The public's role in the evaluation of health care technology. The conflict over ECT. *International Journal of Technology Assessment Health Care*, **12**, 657–72.

Janicak, P.G., Davies, J.M., Preskorn, S.H., & Ayd, F.J. (1993). *Principles and Practice of Psychopharmacotherapy*. PA: Williams & Wilkins. Update Note (1995). *Advances in the Pharmacotherapy of Depressive Disorders*. Vol. 1, No. 2, Spring, 24 pp.

Kane, J.M. (1989). The current status of neuroleptic therapy. *Journal of Clinical Psychiatry*, **50**, 322–8.

Kantor, S.J. & Glassman, A.H. (1977). Delusional depressions: natural history and response to treatment. *British Journal of Psychiatry*, **131**, 351–6.

Kellner, C.H. (ed). (1991). *Electroconvulsive Therapy. Psychiatric Clinics of North America*, **14**, 793–1035.

Kellner, C.H. (ed.). (1993). ECT and drugs: concurrent administration. *Convulsive Therapy*, **9**, 237–351.

Kellner, C.H. & Fink, M. (1996). Seizure adequacy: does EEG hold the key? *Convulsive Therapy*, **12**, 203–6.

Klein, D.F. (1994). The utility of guidelines and algorithms for practice. *Psychiatric Annals*, **24**, 362–7.

Kramer, B.A. (1999). Use of ECT in California, revisited: 1984–1994. *Journal of Electroconvulsive Therapy*, **15**, 245–51.

Kroessler, D. (1985). Relative efficacy rates for therapies of delusional depression. *Convulsive Therapy*, **1**, 173–82.

Lehrmann, T.M. (2000). *Of 2 Minds: The Growing Disorders in American Psychiatry*, ed. Knopf, NY:

Lieberman, J.A., Kane, J.M., & Johns, C.A. (1989). Clozapine: guidelines for clinical management. *Journal of Clinical Psychiatry*, **50**, 329–38.

McCall, W.V., Reboussin, D.M., Weiner, R.D., & Sackeim, H.A. (2000). Titrated moderately suprathreshold vs fixed high-dose right unilateral electroconvulsive therapy. *Archives of General Psychiatry*, **57**, 438–44.

Meyers, B.S. (1995). Late-life delusional depression: acute and long-term treatment. *International Psychogeriatrics*, **7** Suppl., 113–24.

Moise, F.N. & Petrides, G. (1996). Case study: electroconvulsive therapy in adolescents. *Journal of the American Academy for Child and Adolescent Psychiatry*, **35**, 312–18.

Monroe, R.R. (1991). Maintenance electroconvulsive therapy. In *Electroconvulsive Therapy. Psychiatric Clinics of North America*, ed. C.H. Kellner, **14**, 947–60.

Mulsant, B.H., Haskett, R.F., Prudic, J et al. (1997). Low use of neuroleptic drugs in the treatment of psychotic major depression. *American Journal of Psychiatry*, **154**, 559–61.

Nelsen, M.R. & Dunner, D.L. (1995). Clinical and differential diagnostic aspects of treatment-resistant depression. *Journal for Psychiatric Research*, **29**, 43–50.

Palmer, R.L. (1981). *Electroconvulsive Therapy: An Appraisal*. Oxford: Oxford University Press. 316 pp.

Parker, G., Hadzi-Pavlovic, D., Hickie, I. et al. (1991). Psychotic depression: A review and clinical experience. *Australia and New Zealand Journal of Psychiatry*, **25**, 169–80.

Parker, G., Roy, K., Hadzi-Pavlovic, D., & Pedic, F. (1992). Psychotic (delusional) depression: a meta-analysis of physical treatments. *Journal of Affective Disorders*, **24**, 17–24.

Parker, G., Hadzi-Pavlovic, D., Brodaty, H. et al. (1995). Sub-typing depression, II: Clinical distinction of psychotic depression and non-psychotic melancholia. *Psychological Medicine*, **25**, 825–32.

Petrides, G. & Fink, M. (1996). The 'half-age' stimulation strategy for ECT dosing. *Convulsive Therapy*, **12**, 138–46.

Petrides, G., Dhosshe, D., Fink, M., & Francis, A. (1994). Continuation ECT: relapse prevention in affective disorders. *Convulsive Therapy*, **10**, 189–94.

Preskorn, S.H., Janicak, P.G., Davis, J.M., & Ayd, F.J. (1995). Advances in the pharmacotherapy of depressive disorders. Update to *Principles and Practice of Pharmacotherapy*, Vol. 1(2), pp. 1–24. Baltimore: Williams & Wilkins.

Prudic, J., Sackeim, H.A., & Devanand, D.P. (1990). Medication resistance and clinical response to electroconvulsive therapy. *Psychiatry Research*, **31**, 287–96.

Reid, W.H., Keller, S., Leatherman, M., & Mason, M. (1998). ECT in Texas: 19 months of mandatory reporting. *Journal of Clinical Psychiatry*, **59**, 8–13.

Reus, V.I. (1996). Management of treatment-resistant unipolar and chronically depressed patients. *Psychiatric Clinics of North America*, **19**, 201–14.

Rey, J.M. & Walter, G. (1997). Half a century of ECT use in young people. *American Journal of Psychiatry*, **154**, 595–602.

Roose, S.P., Glassman, A.H., Attia, E. et al. (1994). Comparative efficacy of selective serotonin reuptake inhibitors and tricyclics in the treatment of melancholia. *American Journal of Psychiatry*, **151**, 1735–9.

Rothschild, A.J. (1996). Management of psychotic, treatment-resistant depression. *Psychiatric Clinics of North America*, **19**, 237–52.

Rush, A.J., Crismon, M.L., Toprac, M.G. et al. (1998). Consensus guidelines in the treatment of major depressive disorder. *Journal of Clinical Psychiatry*, **59** (Suppl. 20), 73–84.

Sackeim, H.A., Prudic, J., Devanand, D.P. et al. (1990). The impact of medication resistance and continuation pharmacotherapy on relapse following response to electroconvulsive therapy in major depression. *Journal of Clinical Psychopharmacology*, **10**, 96–104.

Sackeim, H.A., Prudic, J., Devanand, D.P. et al. (1993). Effects of stimulus intensity and electrode placement on the efficacy and cognitive effects of electroconvulsive therapy. *New England Journal of Medicine*, **328**, 839–46.

Sackeim, H.A., Prudic, J., Devanand, D.P. et al. (2000). A prospective, randomized, double-blind comparison of bilateral and right unilateral electroconvulsive therapy at different stimulus intensities. *Archives of General Psychiatry*, **57**, 425–34.

Song, F., Freemantle, N., Sheldon, T.A. et al. (1993). Selective serotonin reuptake inhibitors: meta-analysis of efficacy and acceptability. *British Medical Journal*, **306**, 683–7.

Spiker, D.G., Weiss, J.C., Dealy, R.S. et al. (1985). The pharmacologic treatment of delusional depression. *American Journal of Psychiatry*, **142**, 430–6.

Walter, G. & Rey, J.M. (1997). An epidemiological study of the use of ECT in adolescents. *Journal of the American Academy of Child and Adolescent Psychiatry*, **36**, 809–15.

# 12

# Thyroid augmentation

Russell T. Joffe

## Introduction

For the greater part of this century, thyroid hormones have been considered as viable treatments for patients with mood disorders, particularly those with treatment-resistant illness. This interest in the therapeutic effect of thyroid hormones arises from the well-established association between abnormalities of the thyroid axis and psychiatric symptomatology, especially alterations in mood. In particular, the association between clinical thyroid disease, both hyperthyroidism and hypothyroidism and mood disturbance has been well documented. Specifically, hypothyroidism is commonly associated with symptoms of depression (Hall, 1983; Whybrow et al., 1969) whereas, in hyperthyroidism, there is a broader range of psychiatric symptomatology including anxiety, mood lability, cognitive impairment as well as symptoms of mania and psychosis (Fava et al., 1987; MacCrimmon et al., 1979; Weller, 1984; Kathol et al., 1986; Jefferson, 1988). In addition, hyperthyroidism may also be associated with features of depression (Jefferson, 1988). This rich clinical literature (Hall, 1983; Whybrow et al., 1969; Fava et al., 1987; McCrimmon et al., 1979; Weller, 1984; Kathol et al., 1986; Jefferson, 1988) documenting an association between psychiatric illness and thyroid disease has also shown that successful treatment of the thyroid disease is usually although not always associated with resolution of psychiatric symptoms, especially in patients with hypothyroidism (Wolfson & Jefferson, 1985; Loosen, 1986).

The above-mentioned literature in patients with clinical thyroid disease has certainly provided one of the strong clinical and theoretical rationales for the use of thyroid hormones in the treatment of depression. In addition, other clinical and preclinical observations also provided support for treatment of depression with thyroid hormones. First, there is an extensive literature which documents the impact of thyroid hormones on various biogenic amine systems, particularly including norepinephrine (Breese et al., 1974; Whybrow et al., 1972). As abnormalities of norepinephrine are thought to be of etiologic importance in depressive disorder, thyroid hormones, which enhance norepinephrine, were postulated to have some positive antidepressant benefit. Second, it had been observed in animal

experiments that thyroid hormones enhanced the toxicity of tricyclic antidepressants (Breese et al., 1974) and it was therefore concluded that they may, in a similar
manner, enhance therapeutic action in patients with depression. This last rationale provided impetus for the work of Prange and collaborators who pioneered the
modern use of thyroid hormones in the treatment of depression. All hormones of
the thyroid axis have been used for depression therapy. The peripheral hormones,
thyroxine (T4) and triiodothyronine (T3), have been in use in three ways: first, as
monotherapy for depression; second, to accelerate the onset of antidepressant
effect; and last, to enhance therapeutic response in antidepressant non-responders. The first two strategies will only be considered briefly whereas the last will be
considered in greater detail as it is directly pertinent to the theme of this book.

## Thyrotropin releasing hormone (TRH)

TRH is a peptide composed of three amino acids and is broadly distributed in
brain. Hypothalamic TRH has a regulatory effect on the thyroid axis by stimulating thyrotropin (TSH) which, in turn, regulates thyroid hormone synthesis and
release. However, TRH also has direct effects on brain function, which are
independent of its regulatory effect on the thyroid axis (Griffiths, 1985). Administration of exogenous TRH has wide ranging cardiorespiratory, neurologic and
gastrointestinal effects, one of the most well described of which is the reversal of
hypnotic induced sedation or anesthesia (Griffiths, 1985).

Twelve double-blind studies have evaluated the effects of TRH on symptoms of
major depression when administered as monotherapy (Kastin et al., 1972; Prange
et al., 1972; Coppen et al., 1974; Ehrensing et al., 1974; Hollister et al., 1974;
Vandenberg et al., 1975, 1976; Furlong et al., 1976; Vogle et al., 1977; Mountjoy et
al., 1974; Kiely et al., 1976; Karlberg et al., 1978). In these studies, TRH has been
administered either as an intravenous or oral preparation. In the initial studies,
Kastin and collaborators reported a transient but positive antidepressant effect in
four out of five patients where TRH was administered as a single intravenous dose
of 500 micrograms (Kastin et al., 1972). This finding was confirmed by Prange et
al. (1972) in ten patients who has been administered a single intravenous dose of
600 micrograms of TRH. However the remaining studies showed minimal or no
effects of TRH when administered either intravenously (Coppen et al., 1974;
Ehrensing et al., 1974; Hollister et al., 1974; Vandenberg et al., 1975, 1976; Furlong
et al., 1976; Vogle et al., 1977) or as an oral preparation (Mountjoy et al.. 1974;
Kiely et al., 1976; Karlberg et al., 1978) for varying periods of time, from either a
single dose to as long as one month. On balance, the majority of these studies are
negative and suggest that TRH is unlikely to have any substantial therapeutic
benefit. It further raises the issue whether the positive effects noted in some of the

earlier studies (Kastin et al., 1972; Prange et al., 1972) were attributable to a specific antidepressant effect or were more likely the result of the non-specific activating effect of TRH seen in animal studies (Griffiths, 1985).

In a recent study Khan and collaborators (1994) administered 500 micrograms of TRH to eight depressed patients undergoing a course of electroconvulsive treatment using a randomized, double-blind, placebo-controlled crossover design. The investigators noted that there were greater levels of arousal and better cognitive functioning on a neuropsychiatric test battery when TRH infusion prior to ECT treatments were compared to placebo. Although these data are intriguing, they require replication (Khan et al., 1994). Furthermore, as with some of the earlier monotherapy studies of TRH, the issue of the specificity of the effect noted has to be addressed to determine whether these changes are the result of non-specific arousal or a true antidepressant response.

## Thyroid stimulating hormone (TSH)

Only one study has examined the antidepressant effects of TSH administration. Prange and collaborators (1969) administered 10 IU of TSH intramuscularly to 20 depressed women 24 hours before the beginning of an imipramine trial. The study involved a double-blind, placebo-controlled design. The TSH treated women experienced a more rapid response compared to the saline treated women; all subjects then received oral imipramine. The results of the study are of interest but require replication before an assessment of the efficacy and clinical utility of this peptide can be assessed. If TSH has antidepressant efficacy, its mechanism of action remains uncertain. It could act by stimulating thyroid hormone release from the thyroid gland but it may also have direct behavioral effects which to date are poorly understood.

## Triiodothyronine

This is the most widely and extensively studied thyroid hormone for the treatment of depression. It has been employed as monotherapy, to accelerate antidepressant effect and to augment therapeutic effects in antidepressant non-responders.

## Monotherapy

Two early clinical reports suggest that T3 may improve depressive symptoms and increase spontaneous motor activity in a group of psychiatric patients with mixed diagnoses (Feldmesser-Reiss, 1958; Flach et al., 1958). Conclusions from these reports are limited by numerous methodological issues including the heterogeneity of patient samples, the lack of objective criteria to assess response, the open nature of the studies and the variable approach to thyroid hormone treatment. Until these data are replicated in a more homogenous group of depressed patients utilizing more acceptable research designs, the clinical utility of monotherapy with T3 in the treatment of depression has not been proven.

## Acceleration

Earlier studies, done approximately 30 years ago, suggest that, when T3 is used in combination with tricyclic antidepressants at the initiation of the therapeutic trial, the onset of antidepressant response may be accelerated. In several studies, 25 to 50 micrograms/day of T3 started simultaneously with tricyclic treatment accelerated antidepressant response (Prange et al., 1969; Wilson et al., 1970; Wheatley, 1972). These studies employed placebo-controlled designs and response to T3 was significantly more rapid than to placebo. The effect was much more clearly demonstrated in female rather than male patients (Prange et al., 1969; Wilson et al., 1970; Wheatley, 1972). Not all studies have supported these observations (Feighner et al., 1972). It is of interest that no recent published studies have attempted to replicate this finding especially since reducing the lag in onset of therapeutic response with antidepressant remains a desired objective and would be of unquestioned clinical value. One of the difficulties in such studies is determining early response to treatment. Notwithstanding these methodological issues, it would be of considerable interest to attempt to replicate these earlier studies to determine whether T3 may have use as an accelerator of antidepressant effect.

## Augmentation

The augmentation effect of T3 has been widely studied. To date, there are 11 studies (Earle, 1970; Ogura et al., 1974; Banki, 1975, 1977; Tsutsui et al., 1979; Goodwin et al., 1982; Schwarcz et al., 1984; Gitlin et al., 1987; Thase et al., 1989; Joffe & Singer, 1990; Joffe et al., 1993). These are reviewed in Table 12.1. There are six open, uncontrolled studies, four double-blind controlled studies and one open, partially controlled study. The overall response rate is approximately 55%.

With respect to the open studies there has been only one negative trial. Thase and collaborators (1989) observed an antidepressant response in only 5 (25%) of 20 depressed patients. However their study sample was composed of a severely ill group of patients characterized by a highly recurrent major depressive illness and

**Table 12.1.** Triiodothyronine (T3) potentiation of tricyclic antidepressants

| Study | $n$ | Design | Dose Of T3 (mcg/day) | Result |
|---|---|---|---|---|
| Earle (1970) | 25 | Open, uncontrolled | 25 | 14 of 25 |
| Banki (1975) | 52 | Open, uncontrolled | 20–40 | 39 to 52 |
| Banki (1977) | 33 | Open, partially controlled | 20 | 23 to 33 |
| Ogura et al. (1974) | 44 | Open, uncontrolled | 20–30 | 29 of 44 |
| Tsutsui et al. (1979) | 11 | Open, uncontrolled | 5–25 | 10 of 11 |
| Goodwin et al. (1982) | 12 | Double-blind, controlled mirror design | 25–50 | 8 of 12 |
| Schwarcz et al. (1984) | 8 | Open, uncontrolled | 25–50 | 4 of 8 |
| Gitlin et al. (1987) | 16 | Double-blind, controlled, crossover | 25 | T3 and placebo no difference |
| Thase et al. (1989) | 20 | Open, uncontrolled | 25 | 5 of 20 |
| Joffe and Singer (1990) | 38 | Double-blind, controlled randomized | 37.5 | T3 9 of 17 vs. 4 of 21 T4 |
| Joffe et al. (1993) | 51 | Double-blind, controlled lithium and placebo | 37.5 | 10 of 17 T3 |

this may explain the relatively low response to the addition of T3. The five controlled studies, four double-blind and one open provide an overall response rate of about 50% which is consistent with that observed in the open studies. The one negative study (Gitlin et al., 1987) has several methodological limitations. In this study a significant difference between T3 and placebo was not observed when a 2-week double-blind, controlled crossover design was utilized in 16 subjects who had failed to respond to a tricyclic antidepressant. However, it could be argued that this type of design may not be the most appropriate for evaluating the efficacy of antidepressant augmentation effects as the variable delay in onset and offset of action of these treatment strategies may make the data difficult to interpret. Of the listed studies in Table 12.1, we have carried out the two most recent of the double-blind studies. In the first, we directly compared T3 to T4 augmentation in 38 patients with major depressive disorder who had failed to respond to an adequate trial of either desipramine or imipramine (Joffe & Singer, 1990). Using a double-blind, controlled design we showed that 9 of 17 patients responded to T3 whereas 4 of 21 patients responded to T4 within the 3-week duration of the trial. Our data are limited by the absence of a placebo-controlled group. However, this is the first study to directly compare T3 to T4 in a group of euthyroid depressed patients and suggest that T3 may be more effective under these treatment conditions. In our other study, we were the first to directly compare T3 and lithium augmentation of tricyclic antidepressants (Joffe et al., 1993). In this study, 51 patients with primary major depressive disorder who were euthyroid and who had failed an adequate treatment trial with either desipramine or imipramine, were randomly assigned to receive either lithium or T3 using a double-blind, placebo-controlled design. The study extended over a period of 2 weeks. Ten of 17 patients (58.5%) responded to T3, 9 of 17 (52.9%) responded to lithium and only 3 of 16 (18.8%) responded to placebo. Both T3 and lithium were significantly more effective than placebo but the two active treatments did not differ in their rate of treatment response from each other (Joffe et al., 1993).

The findings in the last study (Joffe et al., 1993) are of considerable clinical interest. Lithium is regarded as the gold standard for augmentation strategies and is widely believed to be one of the most effective augmentation treatments. T3 is generally regarded as less effective and is not as widely used. These assumptions, however, were largely based on clinical anecdotal experience and our study was the first to directly compare these two strategies and demonstrate them to be equally effective. Although the overall response rates were comparable between the two treatments, lithium and T3, it is possible that T3 and lithium may be effective in different patients. In fact, case series suggest that non-response to one does not predict non-response to the other (Garbutt et al., 1986; Joffe, 1988a). Furthermore, we have found that there are no useful clinical or biochemical predictors of response to either lithium or T3 in tricyclic antidepressant non-responders (Joffe et al., 1993).

As can be seen in Table 12.1, all trials of T3 augmentation have involved the use of tricyclic antidepressants. However, several case reports suggest the efficacy of T3 augmentation with both monoamine oxidase inhibitors (Hullett & Bidder, 1983; Joffe, 1988b) as well as serotonin reuptake inhibitors (Joffe, 1992). Although these clinical data would support the efficacy of T3 augmentation with antidepressants other than the tricyclics, these data are extremely limited and larger scale controlled trials of T3 augmentation of newer classes of antidepressants, particularly the selective serotonin reuptake inhibitors, are warranted.

In a recent meta-analysis (Aronson et al., 1996), it was observed that patients treated with T3 augmentation were twice as likely to respond as controls treated with placebo. Improvements in depression scores were moderately large with active T3 treatment. It was concluded that T3 augmentation may be an effective method of increasing response rates and decreasing depression severity scores in patients with treatment-resistant depression who have not responded to tricyclic antidepressant therapy (Aronson et al., 1996).

In general, one of the major advantages of T3 augmentation is that it is well tolerated with few side effects. This is particularly the case at doses of 25 micrograms/day or less. At these doses symptoms of hyperthyroidism are extremely unlikely although at 50 micrograms/day these may be more likely to occur.

Symptoms of cardiotoxicity with T3 augmentation have been very rarely reported (Gitlin et al., 1987).

In a recent preliminary study, Stern and collaborators (1991) observed that T3 augmentation led to fewer required treatments and less cognitive impairment in a group of 20 male patients with various subtypes of major depression who received electroconvulsive treatment. Further studies in animals (Stern et al., 1995) suggest that this cognitive sparing effect is a direct effect of the T3 on ECT-related cognitive impairment rather than on cognitive impairment related to anesthesia. These preliminary findings are of considerable interest and await replication in larger scale controlled studies.

## Thyroxine

There are very few studies which have examined the use of T4 to augment antidepressant response. The majority of the earlier studies (see Table 12.1) employed T3 as it was felt that with its short half-life it would be less likely to cause symptoms of toxicity. It was assumed that T4 would be comparable to T3 in augmentation of antidepressant response as both would enhance thyroid hormone levels. In the only study to directly compare T4 to T3 (Joffe & Singer, 1990), the antidepressant augmenting effect of T3 was found to be superior to T4. As previously noted, methodological problems limit conclusions from this study. However these preliminary and provocative findings require replication using an adequately designed, placebo-controlled study. In the only other study of which we are aware to evaluate the efficacy of T4 augmentation of antidepressants, Targum and collaborators (1984) reported a favorable augmentation response to T4 in seven patients with major depression. However, five of the seven patients had evidence of subclinal hypothyroidism so it is difficult to determine whether in fact the therapeutic effect of T4 was a true antidepressant augmentation effect or the result of thyroid replacement therapy in patients with mildly compromised thyroid function. At this time, the antidepressant augmenting effect of T4 remains to be studied. However, in the absence of some degree of hypothyroidism, the antidepressant effect of T4 is uncertain.

In summary, various hormones of the thyroid axis have been used in the treatment of depression. There is virtually no evidence to support the efficacy of any of these hormones as monotherapy for major depression. Although the data on the use of T3 to accelerate antidepressant response is intriguing, modern studies are required employing rigorous research designs. The best evidence for the use of thyroid hormones in the treatment of depression is the use of T3 to augment therapeutic response in antidepressant non-responders. Here, the studies including the relevant meta-analysis (Aronson et al., 1996) as well as clinical experience suggest that T3 is an effective and clinically useful strategy in the approach to the treatment-resistant patient.

## Mechanism of action of thyroid hormones in the treatment of depression

The therapeutic benefit of each of the hormones of the thyroid axis in depression remains unclear. Although hypotheses have been proposed to explain the putative therapeutic effects of TRH and TSH, until such time as their therapeutic benefit is established, their mechanism of action remains highly speculative.

An explanation for the therapeutic effect of T3 also remains elusive although several possibilities have been proposed. First, it has been suggested that T3 may act through potentiation of biogenic amines, particularly catecholamines (Whybrow & Prange, 1981). This is an attractive hypothesis as it clearly links to the potential role of catecholamines in the biological basis of depressive illness. However, further research is required to determine whether indeed this may explain the mechanism of action of T3. Second, it has been suggested that T3 has a therapeutic action by acting as replacement therapy for subtle, often subclinical forms of hypothyroidism associated with major depression (Gold et al., 1981). Although this hypothesis is consistent with widely held views about a relationship between thyroid hypofunction and depression (Hall, 1983; Whybrow et al., 1969), the majority of studies (see Table 12.1) have involved patients who are by conventional thyroid hormone measures, completely euthyroid. Last, a competing hypothesis is that thyroid hormone augmentation may act by correcting a relative increase in thyroid hormone levels associated with depression (Joffe et al., 1984). Further study is required to elucidate the mechanism of action of thyroid hormones in the treatment of depression, particularly the augmentation effect in therapeutic non-responders. Regardless of the mechanism of action, thyroid hormones, particularly T3, may be useful in selective treatment-resistant patients to boost their therapeutic response and reduce their depressive symptomatology.

## Clinical applications

Major depressive disorder is an illness which has a propensity for chronicity and recurrence (Keller et al., 1984). A substantial number of patients who receive optimum antidepressant therapy will fail to respond or have an incomplete antidepressant response to their first antidepressant trial (Joffe & Levitt, 1995). It is estimated that approximately half of patients will have a partial or non-response to their first antidepressant trial and will require some further therapeutic intervention (Joffe & Levitt, 1995). Several options have been proposed for such patients (Joffe et al., 1996). These include electroconvulsive treatment, antidepressant substitution and augmentation or combination treatment. Substitution refers to discontinuation of the first unsuccessful antidepressant and introduction of a second new antidepressant trial. Augmentation/combination refers to the combined use of treatments in an attempt to boost therapeutic response (Joffe et al., 1996). Augmentation/combination may offer several advantages over substitution. Although unlikely to be a more effective treatment strategy, augmentation/combination may improve the efficiency of antidepressants by reducing the time wasted for discontinuation of the first antidepressant trial, a possible washout of the first drug the introduction of a second trial and the lag in onset of therapeutic response to this second antidepressant. Augmentation/combination treatments may work as rapidly as 48 hours although more commonly within 2–3 weeks (de Montigny, 1994). A whole range of augmentation strategies have been described. Two of the most commonly employed antidepressant augmentation strategies are the addition of lithium and T3. Although lithium has achieved widespread therapeutic use and has come to be regarded as the gold standard for augmentation therapy, T3 is less widely regarded as a clinically useful treatment strategy. Review of the literature suggests that in fact T3 is a useful and clinically effective treatment strategy comparable in efficacy to lithium. T3, especially in doses of 25 micrograms or less, is also generally well tolerated and unlikely to cause serious adverse effects. These data would suggest that T3 should be more commonly considered as a useful augmentation strategy in antidepressant non-responders.

The major dilemma in the selection of any augmentation strategy is the paucity of systematic data to arrive at a decision about which treatment is useful under any particular circumstances. Furthermore, prioritizing augmentation or combination strategies also remains problematic because of the lack of systematic and controlled studies. The decision about which treatment to use in any particular circumstance or the order in which augmentation strategies should be employed is largely based on clinical experience or expert opinion rather than empirical data. While this may be useful until such time as the required data are available, the common methodologies for developing algorithms for treatment of treatment-resistant patients is subject to bias and may potentially deprive patients of effective treatments. T3 is not an effective treatment for all antidepressant non-responders. Nor however is it completely ineffective. It should therefore be given reasonable consideration alongside with other augmentation strategies when patients have failed to respond to antidepressants. It may also be used where other augmentation strategies such as lithium are contraindicated, ineffective or poorly tolerated. The thyroid status of a depressed patient is not a good predictor of T3 augmentation response. The efficacy of T3 has been mostly documented in euthyroid depressed patients. However, in patients with subtle degrees of subclinical hypothyroidism, it may be reasonable to attempt T3 augmentation as a preferred strategy. No clinical feature of the depressed patient predicts response to T3. In particular, T3 may be effective in patients with psychomotor retardation as well as agitation so that T3 augmentation may be available to a broad range of subtypes of major depressive disorder.

An algorithm for the treatment of resistant depression remains elusive. While such an algorithm can enumerate the various options available for augmentation or combination treatment, there are no clear empirical data which are reliable and useful to guide the selection of one strategy over another or to prioritize these various strategies so as to produce a standard approach or 'care map' for the treatment of the treatment-resistant depressed patient.

## REFERENCES

Aronson, R., Offman, H.J., Joffe, R.T., & Naylor, C.D. (1996). Triiodothyronine augmentation in the treatment of refractory depression: a meta-analysis. *Archives of General Psychiatry*, **53**, 842–8.

Banki, C.M. (1975). Triiodothyronine in the treatment of depression. *Orvieti Italia*, **116**, 2543–7.

Banki, C.M. (1977). Cerebrospinal fluid amine metabolites after combined amitriptyline-triiodothyronine treatment of depressed woman. *European Journal of Clinical Pharmacology*, **11**, 311–15.

Breese, G.R., Prange, A.J. Jr, & Lipton, M.A. (1974). Pharmacological studies of thyroid–imipramine interactions in animals. In *The Thyroid Axis, Drugs and Behavior*, ed. A.J. Prange Jr, pp. 29–48. New York: Raven Press.

Coppen, A., Montgomery, S., & Pet, M. (1974). Thyrotropin-releasing hormone in the treatment of depression. *Lancet*, **1**, 433–5.

De Montigny, C. (1994). Lithium addition in treatment-resistant depression. *International Clinical Psychopharmacology*, **9**(Suppl.), 31–5.

Earle, B.V. (1970). Thyroid hormone and tricyclic antidepressants in resistant depression. *American Journal of Psychiatry*, **126**, 1667–9.

Ehrensing, R.H., Kastin, A.J., & Schalch, D.S. (1974). Affective state and thyrotropin and prolactin response after repeated injections of thyrotropin-releasing hormone in depressed patients. *American Journal of Psychiatry*, **131**, 714–18.

Fava, G.A., Sonino, N., & Morphy, M.A. (1987). Major depression associated with endocrine disease. *Psychiatric Developments*, **4**, 321–48.

Feighner, J.P., King, L.J., Schuckit, M.A., Croughan, J., & Briscoe, W. (1972). Hormonal potentiation of imipramine and ECT in primary depression. *American Journal of Psychiatry*, **28**, 1230–4.

Feldmesser-Reiss, E.E. (1958). The application of triiodothyronine in the treatment of mental disorders. *Journal of Nervous and Mental Disease*, 127, 540–3.

Flach, F.F., Celian, C.I., & Rawson, R.W. (1958). Treatment of psychiatric disorders with triiodothyronine. *American Journal of Psychiatry*, 114, 841–6.

Furlong, F.W., Brown, G.M., & Beeching, M.F. (1976). Thyrotropin-releasing hormone: Differential antidepressant and endocrinological effects. *American Journal of Psychiatry*, 133, 1187–90.

Garbutt, J.C., Mayo, J.B. Jr, Gillette, G.M., Little, K.Y., & Mason, G.A. (1986). Lithium potentiation of tricyclic antidepressants following lack of T3 potentiation. *American Journal of Psychiatry*, 143, 1038–9.

Gitlin, M.J., Weiner, H., Fairbanks, L., Herschman, J.M., & Friedfeld, N. (1987). Failure of T3 to potentiate tricyclic antidepressant response. *Journal of Affective Disorders*, 13, 267–72.

Gold, M.S., Pottash, A.L.C., & Extein, I. (1981). Hypothyroidism and depression: evidence from complete thyroid function evaluation. *Journal of the American Medical Association*, 242, 1919–22.

Goodwin, F.K., Prange, A.J. Jr, Post, R.M., Muscettola, G., & Lipton, M.A. (1982). Potentiation of antidepressant effects by L-triiodothyronine in tricyclic non-responders. *American Journal of Psychiatry*, 139, 34–8.

Griffiths, E.C. (1985). TRH: endocrine and central effects. *Psychoneuroendocrinology*, 10, 225–35.

Hall, R.C.W. (1983). Psychiatric effects of thyroid hormone disturbance. *Psychosomatics*, 24, 7–14.

Hollister, L.E., Berger, P., & Ogle, F.L. (1974). Protirelin (TRH) in depression. *Archives of General Psychiatry*, 31, 468–70.

Hullett, F.J. & Bidder, T.G. (1983). Phenelzine plus triiodothyronine combination in a case of refractory depression. *Journal of Nervous and Mental Disease*, 171, 318–20.

Jefferson, J.W. (1988). Haldol diaconate and thyroid disease. *Journal of Clinical Psychiatry*, 49, 457–8.

Joffe, R.T. (1988a). Triiodothyronine potentiation of antidepressant effect of phenelzine. *Journal of Clinical Psychiatry*, 49, 409–10.

Joffe, R.T. (1988b). T3 and lithium potentiation of tricyclic antidepressants. *American Journal of Psychiatry*, 145, 1317–18.

Joffe, R.T. (1992). Triiodothyronine potentiation of fluoxetine in depressed patients. *Canadian Journal of Psychiatry*, 37, 48–50.

Joffe, R.T. & Levitt, A.J. (1995). Antidepressant failure: augmentation and substitution. *Journal of Psychiatry and Neuroscience*, 20, 7–9.

Joffe, R.T. & Singer, W. (1990). A comparison of triiodothyronine and thyroxine in the potentiation of tricyclic antidepressants. *Psychiatry Research*, 32, 241–51.

Joffe, R.T., Ry-Byrne, P.P., Uhde, T.W., & Post, R.M. (1984). Thyroid function and affective illness: a reappraisal. *Biological Psychiatry*, 19, 1685–91.

Joffe, R.T., Levitt, A.J., Bagby, R.M., MacDonald, C., & Singer, W. (1993). Predictors of response to lithium and triiodothyronine augmentation of antidepressants in tricyclic non-responders. *British Journal of Psychiatry*, 163, 574–8.

Joffe, R.T., Singer, W., Levitt, A.J., & Macdonald, C. (1993). A placebo-controlled comparison of lithium and triiodothyronine augmentation of tricyclic antidepressants in unipolar refractory depression. *Archives of General Psychiatry*, **50**, 387–93.

Joffe, R.T., Levitt, A.J., & Sokolov, S.T.H. (1996). Augmentation strategies: focus on anxiolytics. *Journal of Clinical Psychiatry*, **57**(Suppl. 7), 25–31.

Karlberg, B.E., Kejellman, B.F., & Kagedal, B. (1978). Treatment of endogenous depression with oral thyrotropin-releasing hormone and amitriptyline. *Acta Psychiatrica Scandinavica*, **58**, 389–400.

Kastin, A.J., Ehrensing, R.H., & Schalch, D.S. (1972). Improvement in mental depression with decreasing thyrotropin response after administration of thyrotropin releasing hormone. *Lancet*, **2**, 740–2.

Kathol, R.G., Turner, R., & Delahunt, J. (1986). Depression and anxiety associated with hyperthyroidism: response to anti-thyroid therapy. *Psychosomatics*, **27**, 501–5.

Keller, M.B., Klerman, G.L., Lavori, P.W., Coryell, W., Endicott, J., & Taylor, J. (1984). Long-term outcome of episodes of major depression: clinical and public health significance. *Journal of the American Medical Association*, **252**, 788–92.

Khan, A., Mirolo, M.H., Claypoole, K. et al. (1994). Effects of low dose TRH on cognitive deficits in the ECT postictal states. *American Journal of Psychiatry*, **151**, 1694–6.

Kiely, W.F., Adrian, A.D., & Lee, J.H. (1976). Therapeutic failure of oral thyrotropin-releasing hormone in depression. *Psychosomatic Medicine*, **38**, 233–41.

Loosen, P.T. (1986). Hormones of the hypothalamic–pituitary–thyroid axis: a psychoneuroendocrine perspective. *Pharmacopsychiatry*, **19**, 401–15.

MacCrimmon, D.J., Wallace, J.E., Goldberg, W.M., & Streiner, D.L. (1979). Emotional disturbance in cognitive deficits in hyperthyroidism. *Psychosomatic Medicine*, **41**, 331–40.

Mountjoy, C.Q., Price, J.S., & Weller, M. (1974). A double-blind cross-over sequential trial of oral thyrotropin-releasing hormone in depression. *Lancet*, **2**, 958–60.

Ogura, C., Okuma, T., Uchida, Y., Imia, S., & Yogi, H. (1974). Combined thyroid (triiodothyronine) – tricyclic antidepressant treatment in depressive states. *Ford Psychiatrica et Neurologica Japonica*, **28**, 189–96.

Prange, A.J. Jr, Wilson, I.C., Raybon, S.M., & Lipton, M.A. (1969). Enhance of the imipramine antidepressant activity by thyroid hormone. *American Journal of Psychiatry*, **12**, 457–69.

Prange, A.J. Jr, Wolfson, I.C., & Lara, P.P. (1972). Effects of thyrotropin-releasing hormone in the treatment of depression. *Lancet*, **2**, 999–1001.

Schwarcz, G., Halaris, A., Baxter, L., Escobar, J., Thompson, M., & Young, M. (1984). Normal thyroid function in desipramine non-responders converted to responders by the addition of ʟ-triiodothyronine. *American Journal of Psychiatry*, **141**, 1614–16.

Stern, R.A., Nevels, C.T., Shelhoic, M.E., Prohaska, M.L., Mason, G.A., & Prange, A.J. Jr (1991). Antidepressant and memory effects of combined thyroid hormone treatment and convulsive therapy: preliminary findings. *Biological Psychiatry*, **30**, 623–7.

Stern, R.A., Whealin, J.M., Mason, G.A. et al. (1995). Influence of ʟ-triiodothyronine on memory following repeated electroconvulsive shock in rats: implications with human electroconvulsive therapy. *Biological Psychiatry*, **37**, 198–201.

Targum, S.D., Greenberg, R.D., Harmon, R.L., Kessler, K., Salerian, A.J., & Fram, D.H. (1984).

Thyroid hormone in the TRH stimulation test in refractory depression. *Journal of Clinical Psychiatry*, **45**, 345–7.

Thase, M.E., Kupfer, D.J., & Jarrett, D.B. (1989). Treatment of imipramine-resistant recurrent depression: I An open clinical trial of adjunctive L-triiodothyronine. *Journal of Clinical Psychiatry*, **50**, 385–8.

Tsutsui, S., Tamazaki, Y., & Namba, T. (1979). Combined therapy of T3 and antidepressants in depression. *Journal of Internal Medicine Research*, **7**, 138–46.

Vandenberg, W., Vanpraag, H.M., Bos, E.R.H., Piers, D.A., Van Zanten, A.K., & Doorenbos, H. (1975). Thyrotropin releasing hormone (TRH) as a possible quick acting but short lasting antidepressant. *Psychological Medicine*, **5**, 404–12.

Vandenberg, W., Vanpraag, H.M., Bos, E.R.H., Piers, D.A., Van Zanten, A.K., & Doorenbos, H. (1976). TRH by slow, continuous infusion: an antidepressant? *Psychological Medicine*, **6**, 393–7.

Vogle, H.P., Benkert, B.F., & Illig, R. (1977). Psychoendocrinological and therapeutic effects of TRH in depression. *Acta Psychiatrica Scandinavica*, **56**, 223–32.

Weller, M.P.I. (1984). Agoraphobia and hyperthyroidism. *British Journal of Psychiatry*, **144**, 553–4.

Wheatley, D. (1972). Potentiation of amitriptyline by thyroid hormone. *Archives of General Psychiatry*, **26**, 229–33.

Whybrow, P.C. & Prange, A.J. Jr (1981). A hypothesis of thyroid-catecholamine-receptor interaction. *Archives of General Psychiatry*, **38**, 106–11.

Whybrow, P.C., Prange, A.J. Jr, & Treadway, C.R. (1969). The mental changes accompanying thyroid gland dysfunction. *Archives of General Psychiatry*, **20**, 48–53.

Whybrow, P.C., Coppen, A., Prange, A.J. Jr, & Lipton, M.A. (1972). Thyroid function and a response to liothyronine in depression. *Archives of General Psychiatry*, **26**, 242–5.

Wilson, I.C., Prange, A.J. Jr, McCalane, T.K., & Raybon, A.M. (1970). Thyroid hormone enhancement of imipramine in nonretarded depression. *New England Journal of Medicine*, **282**, 1063–7.

Wolfson, W.H. & Jefferson, J.W. (1985). Thyroid disease, behavior and psychopharmacology. *Psychosomatics*, **26**, 481–92.

# 13

# Cognitive therapy and psychosocial interventions in chronic and treatment-resistant mood disorders

Jan Scott and Robert J. DeRubeis

## Introduction

During the first half of the twentieth century, chronic mood disorders, such as the condition we now call dysthymia, were viewed as personality disorders for which the treatment of choice was psychotherapy (Scott, 1988; Markowitz, 1994). It was not until the publication of DSM-III (American Psychiatric Association, 1980) that dysthymia was recognized as an affective syndrome that could overlap or coexist with a major depressive disorder, and might respond to treatment with antidepressant medication. This reclassification and the subsequent interest in the nosology of chronic mood disorders led to a number of studies of the phenomenology, prevalence and treatment options available for chronic and treatment-resistant affective syndromes (Guscott & Grof, 1991). Unfortunately, the definitions used and the treatments explored emphasized almost exclusively the biological aspects of chronic disorders (Scott, 1991). Most experts on treatment-resistant mood disorders recommend that the patient be offered a systematic course of somatic treatments, with little or no mention of a need for psychological or social therapy (Greenberg & Spiro, 1987). In this chapter, we highlight the influence of psychosocial factors on the course and outcome of chronic and treatment-resistant mood disorders, and we review the potentially important therapeutic role of psychosocial interventions. We then describe and identify the evidence for the effectiveness of psychosocial approaches with this patient population, with an emphasis on cognitive therapy (CT) in chronic affective disorders.

## The potential role of psychosocial interventions

All professionals working with people experiencing chronic and treatment-resistant mood disorders are psychologically important to those patients. Individuals suffering from persistent symptoms have usually experienced significant disappointments and demoralization following the failure of several previous treatment regimes, and they often perceive that they have been rejected by the clinicians who have offered those treatments. The patients and their 'significant others' may become increasingly skeptical, or lose hope entirely, about the possibility of remission. They may begin to doubt or reject the causal model of the disorder promoted by the clinician and subsequently become ambivalent about adhering to the recommended treatment regimes. A clinician who views his or her role as the intermittent assessment of the patient's mental state and the prescription of sophisticated combinations of medication will rarely achieve good outcomes with this population unless that clinician or a member of the treatment team is able to offer the patient information, education, advice, realistic hope, and psychological support throughout the course of pharmacotherapy (see Table 13.1).

Most of the symptoms of chronic or treatment-resistant mood disorders may be amenable to psychological interventions. For example, hopelessness, suicidal ideation, low self-esteem, poor problem-solving strategies, and avoidant coping styles are highly prevalent in patients with chronic or partially remitted mood disorders (Krantz & Moos, 1988; Scott & Wright, 1996; Cornwall & Scott, 1997). All of these symptoms can be addressed with cognitive and behavioral techniques, either alone or in combination with pharmacotherapy. In addition, non-adherence to medication, which occurs in about 20–50% of this patient population (Klerman, 1990), has been successfully treated through cognitive-behavioral approaches (Cochran, 1984; Rush, 1988).

There are many psychosocial difficulties that may be causes or consequences of chronicity or treatment resistance. Reviews of both unipolar and bipolar mood disorders suggest that lack of social support, poor marital or family relationships, high levels of expressed emotion (EE), and a preponderance of negative life events after the onset of the index illness episode, are associated with chronicity (Akiskal, 1982; Thase & Kupfer, 1987; Scott, 1988, 1995b; Paykel, 1994; Thase, 1994). In some instances, successful treatment with pharmacotherapy allows the patient to draw on his or her own coping skills and resolve these difficulties. However, depressed patients with characteristics such as high levels of premorbid neuroticism and high scores on measures of dysfunctional attitudes are likely to show a poor response to antidepressant monotherapy (Scott, 1988; Paykel, 1994; Thase, 1994). Bothwell and Scott (1997) have similarly shown that in a sample of severely depressed inpatients who received adequate pharmacotherapy, high levels of dysfunctional attitudes (particularly those related to approval) and low self-esteem at admission were the most robust predictors of non-recovery at a two year follow-up. Scott (1997) also reported that, in comparison to age- and gender-matched healthy controls and bipolar patients with good outcome, bipolar patients with poor outcome had significantly higher levels of dysfunctional attitudes, higher levels of the personality trait of sociotropy (where self-worth is determined

**Table 13.1.** Potential role of psychosocial interventions

| Intervention | Aims | Examples |
|---|---|---|
| Supportive therapy | 1. Education about disorder and treatment | Supportive therapy (Greenberg & Spiro,1987) |
| | 2. Remoralization | Clinical Management (Fawcett et al., 1987) |
| | 3. Instillation of hope | |
| Specific cognitive and/or behavioural techniques | 4. Targeting specific psychological symptoms of chronic mood disorder, e.g. hopelessness, suicidal ideation, low self-esteem | CT for low self-esteem (Fennell, 1997) |
| | 5. Enhancing adherence with treatment regime | CT for poor medication adherence (Rush, 1988) |
| | 6. Ameliorating 'drug-resistant' residual symptoms | CT for residual depressive symptoms (Fava et al., 1994) |
| Brief therapy (alone or in combination with medication) | 7. Treatment of comorbidity, e.g. mood disorders with personality or substance misuse disorders | CT for dysthymia (Markowitz, 1994); |
| | 8. Treatment of chronic disorders which fail to respond to any medication regimes | CT for bipolar disorder (Scott, 1996) |
| | | CT milieu therapy (Scott, 1992; Wright et al., 1993) |
| | 9. Treatment of other psychosocial causes or consequences of disorder, e.g. high EE | CT for couples or families (Wright et al., 1993) or IPT (Markowitz, 1994) |
| | 10. Relapse prevention | CT (Evans et al., 1992) or IPT (Frank et al., 1990) |
| Rehabilitation | 11. Overcoming psychological barriers to normal functioning | CT for chronic mood disorders (Wright et al., 1993; Scott & Wright, 1996) |
| | 12. Reintegration with family | CT or IPT |
| | 13. Re-establishing social and work role | CT or IPT |

by the views of others), and lower levels of self-esteem. As these 'drug-treatment resistant' psychological symptoms are often associated with partial remission or increased risk of relapse, there is a strong argument for the simultaneous or sequential use of psychotherapy as an adjunct to pharmacotherapy (Cornwall & Scott, 1997).

There are some instances in which the use of a specific psychological therapy is indicated. For example, only about 50% of patients with chronic minor affective symptoms or dysthymic disorder respond to pharmacotherapy (Markowitz, 1994). These individuals may be candidates for specific approaches such as cognitive therapy or interpersonal therapy. Furthermore, patients with treatment-resistant or chronic affective disorders may have comorbid physical or mental disorders that compound the difficulty of obtaining a satisfactory treatment response. Even if the individual adheres to medication, physical disorders may limit the options for pharmacotherapy, and the presence of a comorbid Axis II disorder is likely to limit the patient's response to medication alone. As personality disorders and substance use disorders each occur in at least 30% of this patient population (Goodwin & Jamison, 1990; Shea et al., 1990; Thase, 1994), there is a need to use a combination of pharmacotherapy and psychosocial interventions. There is also a small literature on the successful use of cognitive therapy, either alone or in combination with medication, for patients with treatment-resistant psychotic symptoms, including paranoid delusions and auditory hallucinations (for a review, see Scott & Wright, 1996).

Finally, many individuals with a chronic or treatment-resistant mood disorder who show a full or partial symptomatic response to pharmacotherapy still exhibit considerable impairment in their social, family and work role functioning. Psychosocial interventions can play a crucial role in rehabilitating these individuals, supporting them through the process of reintegration with their family and community, and preventing future relapse.

## Which psychosocial approaches should be considered?

There is no identified 'best practice' model to use when providing supportive psychotherapy to patients with chronic and treatment-resistant mood disorders. However, these patients tend not to do well with unstructured approaches, as these tend to increase rather than decrease the patient's sense of hopelessness and helplessness (Scott et al., 1991). In the Cambridge-Newcastle Medical Research Council study, we have observed that a medication plus clinical management regime similar to the approach used in the Treatment of Depression Collaborative Research Program (TDCRP; Elkin et al., 1989; see Fawcett et al., 1987) is beneficial to a substantial minority of patients with chronic major depressive disorders.

**Table 13.2.** Characteristics of effective brief psychotherapies

1. The therapy provides the individual with an understandable model of their experiences.
2. Therapeutic interventions are based on a well-planned rationale.
3. Both the therapy and individual treatment sessions are highly structured.
4. Plans for producing change are made in a logical manner.
5. Therapy encourages the independent use of the skills learned outside of the sessions.
6. Any change achieved is attributed to the individual's rather than the therapist's skilfulness.
7. Therapy helps the individual develop a greater sense of self-efficacy.
8. Therapy enhances the individual's ability to independently cope with future adversity.

Structured psychoeducation sessions aimed at describing a causal model of the disorder and the rationale for pharmacotherapy may also enhance both treatment adherence and outcome (Frank et al., 1995; Addis & Jacobson, 1996). As the patient and his or her family usually need help identifying realistic targets and coping with the burden imposed by chronic morbidity, planned follow-up sessions over a period of many months are preferred over irregular or crisis sessions.

If a specific psychotherapy is to be introduced, it is preferable to choose one of the time-limited, 'manualized' (or 'guideline-driven') therapies, such as cognitive therapy or interpersonal therapy, that are of proven efficacy in acute mood disorders (US Department of Health & Human Sciences [US DHHS], 1993; Scott, 1995a). As highlighted in Table 13.2, these approaches share several characteristics which are believed to contribute to their effectiveness (Zeiss et al., 1979; Teasdale, 1985; Scott, 1995a). A manualized therapy provides the individual with an understandable model of their experience. Each therapy has a well-planned rationale and is highly structured. Plans for producing change are made in logical sequences and the therapy encourages the independent use of skills by the patient. Any change that is achieved is attributed to the individual's rather than the therapist's skilfulness. Importantly, the individual develops a greater sense of self-efficacy and belief in their ability to cope with future adversity.

The decision about which manualized therapy to offer a patient will be influenced by the nature of the problems identified, the evidence for the effectiveness of the therapy for the specific treatment targets, and the availability of an experienced therapist who is trained in the use of that particular approach. The importance of the latter should not be underestimated. A pharmacotherapist would not consider a trial of medication to be adequate unless the appropriate drug had been given in an adequate dose for an adequate period of time. Cognitive therapy research has demonstrated a significant correlation ($r = 0.39–0.53$) between therapists' adherence early in therapy to the CT model and symptom change during the course of therapy (DeRubeis & Feeley, 1990, Feeley et al., 1999).

Moreover, individuals treated by an expert CT therapist are less likely to drop out of therapy and are significantly more likely to report symptomatic improvement than those treated by novice therapists (Burns & Nolen-Hoeksema, 1992). Further investigation has established that variation in therapists' skilfulness may account for 20–30% of the variance in patient outcome, and that level of expertise in CT is particularly important when treating individuals with chronic and severe disorders (Roth & Fonagy, 1996; Scott, 1996). O'Malley et al. (1988) have reported similar findings for IPT.

## Outcome research

In this section we briefly review the data on psychosocial interventions and IPT for chronic and treatment-resistant mood disorders. We then explore the use of CT with difficult to treat depressive disorders.

### Psychosocial and psychodynamic approaches

There are several open studies of chronic mood disorders that allude to the benefits of individual, couples, or family psychoeducation sessions (for reviews, see Greenberg & Spiro, 1987; Scott, 1991; Markowitz, 1996). However, the publications reviewed primarily offer descriptive accounts of the content of the course of therapy with few, if any, objective measures of the specific contribution of the psychosocial intervention to patient outcome. Similarly, there are many qualitative discussions of psychoanalytic approaches to depressive personality disorders (see Roth & Fonagy, 1996). On this basis, the use of psychodynamic or psychoanalytic psychotherapies has been advocated for individuals with a dysthymia that appears to have originated from unresolved neurotic conflicts. However, there are no controlled empirical data available regarding the efficacy of these approaches either alone or in combination with drugs.

### Interpersonal therapy

There is a small literature on the use of IPT for individuals with chronic and treatment-resistant disorders. Markowitz (1996) reports that 17 patients with dysthymia (pure dysthymia = 8; double depression = 9) have participated in three pilot studies of IPT. At the end of the acute treatment phase (about 16 weeks of IPT), 11 (65%) patients met criteria for remission (scores on the Hamilton Rating Scale for Depression (HRSD) less than 8), and mean scores on the HRSD had fallen from 21.5 to 7.5. A subgroup of six patients who also received monthly continuation sessions for a further 24 months were reported to have maintained the gains achieved during the acute treatment phase (Markowitz, 1994). In a recent reanalysis of the NIMH study outcome data (Elkin et al., 1995), severely depressed subjects (HRSD > 20) receiving either IPT or imipramine plus clinical management (IMI-CM) were significantly more likely to meet recovery criteria than those receiving placebo plus clinical management (PL-CM). However, chronicity predicted poorer treatment outcome with less symptomatic improvement at 16-week follow-up (Sotsky et al., 1991). There are no published studies on the use of IPT in bipolar disorders, although there are preliminary data suggesting that a combination of interpersonal social rhythm therapy (IPSRT) and medication may be useful to this patient group (Ehlers et al., 1993).

## Cognitive therapy

There is a great deal of evidence that CT is an effective treatment for depression (for reviews of outcome research see: Hollon et al., 1991; US DHHS, 1993; Scott, 1995b). Although most studies have been conducted on outpatient samples that meet research criteria for the diagnosis of acute unipolar major depressive disorder without psychotic features, there are five published studies of the use of CT for dysthymia. In addition, Fava et al. (1994, 1996) have specifically explored the acute and 4-year outcome of patients with residual depressive symptoms who were treated with CT after receiving medication. There are six studies of CT for outpatients or inpatients with severe major depressive disorders, several other researchers undertaking randomized controlled trials of CT for depression have explored the influence of episode severity or chronicity on therapy outcome. There is also a small literature on the use of group and individual CT in bipolar disorder.

### Outpatient CT for dysthymia and residual depressive symptoms

Fennell and Teasdale (1982) reported that when a standard course of outpatient CT was offered to individuals with 'treatment-resistant' dysthymia, only one out of five patients achieved the criteria for recovery, and the reduction in symptom severity between baseline and follow-up assessment was modest (mean HRSD scores fell by 24%). Harpin et al. (1982) reported a statistically significant 37% reduction in mean HRSD scores in 12 patients who had previously failed to respond to medication. Gonzales et al. (1985) undertook the largest study of CT for dysthymia (pure dysthymia = 28; double depression = 26), providing 12 two-hour sessions of either individual or group therapy. Results for group and individual interventions for each patient group were not reported separately, but 19 subjects with dysthymia met recovery criteria (34%), and there was a trend for those with pure dysthymia (47%) to show a greater response than those with double depression (27%). Stravinski et al. (1991) treated six patients with dysthymia with 15 weekly sessions of individual CT and reported that four of them (67%) responded to treatment. Mercier et al. (1992) offered a maximum of 16 weeks of individual CT followed by four booster sessions over the subsequent 6 months to 15 patients with dysthymic disorders (pure dysthymia = 8; double depression = 7) of over 7 years' duration. At 16 weeks, six patients (40%) met recovery criteria (pure dysthymia = 3; double depression = 3), with four patients remaining well at a 10 month follow-up.

Fava and colleagues (1994, 1996) explored the effectiveness of sequential CT or clinical management (CM) for 40 patients who were assessed as having responded to antidepressant medication but who had residual symptoms of major depression. Patients were randomly assigned to CT or CM, and the medication was gradually withdrawn. At 24 months, there was a significant reduction in the level of residual symptoms in the CT group but not in the CM group, and during this period only three CT as compared to seven CM patients experienced a relapse. At the 4-year follow-up, this difference in outcome was significant, with twice as many patients who received CM (70%) as compared to CT (35%) experiencing a depressive relapse.

## Inpatient CT for dysthymia and treatment-resistant major depressive disorders

The only controlled study of CT without medication for inpatients with dysthymia was performed by De Jong et al. (1986; see Table 13.3). This study had significant limitations, including a small number of patients in each treatment condition ($n = 10$) and the use of an outpatient control group. Treatment response was higher in hospitalized patients who received a complete package of CT (60%) as compared to inpatient cognitive restructuring (30%) or supportive outpatient therapy (10%). Although it was reported that gains were maintained at 6-month follow-up, only 50% of the sample took part in this reassessment.

Scott and colleagues (Barker et al., 1987; Scott, 1992) reported two studies of the use of a combined medication plus CT package in chronic treatment-resistant major depression. In the first study, Barker et al. (1987) reported no significant differences in response rate in 20 inpatients randomly assigned to standard inpatient treatment with optimal medication as compared to optimal medication plus CT. However, in a second study of 24 inpatients with treatment-resistant depression of at least four years' duration (see Table 13.3), Scott (1992) noted that inpatient CT plus medication was more effective if given as a 'cognitively oriented hospital milieu' treatment package followed by outpatient CT for 6 months ($n = 16$; recovery rate = 70%) than in a standard individual CT format ($n = 8$; recovery rate = 50%). Furthermore, the percentage change in mean HRSD scores was 57% for CT milieu treatment (mean HRSD fell from 25.5 to 10.6), as compared to 42% for the standard CT approach (mean HRSD fell from 22.5 to 13.1). We also have preliminary data from a 4 year follow-up study of 50 consecutive referrals to this clinic who had chronic treatment-resistant depressive

**Table 13.3.** Outcome research of CT for chronic and refractory depressive disorders

| Study | CT model | Sample size | Recovery rate $n$ | Recovery rate % |
|---|---|---|---|---|
| *Outpatient studies* | | | | |
| Fennell & Teasdale (1982) | 20 sessions over 12–15 weeks | 5 | 1 | 20 |
| Harpin et al. (1982) | 20 sessions over 10 weeks | 12 | 4 | 33 |
| Gonzales et al. (1985) | 12 × 2-hourly group or individual sessions over 8 weeks | 54 | 19 | 34 |
| Stravinski et al. (1991) | 15 weekly sessions | 6 | 4 | 66 |
| Mercier et al. (1992) | Maximum 16 weekly sessions plus four booster sessions over 6 months | 15 | 6 | 40 |
| Total | | 92 | 4 | 37 |
| *Inpatient studies* | | | | |
| DeJong et al. (1986) | 3 months of inpatient CT alone | 10 | 6 | 60 |
| Scott (1992) | | | | |
| *Sample 1* | 15 sessions of individual CT plus medication over 3 months | 8 | 4 | 50 |
| *Sample 2* | Cognitive milieu therapy plus medication over 3 months (about 30–40 hours of CT) | 16 | 11 | 72 |
| Total | | 34 | 21 | 62 |
| Total for inpatient and outpatient studies | | 126 | 55 | 44 |

disorders and who were treated with CT plus medication. In this sample the median time to recovery was 13 months, and 42% of patients met recovery criteria at 48 months (Scott, 1995c).

## Inpatient CT for severe and difficult to treat depressive disorders

Several groups of investigators have explored the effects of CT with or without medication for depressed inpatients. Thase and coworkers (1991) observed a decrease in mean Beck Depression Inventory (BDI) scores from 32.4 to 6.9 in 16 unmedicated hospitalized patients with endogenous depression and HRSD scores of 15 or more, who were offered an average of 13 sessions of CT over 4 weeks. In an expanded study by this same research group, 32 patients with major depression evidenced a response rate of 70% to inpatient CT (Thase, 1994). Bowers (1990) found that moderately to severely depressed inpatients (mean BDI score = 27.3) who received either 12 sessions of CT plus nortriptyline ($n=10$) or a behavioral intervention plus nortriptyline ($n=10$) had significantly lower BDI scores and fewer negative cognitions at the end of treatment than inpatients who received drug alone ($n=10$). Also, patients who were treated with CT were significantly more likely to meet recovery criteria (judged by HRSD score < 6) than other patients (recovery rates: CT = 80%; behavioral intervention = 10%; pharmacotherapy = 20%). Another study of 47 depressed inpatients with HRSD scores of over 17 at intake was reported by Miller et al. (1989). Patients treated with CT plus antidepressant medication improved significantly, but at the end of hospitalization there were no significant differences between 'treatment as usual,' social skills training, and CT (all groups received concomitant antidepressants). Six and 12 months posthospitalization, there was a trend for subjects who received standard treatment to have a higher rate of relapse; the pooled group of psychotherapy patients had a significantly higher rate of recovery (68%) than the standard treatment group (33%). However, it should be noted that there were very high dropout rates from the follow-up phase of this study (medication group = 41%), making interpretation of the results difficult.

### The influence of severity and chronicity of depressive symptoms on response to CT

Investigators who have examined the effect of severity of an acute major depressive episode on response to CT have reported mixed results. Earlier studies by Blackburn et al. (1981), Kovacs et al. (1981), and Teasdale et al. (1984) did not reveal a relation between severity of illness (or endogenous subtype) and treatment outcome with CT. In the TDCRP study, Elkin and colleagues (1989) reported that CT was less effective for severe depression (HRSD > 20) than milder forms of this disorder. However, DeRubeis et al. (1999) have analyzed the data from the TDCRP alongside data from three other CT vs. medication randomized trials (Hollon et al., 1993; Murphy et al., 1984; Rush et al., 1977). They found no advantage of medication over CT in the severe subsamples from these four studies, taken collectively.

Thase and coworkers (1996) found that patients with severe depression were less likely than subjects with less severe disorders to have a full remission after a course of CT. Nevertheless, both patient groups improved substantially, and there were only small differences in end point depression scores. The use of CT for psychotic depression has not been investigated systematically (see Bishop et al., 1986), but in her study of chronic treatment-resistant mood disorders, Scott (1995a) noted that psychotic symptoms predicted a slower response to CT (median time to recovery = 19 months). Robins and Hayes (1993) highlighted that therapists treating individuals with severe depressive disorders tend to target behavioral activation for a prolonged period, rather than cognitive techniques such as hypothesis testing. This means that in time-limited trials of CT, more severely depressed patients may receive less of some of the therapy components that are particularly associated with improvement (DeRubeis & Feeley, 1990).

Gonzales and coworkers (1985) noted that patients with acute major depressive disorders were over twice as likely to respond to 12 weekly 2-hour long sessions of CT ($n = 49$; recovery rate = 76%) as compared to patients with dysthymia ($n = 56$; recovery rate = 34%). Thase et al. (1994) have also reported on the differential response to CT of patients with acute and chronic depressive disorders. Patients who had either major depression superimposed upon dysthymia ('double depression') or chronic major depression were less likely than those with acute depressions to reach full remission (Thase, 1994). But, the group with chronic depressions achieved significant reductions in HRSD and BDI scores nonetheless.

### The use of CT for bipolar disorders

There is a developing body of research on the use of CT in bipolar disorder (Scott, 1995, 1996). The only randomized controlled trial published focused on enhancing adherence to lithium prophylaxis (Cochran, 1984). Twenty-four patients were assigned to standard outpatient treatment or to six sessions of CT plus standard treatment. At follow-up, 57% of patients in the control group as compared to 21% of patients in the intervention group had discontinued lithium. Rehospitalization rates were also significantly higher in the control group.

More recently, manuals have been developed for the use of CT for bipolar disorder (Basco & Rush, 1996) and for rapid cycling disorders (Newman & Beck, 1992). Palmer et al. (1995) reported benefits from group CT for patients with bipolar disorder who had been recently discharged from inpatient treatment. Lam (1997) also reported improved outcomes in patients with bipolar disorder who were assessed as at high risk of relapse despite the use of prophylactic medication. In a pilot study of 12 patients with treatment-resistant bipolar disorder, Scott (1997) reported that CT plus medication led to significant improvements in day-to-day functioning, adherence to pharmacotherapy, and self-esteem in 60% of the sample.

## Overview of CT for chronic and treatment-resistant mood disorders

The CT interventions described in the above outcome studies are based on the approach described by Beck and coworkers (Beck et al., 1979) for less severe conditions. It is apparent that, with few exceptions, the standard CT package of about 12–18 individual sessions is less beneficial to individuals with chronic and treatment-resistant mood disorders. Most of the studies demonstrating significant reductions in levels of severity of depressive symptoms or higher recovery rates

**Table 13.4.** Modifications to CT for clients with chronic and refractory mood disorders

Increase frequency and reduce length of session (e.g. $3 \times 20$ minutes per week)

1. Extend course of therapy (e.g. 30 sessions)
2. Increase interpersonal focus of individual sessions
3. Prolong behavioural focus
4. Introduce conjoint family sessions
5. If hospitalized consider:
   milieu therapy
   predischarge planning and relapse prevention sessions

report modifications to the CT approach to tackle the more pronounced, complex or enduring problems encountered in this patient population (see Table 13.4). These modifications are highlighted in a number of CT manuals produced by clinicians who have worked with patients with severe and chronic unipolar and bipolar disorders (Newman & Beck, 1992; Scott, 1992; Wright et al., 1993; Basco & Rush, 1996; Scott & Wright, 1996; Scott, 1996). The approaches all retain the essential elements of CT with a collaborative–empirical therapeutic relationship at the core of the treatment intervention. The therapy is structured and problem-oriented. Usually, an agenda is set for each session. All patients are socialized to the cognitive model and are then taught how to use cognitive restructuring and behavioral techniques to reduce symptoms. The therapist is quite active, but the patient is encouraged to play a significant role in designing and monitoring any agreed upon homework assignments.

With cases of severe depression, both cognitive and behavioral techniques are used for acute symptom relief, but treatment techniques may be adjusted to help deal with high levels of agitation, insomnia, difficulties with concentration, or profound hopelessness. For example, sessions may be reduced in length but held more frequently, or the overall course of treatment may be extended (Thase et al., 1991a,b; Scott, 1992). Scott (1992) recommended an extended behavioral emphasis often accompanied by 'overlearning' (repetition of behavioral assignments in different situations) during the initial stages of CT with inpatients. More complex cognitive interventions (such as identifying and challenging dysfunctional underlying beliefs) may be delayed until the patient is better able to concentrate on and address psychological issues. It should be emphasized, however, that severely depressed people can often do at least some cognitive restructuring early in treatment. For example, a patient with marked sleep problems not fully responsive to pharmacotherapy might be taught relaxation and imagery procedures in addition to methods of reducing intrusive negative thoughts. This early use of methods to tackle negative cognitive bias is very important, as two of the most significant features of severe or treatment-resistant disorders are hopelessness and suicidal ideation. Cognitive interventions to curb hopelessness and reduce the risk of self-harm are often needed at the outset of treatment.

More intensive inpatient CT approaches have been advocated for severe or chronic and treatment-resistant depressive disorders. These include the use of a 'cognitive milieu' where staff members are trained in CT techniques so that the patient can be exposed to multiple opportunities to learn cognitive and behavioral procedures. Highly developed inpatient cognitive therapy programs usually include psychoeducation, individual therapy, and group CT. Staff members may be assigned to assist with homework assignments, behavioral interventions, or other components of treatment. Before discharge, patients often participate in relapse prevention exercises such as cognitive–behavioral rehearsal. Most cognitive milieu units adopt a cognitive–biological model in which CT and psychopharmacology are the predominant therapies. In addition, it has been noted that enhancing the interpersonal focus of CT or introducing couples or family CT sessions may be associated with greater improvement at the end of therapy (Scott, 1992; Markowitz, 1994).

Although CT has been described as a 'manualized' approach, most cognitive therapists employ considerable flexibility in developing a customized case conceptualization and treatment plan for each patient. For patients with chronic and treatment-resistant disorders, the overall strategy is to look for possible roadblocks to recovery and to design interventions to help the patient revise long-standing negative self-constructs or patterns of behaviour. However, the therapist may focus on specific targets at different phases of the therapy. For example, in severe disorders, CT addresses the need for rapid symptom relief from the first session and only later tackle issues such as improving interpersonal functioning, developing social skills, and modifying of dysfunctional underlying beliefs. In contrast, in the treatment of dysthymia or mild depressions superimposed on a pre-existing personality disorder, the therapist may introduce intensive work on restructuring underlying dysfunctional attitudes at an early stage of the therapy process.

## Conclusions

Patients with chronic and treatment-resistant affective disorders present a challenge for any form of therapy. The overall results of research on psychosocial interventions indicate that these individuals have a more difficult treatment course than those with acute or less extreme symptoms. However, there is evidence to support the effectiveness of CT for both severe and mild chronic depressions, and preliminary data support the use of CT as an adjunct to medication for patients with bipolar disorders.

Most of the outcome research of CT for dysthymia comprises open studies with small sample sizes. However, it should be noted that these studies are comparable in size and design to many studies of pharmacotherapy for this patient population, and the mean recovery rate (40%) is also similar (Price et al., 1986). Given that patients with dysthymia are known to have a low placebo response rate of about 15% (Roth & Fonagy, 1996) and often refuse to take antidepressant medication (Markowitz, 1994), these results should perhaps instill hope rather than despair in clinicians who work with more chronic or treatment-resistant patients. The limited data on inpatients indicate that CT can work without antidepressants for milder disorders, but that inpatient followed by outpatient CT plus optimal pharmacotherapy leads to acceptable recovery rates (Scott, 1992). A 4-year follow-up of this population (Scott, 1995) revealed that fewer than half of the sample had relapsed, and none had developed a further chronic or treatment-resistant episode. Given that maintenance CT or IPT is now being advocated, it may be that these encouraging findings can be built upon in the future.

## REFERENCES

Addis, M. & Jacobson, N. (1996). Reasons for depression and the process and outcome of cognitive-behavioral psychotherapies. *Journal of Consulting and Clinical Psychology*, **64**, 1417–24.5.

Akiskal, H. (1982). Factors associated with incomplete recovery in primary depressive illness. *Journal of Clinical Psychiatry*, **43**, 266–71.

American Psychiatric Association (1980). *Diagnostic and Statistical Manual of Mental Disorders: 3rd edn*. Washington: APA Press.

Barker, W., Scott, J., & Eccleston, D. (1987). The Newcastle chronic depression study: results of a treatment regime. *International Clinical Psychopharmacology*, **2**, 261–72.

Basco, M. & Rush, A. (1996). *Cognitive-behavioral treatment of manic-depressive disorder*. New York: Guilford Press.

Beck, A., Rush, A., Shaw, B., & Emery, G. (1979). *Cognitive Therapy of Depression*. New York: Guilford Press.

Bishop, S., Miller, I., Norman, W., Buda, M., & Foulke, M. (1986). Cognitive therapy of psychotic depression: a case report. *Psychotherapy*, **23**, 167–73.

Blackburn, I., Bishop, S., Glen, I., Whalley, L., & Christie, J. (1981). The efficacy of cognitive therapy in depression: a treatment trial using cognitive therapy and pharmacotherapy, each alone and in combination. *British Journal of Psychiatry*, **139**, 181–9.

Bothwell, R. & Scott, J. (1997). The influence of cognitive variables on recovery in depressed inpatients. *Journal of Affective Disorders*, **43**, 207–12.

Bowers, W. (1990). Treatment of depressed inpatients: cognitive therapy plus medication, relaxation plus medication and medication alone. *British Journal of Psychiatry*, **156**, 73–8.

Burns, D. & Nolen-Hoeksema, S. (1992). Therapeutic empathy and recovery from depression in cognitive-behavioral therapy: a structural equation model. *Journal of Consulting and Clinical Psychology*, **60**, 441–9.

Cochran, S. (1984). Preventing medical non-compliance in the outpatient treatment of bipolar affective disorder. *Journal of Nervous and Mental Diseases*, **176**, 45–54.

Cornwall, P. & Scott, J. (1997). Partial remission in depressive disorders. *Acta Psychiatrica Scandinavica*, **95**, 265–71.

de Jong, R., Trieber, R., & Henrich, G. (1986). Effectiveness of two psychological treatments for inpatients with severe and chronic depressions. *Cognitive Therapy and Research*, **10**, 64553.

DeRubeis, R, & Feeley, M. (1990). Determinants of change in cognitive therapy for depression. *Cognitive Therapy and Research*, **14**, 469–82.

DeRubeis, R., Evans, M., Hollon, S., Garvey, M., Grove, W., & Tuason, V. (1990). How does cognitive therapy work? Cognitive change and symptom change in cognitive therapy and pharmacotherapy of depression. *Journal of Consulting and Clinical Psychology*, **58**, 86–9.

DeRubeis, R., Gelfand, L., Tang, T., & Simons, A. (1999). Medications versus cognitive behavioral therapy for severely depressed outpatients: mega-analysis of four randomized comparisons. *American Journal of Psychiatry*, **156**, 1007–13.

Ehlers, C., Kupfer, D., Frank, E., & Monk, T. (1993). Biological rhythms in depression: the role of zeitgebers and zeitstorers. *Depression*, **1**, 285–93.

Elkin, I., Shea, M., Watkins, J. et al. (1989). NIMH treatment of depression collaborative program: general effectiveness of treatments. *Archives of General Psychiatry*, **46**, 971–82.

Elkin, I., Gibbons, R., Shea, M. et al. (1995). Initial severity and differential treatment outcome in the NIMH treatment of depression collaborative research program. *Journal of Consulting and Clinical Psychology*, **63**, 841–7.

Evans, M., Hollon, S., DeRubeis, R. et al. (1992). Differential response following cognitive therapy and pharmacotherapy for depression. *Archives of General Psychiatry*, **49**, 802–8.

Fava, G., Grandi, S., Zielezny, M., Canestrari, R., & Morphy, M. (1994). Cognitive behavioral treatment of residual symptoms in primary major depressive disorder. *American Journal of Psychiatry*, **151**, 1295–9.

Fava, G., Grandi, S., Zielezny, M., Rafanelli, C., & Canestrari, R. (1996). Four year outcome of cognitive behavioral treatment of residual symptoms in major depression. *American Journal of Psychiatry*, **153**, 945–7.

Fawcett, J., Epstein, P., & Feister, S. (1987). Clinical management – imipramine/placebo administration manual. *Psychopharmacology Bulletin*, **23**, 309–24.

Feeley, M., DeRubeis, R.J., & Gelfand, L.A. (1999). The temporal relation of adherence and alliance to symptom change in cognitive therapy for depression. *Journal of Consulting and Clinical Psychology*, **67**, 578–82.

Fennell, M. (1997). Low self-esteem: a cognitive perspective. *Behavioral and Cognitive Psychotherapy*, **25**, 1–26.

Fennell, M. & Teasdale, J. (1982). Cognitive therapy with chronic drug refractory depressed outpatients: a note of caution. *Cognitive Therapy and Research*, **6**, 455–460.

Frank, E., Kupfer, D., Perel, J. et al. (1990). Three year outcomes for maintenance therapies of recurrent depression. *Archives of General Psychiatry*, **47**, 1093–9.

Frank, E., Kupfer, D., & Siegel, L. (1995). Alliance not compliance: a philosophy of outpatient care. *Journal of Clinical Psychiatry*, **56**, 11–16.

Frank, E., Kupfer, D., Jacob, M., & Jarrett, R. (1987). Personality features and response to acute treatment in recurrent depression. *Journal of Personality Disorders*, **1**, 14–26.

Gonzales, L., Lewinsohn, P., & Clarke, G. (1985). Longitudinal follow-up of unipolar depressives: An investigation of predictors of relapse. *Journal of Consulting and Clinical Psychology*, **53**, 461–9.

Goodwin, F. & Jamison, K. (1990). *Manic Depressive Illness.* Oxford: Oxford University Press.

Greenberg, D. & Spiro, H. (1987). Psychological management of resistant depression. In *Treating Resistant Depression*, ed. J. Zohar & R. Belmaker, pp. 47–64. New York: PMA Publishing Corp.

Guscott, R. & Grof, P. (1991). The clinical meaning of refractory depression: a review for the clinician. *American Journal of Psychiatry*, **148**, 695–704.

Harpin, R., Liberman, R., Marks, I., Stern, S., & Bohannon, W. (1982). Cognitive behaviour therapy for chronically depressed patients: a controlled pilot study. *Journal of Nervous and Mental Diseases*, **170**, 295–301.

Hollon, S., DeRubeis, R., Evans, M., Weimer, M., Garvey, M. et al. (1991). Cognitive therapy and pharmacotherapy for depression: singly and in combination. *Archives of General Psychiatry*, **49**, 774–81.

Hollon, S., Shelton, R., & Davies, D. (1993). Cognitive therapy for depression: conceptual issues and clinical efficacy. *Journal of Consulting and Clinical Psychology*, **61**, 270–5.

Klerman, G. (1990). Treatment of recurrent unipolar major depressive disorder. *Archives of General Psychiatry*, **47**, 11, 58–62.

Kovacs, M., Rush, A., Beck, A., & Hollon, S. (1981). Depressed outpatients treated with cognitive therapy or pharmacotherapy: a one-year follow-up. *Archives of General Psychiatry*, **38**, 33–41.

Krantz, S. & Moos, R. (1988). Risk factors at intake predict non-remission among depressed patients. *Journal of Consulting and Clinical Psychology*, **56**, 863–9.

Lam, D. (1997). Cognitive therapy for manic-depression: a pilot study. *Abstracts of Posters from the 2nd International Conference on Bipolar Disorder*, Pittsburg, USA.

Markowitz, J. (1994). Psychotherapy of dysthymia. *American Journal of Psychiatry*, **151**, 1114–21.

Markowitz, J. (1996). Psychotherapy for dysthymic disorder. *Psychiatric Clinics of North America*, **19**, 133–50.

Mercier, M., Stewart, J., & Quitkin, F. (1992). A pilot sequential study of cognitive therapy and pharmacotherapy of atypical depression. *Journal of Clinical Psychiatry*, **53**, 166–70.

Miller, I., Norman, W., Keitner, G., Bishop, S., & Dow, M. (1989). Cognitive behavioral treatment of depressed inpatients. *Behaviour Therapy*, **20**, 25–7.

Murphy, G., Simons, A., Wetzel, R., & Lustman, P. (1984). Cognitive therapy and nortriptyline, singly, and together, in treatment of depression. *Archives of General Psychology*, **41**, 33–41.

Newman, C. & Beck, A. (1992). *Cognitive Therapy in Rapid Cycling Disorder: A Treatment Manual.* Center for Cognitive Therapy, University of Pennsylvania: Philadelphia.

O'Malley, S., Foley, S., Rounsaville, B. et al. (1988). Therapist competence and patient outcome in interpersonal psychotherapy of depression. *Journal of Consulting and Clinical Psychology*, **56**, 496–501.

Palmer, A., Williams, H., & Adams, M. (1995). Cognitive behaviour therapy in a group format for bipolar affective disorder. *Behavioral and Cognitive Psychotherapy*, **23**, 153–68.

Paykel, E. (1994). Epidemiology of refractory depression. In *Refractory Depression: Current Strategies and Future Directions*, ed. W. Nolen, J. Zohar, S. Roose, & J. Amsterdam, pp. 3–18. Chichester, UK: John Wiley.

Price, L., Charney, D., & Heninger, G. (1986). Variability of response to lithium augmentation in refractory depression. *American Journal of Psychiatry*, **143**, 1387–92.

Robins, C. & Hayes, A. (1993). An appraisal of cognitive therapy. *Journal of Consulting and Clinical Psychology*, **61**, 205–14.

Roth, A. & Fonagy, R. (1996). *What works for whom?* New York: Guilford Press.

Rush, A. (1988). Cognitive approaches to adherence. In *Review of Psychiatry: Volume 8*, (ed. A. Frances and R. Hales). Washington: APA Press.

Rush, J., Beck, A., Kovacs, M., & Hollon, S. (1977). Comparative efficacy of cognitive therapy and pharmacotherapy in the treatment of depressed outpatients. *Cognitive Therapy and Research*, **1**, 17–37.

Scott, J. (1988). Chronic depression. *British Journal of Psychiatry*, **153**, 287–97.

Scott, J. (1991). Chronic depression: epidemiology, demography and definitions. *International Clinical Psychopharmacology*, **6**, 41–9.

Scott, J. (1992). Chronic depression: can cognitive therapy succeed when other treatments fail? *Behavioral and Cognitive Psychotherapy*, **20**, 25–36.

Scott, J. (1995a). Psychological treatments of depression: an update. *British Journal of Psychiatry*, **167**, 289–92.

Scott, J. (1995b). Psychotherapy for bipolar disorder: an unmet need?. *British Journal of Psychiatry*, **167**, 581–8.

Scott, J. (1995c). Immediate and four year outcome of CT for chronic, treatment refractory major depression. Paper presented at the World Congress of Cognitive and Behaviour, Therapies, Copenhagen, Denmark.

Scott, J. (1996). Cognitive therapy in bipolar disorder. *Cognitive and Behavioral Practice*, **3**, 1–23.

Scott, J. (1997). Cognitive therapy for individuals suffering from bipolar disorder. *Abstracts of Posters from the 2nd International Conference on Bipolar Disorder*, Pittsburg, USA.

Scott, J. & Wright, J. (1996). Cognitive therapy for individuals with severe and chronic mental disorders. *American Psychiatric Association Review of Psychiatry*, Vol. 16, pp. 153–201. Washington: APA.

Scott, J., Cole, A., & Eccleston, D. (1991). Dealing with persisting abnormalities of mood. *International Review of Psychiatry*, **3**, 19–33.

Shea, T., Pilkonis, P., Beckham, E. et al. (1990). Personality disorders and treatment outcome in the NIMH treatment of depression collaborative outcome study. *American Journal of Psychiatry*, **147**, 711–18.

Shea, T., Elkin, I., Imber, S. et al. (1992). Course of depressive symptoms over follow-up: findings from the NIMH treatment of depression collaborative research program. *Archives of*

*General Psychiatry* **49**, 782–7.

Sotsky, S., Glass, D., Shea, T. et al. (1991). Patient predictors of response to psychotherapy and pharmacotherapy: Findings in the NIMH treatment of depression collaborative research program. *American Journal of Psychiatry*, **148**, 997–1008.

Stravinski, A., Sahar, A., & Verreault, R. (1991). A pilot study of cognitive treatment of dysthymic disorder. *Behavioral Psychotherapy*, **4**, 387–94.

Teasdale, J. (1985). Psychological treatments for depression – how do they work? *Behaviour Research and Therapy*, **23**, 157–65.

Teasdale, J., Fennell, M., & Hibbert, G. (1984). Cognitive therapy for major depressive disorder in primary care. *British Journal of Psychology*, **144**, 400–6.

Thase, M. (1994). The roles of psychosocial factors and psychotherapy in refractory depression. In *Refractory Depression: Current Strategies and Future Directions*, ed. W. Nolen, J. Zohar, S. Roose, & J. Amsterdam, pp. 83–95. Chichester, UK: John Wiley.

Thase, M. & Kupfer, D. (1987). Characteristics of treatment resistant depression. In *Treating Resistant Depression*, ed. J. Zohar & R. Belmaker, pp. 23–45. New York: PMA Publishing Corp.

Thase, M., Bowler, K., & Harden, T. (1991a). Cognitive behaviour therapy of endogenous depression: Preliminary findings in 16 unmedicated inpatients. *Behaviour Therapy*, **22**, 469–77.

Thase, M., Simons, A., Cahalance, J., McGreary, J., & Hardin, T. (1991b). Severity of depression and response to cognitive therapy. *American Journal of Psychiatry*, **148**, 784–9.

Thase, M., Reynolds, C., & Frank, E. (1994). Response to cognitive therapy in chronic depression. *Journal of Psychotherapy Practice and Research*, **3**, 204–14.

Thase, M., Simons, A., & Reynolds, C. (1996). Psychobiological correlates of poor response to cognitive behaviour therapy: Potential indications for antidepressant pharmacotherapy. *Psychopharmacology Bulletin*, **29**, 293–301.

US DHHS (1993). *Depression in Primary Care. Volume 2: Treatment of Major Depression.* Rockville: AHCPR Publications.

Wright, J., Thase, M,. Beck, A., & Ludgate, J. (1993). *Cognitive Therapy with Inpatients*. New York: Guilford Press.

Zeiss, A., Lewinsohn, P., & Munoz, R. (1979). Non-specific improvement effects in depression using interpersonal skills training, pleasant activity schedules, or cognitive training. *Journal of Consulting and Clinical Psychology*, **47**, 427–39.

**Part IV**

# Special patient populations

# 14

# Chronic and refractory mood disorders in childhood and adolescence

Adelita Segovia, Kelly N. Botteron, and Barbara Geller

## Introduction

Because the study of pharmacologic and non-pharmacologic treatments of childhood depression is several decades behind that of depression occurring later in the lifespan, the definition of 'refractory depression' needs to be modified for the pediatric age group in accordance with this dearth of scientific data (Geller et al., 1996). At the present time there is only one double-blind placebo-controlled study published that establishes superiority of active vs. placebo medication for children and adolescents (Emslie et al., 1997). That study used fluoxetine. Six recent double-blind placebo-controlled studies examining various TCAs using DSM-III or higher diagnoses to characterize subjects were all negative. Based on the above, it can be argued currently that all childhood and adolescent depression can be characterized as 'refractory' if the measurement used is scientific evidence of efficacious treatments.

Nevertheless, the severity and chronicity of child and adolescent depression necessitate interventions which at the moment, unfortunately, cannot be developmentally based and have to largely be extrapolated from work done at older age groups. The problem with extrapolation is that there are clear developmental differences in response to treatment such as the negative TCA studies (Birmaher, 1998; Geller et al., 1999a); neurobiological differences in sleep parameters (Emslie et al., 1994; Dahl et al., 1996; Rao et al., 1996); cortisol metabolism (Puig-Antich et al., 1989) and heart rate variability (Walsh et al., 1994); and in the clinical picture which includes fewer and less prominent vegetative signs with decreasing age (Ryan et al., 1987). Further evidence of developmental differences appear in side effect profiles. Thus, anticholinergic effects usually do not appear in children and adolescents (Geller et al., 1992a,b) while marked obesity and polycystic ovaries have been reported in over 80% of females who received valproate for epilepsy before they were 20 years old, in contrast to a lower rate if treatment was started later in life (Isojarvi et al., 1993). Until age-specific data is available, extrapolation from adult studies and awareness of known and unknown developmental differences is the best that can be done to provide clinical interventions currently.

## Historical perspective

It may seem counter-intuitive that drug rather than non-drug modalities were initially studied for child and adolescent depression because of the possible impingement of biological interventions on normal developmental processes. Pharmacologic interventions, however, were the ones initially proposed and accepted for scientific study with federal support in the late 1970s and through the 1980s. A historical perspective provides the background for how this came to be. First, the hypothesis at that time was that major depressive disorder (MDD) was the same illness across the age span and therefore should have a similar response to treatment. This developmental approach ignored the pediatric adage that 'children are not miniature adults.' However, as a working hypothesis for where to begin studying MDD and for bringing child psychiatry into the main frame of general psychiatry it was visionary, and Puig-Antich's work (Puig-Antich et al., 1980) has shaped the field until the present time. The Puig-Antich (Puig-Antich et al., 1980) vision was that child psychiatry, like adult psychiatry, would fit the medical model; could use DSM-III and higher criteria; and that children could be interviewed using research assessments similar to those used for adults. The latter led to the development of the Kiddie Schedule for Affective Disorders and Schizophrenia (KSADS) and paved the way for interviewing children about their symptoms rather than just interviewing parents and observing children in play therapy. These pioneering developments permitted the determination of suicidality and other ideation and behaviors in children. Such issues ordinarily would not come to light because children do not spontaneously talk about these issues to parents or others. The ability to establish the diagnosis of MDD in children and adolescents was an important aspect of developing scientifically rigorous treatment studies. The use of pharmacologic prior to non-pharmacologic interventions was thus consistent with the zeitgeist that MDD at any age was an illness associated with altered neurochemistry that should respond to a pharmacological intervention. It was only later that investigations (Baxter et al., 1992) provided scientific data that biologic changes could occur in the treatment of some disorders even with non-pharmacologic interventions.

A final reason for pharmacologic preceding non-pharmacologic interventions came from the public health point of view that biologic interventions would entail less costly visits because they would require less time than psychotherapy. Also, drug treatments would be more available in rural and lower socioeconomic areas because they could be provided by non-specialists.

## Tricyclic antidepressant studies

Compared to the virtually hundreds of studies done on adults using multiple TCA preparations, there are seven rigorously designed double-blind placebo-controlled studies of TCAs for children and adolescents (Puig-Antich et al., 1987; Geller et al., 1990, 1992a,b; Kutcher et al., 1994; Kye et al, 1996; Klein et al., 1998; Birmaher et al., 1998). Two of these were for children (Puig-Antich et al., 1987; Geller et al., 1992a,b) and five were for adolescents (Geller et al., 1990; Klein et al., 1998; Birmaher et al., 1998; Kutcher et al., 1994; Kye et al., 1996). Three of these studies were stopped at midpoint because there was virtually no statistical possibility of finding a significant difference between active and placebo groups (Puig-Antich et al., 1987; Geller et al., 1990, 1992a,b). Even after offsetting the high placebo response rate in the Puig-Antich et al. (1987) study by using a single-blind placebo washout phase before randomization to active and placebo groups, there were still no difference between active and placebo subjects in subsequent TCA studies (Geller et al., 1990, 1992a,b). Thus, unlike the approximately two-thirds rate of positive studies in adults (Klein et al., 1980), there is not yet a positive TCA study for the pediatric age group.

There has been much speculation on possible reasons for this poor outcome (Geller et al., 1996). First among these reasons again has to be set in historical context. At the time that the initial TCA studies were developed for children in the late 1970s and 1980s, it was still not widely accepted that it was appropriate to use pharmacologic interventions for psychiatric disorders during the pediatric years. Thus, populations were selected to be severe and chronic so that there could be a general consensus that these very ill young subjects should get the benefit of pharmacologic intervention studies. The characteristics of the subjects in the initial childhood studies and in the adolescent studies was that they were severe, chronic, and highly comorbid, i.e. the same profile that has been associated with poorer response in studies of TCAs in adults (Kocsis et al., 1989).

In addition to the issue of clinical characteristics that might influence poorer outcome, the differences in neurobiology may also have been associated with differences in response. Thus, as noted above, evidence for different catecholamine mechanisms developmentally are supported by differences in heart rate variability, anticholinergic side effects and vegetative manifestations of MDD in children versus adults. Because the single positive study available (Emslie et al., 1997) used fluoxetine, a serotonergic drug may be more appropriate developmentally.

Another issue that needs to be considered as a biological difference is that when children are seen for an initial episode it cannot yet be known if their future course will be unipolar MDD or a bipolar picture. The rate of switch to bipolarity among prepubertal MDD subjects was 32% (80% switched while they were still prepubertal) (Geller et al., 1994). This is higher than the 5–20% reported for adolescents and adults (Clayton, 1981; Strober, 1982; Andreasen et al., 1988). It is possible that giving TCAs to children who are actually early in the course of bipolar disorder

**Table 14.1.** Pharmacotherapy studies in child and adolescent depression

| Author | Year | Age range | Mean age | Depressed subjects | Dosing medication | Study strategy | Design | Conclusion |
|---|---|---|---|---|---|---|---|---|
| Puig-Antich et al. | 1987 | Child | 9.1 | 38 | IMI | Fixed dose ≤ 5 mg/kg/d | DBPC – 6-week outpatient | n.s. |
| Geller et al. | 1989 | Child | 9.7 | 50 | NT | Fixed plasma level 89.9 ± 14.4 | DBPC – 2-week PLWO 8-week trial | n.s. |
| Geller et al. | 1990 | Adolescent | 14.3 | 31 | NT | Fixed plasma level 91.1 ± 18.3 | DBPC – 2-week PLWO 8-week trial | n.s. |
| Simeon et al. | 1990 | Adolescent | | 40 | FLX | 60 mg/d | DBPC – 7-week trial | Approx. two-thirds of both groups improved n.s. difference |
| Geller et al.* | 1997 | Child | | 30 | LI | To Li level 0.9 ± 0.2 meq/l | DBPC – 6-week trial | n.s. |
| Kutcher et al. | 1994 | Adolescent | 17.8 | 60 | DMI | 200 mg/d | DBPC – 1-week PLWO 6-week trial | n.s. |
| Kye et al. | 1996 | Adolescent | 14.9 | 31 | AMI | ≤ 5 mg/kg/d | DBPC – 2-week PLWO – 8-week trial | Mixed – CGI data suggested AMI > Pl, KSADS data n.s. |
| Emslie et al. | 1997 | Child and adolescent | | 96 | FLX | 20 mg/d | DBPC – 8-week trial | Fluoxetine superior to placebo |
| Klein et al. | 1998 | Adolescent | | 45 | DMI | | DBPC – 2-week PLWO – 6-week trial | n.s. |
| Birmaher et al. | 1998 | Adolescent | 16.2 | 27 | AMI | To max. of 300 mg/day or level ≤ 300 mg/ml | DBPC – 10-week trial | n.s. |

*Key:* * depressed children with family history of future bipolarity; IMI – imipramine; AMI – amitriptyline; NT – nortriptyline; FLX – fluoxetine; Li – lithium; DBPC – double-blind placebo controlled trial; PLWO – placebo washout; n.s. – not statistically significant.

(Adopted from Botteron & Geller, 1997.)

may hinder responsiveness, because the children may have bipolar depression (Himmelhoch & Garfinkel, 1986). Recognition of prepubertal and early adolescent BP is thus important for clinicians (Geller et al., in press).

There is also a question as to whether MDD actually is the same illness across the age span. The models that need to be considered here are whether MDD will be similar to juvenile and adult onset diabetes (i.e. similar phenotypes with differing genetic mechanisms) or whether it will be similar to collagen diseases which are more severe in children but are believed to have a similar pathogenesis. Familial genetic studies at this point in time are in agreement that there is greater familial aggregation for both mood disorders and substance use disorders when the child with a mood disorder is the proband (Puig-Antich et al., 1989b; Todd et al., 1993). By comparison to other illnesses with an etiologically genetic component, greater familial aggregation is often associated with earlier onset, greater severity, and more treatment resistance (Childs & Scriver, 1986).

## Serotonin reuptake inhibitor studies

There have been two published studies of specific serotonin reuptake inhibitors (see Table 14.1). The Emslie et al. (1997) federally funded study used double-blind placebo-controlled methodology following a lead-in period. Subjects could be 8–18 years old and needed DSM-III-R major depressive disorder. On the whole, this sample was less clinically severe than subjects studied in the imipramine and nortriptyline studies (Puig-Antich et al., 1987; Geller et al., 1990, 1992a,b). All subjects were randomized either to placebo or to a fixed 20 mg dose of fluoxetine. On both clinical global impression ratings and the Revised Children's Depression Rating Scale total scores, there were significant differences between active and placebo subjects which became apparent at week five. There was a wide standard deviation in outcomes showing that there was a wide variation in clinical recovery comprising the few who had complete recovery to many who had only partial or little improvement. A double-blind placebo-controlled study done earlier by Simeon et al. (1990) did not find a significant difference between active and placebo subjects, with two-thirds of both groups demonstrating marked to moderate improvement. However, this study did not include the rigorous methodology including a long lead-in period and was an acute trail of 8 weeks' duration.

The findings by Emslie et al. (1997) support the need for continued study of serotonin reuptake inhibitors as potentially important agents for children.

## Lithium study

Based on the high switch rate of subjects with prepubertal MDD to prepubertal

**Table 14.2.** Psychotherapy studies in child and adolescent depression

| Author | Year | Mean age | Subject population | Assessment | Number of subjects | Type of therapy | Control group | Duration | Conclusion |
|---|---|---|---|---|---|---|---|---|---|
| Reynolds & Coates | 1986 | 15.7 | Screened high school students | Self-rating non-DSM BDI, BID, RADS | 30 | Group CBT group relaxation training | Waiting list | 5 weeks (2 × week) 5 weeks FU | Both group treatments significant improvement vs. controls |
| Stark et al. | 1987 | 11.2 | Screened elementary school students | Self-rating non-DSM CDI | 29 | Group self-control therapy problem-solving therapy | Group behavioral | 5 weeks active | Improvement in both groups self ratings |
| Kahn et al. | 1990 | 7th graders | Middle school students with 'depression' | Self-rating | 68 | Three types waiting list group CBT | | 6–8 weeks (2 × week) 1 month FU | All three groups CBT CBT significant > control |
| Lewinson et al. | 1994 | 16.2 | Non-referred high school subjects | KSADS-E | 54 | Group CBT group relaxation training | Waiting list | 7 weeks 2 × weeks 2 year FU | Both group therapies significantly superior to waiting list |
| Mufson et al. | 1994 | 14.2 | Referred adolescents | KSADS-E HRSD; BDI | 14 | Individual IPT | None | 14 weeks | |
| Wood et al. | 1996 | 14.2 | Clinically referred KSADS | KSADS | 48 | CBT | Relaxation therapy | 6 sessions | CBT > relaxation |
| Brent et al. | 1997 | 15.7 | Clinically referred children KSADS | KSADS-EBP; BDI; CBCL | 78 | Individual CBT; systemic, family behavior therapy | Individual supportive therapy | 12–16 weeks | CBT > SBPT OBT > NST |

*Key:* BDI – Beck Depression Inventory; BID – Bellevue Index of Depression; RADS – Reynolds Adolescent; CDI – Children's Depression Inventory; HRSD – Hamilton Rating Scale for Depression; CBCL – Childhood Behavior Checklist

(Adopted from Botteron & Geller, 1997.)

bipolarity noted above (Geller et al., 1994), a double-blind placebo-controlled study was performed to test whether lithium would be effective for MDD in children who had MDD with family history predictors of future bipolarity (Geller et al., 1999b). This was a 6-week study in which the level of lithium was fixed by using a pharmacokinetic design. All subjects received a single 600 mg dose at baseline and subsequently had their dose adjusted using the Cooper et al. (1973) nomogram, which had been shown to work for children and adolescents to more rapidly achieve a therepeutic serum level (Geller et al., 1992a,b). Subjects had a mean age of 10.7 ± 1.2 years. Using intent to treat and completer analyses, there were no significant differences between active and placebo subjects on any of the continuous or categorical variables. Families were highly loaded including 40% of parents with bipolar disorder. Eighty percent of subjects had bipolar disorder in at least one first or second degree relative. The mean lithium level was 0.99 ± 0.16 meq/l. Of note, four subjects in the active group needed to be discontinued because of side effects, one for impairing nausea and vomiting and three for impairing cognitive difficulties which reversed when the lithium was discontinued. The negative outcome in addition to the poor side effect profile suggested that further study of lithium for prepubertal MDD with family history predictors of future bipolarity was not warranted at this time.

## Psychotherapy trials

There have been a small number of systematic studies reported examining the efficacy of psychotherapy interventions for child and adolescent depression. A number of these early trials, however, were completed in population samples identified through school surveys (see Table 14.2). Three groups (Reynolds & Coates, 1986; Stark et al., 1987; Kahn et al., 1990) identified late childhood and adolescent subjects through self-ratings on depression inventories and enrolled subjects with high scores in controlled therapy trials. Reynolds and Coates (1986) compared group cognitive behavioral therapy (CBT) to group relaxation training and a waiting list control group and demonstrated that both treatment groups had a significant reduction in self-reported depressive symptoms in comparison to the controls and the conclusion of treatment and at 5-week follow-up. Stark et al. (1987) examined group self-control therapy in comparison to group problem solving therapy and reported significant improvement in both groups at the conclusion of treatment. Kahn et al. (1990) in the largest school study, compared three types of group CBT in comparison to a waiting list control group and found all three groups to be superior to the waiting list at the conclusion of treatment and at 1-month follow-up. Although these initial reports are promising, it is unclear how these results will generalize to clinically referred populations.

Recently, several randomized controlled trials have been reported for clinically identified populations with depression and thus far the results have been encouraging (see Table 14.2). Mufson et al. (1994) compared a small group of clinically referred subjects who were randomized to either individual interpersonal therapy (IPT) or no psychotherapy and reported significant improvement in the IPT subjects. Wood et al. (1996) studied 48 adolescents who were randomized to either individual CBT or relaxation therapy and found a short course (six sessions) of CBT to be significantly superior to relaxation therapy in reduction of depressive symptoms. They subsequently examined clinical features which predicted response vs. non-response and reported (Jayson et al., 1998) that higher levels of social impairment as measured by the Social Adjustment Inventory for Children and Adolescents (SAICA) and older age (older adolescent vs. younger adolescent) predicted poorer response to a short course of CBT. In the largest study reported to date, Brent et al. (1997) enrolled 107 adolescents with DSM-III-R MDD in a randomized controlled trial comparing individual CBT, systematic behavior family therapy (SBFT) or individual non-directive supportive therapy (NST). Seventy-eight subjects completed the study. There was a clear and significantly superior result for CBT in comparison to the SBFT and NST; 64.7% of the CBT group demonstrated remission of MDD in comparison to 37.9% for the SBFT and 39.4% for the NST groups. The rate of symptomatic improvement and the parent's ratings of treatment credibility were also significantly higher for the CBT group. The Wood et al. (1996) and Brent et al. (1997) studies both demonstrated a differential treatment effect between psychotherapy types in contrast to non-specific positive findings in several earlier studies. These two studies were also the most scientifically rigorous. Both included standardized subject characterization of clinically referred individuals, and are probably most applicable to clinically referred adolescents.

Two recent meta-analyses of child and adolescent CBT studies have both supported the potential effectiveness of this intervention in mild to moderate depression. Reinicke et al. (1998) reported an effect size of $-1.02$ post-treatment and $-0.61$ follow up. Using a different meta-analytic approach, Harrington et al. (1998) reported a pooled odds ratio of 3.2 (95% confidence interval 1.9–5.2) for the rate of remission from depression in CBT groups vs. comparison groups. It should be noted that the majority of psychotherapy studies to date have been completed on adolescents with mild to moderate depression, and all of the early studies were completed on non-clinically referred children without complete standardized assessment. More recent trials have begun to address clinically relevant issues. These trials are encouraging, but there is a need for further double-blind randomized controlled trials. It is unclear how these results will apply to children or adolescents who are treatment resistant or refractory to pharmacotherapy trials. As is the case with many treatment resistant cases, we generally recommend a combination of pharmacotherapy along with individual CBT in children and adolescents who are not responding adequately to one modality or the other.

## Differential diagnosis before beginning medication

Although family studies of children with MDD (Puig-Antich et al., 1989b; Weller et al., 1994; Neuman et al., 1997) have shown highly loaded family histories for affective disorder which helps with the differential diagnosis in a child, phenotypic MDD can appear for reasons other than genetic familial transmission. Important in the differential are over the counter cold and allergy preparations; steroids, especially as the prevalence of asthma is increasing; and hypothyroidism. The latter, although rare, will occasionally be seen. Children who are in a situation that can produce severe grief such as an abusive or neglectful home, having an ill parent, or when a single parent has found a new significant other, may also present with serious sadness that requires differentiation from a major depressive disorder. Current data from the seminal work by Weller et al. (1991) suggests that the course of grief is similar in children to adults and that prolonged grief will generally occur in those children who have significantly greater familial loading for affective disorder. Thus, prolonged grief with a positive family history should be considered as a possible indication for beginning pharmacotherapy.

## Clinical management of treatment refractory child and adolescent depression

As noted early in this chapter, treatment resistance is a difficult concept to operationalize in young populations, and may apply to a substantial proportion of children and adolescents who are seen clinically. It is clearly established that pediatric major depression is a valid diagnostic entity which as clinical continuity with adult affective disorders. Children and adolescents with major depression present with substantial functional impairment in interpersonal, familial, academic and other domains and often progress to recurrent depressive episodes or the onset of mania. They are at substantial risk for the development of substance abuse and at high risk for suicide attempts and completion. Although it is generally very clear that they are in need of definitive clinical intervention, currently available research only provides a crude basis for treatment algorithms. Based on the previously cited research investigations and our clinical experience, some treatment recommendations are outlined below.

First to recapitulate a few points mentioned earlier: (i) There are clear neurodevelopmental differences from child and adolescent to adult populations and treatment responses and side effect profiles do not necessarily generalize from adult to pediatric populations. (ii) Family and genetic studies have established a high familial loading for affective disorders and substance abuse in the first and second degree relatives of children with major depression. Thus, many parents of children presenting may currently be experiencing an episode of illness. As it is clear that family psychopathology can affect treatment outcome, it is important to assess the primary caretakers and potentially recommend treatment for them if indicated. Treatment of the extended family may be critical to the clinical progress of the child or adolescent.

Family and patient psychoeducation and support are essential in the initial phases of treatment. Education about the nature of affective disorders and potential treatment options should be discussed. Even in early meetings it may be important to discuss the potential longitudinal course, including a discussion of symptoms of mania which may begin spontaneously, or be related to the use of pharmacotherapeutic agents. The choice of initial treatment, either psychotherapy or pharmocotherapy is not easily established and is dependent on multiple familial and clinical factors in individual cases.

## A comparison of SSRIs vs. TCAs for children

Comparison of the side effect profile for SSRIs vs. TCAs favors SSRIs. Potential for overdose is a significant concern in the treatment of mood disordered children and adolescents. SSRIs have a very low potential of lethality, while the lethality of TCAs is very high. This is especially important for adolescents who have been known to overdose on their TCA prescriptions even when it was prescribed one week at a time. SSRIs require no monitoring of EKG or blood levels, while these must be monitored with TCAs to avoid toxicity. Dosing regime with SSRIs can be once daily but because of the shorter half-life with TCAs, usually twice a day dosing is necessary. The latter is important when both parents work or the family has a single parent. Thus the less complicated the regime, the more likely there will be compliance. Finally, there has been the issue of unexplained sudden death occurring in children receiving TCAs (Geller, 1991b; Riddle et al., 1991). Although a statistical association has not been found for this fortunately rare event, it nevertheless needs to be considered in deciding which drug to use (Biederman, 1991). At the present time, perhaps the best clinical use of TCAs is for subjects who come to your office already on this medication and are doing well; who have reasonable plasma levels and EKGs that do not have prolongation of the QT interval; whose family has been informed of the sudden death literature and accepts this unlikely but possible outcome; and whose family members have done well on TCAs.

## Choosing a SSRI

One of the main differences between fluoxetine and its more recent counterparts, paroxetine and sertraline, are pharmacokinetic. Fluoxetine can take weeks or more to reach steady state while for paroxetine and sertraline this is a matter of days. Both types of SRIs have non-linear pharmacokinetics so that this is not a distinguishing feature. The potential problems with the long half-life of fluoxetine are that if the child overdoses it will take a long time for the medication to disappear; if an adverse drug–drug interaction occurs, again it will be a long time before the medication is eliminated; if it is ineffective, one has to then gauge when a more effective medication can be added; and finally, because again we do not know if the episode of MDD in a child or adolescent is the beginning of a unipolar or bipolar course, if a child should switch to mania on fluoxetine, it will be some days before the medication will clear. A potential advantage of the long half-life, across the age span, is that it can be given once daily and that if a subject is non-compliant there is less threat to stable recovery. SSRIs have potential drug–drug interactions with thioridazine, TCAs, and terfenadine (recently removed from the US market).

## How long to wait before changing medications

As demonstrated in the Emslie et al. study (1997), it was 5 weeks before significant differences between active and placebo groups were evident. Thus, it is important to inform families at the beginning that unlike the advertisements on TV that show medications working before the commercial is over, the SSRIs may take longer. A useful analogy with children is to the story of the rabbit and the turtle. Families can be informed that 'we're like the turtle; we're slow, but we win the race.'

Increasing the dose has to also take into account genetic variation in metabolism. Findling (1996) has shown for paroxetine that low CYP450 2D6 is associated with high rates of side effects. Similarly, if no side effects and no response is seen, it may be because CYP450 2D6 is high and the child is a rapid metabolizer. Given the above, usually with children a dose of 10 mg of paroxetine or fluoxetine can be begun or 25 mg of sertraline and one can then wait a few weeks before deciding on an increase. Families must be given careful instruction on how to recognize mania so that they can contact the physician immediately should this occur.

## Conclusions

In summary, treatment resistance is a significant problem in child and adolescent affective disorders, and unfortunately pharmacotherapeutic and psychotherapeutic intervention trials have been less prevalent than in the adult literature.

However, there have been a number of rigorous, systematic studies which are beginning to inform treatment decdisions for this potentially difficult population. Current evidence suggests that children and adolescents are likely to be refractory to tricyclic antidepressants, but may be more responsive to serotonergic reuptake inhibitors. The role for psychotherapy is supported in a small number of recent studies. However, clearly there is a huge need for further pharmacotherapeutic and psychotherapeutic research to more clearly define effective treatment strategies, in not only acute trials, but also to establish the potential long term effect on mediating future recurrences and progression to mania, substance abuse or other comorbid disorders. Progress for treatment strategies in child and adolescent populations will also depend on advancing or understanding of the neuropathophysiology and the neurodevelopmental consequences and correlates of early onset affective disorder. Such knowledge may play a critical role in developing treatments which are specifically tailored to pediatric populations and aimed at mediating neurodevelopmental consequences, rather than simply extrapolated from symptomatic, therapeutic treatment trials of mature adult populations.

## REFERENCES

Andreasen, N.C., Grove, W.M., Coryell, W.H., Endicott, J., & Clayton, P.J. (1988). Bipolar versus unipolar and primary versus secondary affective disorder: which diagnosis takes precedence? *Journal of Affective Disorders*, **15**(1), 69–80.

Baxter, L., Schwartz, J., & Bergman, K. (1992). Caudate glucose metabolic rate changes with both drug and behavior therapy for obsessive-compulsive disorder. *Archives of General Psychiatry*, **49**, 681–9.

Biederman, J. (1991). Sudden death in children treated with a tricyclic antidepressant. *Journal of the American Academy of Child and Adolescent Psychiatry*, **30**(3), 495–8.

Birmaher, B. (1998). Should we use antidepressant medications for children and adolescents with depressive disorders? *Psychopharmacology Bulletin*, **34**(1), 35–9.

Birmaher, B., Waterman, G.W., Ryan, N.D.. et al. (1998). Randomized, controlled trial of amitriptyline versus placebo for adolescents with 'treatment-resistant' major depression. *Journal of the American Academy of Child and Adolescent Psychiatry*, **37**(5), 527–35.

Botteron, K.N. & Geller, B. (1997). Treatment resistant depression in children and adolescents. *Depression and Anxiety*, **4**, 212–23.

Brent, D.A., Holder, D., Kolko, D. et al. (1997). A clinical psychotherapy trial for adolescent depression comparing cognitive, family, and supportive therapy. *Archives of General Psychiatry*, **54**, 877–85.

Childs, B. & Scriver, C.R. (1986). Age at onset and causes of disease. *Perspectives in Biology and Medicine*, **29**, 437–60.

Clayton, P.J. (1981). The epidemiology of bipolar affective disorder. *Comprehensive Psychiatry*, **22**(1), 31–43.

Cooper, T.B., Bergner, P.E., & Simpson, G.M. (1973). The 24-hour serum lithium level as a prognosticator of dosage requirements. *American Journal of Psychiatry*, **130**(5), 601–3.

Dahl, R.E., Ryan, N.D., Matty, M.K. et al. (1996). Sleep onset abnormalities in depressed adolescents. *Biological Psychiatry*, **39**(6), 400–10.

Emslie, G.J., Rush, A.J., Weinberg, W.A., Rintelmann, J.W., & Roffwarg, H.P. (1994). Sleep EEG features of adolescents with major depression. *Biological Psychiatry*, **36**(9), 573–81.

Emslie, G., Rush, A.J., Weinberg, A.W. et al. (1997). A double-blind, randomized placebo-controlled trial of fluoxetine in children and adolescents with depression. *Archives of General Psychiatry*, **54**, 1031–7.

Findling (1996). Putative determinants of paroxetine response in pediatric patients with major depression. *Psychopharmacology Bulletin*, **32**(446).

Geller, B. (1991a). Psychopharmacology of children and adolescents: pharmacokinetics and relationships of plasma/serum levels to response. *Psychopharmacology Bulletin*, **27**(4), 401–9.

Geller, B. (1991b). Commentary on unexplained death of children on Norpramin. *Journal of the American Academy of Child and Adolescent Psychiatry*, **30**(4), 682–4.

Geller, B., Cooper, T., Graham, D., Marstellar, F., & Bryand, D. (1990). Double-blind placebo-controlled study of nortriptyline in depressed adolescents using a 'fixed plasma level' design. *Psychopharmacology Bulletin*, **26**, 85–90.

Geller, B., Cooper, T., Graham, D., Fetner, H., Marsteller, F. & Wells, J. (1992a). Pharmacokinetically designed double-blind placebo-controlled study of nortriptyline in 6–12 year olds with major depressive disorder. *Journal of the American Academy of Child and Adolescent Psychiatry*, **31**, 34–44.

Geller, B., Fox, L.W., Cooper, T.B., & Garrity, K. (1992b). Baseline and 2–3-year follow-up characteristics of placebo-washout responders from the nortriptyline study of depressed 6–12-year-olds. *Journal of the American Academy of Child and Adolescent Psychiatry*, **31**(4), 622–8.

Geller, B., Fox, L.W., & Clark, K.A. (1994). Rate and predictors of prepubertal bipolarity during follow-up of 6–12-year-old depressed children. *Journal of the American Academy of Child and Adolescent Psychiatry*, **33**(4), 461–8.

Geller, B., Todd, R.D., Luby, J., & Botteron, K.N. (1996). Treatment-resistant depression in children and adolescents. *Psychiatric Clinics of North America*, **19**(2), 253–67.

Geller, B., Biederman, J., Leonard, H. et al. (1999a). Critical review of tricyclic antidepressant use in children and adolescents. *Journal of the American Academy of Child and Adolescent Psychiatry*, **38**, 513–16.

Geller, B., Cooper, T.B., Zimerman, B. et al. (1999b). Lithium for prepubertal depressed children with family history predictors of future bipolarity: a double-blind, placebo-controlled study. *Journal of Affective Disorders*, **51**, 165–75.

Geller, B., Williams, M., Zimerman, B., Frazier, J., Beringer, L., & Warner, K.L. (in press). Prepubertal and early adolescent bipolarity differentiate from ADHD by manic symptoms, grandiose delusions, ultra-rapid or ultradian cycling. *Journal of Affective Disorders*.

Harrington, R., Whittaker, J., Shoebridge, P., & Campbell, F. (1998). Systematic review of efficacy of cognitive behavior therapies in childhood and adolescent depressive disorder. *British Medical Journal*, **316**(7144), 1559–63.

Himmelhoch, J.M. & Garfinkel, M.E. (1986). Sources of lithium resistance in mixed mania. *Psychopharmacol Bulletin*, **22**(3), 613–20.

Isojarvi, J.I., Laatikainen, T.J., Pakarinen, A.J., Juntunen, K.T., & Myllyla, V.V. (1993). Polycystic ovaries and hyperandrogenism in women taking valproate for epilepsy. *New England Journal of Medicine*, **329**(19), 1383–8.

Jayson, D., Wood, A., Kroll, L., Fraser, J., & Harrington, R. (1998). Which depressed patients respond to cognitive-behavioral treatment? *Journal of the American Academy of Child Adolescent Psychiatry*, **37**(1), 35–9.

Kahn, J., Kehle, T., Jenson, W., & Clark, E. (1990). Comparison of cognitive-behavioral relaxation and self-modeling interventions for depression among middle-school students. *School Psychology Review*, **19**, 196–211.

Klein, D.F., Gittelman, R., Quitkin, F., & Rifkin, A. (1980). *Diagnosis and Drug Treatment of Psychiatric Disorders: Adults and Children*, pp. 268–408. Baltimore, MD: Williams & Wilkins.

Klein, R.G., Mannuzza, S., Koplewicz, H.S. et al. (1998). Adolescent depression: controlled desipramine treatment and atypical features. *Depression and Anxiety*, **7**(1), 15–31.

Kocsis, J.H., Mason, B.J., Frances, A.J., Sweeney, J., Mann, J.J., & Marin, D. (1989). Prediction of response of chronic depression to imipramine. *Journal of Affective Disorders*, **17**(3), 255–60.

Kutcher, S., Boulos, C., Ward, B. et al. (1994). Response to desipramine treatment in adolescent depression: a fixed dose, placebo-controlled trial. *Journal of the American Academy of Child and Adolescent Psychiatry*, **33**, 686–94.

Kye, C.H., Waterman, G.S., Ryan, N.D. et al. (1996). A randomized, controlled trial of amitriptyline in the acute treatment of adolescent major depression. *Journal of the American Academy of Child and Adolescent Psychiatry*, **35**(9), 1139–44.

Mufson, L., Moreau, D., Weissman, M.M, Wickramaratne, P., Martin, J., & Samoilov, A, (1994). Modification of interpersonal psychotherapy with depressed adolescents (IPT-A): phase I and II studies. *Journal of the American Academy of Child and Adolescent Psychiatry*, **33**(5), 695–705.

Neuman, R.J., Geller, B., Rice, J.P., & Todd, R.D. (1997). Increased prevalence and earlier onset of mood disorders among relative of prepubertal versus adult probands. *Journal of the American Academy of Child and Adolescent Psychiatry*, **36**(4), 466–73.

Puig-Antich, J. (1987). Sleep and neuroendocrine correlates of affective illness in childhood and adolescence. *Journal of Adolescent Health Care*, **8**, 505–29.

Puig-Antich, J., Orvaschel, H., Tabrizi, M., & Chambers, W. (1980). The Schedule for Affective Disorders and Schizophrenia for School-age Children – Epidemiologic version. *New York, NY: New York State Psychiatric Institute and Yale University School of Medicine:*

Puig-Antich, J., Perel, J.M., Lupatkin, W. et al. (1987). Imipramine in prepubertal major depressive disorders. *Archives of General Psychiatry*, **44**(1), 81–9.

Puig-Antich, J., Dahl, R., Ryan, N. et al. (1989a). Cortisol secretion in prepubertal children with major depressive disorder. *Archives of General Psychiatry*, **46**, 801–9.

Puig-Antich, J., Goetz, D., Davies, M. et al. (1989b). A controlled family history study of prepubertal major depressive disorder. *Archives of General Psychiatry*, **46**, 406–18.

Rao, U., Dahl, R.E., Ryan, N.D. et al. (1996). The relationship between longitudinal clinical course and sleep and cortisol changes in adolescent depression. *Biological Psychiatry*, **40**(6), 474–84.

Reinecke, M., Ryan, N., & Dubois, D. (1998). Cognitive-behavioral therapy of depression and depressive symptoms during adolescence: a review and meta-analysis. *Journal of the American Academy of Child and Adolescent Psychiatry*, **37**(1), 26–34.

Reynolds, W. & Coates, K. (1986). A comparison of cognitive-behavioral therapy and relaxation training for the treatment of depression in adolescents. *Journal of Consulting and Clinical Psychology*, **54**(5), 653–60.

Riddle, M., Geller, B., & Ryan, N. (1993). Another sudden death in a child treated with desipramine. *Journal of the American Academy of Child and Adolescent Psychiatry*, **32**(4), 792–7.

Ryan, N.D., Puig-Antich, J., Ambrosini, P. et al. (1987). The clinical picture of major depression in children and adolescents. *Archives of General Psychiatry*, **44**, 854–61.

Simeon, J.G., Dinicola, V.F., Ferguson, H.B., & Copping, W. (1990). Adolescent depression: a placebo-controlled fluoxetine treatment study and follow-up. *Progress in Neuro-Psychopharmacology and Biological Psychiatry*, **14**, 791–5.

Stark, K., Reynolds, W., & Kaslow, N. (1987). A comparison of the relative efficacy of self-control therapy and a behavioral problem-solving therapy for depression in children. *Journal of Abnormal Child Psychology*, **15**, 91–113.

Strober, M. (1982). Relevance of early age-of-onset in genetic studies of bipolar affective disorder. *Journal of the American Academy of Child and Adolescent Psychiatry*, **4**, 606–10.

Todd, R.D., Neuman, R., Geller, B., Fox, L.W., & Hickok, J. (1993). Genetic studies of affective disorders: should we be starting with childhood onset probands? *Journal of the American Academy of Child and Adolescent Psychiatry*, **32**(6), 1164–71.

Walsh, B., Giardina, E.G., & Sloan, R. (1994). Effects of desipramine on autonomic control of the heart. *Journal of the American Academy of Child and Adolescent Psychiatry*, **33**, 191–7.

Weller, R.A., Weller, E.B., Fristad, M.A., & Bowes, J.M. (1991). Depression in recently bereaved prepubertal children. *American Journal of Psychiatry*, **148**(11), 1536–40.

Weller, R., Kapadia, P., Weller, E., Fristad, M., Lazaroff, L., & Preskorn, S. (1994). Psychopathology in families of children with major depressive disorders. *Journal of Affective Disorders*, **31**, 247–52.

Wood, A., Harrington, R., & Moore, A. (1996). Controlled trial of a brief cognitive-behavioral intervention in adolescent patients with depressive disorders. *Journal of Child Psychology and Psychiatry*, **35**, 1156–61.

# 15

# Treatment-resistant depression in the elderly

Paul A. Newhouse and Jaskaran Singh

## Introduction

Surveys of healthy elderly individuals have revealed that 15% of community dwelling elderly report clinically significant degrees of depressed mood, 4% suffer from a major depressive disorder, and 6.5% have depression associated with a significant medical illness (Blazer & Williams, 1980). However, in special settings, the prevalence rates of depressive disorders may be much higher. Major depressive disorders have been reported in from 17% (Van Marwijk et al., 1990) to 31% of elderly medical patients in a clinic (Okimoto et al., 1982), and up to 45% in hospitalized elderly (Kitchell et al., 1982). Rapp and colleagues (Rapp et al., 1988) reported that 27% of elderly male patients in a general hospital had a diagnosable psychiatric disorder, most commonly depression. Depression may also contribute to higher overall mortality rates through poor self-care, inadequate compliance with medical treatment, and poorer physical functioning. It has been estimated that up to 20% of non-cognitively impaired individuals in nursing homes suffer from major depressive disorder (Blazer, 1989). The rate among cognitively impaired individuals may be even higher.

The consequences of untreated or inadequately treated depressive disorder in the elderly are serious. Suicide rates rise over the life cycle and increase dramatically in old age. In 1986, the suicide rate for the elderly was 21.6 per 100 000 compared to 12.8 per 100 000 for the general population (Allen & Blazer, 1991). For elderly white males, this rate increases to 40–75 per 100 000 (Katz et al., 1988). Suicide rates for elderly men are five times higher than those for elderly women. In addition, morbidity from these disorders is not limited to suicide. Increased rate of utilization of medical services, increased morbidity and mortality from medical illnesses, polypharmacy, and inappropriate institutionalization are all well-studied consequences of untreated depressive disorders in the elderly (Katz et al., 1988; Borson et al., 1986; Berkman et al., 1986). A study of medical outcomes (Wells et al., 1989) revealed that the physical disability of patients with major depressive illness was worse than that of other chronic diseases of the elderly including diabetes, arthritis, and hypertension.

Despite the evidence for significant morbidity and mortality resulting from depressive illness, this disorder is inadequately recognized and treated by clinicians. Recognition is hampered by misconceptions about depression and the aging process, an unjustified nihilistic attitude about the treatment of depression in the elderly (Brodaty et al., 1993), inadequate attention to psychological symptoms and an exclusive focus on somatic complaints. Symptomatic depression in the elderly is recognized as little as 10% of the time (Borson et al., 1986). In one study of a Virginia general medical clinic, less than 1% of clinically depressed medical outpatients were referred for treatment (Borson et al., 1986). Even when recognized, the depressed elderly are often treated suboptimally. Reasons for this include poorer tolerance of side effects, poorer compliance with treatment, and inadequate dosage (Dunner, 1994).

The effective treatment of depression in the elderly is complicated by a number of factors. Inadequate recognition of the biomedical nature of major depressive disorder in the elderly may lead to an improper choice of treatment or no treatment at all. When medications are chosen, biological changes in drug absorption, distribution, and metabolism complicate the choice of dose level and dosing interval. Comorbidity associated with other medical conditions associated with aging complicate the choice of antidepressant (Cavanaugh et al., 1983). For example, the treatment of patients with concomitant cardiovascular disease may be problematic, especially with tricyclic antidepressants (Glassman et al., 1990). Treatment often has to be modified to account for other medical illnesses and medication, and the reduced ability of the elderly person's body to metabolize the medication. Duration of treatment may have to be longer than with younger individuals as patients may respond more slowly to antidepressant medication than younger individuals. Concomitant anxiety is more common among elderly depressed patients than in younger depressed patients and may require simultaneous treatment (Abrams, 1991).

In an examination of the detection and treatment of depression in hospitalized elderly men, Koenig and coauthors (1988) found that over 85% of the patients had a relative or absolute medical contraindication to the use of older tricyclic antidepressants. Such contraindications may include cardiac rhythm disturbances (Glassman & Roose, 1994), prostatic hypertrophy with urinary difficulties, evidence of significant autonomic dysfunction, and mild cognitive dysfunction (Marcopulos & Graves, 1990). The existence of these contraindications have led many primary care practitioners to be reluctant to treat geriatric depression aggressively. Even with successful treatment, the adverse effects may make it difficult for patients to sustain their treatment and/or prophylaxis. Older individuals appear reluctant and unaccustomed to seeking help for these disorders for a variety of reasons, including the belief that nothing can be done to help them, the stigmatization of mental illness (i.e. that those who seek psychiatric help are 'crazy'), the difficulty in obtaining appropriate referrals from primary practitioners, the physical and logistical difficulties in accessing services, particularly in rural areas, the reluctance of the community mental health system to provide targeted services, and inadequate reimbursement for those services.

In spite of the enormous need, very few specialty services exist that are devoted to treating depression and other psychiatric disorders in geriatric patients. Few private mental health practitioners provide such services. In part, the paucity of such services reflects the increased complications associated with assessing, diagnosing, and treating depression in the elderly. Elderly patients often have complicating medical illnesses, take multiple medications with complex interactions, and have significant psychosocial problems. The diagnostic workup of an elderly patient suffering from depression who may have accompanying cardiac disease, arthritis, vision problems and mild neurological impairment can be a daunting task for the non-specialist. The potential medical complications of aggressive treatment of depression in elderly, medically frail patients lead to a reluctance of non-specialist physicians to treat depression. Finally, there is an attitude among some health-care providers that depressive disorders are a 'normal' part of aging, that there is nothing that can be done to treat them, and that the treatment of them is not important. These beliefs are incorrect, and impair adequate treatment of depressive disorders in the elderly. Finally, depression and depressive disorders degrade the quality as well as the quantity of life. Elderly patients who suffer from depression cannot proceed with the normal adjustments that must be made to getting older. Their capacity to enjoy their later years is impaired or extinguished, and capacity to perform work or self-care is severely impaired.

Treatments that are effective in younger individuals for depression are effective in elderly individuals, although treatment details are often different. However effective, medication treatment alone is not always sufficient to fully address depressive illness in elderly patients. The complicated psychosocial and psychological issues that are pertinent to the aging process must often be dealt with. Involvement of spouses and families is often crucial to the success of treating depression in the elderly, more so than with younger adults. Comprehensive treatment of biomedical, psychological, and social issues provides the most effective treatment approach for the depressed elderly (Allen & Blazer, 1991).

## Treatment resistance

In spite of effective treatment for many patients, some patients will be resistant to straightforward treatment or will be difficult to treat for other reasons. The concept of treatment resistance will be explored here as it may apply more specifically to elderly patients. General concepts are covered in Chapter 1. The true prevalence of treatment-resistant depression in elders has been estimated to range from 18 to 40%, although the latter figure especially is almost certainly too high (Bonner & Howard, 1995). The greater difficulties involved in treating elderly individuals and a certain degree of therapeutic nihilism in clinicians and patients may explain the higher figure (Collins et al., 1995). For example, in a study of antidepressant treatment by primary care physicians, physicians were informed by the research team of the depression scores of their patients after a careful clinical interview. Nonetheless, fewer patients were placed on antidepressants by their physicians than would have been predicted by the scores (Callahan et al., 1996). The investigators concluded that physician and perhaps patient negative attitudes regarding the efficacy and utility of treatment may have contributed to undertreatment. The phenomenon of non-response or unresponsiveness to antidepressant treatment may, especially in geriatric patients, disguise or be accounted for by a number of other problems and concerns which may either go unrecognized or unaddressed by physicians (Heston et al., 1992).

### Treatment resistant or misdiagnosis?

A major concern when treating all patients but especially elderly ones is whether the diagnosis is correct and/or complete. Other illnesses may produce depressive symptoms and signs or may be mistaken for symptoms of a major depressive disorder (Baker, 1995). However, treatment of those signs and symptoms with a conventional approach may often be unsuccessful.

One of the most common examples is alcohol abuse. Alcohol abuse is often unrecognized and untreated in older adults. Many individuals may escape clinical detection for long periods of time because the pattern of drinking often does not resemble the binge drinking seen in younger individuals; often these patients do not come to medical attention primarily for direct consequences of alcohol use until quite late. DSM criteria may be difficult to apply to the elderly who often do not show the common social consequences of alcohol abuse. Because many elderly patients are not working and may lead fairly isolated lives, the manifest signs of alcohol abuse may be more subtle than in younger patients. Many individuals, especially women may consume large amounts of alcohol over long periods of time without arousing suspicion of families or physicians because they may rarely appear obviously intoxicated. Further, these individuals may often have the onset of alcoholism at later age. Robins and colleagues (1988) reported that, for an older (60 + ) alcoholic cohort, the average age of onset was 31.0 years in men and 40.6 years in women. Alcohol abuse and dependence can arise *de novo* in old age, perhaps related to particular psychosocial factors peculiar to aging (Vaillant, 1983, Atkinson et al., 1985). Increasing age does not generally bring about a decrease in drinking problems (Robins et al., 1988). The prevalence of alcohol abuse in general medical populations is estimated to be upwards of 25% (Miller & Gold, 1989). Despite this, the diagnosis of alcohol abuse in the elderly is made much less often than epidemiologic studies suggest that it should (Koch & Knapp, 1987; Whitcup & Miller, 1987).

Little specific data exist regarding the incidence of depressive symptoms in geriatric alcohol abusers; however, other studies of alcoholics in general suggest prevalence rates as high as 59%, averaging at least 15% with higher rates for women (Schuckit et al., 1983). In a study of depressive symptoms in male alcoholics, age was found to have the strongest relationship to those symptoms (Hyer et al., 1987). These signs and symptoms may bring the patient to clinical attention independent of the alcohol abuse. If a reliable informant is not available, the extent of alcohol intake may not be appreciated by the clinician. A diagnosis of depressive disorder may be made and treatment prescribed. Because of the alcohol intake, antidepressant therapy may be ineffective. It is clinical lore that it is essentially impossible to treat depression successfully in the face of continued significant alcohol intake; the patient must be assisted to cease drinking alcohol before the clinician embarks on aggressive antidepressant therapy.

Therapeutic difficulty may also result from a wide variety of concomitant medical diagnoses that occur more or less commonly in the elderly. Endocrine dysfunctions are particularly prominent in this regard. Thyroid disease (usually hypothyoidism, but occasionally apathetic hyperthyroidism) may produce antidepressant resistance (Hickie et al., 1996). Many elderly depressed patients appear to present with compensated hypothyroidism (i.e. elevated TSH with normal or borderline $T_4$ and FTI). Such patients may progress to frank hypothyroidism. In the study by Hickie and colleagues (1996), 22% of the treatment-resistant patients were at least subclinically hypothyroid compared to only 2% of non-treatment-resistant patients. If such patients are unresponsive to antidepressant, the addition of thyroxine may convert them to responders. Other rarer abnormalities of the endocrine system, e.g. Cushing's disease, have a well-known association with depression and inhibitors of cortisol synthesis such as metyrapone have been shown to improve resistant depression (Iizuka et al., 1996). Non-insulin-dependent diabetes mellitus (type II) appears to be an important positive risk factor for depression in the elderly independent of gender, cognitive impairment, other chronic medical conditions, and living situation (Amato et al., 1996). Poorly controlled blood sugar may be a symptom of and contribute to poor response to antidepressant treatment. A study of the androgenic steroid dehydroepiandrosterone sulfate (DHEAS) levels in elderly individuals in a community-based study showed that not only did DHEAS levels decline with age in both genders, but that in women low levels were significantly associated with depressive symptoms, poor subjective perception of health, and functional impairment (Berr et al., 1996).

Neoplasms, particularly solid-tissue tumors, can produce both diagnostic confusion and therapeutic resistance if unrecognized. Perhaps the most well-known example is pancreatic carcinoma where it has been reported that the clinical presentation of depression often precedes the discovery of the tumor (Hornig-Rohan & Amsterdam, 1994). Following excision of the tumor, therapeutic response is sometimes restored (Pomara & Gershon, 1984). Infections, particularly indolent or chronic ones (e.g. AIDS, tuberculosis, Lyme disease) may make depression unresponsive or treatment-resistant (Kamholz & Mellow, 1996). Sleep apnea has been reported to produce treatment-resistant depression, with substantial improvement in mood symptoms following correction of the apnea (Hornig-Rohan & Amsterdam, 1994; Kamholz & Mellow, 1996).

Neurologic illnesses are, not surprisingly, one of the most common and significant comorbidities associated with difficult to treat depression in the elderly. Cerebral vascular accidents are no doubt the most frequent example of this association. There is an anatomic correlation between the degree of depressive signs and symptoms post-stroke and the location and size of the lesion(s). Some investigators have found that depression scores tend to be higher with left-sided lesions and those lesions nearer the frontal pole (Robinson et al., 1983), but others find no anatomic differences (Agrell & Dehlin, 1994). Upwards of 50% of post-stroke patients will develop depression within a year (Robinson et al., 1984). Unsuccessful initial rehabilitation following stroke, coupled with depression, may lead to a downward spiral of worsening depression, inadequate effort at rehabilitation leading to failure, increased dependency, excess functional disability, and intractable depression and physical deficits. Parkinson's disease patients have a high (30–70%) rate of depression (Cummings, 1992). A recent outpatient study in Norway showed that at least 45% had significant depressive symptoms and 24% showed Beck Depression Inventory scores over 18, suggesting significant depression compared to 11% of patients with diabetes and 4% of elderly controls (Tandberg et al., 1996). Many patients may not be optimally managed with anti-parkinsonian medications. Inadequate control of extrapyramidal symptoms may lead to depressive symptoms that do not resolve with standard treatment. Symptoms of freezing and bradykinesia seem particularly troubling to patients and may produce considerable distress. Adequate control of motor abnormalities in disorders such as Parkinson's disease or Huntington's disease may be critical to ensuring successful treatment of concomitant depression.

The relationship of depression to dementia deserves consideration as well when assessing treatment failure or difficulties. While patients with cortical dementias such as Alzheimer's disease may not initially show high rates of depression, the functional impairment of patients with a cortical dementia and depression-induced dementia may be similar (Yesavage, 1993). In a not uncommon scenario, the clinician may interpret patient or family complaints of cognitive impairment and memory loss as depression and treat the patient with antidepressants without a formal assessment of the patient's cognitive and functional status.

If the patient is suffering from a degenerative neuropsychiatric disorder, the antidepressants will be ineffective in resolving these complaints (Jones & Reifler, 1994). Definitive assessment and treatment is often delayed because of the usually fruitless antidepressant trial. The neuropsychologic profile of the cognitive impairment of depression and cortical dementia can generally be distinguished by formal testing (Albert, 1991). However, this usually requires more than simple screening instruments (e.g. the Mini Mental State Exam). In an elderly patient who presents with significant functional impairment, the diagnosis of a cortical dementia should be considered and the diagnostic evaluation broadened to assess this possibility more fully.

More acute mental status changes may also be mistaken for depression. In a study of hospitalized elderly patients, Farrell and Ganzini (1995) found that 42% of 67 patients referred for treatment of depression were found to be delirious. The delirious subjects often endorsed depressive symptoms including low mood (60%), worthlessness (68%) and thoughts of death (52%). Such subjects tended to be older and more impaired in activities of daily living. Intriguingly, the diagnosis of delirium had been considered in only three subjects out of the 67.

### Treatment resistance vs. slow responders?

A further complication is the possibility that elderly patients may be slower to respond to treatment than younger patients (Kamholz & Mellow, 1996). Thompson and Thompson (1991) have questioned whether non-responsive patients are 'treatment resistant or irresolutely treated'. Several authors have noted an increased response rate if treatment is extended past the usual 4–6 week trial. Georgatas and McCue (1989) noted increased benefit from increasing the length of a treatment trial past 7 weeks. Reynolds and colleagues (1994) noted in a study of the treatment of consecutive depressive episodes that the best results from antidepressants were seen after as much as 3 months of drug administration. In a study of time to stabilization after antidepressive treatment, Greenhouse and colleagues (1987) noted a 25% increase in response to therapy if the trial was extended from 10 to 17 weeks. Newhouse et al. (2000) studied the effects of blind administration of sertraline or fluoxetine over 12 weeks in depressed geriatric outpatients. While both drugs were similarly effective, what was notable was that the improvement in mean Hamilton Depression Rating Scale scores was linear, i.e. patients continued to improve over the entire period and a plateau of depression scores was not seen.

## Biologic changes with aging that may contribute to treatment resistance

Biologic changes that occur as a consequence of normal aging may contribute significantly to treatment difficulties and intolerance or ineffectiveness, especially if not fully appreciated. These changes are briefly reviewed below.

### Absorption

Age-related factors that may alter drug absorption include reduced gastric motility (Evans et al., 1981), increased gastric pH (Geokas & Haverback, 1969), reduced portal circulation (Bradley et al., 1945), and decreased intestinal motility. Oral administration of drugs is by far the most common portal of entry and unfortunately is also the most unpredictable in terms of final bioavailability. Little information is available regarding the effect of age on the absorption of antidepressant medications, although there are several theoretical considerations outlined above which may effect drug absorption. A drug with anticholinergic properties, e.g. tricyclic antidepressants (TCAs), may further decrease intestinal motility, leading to decreased absorption. There are no studies that show that the maximum concentration of a drug after oral dosing is affected by age (Montamet et al., 1989). However, concomitant medical conditions such as congestive cardiac failure, inflammatory bowel diseases and diabetic gastroparesis may retard drug absorption (Abernathy, 1992). Failure of a drug to be absorbed may result in decreased bioavailability at the final receptor site.

### Drug distribution

The apparent volume of distribution ($V_d$) reflects a balance between binding to tissues and binding to plasma proteins. Changes in either tissue or plasma binding can change the apparent volume of distribution determined from plasma concentration measurement. Factors affecting drug distribution with aging are decreased plasma proteins, decreased lean-body mass, increase in fatty tissue and decreased plasma volume. As a result, lipophilic drugs such as tricyclic antidepressants would have a larger volume of distribution and be preferentially diverted to fatty tissues. The effects of this have not been systematically studied to determine if this decreases the drug bioavailabilty, but in a case of a toxic level, it would make hemodialysis relatively ineffective. Since the elimination half-life is directly proportional to the $V_d$, given equal clearance, this shift would tend to lead to a longer half-life (Jenike, 1989). Drugs that are highly bound to proteins such as sertraline and phenytoin may result in greater free drug concentrations with aging and thus raise the potential for increased toxicity at a similar total plasma concentration. For example, alpha 1 acid glycoprotein is an important binding site for drugs such as TCAs. With aging, alpha 1 acid glycoprotein decreases, and is increased in inflammatory conditions, which may cause changes in plasma levels of unbound drug.

## Metabolism

The ability of the liver to metabolize drugs decreases with age (Greenblatt et al., 1982). Most psychotropic agents, with the exception of lithium, are lipophilic, and they must be converted to a water soluble compound before elimination by the kidney. With age, there is a decrease in hepatic mass, decreased hepatic blood flow, as well as evidence for decrease in metabolic capacity (phase I reactions: hydroxylation and demethylation). This may result in a delay in clearance of medications that undergo extensive first pass metabolism and a marked increase in the maximum concentration of the drug (Abernathy, 1992). The effect of these hepatic changes may prolong elimination half-life of drugs by as much as two to three times (Young & Myers, 1991). Studies have shown that 5–10% of Caucasians are 'poor hydroxylators,' and thus run an additive risk of developing potentially toxic levels of drugs metabolized by this enzymatic system (Tacke et al., 1992) .

## Renal drug excretion

Blood flow and glomerular filtration decrease by 6–10% per decade of life after the age of 40 (Davis & Shock, 1950). By the age of 70 total renal function may have decreased by 40–50%, even in the absence of renal disease (Turner et al., 1992). This results in prolongation of half-life as well as a potential for toxicity of active drugs that are excreted by the kidney, e.g. lithium, as well as active metabolites of drugs. For example, desipramine is metabolized to 2-hydroxydesipramine, which has both therapeutic efficacy and cardiovascular toxicity. The level of metabolites is usually not measured during clinical assays and therefore, plasma drug levels may mislead the clinician into believing that a larger safety margin exists than actually does (Salzman, 1985). Serum creatinine levels may overestimate GFR in elderly patients, because decreased muscle mass causes decreased creatinine production (Molholm et al., 1970).

## Cognitive and social factors with aging that may contribute to treatment resistance

Not all of the factors that produce complications in treating depression in the elderly have biologic or physical changes as their source. This was most clearly shown by Beekman and colleagues (1995) in a study of the association of depressive symptoms and physical health in older adults. Their study showed that there was only a relatively weak association between depression symptoms and reports of physical problems or infirmities. Marital status appeared to be an independent risk factor for the development of depressive symptoms. When marital status was controlled, there was no significant association between self-report measures of physical health and depression in women. In the oldest men, however, the association between perceived physical health and non-somatic symptoms of depression was significant.

The relationship of cognitive functioning to depression is complex. There are significant cognitive changes that are associated with normal aging including slower central processing, slower decision making, less efficient transfer of information to long-term storage, and decreased psychomotor speed. However, these changes do not normally produce any significant functional impairment. Nonetheless, depression may be accompanied by significant cognitive impairment and functional decline, especially in the elderly (Lichtenberg et al., 1995). This cognitive impairment in and of itself may make treatment problematic. Impaired concentration and poor attention with subsequent loss of short-term memory will increase compliance problems, impair nutrition, and increase the likelihood of adverse drug reactions and drug interactions. Although data is limited, it is likely that treatment of cognitively impaired depressed elderly outpatients is not as successful as with non-cognitively impaired individuals, in part because of the greater difficulties associated with treating such patients, rather than inherent treatment resistance. This suggests that cognitive assessment should be part of any evaluation for depression in the elderly. If significant cognitive deficits are identified or suspected, the clinician may have to adjust for this in treatment planning. Supervision of medication administration and nutrition may be necessary. In more severe cases, supervision of basic instrumental activities of daily living (ADLs) may also be required. The use of visiting nurse or similar services may be a very useful adjunct and may be required for treatment to be successful, especially if no family is present.

Functional impairment may also be exacerbated by social factors that make effective treatment difficult. Social isolation may be a significant factor leading to a decline in self-care, may greatly complicate effective treatment, and may be an independent risk factor for poor outcomes (Sarkisian & Lachs, 1996), including institutionalization (Steinbach, 1992) and death (Hanson et al., 1989). Those without social and community ties are more likely to die within a fixed period than those with such contacts (Berkman & Syme, 1979). Malnutrition may occur in part because of social isolation combined with depression and may be a significant overlooked factor in decreasing the effectiveness of treatment. It is estimated that 55% of geriatric inpatients are protein-calorie undernourished, even though most of the time, this condition is neither diagnosed nor treated (Mowe & Bohmer, 1991). Undernutrition is an independent risk factor for death in the elderly (Sullivan et al., 1991). Assessment of this potential problem may be aided by examining levels of albumin and cholesterol, which, if low, may be associated with inadequate nutrition (Rudman & Feller, 1989). An intriguing finding is that low cholesterol appears to be associated with depressive illness, particularly in males (Morgan et al., 1993). In this study, low cholesterol appeared to precede the onset of depression and was a risk factor independent of age, health status, number of chronic illnesses, and exercise. These data suggest a mechanism whereby poor nutrition may contribute significantly to non-remission. There may be an association between low cholesterol and decreased serotonin function through several mechanisms, including increased platelet serotonin uptake velocity (Guicheney et al., 1988), and potentially increased serotonin uptake in the brain (Meltzer, 1989). These may lead to an increased susceptibility to depression in the aged, who show reductions in some amine neurotransmitters (Morgan et al., 1993).

Certain social circumstances that are more common in the elderly may also complicate the assessment and treatment of depression. Dealing with loss of other people close to them is a pervasive developmental task that older adults face. One-half of all women over 65 are widows; among those over 75, the percentage is two-thirds (Warheit et al., 1991). The higher suicide rate of elderly males has been in part ascribed to a greater difficulty in connecting to social networks (Allen & Blazer, 1991). Additionally, the loss of other family, but more particularly friends and social contacts may be critical losses. Nelson (1989) has investigated the role of social supports and depression among the institutionalized elderly. The perception of social support was significantly correlated with the degree of depression in these residents, suggesting that even within a structured institution, the degree of social support may vary. Nelson further found that the frequency of religious participation may also interact with the degree of depression present. Lee and colleagues (1996) found in a sample of Korean immigrant elders that social support was more important than instrumental support in preventing depressive symptoms. This finding is also supported by the cross-national study of Lamb (1996) who found a correlation between lack of social support and depression. Studies such as these support the importance of considering the social ecology of a patient's life when assessing the reasons for treatment refractoriness or failure.

Bereavement is an additional social risk factor that may complicate treatment. While grief resulting from loss of a loved one is a normal life experience, prolonged grief may result in a necessity for treatment. However, Prigerson and colleagues (1995) have identified a complex of symptoms that may constitute a separate entity from depression that they call 'complicated grief.' Their analysis revealed seven symptoms that constitute this syndrome: searching, yearning, preoccupation with thoughts of the deceased, crying, disbelief regarding the death, feeling stunned by the death, and lack of acceptance. Scores on these items were significantly associated with impairments in global functioning, mood, sleep, and self-esteem. These investigators suggest that this entity may require specialized treatment. If further research bears out the validity of this syndrome, it suggests that standard treatment for depression may be inappropriate or ineffective. Tailoring treatment to focus on issues of grief and loss may be vital in assisting elderly patients in surmounting this developmental crisis.

## Managing treatment refractoriness/resistance

### Diagnostic reassessment

The management of resistant depression in elderly patients remains a clinical challenge. Age-related social, biologic, and medical complications create challenges that differ from the treatment of younger individuals. As the sections above have made clear, proper assessment of such patients is crucial prior to concluding that the patient is treatment-resistant. When faced with a patient who is not responding to treatment, the first step should be a complete reassessment to ensure that the correct diagnosis has been made. A review of the patient's history, including an assessment of the patient's level of functioning, social contacts, life stressors, family relationships, and living environment should be completed. In addition to the history, a full mental status exam with cognitive testing should be done. Such testing should, at a minimum, utilize a broad screening battery such as the Mini Mental State Exam (Folstein et al., 1975), but may also include further testing to more carefully define the cognitive status of the patient, as some patients with high premorbid intelligence and/or significant education may score normally on screening batteries yet be substantially cognitively impaired. Consultation with a neuropsychologist is usually required to obtain a more detailed cognitive assessment.

A physical exam is often indicated, including a detailed neurological exam. The primary goal of such an exam is to evaluate whether the patient may have an unsuspected physical illness that is contributing to or causing treatment resistance. Many elderly patients will not have had a comprehensive medical evaluation in the recent past, therefore such an evaluation will not often be duplicative. The neurologic exam should focus on ruling out complicating neuropsychiatric disorders such as Parkinson's disease, examining the nervous system for evidence of systemic disease (e.g. peripheral neuropathy secondary to diabetes), and looking for localizing signs that might point to intracerebral pathology. A broad-based laboratory assessment should be completed including a complete blood count, plasma chemistries, electrolytes, and enzymes, thyroid studies (TSH, Free $T_4$), and urinalysis. Additional specialized tests should be performed as indicated, e.g. syphilis serology, blood alcohol. Brain imaging studies are probably not indicated routinely, as the yield from such studies is generally low in unselected cases, but may be helpful where intracerebral pathology is suspected, especially cerebrovascular disease. If general cerebral morphology is to be assessed, then a computerized tomography (CT) scan is usually sufficient. However, if the presence of old infarcts is suspected, or if it is desired to examine subcortical structures in detail, then a magnetic resonance imaging (MRI) study will be more useful.

## Optimizing management of other medical problems

Once other acute or chronic medical problems are identified, it is necessary to ensure that these problems are either resolved or managed. The psychiatrist must work closely with the patient's primary health-care provider to ensure that such management occurs. Systemic diseases that are particularly important in this regard include diabetes, rheumatoid disorders, thyroid disturbances, congestive heart failure, chronic obstructive pulmonary disease, renal insufficiency, and bowel disorders. Diagnosis and treatment of these disorders is particularly important to help distinguish their symptoms from those of depressive illness. However, there can be a complex interaction between depressive symptoms and physical illness. Penninx and colleagues (1996) examined the psychological effects of chronic diseases on elders and found that psychological stress was most common with osteoarthritis, rheumatoid arthritis, and stroke, whereas it was less common with diabetes and cardiac disorders. In addition, Wassertheil-Smoller and coworkers (1995) found that the presence of depressive symptoms in elders was associated with a significantly increased risk of stroke, myocardial infarction, and death. Carney and colleagues (1995) showed that depressed elders were less likely to adhere to prophylactic cardiac medication than patients who were not depressed. In a study of the impact of depressive symptoms on physical disability, Bruce and colleagues (1994) found evidence that depressive symptoms and physical disability can initiate a spiraling decline in physical and psychological health in elderly individuals. These studies suggest that collaborative management with the patient's primary health-care provider is necessary to reduce long-term risk.

A common complication in elderly patients is the management of chronic pain. Although a full review of this topic is beyond the scope of this chapter, the effects of chronic pain may intertwine with depression, and the treatment of depression may become confounded by the pain disorder. Parmelee and colleagues (1991) examined the relationship between pain and depression in depressed and non-depressed elderly subjects. They found that depression scores explained much of the variance in pain reports, even controlling for functional disability and health status. Their work suggests that, even when a physical source is found, depression complicates the treatment of pain.

## Drug therapy

Medication remains the mainstay of treatment for treatment-resistant depression in the elderly. An overview of strategy will be given here, as well as details regarding specific combinations and less orthodox treatments. For a comprehensive review of the treatment of geriatric patients with the different antidepressant drug classes, the reader is referred to reviews by McCue (1992), Bressler and Katz (1993), Flint (1994), Kamholz and Mellow (1996), and Newhouse (1996).

Choice of the appropriate medication remains problematic. Once an accurate diagnosis is made and the symptom complex identified, the choice of medication by the physician is not always based on entirely quantifiable or logical criteria. Use of the response to a single dose of a stimulant medication has been re-examined for its predictive value in elderly patients (Spar & LaRue, 1985). The response of elderly patients to 20 mg of methylphenidate was predictive of the therapeutic response to desipramine, but not amitriptyline, suggesting that there may be some utility to using this maneuver, particularly in inpatient settings. In general, however, medication choice usually involves the balancing of side effect profiles with the desire for specific symptom relief. Without evidence for differential efficacy, other properties of the medications available must be examined. Therefore, for the patient that is not sleeping, a more sedating antidepressant is usually chosen; for a patient that is very lethargic and apathetic, a more energizing medication may be used. Once a choice of medication has been made, it is a long-established principle of initiating therapy in older patients to begin at lower doses and increase the dose more slowly than in younger patients. A common reason for treatment failure in the elderly appears to be too high a starting dose and/or too rapid a titration. Starting the patient at doses that might be routine for younger patients is more likely to provoke reports of difficulty tolerating side effects. This appears to be a common reason in primary care settings for treatment failure and referral to specialty clinics. What therefore may be interpreted as treatment failure may be treatment intolerance. It seems prudent to start elderly patients at one-half to one-quarter of the usual clinically effective doses, particularly if the patient is very old ( > 75), has significant medical comorbidity, or has a history of being intolerant to medication. A gradual run-in to an effective dose can be done over several weeks, especially with outpatients. This strategy will increase compliance and the likelihood of tolerability. This strategy seems as important with newer agents as with the older medications. For example, with SSRIs, the anxiety that can be produced early in the course of treatment may be a direct result of increased serotonin availability. Lawlor et al. (1991) showed that administration of the direct serotonin agonist MCPP produced considerable anxiety, agitation, and disrupted sleep in normals. This anxiety/agitation appears to be a frequent reason given by elderly depressed patients for discontinuing medication.

This complaint, as well as gastrointestinal complaints are minimized by starting at lower than routine clinical doses. Starting doses of SSRIs should be no more than one-half the routine clinical dose, e.g., fluoxetine and paroxetine at 10 mg/day, sertraline at 25 mg/day, and fluvoxamine at 25–50 mg/day. The patient should be maintained on this dose for at least 4–7 days before consideration is given to raising the dose.

The issue of target dose seems less in doubt. There is little evidence that elderly patients need lower doses of antidepressant medications, or perhaps more accurately, they appear to need equivalent doses, i.e. those doses that produce similar plasma and/or brain levels of drug to those of younger patients (Georgotas et al., 1986; Nelson et al., 1985). This may require lower doses. The inability to tolerate clinically effective doses of some antidepressants is a major limitation of their use in the elderly, particularly the oldest-old. Monitoring of plasma levels of older agents, e.g. nortriptyline and desipramine, is a valuable adjunct to their use in the elderly as the values may help clarify whether a clinically effective dose can be reached and tolerated by the patient. Knowledge of levels of newer agents such as the SSRIs has less clear value. By contrast, elderly patients do not appear to need higher doses of antidepressants than younger individuals due to any inherent or hypothesized impaired plasticity. Newhouse et al. (2000) showed in a study of the effects of fluoxetine and sertraline in depressed geriatric outpatients that there was no difference in the proportion of patients on either drug who improved on a higher or lower dose in this flexible dose study. Equal numbers of patients improved on 50 mg of sertraline or 20 mg of fluoxetine as on doses twice as large. In general, it appears that beyond minimally effective doses, the dose–response curve is not linear, but the dose–side effect curve is. Treatment failure may be secondary to too high a dose in addition to an inadequate dose.

No particular agent appears to have unique efficacy in treatment-resistant patients and the choice of initial mediation is made on the basis of the symptoms of the patients combined with side effect profile of the agents under consideration. It has been suggested that newer agents such as venlafaxine may be more effective in treatment-resistant patients (Nierenberg et al., 1994), although its long-term efficacy is unclear. This agent is associated with significant problematic side effects in some elderly patients, although most appear to tolerate the side effects if carefully managed (Kahn et al., 1995).

## Concomitant neuropsychiatric symptoms and comorbidity

The proper treatment of associated symptoms is critical to success in treating resistant geriatric depression. Perhaps the most common is anxiety. Anxiety symptoms have a very high comorbidity with depression in elderly patients; rates of concomitant anxiety disorder diagnoses as high as 38% have been documented

(Alexopolous, 1989). As noted above, certain antidepressants may actually increase anxiety symptoms early in treatment, especially if the dose is accelerated rapidly. The co-occurrence or worsening of such symptoms may lead to non-compliance or discontinuation, particularly newer, less sedating agents. Concomitant anxiolytic medication may be valuable in leading to rapid relief of anxiety and continued acceptance and tolerance of antidepressant treatment. Treatment with short-acting benzodiazepines (e.g. lorazepam) at low doses is often useful until antidepressant effects become manifest and anxiety symptoms begin to resolve as part of the depression lifting. However, elderly depressed patients may be inappropriately over- or mistreated with these agents. Zisselman and colleagues (1996) found that 40% of hospitalized elderly depressed patients had received solely benzodiazepines as treatment for depression while an outpatient. Some patients may require more chronic anxiolytic therapy however, and short-acting agents may not be optimal for those patients. Unless there is evidence for significantly impaired hepatic function, long-acting benzodiazepines can be used in low doses. Clonazepam may be particularly useful in this regard because of its long half-life, which reduces patients' clock watching, and its metabolism by nitro-reduction (in addition to oxidative hydroxylation), which does not appear to be as significantly interfered with by antidepressants which are cytochrome oxidase inhibitors as other agents in this class. However, this drug, like many drugs in its class, can produce significant sedation and ataxia which, if not monitored closely, can cause additional morbidity.

Concomitant psychotic symptoms can be particularly problematic in the elderly. The presence of psychosis, if not recognized and adequately treated, is a common reason for treatment failure. Studies of late life delusional depression (Meyers, 1995) suggest that this disorder shows poorer medical and psychiatric outcome and an increased risk for medication-related side effects. Effective therapy usually requires either combined antidepressant-neuroleptic therapy or electroconvulsive therapy (ECT). Elderly patients are more vulnerable to difficulties with this combination, yet the availability of newer neuroleptic agents such as risperidone and olanzapine have increased treatment options. Low dose neuroleptic therapy added to antidepressants may bring about clinical improvement in patients who have failed conventional monotherapy and a low threshold should be considered in elderly patients whose depression appears to have nihilistic, severely self-deprecatory, or delusional elements. The coexistence of a dementing disorder along with depression may also suggest the use of neuroleptics.

Cognitively impaired elderly patients with depression represent a special challenge to clinicians. Such patients may be particularly vulnerable to the side effects of antidepressants even at nominal clinical doses, making effective treatment problematic (Knegtering et al., 1994). It is unclear whether doses or plasma levels found to be necessary in non-impaired patients are useful as guides to therapy in patients with significant cerebral damage. The advent of relatively easy to use specific antidementia drugs, such as the anticholinesterase donepezil, offers new therapeutic opportunities. Preliminary studies suggest that agents which improve cholinergic function may improve behavioral problems in Alzheimer's disease patients, including depressive symptoms and/or apathy and agitation (Cummings & Kaufer, 1996). Symptoms in such patients which may have the appearance of an agitated depression may respond positively to such agents. Unless a patient with Alzheimer's disease clearly shows a full symptom picture consistent with a major depression, it may be advisable to administer a trial of an agent such as donepezil first to see if behavioral problems improve. Depressed patients with Alzheimer's disease have been successfully treated with tricyclic antidepressants (Reifler et al., 1989; Petracca et al., 1996) but the advent of newer agents allows better therapeutic options with drugs that have little or no antimuscarinic cholinergic receptor activity, such as the SSRIs (Volicer et al., 1994; Corey-Bloom & Galasko, 1995; Alexopolous, 1996). Combined treatment with procholinergic agents and antidepressants, particularly agents without antimuscarinic activity should be attempted in patients who have persisting depressive symptoms or in whom the diagnosis of depression is unclear.

Depression following stroke is a common and often difficult-to-treat disorder (Gustafson et al., 1995) with ominous implications for long-term rehabilitation (Angeleri et al., 1993). Although tricyclic antidepressants have been shown to be helpful (Lauritzen et al., 1994), side effects often limit their effectiveness or applicability. Newer agents may be more useful, better tolerated and have a higher response rate (Andersen et al., 1994; Dam et al., 1996; Stamenkovic et al., 1996), including stimulants (Lazarus et al., 1994). However, Robinson and colleagues (2000) have recently shown that nortriptyline was more effective than fluoxetine in the short-term treatment of poststroke depression. Poststroke patients may also demonstrate pathological laughing and crying (emotional incontinence) which may be confused with depression. Antidepressants such as SSRIs seem particularly helpful in alleviating this condition (Andersen et al., 1993; Mukand et al., 1996).

### Augmentation/combinations

Lithium augmentation is a common therapeutic maneuver in younger treatment-resistant patients. Results in elderly patients have been mixed, with improvement noted but also increased toxicity. Flint and Rifat (1994) examined the efficacy of lithium augmentation in an open, prospective study of elderly treatment failures. Less than half responded after 2 weeks, and many developed dose-limiting side effects. Other studies which are more positive in terms of response rates (Van Marwijk et al., 1990) still showed evidence of significant toxicity, especially in the older-old patient. Lafferman and associates (1998) found over a 50% response to lithium augmentation in previously treatment-resistant elderly patients. Zimmer and colleagues (1991) reported that 10 out of 15 severely depressed elderly inpatients responded to lithium augmentation of nortriptyline, but they concluded that the effect of lithium may not have been specific. However, follow-up studies suggesting that discontinuation of lithium following improvement may lead to increased risk of relapse (Reynolds et al., 1996) and refractoriness to further lithium treatment (Hardy et al., 1997) which have been used to argue for a specific beneficial effect of lithium augmentation of unipolar depression in the elderly. Lithium augmentation has been successfully used in combination with several SSRIs in the elderly (paroxetine, sertraline, and fluvoxamine), although toxicity has been seen as well (Kamholz & Mellow, 1996). Whether lithium toxicity is enhanced by the presence of the SSRI is unclear. When lithium is used as an augmentative agent, doses should be kept low, especially for initiation. In frail or small patients, 150 mg is an appropriate starting dose, and generally doses greater than 450 mg are rarely helpful or necessary (Kushnir, 1986). A trial of up to 4 weeks is recommended by most authors and, if a response occurs, continuation of the treatment is required.

### Combinations of antidepressants

This is an increasingly common maneuver in treatment-resistant patients, particularly SSRI–tricyclic combinations (Zajecka et al., 1995) and has been used successfully in elderly patients. Seth and colleagues (1992) reported on eight patients who had failed monotherapy with a variety of agents or ECT, successfully treated with combined SSRI and nortriptyline, seven of whom were elderly. The combination was well tolerated and successful. Weilburg and associates (1989) reported that fluoxetine added to non-MAOI antidepressant regimens in 30 poorly responsive outpatients converted 26 to full responders. It is possible that, in some cases, the effect of adding the SSRI is simply to raise the blood level of the tricyclic antidepressant into the therapeutic range, but this is unlikely to be the sole therapeutic action of this combination. It is important to add small doses of the tricyclic if the SSRI has been started first and to monitor blood levels, as enzyme inhibition by the SSRI will produce higher blood levels for a given dose than would be expected otherwise. Dosage of the tricyclic may have to be lowered if the SSRI is added second. Combining SSRIs with MAO inhibitors is contraindicated because of the significant potential for serious adverse events presumably due to an exaggerated serotonin effects (the so-called serotonin syndrome).

Monoamine oxidase inhibitors (MAOIs) have been reported to be helpful for treatment-resistant elderly depressed patients (Georgotas et al., 1983). Reversible MAOIs such as moclobemide have been reported to be helpful in the elderly (Nair et al., 1995), but no studies exist with treatment-resistant patients. Combined MAOI–tricyclic therapy has been safely used over an extended period in some treatment-resistant patients (Berlanga & Ortega-Soto, 1995), although no studies exist in the elderly.

## Other combination treatments

Either anticonvulsants alone or combinations of antidepressants and anticonvulsants have been reported to be helpful in the treatment of treatment-resistant patients (Cullen et al., 1991; Ketter et al., 1995), although the rate of complications was higher in older patients, with 71% of responders in the Cullen study who used carbamazepine discontinuing therapy. Sodium valproate may be better tolerated in combination (Corrigan, 1992), although even this agent can produce substantial sedation.

Schneider and colleagues have recently noted (1997) that elderly women who were receiving estrogen replacement therapy while participating in trial of fluoxetine vs. placebo for depression had significantly greater clinical improvement than those women who were not receiving estrogen, suggesting an interaction between hormone status and antidepressant treatment. However, a prospective study of the effect of estrogen over 2 weeks on the response to imipramine in mostly postmenopausal severely depressed patients found no effect (Shapira et al., 1985). Therapeutic effects of an estrogen–antidepressant combination may take longer to appear or may be only helpful in milder depression.

Bell and associates (1992) reported that vitamins B1, B2, and B6 were helpful in augmenting the effects of tricyclic antidepressants in depressed geriatric inpatients with improvements both in depression and cognitive function scores.

## Non-traditional agents

Clomipramine is not widely used as an antidepressant in the United States. Nonetheless, it has significant antidepressive effects and has been studied in the elderly. Kunik and colleagues (1994) studied five treatment-resistant depressed elderly females and found that clomipramine was well tolerated and decreased depression scores and the frequency of somatic complaints. They suggest that plasma monitoring is necessary as steady state was reached at lower doses than in younger individuals. Intravenous clomipramine has been proposed as an effective treatment for treatment-resistant depression under controlled conditions (Kielholz et al., 1982).

Stimulants have had a checkered history in the psychiatric pharmacopoeia. However, stimulants may be underutilized, particularly in the elderly (Warneke, 1990). Stimulants have antidepressive and/or energizing effects on their own, especially in medically ill debilitated patients (Wallace et al., 1995). Lazarus and colleagues (1994) found that methylphenidate was superior to nortriptyline in the rapid amelioration of depressive symptoms in poststroke patients with an average speed of response of 2.4 days compared to 27 days for nortriptyline. Stimulants may be particularly helpful in patients for whom the diagnosis of major depression may be obscure because of a debilitating illness such as cancer. Such patients may have many of the somatic symptoms of depression along with fatigue or malaise; however, their mood may not be congruent with the somatic picture. Stimulants may be very effective in mobilizing such patients although long-term efficacy is unclear. Stimulants have been used to hasten the onset of the effects of tricyclic antidepressants (Gwirtsman et al., 1994), augment the effects of SSRIs, and to potentiate MAOIs safely in younger treatment resistant patients (Fawcett et al., 1991). Combinations of stimulants with other antidepressant agents in the elderly do not seem to have been systematically studied, but appear to be in fairly common use by clinicians (Feighner et al., 1985).

## Electroconvulsive therapy (ECT)

ECT remains the primary choice for non-drug responsive depression, especially in older patients, with response rates up to 92% in some case series (Kramer, 1987). However, treatment-resistant status appears to result in a lower response rate to ECT of around 50% (Prudic et al., 1990). ECT may be appropriate as a first-line treatment in patients who are highly suicidal, malnourished, or for whom medical complications preclude effective drug therapy (Kamholz & Mellow, 1996; Greenberg & Fink, 1992). Some authors suggest that patients with high risk for cerebrovascular disease due to prior events or risk factors should not be given ECT due to the risk of exacerbating the condition secondary to ECT-induced hypoperfusion (Blackburn & Decalmer, 1994). Studies have suggested that the very old and frail elderly are at increased risk of complications from ECT and must be monitored carefully (Hay, 1991). Outpatient ECT is a useful maintenance treatment in patients who are unable to be maintained successfully in remission with medication.

## Psychosurgery

For completely treatment-resistant patients, psychosurgical procedures have been utilized in rare instances. The most recent case series of Lovett and colleagues (1989) showed that two-thirds of a mixed age group of 15 patients showed improvement in the severity of depressive symptoms after subcaudate stereotactic tractotomy, but that only one-third showed a decrease in the frequency of episodes.

## Psychotherapy

While it seems abundantly clear that psychotherapeutic approaches should be valuable in treatment-resistant depression in the elderly, there are few systematic

data. Reynolds and associates (1992) have studied the effects of combined pharmacotherapy with nortriptyline and interpersonal psychotherapy in elderly patients with recurrent (but not treatment resistant) major depression. Seventy-nine
percent of patients achieved a full remission on the combination therapy by a
median of 9 weeks, but 24% of patients blindly switched to placebo during the
16-week continuation phase relapsed despite continued psychotherapy; none
relapsed in the drug and psychotherapy continuation group. Wilson and colleagues (1995) showed that cognitive-behavioral therapy was a valuable adjunct to
medication in the maintenance phase of depression treatment. A variety of
psychotherapeutic and/or family-centered approaches may be valuable in the
treatment-resistant elderly patient in both outpatient and institutional settings,
especially cognitive-behavioral therapy (Thompson, 1996) and interpersonal therapy (Mossey et al., 1996), but a full review of this topic is beyond the scope of this
chapter. The reader is referred to further reviews on this topic (Sadavoy, 1994).

## Management algorithm

Confronted with an apparently treatment-resistant elderly patient, management
should proceed in a logical stepwise manner. Revisiting the history from the
beginning and performing a diagnostic reassessment is critical. In patients with
complex medication histories, it is often helpful to prepare a chronological
summary of the treatment as far as records or memories permit. Additional family
members should be enlisted if available for an expanded psychosocial and/or
medical history. Within institutional settings, consultation with staff is crucial, as
they are not only the best source of information about the patient, but essentially
represent the environment in which the patient lives. It is at this point that
additional diagnostic studies and procedures or consultations with medical colleagues can be obtained. Once an appropriate diagnosis or diagnoses have been
made, concomitant conditions can then be managed or corrected and the effects
of comedication assessed.

Medication trials should be extended. As data reviewed above indicate, medication trials in the elderly should be carried beyond what is typical in younger
patients before it is concluded that the chosen medication is ineffective. Trials of
initial agents in treatment-resistant patients should be up to 12 weeks. Generally
speaking, patients for whom sleep difficulties and anxiety are significant problems
may benefit from tricyclics alone or other agents combined with anxiolytics.
Non-anxious patients, and those with prominent apathy, abulia, or anergia may
benefit from SSRIs, bupropion, or venlafaxine. MAOIs are generally reserved for
second-line treatment and require a co-operative responsible patient or an institutional setting. Dose increases are reasonable after 4 weeks if no improvement is

seen, although it should be kept in mind that the elderly are more vulnerable to adverse effects, even at so-called therapeutic doses or plasma levels.

Augmentation is called for if only partial or no improvement is seen after 6–8 weeks. Anxiety symptoms that persist may require concomitant anxiolytics. Short half-life agents are suitable for limited use; for chronic use, longer half-life agents in low doses may be more useful. Lithium is a reasonable choice for direct antidepressant augmentation, although CNS toxic effects can occur even without the obvious signs of clinical toxicity. Plasma levels are less useful as a guide to therapy than in younger patients. Neuroleptics are generally a necessary adjunct for patients in whom psychotic thinking is present. The elderly are exquisitely sensitive to the adverse effects of these agents, so doses must be carefully monitored. Thyroid hormone may be useful in patients who have marginal thyroid function. Combinations of different classes of agents (e.g. tricyclics and SSRIs) may be useful in resistant patients and may be complementary in terms of symptom relief. Attention must be paid to the potential for adverse drug interactions, particularly through inhibition of metabolism of one drug by another, leading to unexpectedly elevated plasma levels. Stimulants may be helpful, either as monotherapy for certain conditions, or as adjuncts, particularly in patients with debilitating illnesses.

If an adequate trial at substantial dosage with augmentation of a single agent is ineffective, then consideration should be given to the reasons for failure, including diagnostic reassessment, re-examination of potential confounding medical conditions or medications, and the psychosocial situation, looking for potential contributing factors to treatment failure. Second-line treatment may then commence with a different class of medication, followed by a second round of augmentation. Triple drug combinations may be justified in unusual cases and may be quite successful if carefully monitored. ECT should be considered after the first treatment failure if the patient is suicidal, debilitated, or intolerant of nominally therapeutic doses of medication. ECT trials should also be sustained, particularly in treatment-resistant patients, and may require more than the typical six to ten unilateral treatments. Outpatient ECT maintenance should be considered in successfully remitted patients who have shown recurrent disease or multiple drug failures. A trial of intensive short-term inpatient treatment may have significant positive impact on the treatment-resistant elderly patient (Zubenko et al., 1994).

Unusual treatment or augmentation schemes as outlined above can be considered in patients who remain poorly or unresponsive to the above regimens. It is recommended that the clinician obtain consultation from a colleague to assist with confirmation of the diagnostic assessment and proposed course of action, along with informed consent from the patient and family. In patients with significant cognitive impairment secondary to Alzheimer's disease or related

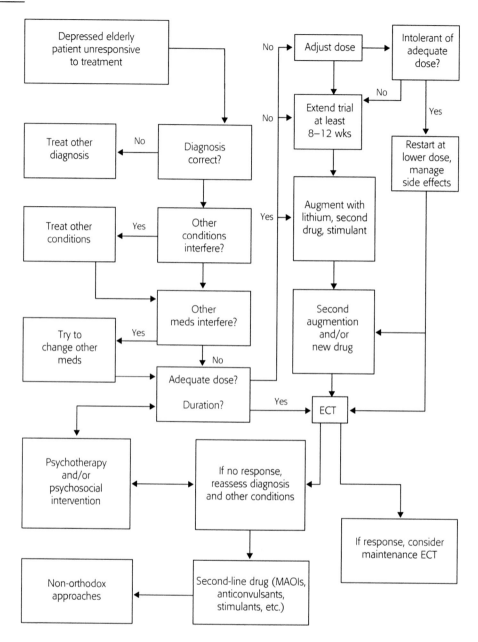

Fig. 15.1.    Management algorithm for depressed elderly patient unresponsive to treatment. This algorithm is meant for general guidance only; treatment must be individualized. The algorithm assumes that continuing from one box to another indicates continued non-response or inadequate response to treatment. Some decision points may have more than one acceptable choice.

dementias, consideration should be given to cognitive enhancement therapy, such as with donepezil. Psychotherapeutic approaches should also be integrated into the treatment plan of the patient. Consultation with practitioners who are expert in either cognitive-behavioral or interpersonal approaches may be very helpful. Working directly with families, spouses, and/or institutional staff may be vital to treatment success.

The flow-chart (Fig. 15.1) is provided to summarize the treatment path recommended. This flow-chart gives general recommendations only and treatment must be individualized, especially for medically complex patients.

## Prognosis

Finally, an attitude of therapeutic nihilism must be avoided. With elderly patients, especially the debilitated or the very old, it may be possible for the clinician to succumb to therapeutic fatigue or resignation about the hopelessness of the patient's condition. This is especially a risk in long-term care institutions, where clinicians may unwittingly collude with the staffs' therapeutic fatigue and avoid treating certain patients aggressively or in a sustained manner.

The prognosis for depressed elderly patients is better than commonly believed. Bonner and Howard (1995) suggest that the 18–40% rate of treatment-resistant elderly patients is an overestimation if patients are vigorously treated. Stoudemire and colleagues (1993) followed 17 elderly treatment-resistant patients at 15 months and 4 years after initial treatment. Forty-seven percent were improved at 15 months and 71% were improved at 4 years. Studies by Alexopolous and associates (1996) show that the recovery rate of elderly depressed patients is similar to that of younger patients. Patients with onset of depression in late life had a higher risk for chronicity. In the follow-up study by Brodaty and colleagues (1993), although the recovery rate of elders overall was no different from younger patients, late-onset patients had a better prognosis. These data suggest that elderly patients do respond to sustained, vigorous treatment. Although full remission may not be achieved in all cases, substantial and meaningful clinical improvement is almost always possible. As clinicians, we now have the tools to greatly improve the quality and quantity of life for our elderly patients.

## REFERENCES

Abernathy, D.R. (1992). Psychotropic drugs and aging process: pharmacokinetics and phar-macodynamics. In *Clinical Geriatric Psychopharmacology 2nd edn.*, ed. C. Salzman, pp. 61–76. Baltimore, MD: Williams and Wilkins.

Abrams, R. (1991). Anxiety and personality disorders. In *Comprehensive Review of Geriatric Psychiatry*, ed. J. Sadavoy, L.W. Lazarus, & L.F. Jarvik, pp. 369–86. Washington DC: American Psychiatric Association Press.

Agrell, B. & Dehlin, O. (1994). Depression in stroke patients with left and right hemisphere lesions. A study in geriatric rehabilitation in-patients. *Aging (Milano)*, **6**, 49–56.

Albert, M.S. (1991). Neuropsychological testing. In *Comprehensive Review of Geriatric Psychiatry*, ed. J. Sadavoy, L.W. Lazarus, & L.F. Jarvik, pp. 222–44. Washington DC: American Psychiatric Association Press.

Alexopolous, G. (1989). Anxiety and depression in the elderly. Paper presented at the Harvard–NIMH Conference on Anxiety and the Elderly, Boston, January 9–10.

Alexopoulos, G.S. (1996). The treatment of depressed demented patients. *Journal of Clinical Psychiatry*, **57** Suppl. 14, 14–20.

Alexopoulos, G.S., Meyers, B.S., Young, R.C. et al. (1996). Recovery in geriatric depression. *Arhives of General Psychiatry*, **53**, 305–12.

Allen, A. & Blazer, D. (1991). Mood disorders. In *Comprehensive Review of Geriatric Psychiatry*, ed. J. Sadavoy, L.W. Lazarus, & L.F. Jarvik, pp. 337–52. Washington DC: APA Press.

Amato, L., Paolisso, G., Cacciatore, F. et al. (1996). Non-insulin-dependent diabetes mellitus is associated with a greater prevalence of depression in the elderly. The Osservatorio Geriatrico of Campania Region Group. *Diabetes Metabolism*, **22**, 314–18.

Andersen, G., Vestergaard, K., & Riis, J.O. (1993). Citalopram for post-stroke pathological crying. *Lancet*, **342**(8875), 837–9.

Andersen, G., Vestergaard, K., & Lauritzen, L. (1994). Effective treatment of poststroke depression with the selective serotonin reuptake inhibitor citalopram *Stroke*, **25**, 1099–104.

Angeleri, F., Angeleri, V.A., Foschi, N. et al. (1993). The influence of depression, social activity, and family stress on functional outcome after stroke. *Stroke*, **24**, 1478–83.

Atkinson, R.M., Turner, J.A., Kofoed, L.I. et al. (1985). Early versus late onset alcoholism in older persons. *Alcoholism: Clinical and Experimental Research*, **9**, 513–15.

Baker, F.M. (1995). Misdiagnosis among older psychiatric patients. *Journal of the National Medical Association*, **87**, 872–6.

Beekman, A.T., Kriegsman, D.M., Deeg, D.J., & van Tilburg, W. (1995). The association of physical health and depressive symptoms in the older population: age and sex differences. *Society of Psychiatry and Psychiatric Epidemiology*, **30**, 32–8.

Bell, I.R., Edman, J.S., Morrow, F.D. et al. (1992). Brief communication. Vitamin B1, B2, and B6 augmentation of tricyclic antidepressant treatment in geriatric depression with cognitive dysfunction. *Journal of the American College of Nutrition*, **11**, 159–63.

Berkman, L.F. & Syme, S.L. (1979). Social networks, host resistance, and mortality: a nine year follow-up study of Alameda county residents. *American Journal of Epidemiology*, **109**, 186–204.

Berkman, L.F., Berkman, C.S., & Kasl, S. (1986). Depressive symptoms in relation to physical health and functioning in the elderly. *American Journal of Epidemiology*, **124**, 372–88.

Berlanga, C. & Ortega-Soto, H.A. (1995). A 3-year follow-up of a group of treatment-resistant depressed patients with a MAOI/tricyclic combination. *Journal of Affective Disorders*, **34**, 187–92.

Berr, C., Lafont, S., Debuire, B. et al. (1996). Relationships of dehydroepiandrosterone sulfate in the elderly with functional, psychological, and mental status, and short-term mortality: a French community-based study. *Proceedings of the National Academy of Sciences, USA*, 12(93), 13410–15.

Blackburn, P.A. & Decalmer, P. (1994). Case report: Is ECT safe in patients with cerebrovascular disease? *International Journal of Geriatric Psychiatry*, 9, 757–61.

Blazer, D. (1989). Depression in the elderly. *New England Journal of Medicine*, 320, 164–6.

Blazer, D. & Williams, C.D. (1980). Epidemiology of dysphoria and depression in an elderly population. *American Journal of Psychiatry*, 139, 439–44.

Bonner, D. & Howard, R. (1995). Treatment-resistant depression in the elderly. *International Psychogeriatrics*, 7 Suppl, 83–94.

Borson, S., Barnes, R.A., & Kukull, W.A. (1986). Symptomatic depression in elderly medical outpatients: I. Prevalence, demography, and health service utilization. *Journal of the American Geriatric Society*, 34, 341–7.

Bradley, S.E., Ingelfinger, F.J., Bradley, G.P. et al. (1945). The estimation of hepatic blood flow in man. *Journal of Clinical Investigations*, 24, 890–7.

Bressler, R. & Katz, M.D. (1993). Drug therapy for geriatric depression. *Drugs Aging*, 3, 195–219.

Brodaty, H., Harris, L., Peters, K. et al. (1993). Prognosis of depression in the elderly: a comparison with younger patients. *British Journal of Psychiatry*, 163, 589–596.

Bruce, M.L., Seeman, T., Merrill, S.S. et al. (1994). The impact of depressive symptomatology on physical disability: MacArthur Studies of Successful Aging. *American Journal of Public Health*, 84, 1796–9.

Callahan, C.M., Dittus, R.S., & Tierney, W.M. (1996). Primary care physicians' medical decision making for late-life depression. *Journal of General Internal Medicine*, 11, 218–25.

Carney, R.M., Freedland, K.E., Eisen, S.A. et al. (1995). Major depression and medication adherence in elderly patients with coronary artery diseae. *Health Psychology*, 14, 88–90.

Cavanaugh, S., Clark, D.C., & Gibbons, R.D. (1983). Diagnosing depression in the hospitalized medically ill. *Psychosomatics*, 24, 809–15.

Collins, E., Katona, C., & Orrell, M. (1995). Management of depression in the elderly by general practitioners: II. Attitudes to aging and factors affecting practice. *Family Practice*, 12, 12–17.

Corey-Bloom, J. & Galasko, D. (1995). Adjunctive therapy in patients with Alzheimer's disease. A practical approach. *Drugs Aging*, 7, 79–87.

Corrigan, F.M. (1992). Sodium valproate augmentation of fluoxetine or fluvoxamine effects [letter]. *Biological Psychiatry*, 31, 1178–9.

Cullen, M., Mitchell, P., Brodaty, H. et al. (1991). Carbamazepine for treatment-resistant melancholia. *Journal of Clinical Psychiatry*, 52, 472–6.

Cummings, J.L. (1992). Depression and Parkinson's disease: a review. *American Journal of Psychiatry*, 149, 443–54.

Cummings, J.L. & Kaufer, D. (1996). Neuropsychiatric aspects of Alzheimer's disease: the cholinergic hypothesis revisited. *Neurology*, 47, 876–83.

Dam, M., Tonin, P., De Boni, A. et al. (1996). Effects of fluoxetine and maprotiline on functional recovery in poststroke hemiplegic patients undergoing rehabilitation therapy. *Stroke*, 27, 1211–14.

Davis, D.F. & Shock, N.W. (1950). Age changes in glomerular filtration rate, effective renal plasma flow, and tubulary capacity in adult males. *Journal of Clinical Investigations*, **29**, 496–506.

Dunner, D.L. (1994). An overview of paroxetine in the elderly. *Gerontology*, **40**, 21–7.

Evans, M.A., Triggs, E.J., Cheung, M. et al. (1981). Gastric emptying rates in the elderly: implications for drug therapy. *Journal of the American Geriatric Society*, **29**, 201–5.

Farrell, K.R. & Ganzini, L. (1995). Misdiagnosing delirium as depression in medically ill elderly patients. *Archives of Internal Medicine*, **155**, 2459–64.

Fawcett, J., Kravitz, H.M., Zajecka, J.M. et al. (1991). CNS stimulant potentiation of monoamine oxidase inhibitors in treatment-refractory depression. *Journal of Clinical Psychopharmacology*, **11**, 127–32.

Feighner, J.P., Herbstein, J., & Damlouji, N. (1985). Combined MAOI, TCA, and direct stimulant therapy of treatment-resistant depression. *Journal of Clinical Psychiatry*, **46**, 206–9.

Flint, A.J. (1994). Recent developments in geriatric psychopharmacology. *Canadian Journal of Psychiatry*, **39**(8 Suppl. 1), S9–18.

Flint, A.J. & Rifat, S.L. (1994). A prospective study of lithium augmentation in antidepressant-resistant geriatric depression. *Journal of Clinical Psychopharmacology*, **14**, 353–6.

Folstein, M.F., Folstein, S.E., & McHugh, P.R. (1975). Mini-Mental State: a practical method for grading the cognitive state of patients for the clinician. *Journal of Psychiatric Research*, **12**, 189–98.

Geokas, M.C. & Haverback, B.J. (1969). The aging gastrointestinal tract. *American Journal of Surgery*, **117**, 881–92.

Georgotas, A. & McCue, R.C. (1989). The additional benefit of extending an antidepressant trial past seven weeks in the depressed elderly. *International Journal of Geriatric Psychiatry*, **4**, 191–5.

Georgotas, A., Friedman, E., McCarthy, M. et al. (1983). Resistant geriatric depressions and therapeutic response to monamine oxidase inhibitors. *Biological Psychiatry*, **18**, 195–205.

Georgotas, A., McCue, R.C., Hapworth, W. et al. (1986). Comparative efficacy and safety of MAOIs versus TCAs in treating depression in the elderly. *Biological Psychiatry*, **21**, 1155–66.

Glassman, A.H. & Roose, S.P. (1994). Risks of antidepressants in the elderly: tricyclic antidepressants and arrhythmia-revising risks. *Gerontology*, **40** (Suppl), 15–20.

Glassman, A.H., Dietch, J.T., & Fine, M. (1990). The effect of nortriptyline in elderly patients with cardiac conduction disease. *Journal of Clinical Psychiatry*, **51**, 65–7.

Greenberg, L. & Fink, M. (1992). The use of electroconvulsive therapy in geriatric patients. *Clinical Geriatric Medicine*, **8**, 349–54.

Greenblatt, D.J., Sellers, E.M., & Shader, R.I. (1982). Drug disposition in old age. *New England Journal of Medicine*, **306**, 1081–8.

Greenhouse, J.B., Kupfer, D.J., Frank, E. et al. (1987). Analysis of time to stabilization in the treatment of depression: Biological and clinical correlates. *Journal of Affective Disorders*, **13**, 259–66.

Guicheney, P., Devynck, M.A., Cloix, J.F. et al. (1988). Platelet 5-HT content and uptake in essential hypertension: role of endogenous digitalis-like factors and plasma cholesterol. *Journal of Hypertension*, **6**, 115–26.

Gustafson, Y., Nilsson, I., Mattsson, M. et al. (1995). Epidemiology and treatment of post-stroke depression. *Drugs Aging*, **7**, 298–309.

Gwirtsman, H.E., Szuba, M.P., Toren, L. et al. (1994). The antidepressant response to tricyclics in major depressives is accelerated with adjunctive use of methylphenidate. *Psychopharmacology Bulletin*, **30**, 157–64.

Hanson, B.S., Isacsson, S.O., Janzon, L. et al. (1989). Social network and social support influence mortality in elderly men. The prospective population study of men born in 1914, Malmo, Sweden. *American Journal of Epidemiology*, **130**, 100–1.

Hardy, B., Shulman, K.I., & Zucchero, C. (1997). Gradual discontinuation of lithium augmentation in elderly patients with unipolar depression. *Journal of Clinical Psychopharmacology*, **17**, 22–6.

Hay, D.P. (1991). Electroconvulsive therapy. In *Comprehensive Review of Geriatric Psychiatry*, ed. J. Sadavoy, L.W. Lazarus, & L.F. Jarvik, pp. 469–86. Washington DC: APA Press.

Heston, L.L., Garrard, J., Makris, L. et al. (1992). Inadequate treatment of depressed nursing home elderly. *Journal of the American Geriatric Society*, **40**(11), 1117–22.

Hickie, I., Bennett, B., Mitchell, P., Wilhelm, K., & Orlay, W. (1996). Clinical and subclinical hypothyroidism in patients with chronic and treatment-resistant depression. *Australia and New Zealand Journal of Psychiatry*, **30**, 246–52.

Hornig-Rohan, M. & Amsterdam, J.D. (1994). Clinical and biological correlates of treatment-resistant depression: an overview. *Psychiatric Annals*, **24**, 220–7.

Hyer, L., Carson, M., Nixon, D. et al. (1987). Depression among alcoholics. *International Journal of Addiction*, **22**, 1235–41.

Iizuka, H., Kishimoto, A., Nakamura, J., & Mizukawa, R. (1996). Clinical effects of cortisol synthesis inhibition on treatment-resistant depression. *Nihon Shinkei Seishin Yakurigaku Zasshi*, **16**, 33–6.

Jenike, M.A. (1989). *Geriatric Psychiatry and Psychopharmacolgy, A Clinical Approach*. Chicago: Year Book Medical Publishers.

Jones, B.N. & Reifler, B.V. (1994). Depression coexisting with dementia. Evaluation and treatment. *Medical Clinics of North America*, **78**, 823–40.

Kahn, A., Rudolph, R., Baumel, B. et al. (1995). Venlafaxine in depressed geriatric outpatients: an open-label clinical study. *Psychopharmacology Bulletin*, **31**, 753–8.

Kamholz, B.A. & Mellow, A.M. (1996). Management of treatment resistance in the depressed geriatric patient. *Psychiatric Clinics of North America*, **19**, 269–86.

Katz, I.R., Curlik, S., & Nemetz, P. (1988). Functional psychiatric disorders in the elderly. In *Essentials of Geriatric Psychiatry*, ed. L.F. Jarvik, J.R. Foster, J.D. Lieff, & S.R. Mershon, pp. 113–37. New York: Springer.

Ketter, T.A., Post, R.M., Parekh, P.I. et al. (1995). Addition of monoamine oxidase inhibitors to carbamazepine: preliminary evidence of safety and antidepressant efficacy in treatment-resistant depression. *Journal of Clinical Psychiatry*, **56**, 471–5.

Kielholz, P., Terzani, S., Gastpar, M. et al. (1982). Treatment of therapy-resistant depressions. Results of combined infusion treatment. *Schweizerische Medizinische Wochenschrift*, **112**, 1090–5.

Kitchell, M.A., Barnes, R.F., & Veith, R.C. (1982). Screening for depression in hospitalized geriatric medical patients. *Journal of the American Geriatric Society*, **30**, 174–7.

Knegtering, H., Eijck, M., & Huijsman, A. (1994). Effects of antidepressants on cognitive functioning of elderly patients. A review. *Drugs Aging*, **5**, 192–9.

Koch, H. & Knapp, D.E. (1987). Highlights of drug utilization in office practice, *National Ambulatory Medical Survey 1985. Advance Data from Vital and Health Statistics*, No. 134 (DHHS pub no. (PHS) 87–1250) Hyattsville, MD: National Center for Health Statistics.

Koenig, H.G., Meador, K.G., Cohen, H.G. et al. (1988). Detection and treatment of major depression in older medically ill hospitalized patients. *International Journal of Psychiatry Medicine*, **18**, 17–31.

Kramer, B.A. (1987). Electroconvulsive therapy use in geriatric depression. *Journal of Nervous and Mental Diseases*, **175**, 233–5.

Kunik, M.E., Pollock, B.G., Perel, J.M. et al. (1994). Clomipramine in the elderly: tolerance and plasma levels. *Journal of Geriatric Psychiatry and Neurology*, **7**, 139–43.

Kushnir, S.L. (1986). Lithium-antidepressant combinations in the treatment of depressed, physically ill geriatric patients. *American Journal of Psychiatry*, **143**, 378–9.

Lafferman, J., Solomon, K., & Ruskin, P. (1988). Lithium augmentation for treatment-resistant depression in the elderly. *Journal of Geriatric Psychiatry and Neurology*, **1**, 49–52.

Lamb, V.L. (1996). A cross-national study of quality of life factors associated with patterns of elderly disablement. *Social Science and Medicine*, **42**, 363–77.

Lauritzen, L., Bendsen, B.B., Vilmar, T. et al. (1994). Post-stroke depression: combined treatment with imipramine or desipramine and mianserin. A controlled clinical study. *Psychopharmacology (Berl.)* **114**, 119–22.

Lawlor, B.A., Newhouse, P.A., Balkin, T. et al. (1991). A preliminary study of the effects of the serotonin agonist m-CPP on sleep architecture and behavior in healthy volunteers. *Biological Psychiatry*, **29**, 281–6.

Lazarus, L.W., Moberg, P.J., Langsley, P.R. et al. (1994). Methylphenidate and nortriptyline in the treatment of poststroke depression: a retrospective comparison. *Archives of Physical Medicine and Rehabilitation*, **75**, 403–6.

Lee, M.S., Crittenden, K.S., & Yu, E. (1996). Social support and depression among elderly Korean immigrants in the United States. *International Journal of Aging and Human Development*, **42**, 313–27.

Lichtenberg, P.A., Ross, T., Millis, S.R., & Manning, C.A. (1995). The relationship between depression and cognition in older adults: a cross-validation study. *Journals of Gerontology, B Psychological Sciences and Social Sciences*, **50**, P25–P32.

Lovett, L.M., Crimmins, R., & Shaw, D.M. (1989). Outcome in unipolar affective disorder after stereotactic tractotomy. *British Journal of Psychiatry*, **155**, 547–50.

McCue, R.E. (1992). Using tricyclic antidepressants in the elderly. *Clinical Geriatric Medicine*, **8**, 323–34.

Marcopulos, B.A. & Graves, R.E. (1990). Antidepressant effect on memory in depressed older patients. *Journal of Clinical and Experimental Neuropsychology*, **12**, 655–63.

Meltzer, H. (1989). Serotonergic function in depression. *British Journal of Psychiatry*, **155** (Suppl. 8), 25–31.

Meyers, B.S. (1995). Late-life delusional depression: acute and long-term treatment. *Interna-*

*tional Psychogeriatrics*, **7** Suppl, 113–24.

Miller, N.S. & Gold, M.S. (1989). Suggestions for changes in DSM-III-R criteria for substance use disorders. *American Journal of Drug and Alcohol Abuse*, **2**, 223–30.

Molholm, H.J., Hansen, J., Kampmann, J., & Lauson, H. (1970). Renal excretion of drugs in the elderly. *Lancet*, **1**, 1170.

Montamet, S., Cusack, B., & Vestal, R.E. (1989). Management of drug therapy in the elderly. *New England Journal of Medicine*, **321**, 303–9.

Morgan, R.E., Palinkas, L.A., Barrett-Connor, E.L. et al. (1993). Plasma cholesterol and depressive symptoms in older men. *Lancet*, **341**, 75–9.

Mossey, J.M., Knott, K.A., Higgins, M. et al. (1996). Effectiveness of a psychosocial intervention, interpersonal counseling, for subdysthymic depression in medically ill elderly. *Journal of Gerontology, A Biological Sciences and Medical Sciences*, **5**, M172–8.

Mowe, M. & Bohmer, T. (1991). The prevalence of undiagnosed protein-calorie undernutrition in a population of hospitalized elderly patients. *Journal of the American Geriatric Society*, **39**, 1089–92.

Mukand, J., Kaplan, M., Senno, R.G. et al. (1996). Pathological crying and laughing: treatment with sertraline. *Archives of Physical Medicine and Rehabilitation*, **77**, 1309–11.

Nair, N.P., Ahmed, S.K., Kin, N.M. et al. (1995). Reversible and selective inhibitors of monamine oxidase A in the treatment of depressed elderly patients. *Acta Psychiatrica Scandinavica*, **386** (Suppl.) 28–35.

Nelson, P.B. (1989). Social support, self-esteem, and depression in the institutionalized elderly. *Issues Mental Health Nursing*, **10**, 55–68.

Nelson, J.C., Jatlow, P., & Mazure, C. (1985). Desipramine plasma levels and response in elderly melancholic patients. *Journal of Clinical Psychopharmacology*, **5**, 217–20.

Newhouse, P.A. (1996). Use of serotonin selective inhibitors in geriatric depression. *Journal of Clinical Psychiatry*, **57** (Suppl.), 12–22.

Newhouse, P.A., Krishnan, K.R.R., Doraiswamy, P.M., Richter, E.M., Batzar, E.D., & Clary, C.M. (2000). A double-blind comparison of sertraline and fluoxetine in depressed elderly outpatients. *Journal of Clinical Psychiatry* **61**, 559–68.

Nierenberg, A.A., Feighner, J.P., Rudolph, R. et al. (1994). Venlafaxine for treatment-resistant unipolar depression. *Journal of Clinical Psychopharmacology*, **14**, 419–23.

Okimoto, J.T., Barnes, R.F., & Veith, R.C. (1982). Screening for depression in geriatric medical patients. *American Journal of Psychiatry*, **139**, 799–802.

Parmelee, P.A., Katz, I.R., & Lawton, M.P. (1991). The relation of pain to depression among institutionalized aged. *Journal of Gerontology*, **46**, P15–21.

Penninx, B.W., Beekman, A.T., Ormel, J. et al. (1996). Psychological status among elderly people with chronic diseases: does type of disease play a part?. *Journal of Psychosomatic Research*, **40**, 521–34.

Petracca, G., Teson, A., Chemerinski, E. et al. (1996). A double-blind placebo-controlled study of clomipramine in depressed patients with Alzheimer's disease. *Journal of Neuropsychiatry and Clinical Neuroscience*, **8**, 270–5.

Pomara, N. & Gershon, S. (1984). Treatment-resistant depression in an elderly patient with pancreatic carcinoma: case report. *Journal of Clinical Psychiatry*, **45**, 439–40.

Prigerson, H.G., Frank, E., Kasl, S.V. et al. (1995). Complicated grief and bereavement-related depression as distinct disorders: preliminary empirical validation in elderly bereaved spouses. *American Journal of Psychiatry*, **152**, 22–30.

Prudic, J.M., Sackheim, H.A., & Devanand, D.P. (1990). Medication resistance and clinical response to electroconvulsive therapy. *Psychiatry Research*, **31**, 287–96.

Rapp, S.R., Parisi, S.A., Walsh, D., & Wallace, C.E. (1988). Detecting depression in elderly medical inpatients. *Journal of Consulting and Clinical Psychology*, **56**, 509–13.

Reifler, B.V., Teri, L., Raskind, M. et al. (1989). Double-blind trial of imipramine in Alzheimer's disease patients with and without depression. *American Journal of Psychiatry*, **146**, 45–9.

Reynolds, C.F. 3rd, Frank, E., Perel, J.M. et al. (1992). Combined pharmacotherapy and psychotherapy in the acute and continuation treatment of elderly patients with recurrent major depression: a preliminary report. *American Journal of Psychiatry*, **149**, 1687–92.

Reynolds, C.F., Frank, E., Perel, J.M. et al. (1994). Treatment of consecutive episodes of major depression in the elderly. *American Journal of Psychiatry*, **151**, 1740–3.

Reynolds, C.F. 3rd, Frank, E., Perel, J.M. et al. (1996). High relapse rate after discontinuation of adjunctive medication for elderly patients with recurrent major depression. *American Journal of Psychiatry*, **153**, 1418–22.

Robins, L.N., Helzer, J.E., Przybeck, T.R. et al. (1988). Alcohol disorders in the community: a report from the Epidemiologic Catchment Area. In *Alcoholism: Origins and Outcome*, ed. R. Rose & J. Barret, pp. 15–29. New York: Raven.

Robinson, R.G., Kubos, K.L., Starr, L.B. et al. (1983). Mood changes in stroke patients: relationship to lesion location. *Comprehensive Psychiatry*, **24**, 555–66.

Robinson, R.G., Starr, L.B., & Price, T.R. (1984). A two year longitudinal study of mood disorders following stroke: prevalence and duration at six months follow-up. *British Journal of Psychiatry*, **144**, 256–62.

Robinson, R.G., Schultz, S.K., Castillo, C. et al. (2000). Notriptyline versus fluoxetine in the treatment of depression and in short-term recovery after stroke: a placebo-controlled, double-blind study. *American Journal of Psychiatry*, **157**, 351–9.

Rudman, D. & Feller, A.G. (1989). Protein-calorie undernutrition in the nursing home. *Journal of the American Geriatric Society*, **37**, 173–83.

Sadavoy, J. (1994). Integrated psychotherapy for the elderly. *Canadian Journal of Psychiatry*, **39**(8 suppl. 1), S19–26.

Salzman, C. (1985). Clinical use of antidepressant blood levels and the electrocardiogram. *New England Journal of Medicine*, **313**, 512–13.

Sarkisian, C.A. & Lachs, M.S. (1996). 'Failure to thrive' in older adults. *Annals of Internal Medicine*, **15**(124), 1072–8.

Schneider, L.S., Small, G.W., Hamilton, S.H. et al. (1997). Estrogen replacement and response to fluoxetine in a multicenter geriatric depression trial. *American Journal of Geriatric Psychiatry*, **5**, 97–106.

Schuckit, M.A. (1983). A clinical review of alcohol, alcoholism, and the elderly patient. *Journal of Clinical Psychiatry*, **43**, 396–9.

Seth, R., Jennings, A.L., Bindman, J., Phillips, J., & Bergmann, K. (1992). Combination treatment with noradrenalin and serotonin reuptake inhibitors in resistant depression. *British*

*Journal of Psychiatry*, **161**, 562–5.

Shapira, B., Oppenheim, G., Zohar, J. et al. (1985). Lack of efficacy of estrogen supplementation to imipramine in resistant female depressives. *Biological Psychiatry*, **20**, 576–9.

Spar, J.A. & LaRue, A. (1985). Acute response to methylphenidate as a predictor of outcome of treatment with TCAs in the elderly. *Journal of Clinical Psychiatry*, **46**, 466–9.

Stamenkovic, M., Schindler, S., & Kasper, S. (1996). Therapy of post-stroke depression with fluoxetine. A pilot project. *Nervenarzt*, **67**, 62–7.

Steinbach, U. (1992). Social networks, institutionalization, and mortality among elderly people in the United States. *Journal of Gerontology*, **47**, S183–90.

Stoudemire, A., Hill, C.D., Morris, R. et al. (1993). Long-term outcome of treatment-resistant depression in older adults. *American Journal of Psychiatry*, **150**, 1539–40.

Sullivan, D.H., Walls, R.C., & Lipschitz, D.A. (1991). Protein-energy undernutrition and the risk of mortality within 1 year of hospital discharge in a select population of geriatric rehabilitation patients. *American Journal of Clinical Nutrition*, **53**, 599–605.

Tacke, U., Leinonen, E., Lillsunde, P. et al. (1992). Debrisoquine hydroxylation phenotypes of patients with high versus low to normal serum antidepressant concentration. *Journal of Clinical Psychopharmacology*, **12**, 262–7.

Tandberg, E., Larsen, J.P., & Aarsland, D. (1996).The occurrence of depression in Parkinson's disease. A community-based study. *Archives of Neurology*, **53**, 175–9.

Thompson, C. & Thompson, C.M. (1991). Treatment resistant or irresolutely treated?. *International Clinical Psychopharmacology*, **6** (Suppl. 1), 31–8.

Thompson, L.W. (1996). Cognitive-behavioral therapy and treatment for late-life depression. *Journal of Clinical Psychiatry*, **57** (Suppl. 5), 29–37.

Turner, N., Scarpace, P.J., & Lowenthal, D.T. (1992). Geriatric pharmacology: basic and clinical consideration. *Annual Review of Pharmacology and Toxicology*, **32**, 271–302.

Vaillant, G.E. (1983). *The Natural History of Alcoholism.* Boston MA: Harvard University Press.

Van Marwijk, H.W., Bekker, F.M., Nolen, W.A. et al. (1990). Lithium augmentation in geriatric depression. *Journal of Affective Disorders*, **20**, 217–23.

Volicer, L., Rheaume, Y., & Cyr, D. (1994). Treatment of depression in advanced Alzheimer's disease using sertraline. *Journal of Geriatric Psychiatry and Neurology*, **7**, 227–9.

Wallace, A.E., Kofoed, L.L., & West, A.N. (1995). Double blind, placebo-controlled trial of methylphenidate in older depressed medically ill patients. *American Journal of Psychiatry*, **152**, 929–31.

Warheit, G.J., Longino, C.F., & Bradsher, J.E. (1991). Sociocultural Aspects. In *Comprehensive Review of Geriatric Psychiatry*, ed. J. Sadavoy, L.W. Lazarus, and L.F. Jarvik, pp. 99–116. Washington DC: APA Press.

Warneke, L. (1990). Psychostimulants in psychiatry. *Canadian Journal of Psychiatry*, **35**, 3–10.

Wassertheil-Smoller, S., Applegate, W.B., Berge, K. et al. (1995). Change in depression as a precursor of cardiovascular events. SHEP Cooperative Research Group (Systolic Hypertension in the Elderly). *Archives of Internal Medicine*, **156**, 553–61.

Weilburg, J.B., Rosenbaum, J.F., Biederman, J. et al. (1989). Fluoxetine added to non-MAOI antidepressants converts nonresponders to responders: a preliminary report. *Journal of Clinical Psychiatry*, **50**, 447–9.

Wells, K.B., Stewart, A., Hays, R.D. et al. (1989). The functioning the well-being of depressed patients: results from the medical outcomes study. *Journal of the American Medical Society*, **262**, 914–19.

Whitcup, S.M. & Miller, F. (1987). Unrecognized drug dependence in psychiatrically hospitalized elderly patients. *Journal of the American Geriatric Society*, **35**, 297–301.

Wilson, K.C., Scott, M., Abou-Saleh, M. et al. (1995). Long-term effects of cognitive-behavioural therapy and lithium therapy on depression in the elderly. *British Journal of Psychiatry*, **167**, 653–8.

Yesavage, J. (1993). Differential diagnosis between depression and dementia. *American Journal of Medicine*, **24**, 94(5A), 23S–28S.

Young, R.C. & Myers, B.S. (1991). Psychopharmacology. In *Comprehensive Review of Geriatric Psychiatry*, ed. J. Sadavoy, L.W. Lazarus, & L.F. Jarvik, pp. 435–68. Washington: American Psychiatric Association Press.

Zajecka, J.M., Jeffries, H., & Fawcett, J. (1995). The efficacy of fluoxetine combined with a heterocyclic antidepressant in treatment-resistant depression: a retrospective analysis. *Journal of Clinical Psychiatry*, **56**, 338–43.

Zimmer, B., Rosen, J., Thornton, J.E. et al. (1991). Adjunctive lithium carbonate in nortriptyline-resistant elderly depressed patients. *Journal of Clinical Psychopharmacology*, **11**, 254–6.

Zisselman, M.H., Rovner, B.W., & Shmuely, Y. (1996). Benzodiazepine use in the elderly prior to hospitalization. *Psychosomatics*, **37**, 38–42.

Zubenko, G.S., Mulsant, B.H., Rifai, A.H. et al. (1994). Impact of acute psychiatric inpatient treatment on major depression in late life and prediction of response. *American Journal of Psychiatry*, **151**, 987–94.

# 16

# Management of treatment-resistant depression during pregnancy and the postpartum period

Zachary N. Stowe, Pamela McCreary, Amy Hostetter, Claudia Baugh, and Alexis Llewellyn

## Introduction

The management of pregnant and postpartum women with major depression may be complicated, especially when pharmacological therapies are involved. Many clinicians will encounter this situation at some point due to the high incidence of major depression during the childbearing years and the growing number of women who plan to nurse. The prevalence of this clinical situation has resulted in the comprehensive review of the available data on the use of psychotropic medications during pregnancy and lactation (Altshuler et al., 1996; Cohen, 1989; Kerns, 1986; Miller, 1991; 1994a; Robinson et al., 1986; Stowe & Nemeroff, 1995a,b; Stowe et al., 1998; Wisner & Perel, 1988; Llewellyn & Stowe, 1998). Numerous confounds in much of this literature make the development of definitive treatment guidelines for this period difficult. The literature on cases of treatment-resistant depression is sparse, requiring empirical interpretation of previous case reports and registries. The proportion of women with major depression in pregnancy or postpartum that are resistant to treatment is unknown, and there are no formal studies on the use of potential augmentation strategies involving multiple medications during pregnancy or postpartum. The lack of information on these topics may be due to a lack of documentation of multiple medication use in the literature. Equally plausible, treatment-resistant depressive episodes during this specific time period may not be identified as such, with professionals and patients more willing to tolerate symptoms without employing more aggressive treatment strategies. The most common situations that the clinician will encounter in the management of reproductive age women with treatment-resistant depression include: (i) inadvertent conception during treatment; (ii) prepregnancy consultation; (iii) exacerbation of psychiatric symptoms during pregnancy and/or the postpartum period; and/or (iv) prophylactic treatment planning for women at high risk for a postpartum mental illness.

To address these issues, we provide a brief review of the available data; emphasize the components of an individualized comprehensive risk–benefit assessment; and propose general algorithms for systematically approaching these situations. With the complexity of these issues, one must remember that the clinician's primary goal of treatment is to: 'minimize fetal and neonatal exposure to psychotropic medications while maintaining maternal mental health; and not sacrificing one for the other.'

# Incidence

## Pregnancy

Early studies (Pugh et al., 1963) suggest a decrease in psychiatric hospitalizations during pregnancy, and some groups report a decrease in symptoms and/or severity of depression during pregnancy (Zajick, 1981; Sim, 1963; Rosenberg & Silver, 1965). Recent studies fail to support the position that pregnancy confers any protection from major depression. Several studies show similar rates of major depression between gravid and non-gravid women (O'Hara et al., 1984, 1990; Watson et al., 1984; Kumar & Robson, 1984). On depression rating scales, such as the Beck Depression Inventory (BDI), up to 70% of pregnant women endorse depressive symptoms, and 10–16% of women meet full diagnostic criteria (Affonson et al., 1990; Beck, 1995; Kumar & Robson, 1984; Weissman & Olfson, 1995). The overlap of symptoms between the normal sequela of pregnancy and those of major depression, renders an accurate determination of illness prevalence difficult. There appears to be both a professional and societal propensity to dismiss depressive symptoms such as changes in appetite, body weight, sleep, libido, and energy as solely related to pregnancy (Klein & Essex, 1995). Further confounding the assessment of major depression during pregnancy is a failure to check for medical illness that could potentially contribute to depressive symptoms, including: anemia, gestational diabetes, and/or thyroid dysfunction (Pedersen et al., 1993). Mounting evidence indicates that antithyroglobulin antibodies appear in mid to late pregnancy (Harris, 1993; Harris et al., 1993); the clinical significance of this is unclear with respect to depression. The possibility for medical illness contributing to depression during pregnancy underscores the need for appropriate laboratory evaluation, especially in treatment-resistant cases.

The severity of depression during pregnancy compared to non-gravid states remains unknown. Retrospective data demonstrates a decrease in the incidence of suicide during pregnancy (Appleby, 1991). In contrast, our group (Llewellyn et al., 1998) found that more than 40% of pregnant women referred to our program (a tertiary referral center) endorse suicidal thoughts. The strongest predictor of this suicidal ideation during pregnancy is a history of early sexual abuse. The incidence of treatment-resistant depression during pregnancy is unknown, and no treatment studies or specific case reports exist. Comorbid states of depression and one or more other psychiatric diagnosis may be mistaken for a treatment-resistant depression rather than two separate illnesses that need treatment planning. Pregnancy data on other diagnoses shows possible improvement in panic disorder and typical onset or worsening in OCD and disorders with a psychotic component (schizophrenia, schizoaffective disorder, etc.) (McNeil et al., 1984 a,b; Neziroglu et al., 1992). Proper diagnosis of other illnesses is pivotal in ruling out, or identifying, a case of treatment-resistant depression in this population.

## Postpartum

Childbirth is a time of copious biological, psychosocial, and economic alterations that may pose significant risk for relapse of pre-existing psychiatric conditions, or may serve as a precipitant for 'index' episodes of depression. Official recognition of postpartum onset mental illness has only recently occurred. DSM-IV now includes a modifier for 'postpartum onset' of mood disorders in which symptoms start within the first 4 weeks postpartum (APA, 1994). Kendall and colleagues (1987) illustrate a marked increase in both general and psychotic psychiatric hospitalizations for up to 2 years postpartum. They find the greatest risk of admisssion in the first 3 months postpartum (Kendall et al., 1987). A second study demonstrates that up to 12.5% of all psychiatric hospital admissions of women occur during the first postpartum year (Duffy, 1983). The pathological categories of postpartum mood disorders that are generally recognized by the professional community include: postpartum psychosis (PPP) and postpartum depression (PPD) (O'Hara, 1991). There are also case reports of postpartum onset of OCD and panic disorder (Sichel et al., 1993). The clinical presentation of a postpartum mental illness may include both affective and anxiety symptoms (DSM-IV).

Postpartum psychosis is a rare condition that occurs in 1–2 of every 1000 live births, typically with onset in the first 6 weeks postpartum (McGorry & Conell, 1990; Sibert, 1993; Weissman & Olfson, 1995) . The majority of these psychoses represent affective disorders (bipolar disorder or unipolar major depression) (McGorry & Conell, 1990). Postpartum depression is a major depressive episode that affects between 10 and 22% of women, and up to 26% of adolescent women (Cooper & Murray, 1995; Duffy, 1983; Richards, 1990; Stowe & Nemeroff, 1995a,b; Troutman & Cutrona, 1990) during the first postpartum year. Several risk-factors have been identified for PPD (Stowe & Nemeroff, 1995a,b): a personal or familial history of depression, especially of PPD (Playfair & Gowers, 1981; Richards, 1990); a previous episode of PPD; and a history of depression prior to conception (Kitamura et al., 1993). Anxiety and depression during pregnancy are also reported indicators for a future PPD (O'Hara et al., 1982; O'Hara, 1986).

The limited treatment studies in women with postpartum depression (Appleby et al., 1997; Stowe et al., 1995) demonstrate a remarkably high rate of treatment response. A second group demonstrates the utility and efficacy of interpersonal psychotherapy (IPT) (Stuart & O'Hara, 1995). Our group details a treatment response analysis using a combined treatment protocol (SSRI monotherapy, supportive psychotherapy, behavioral modification, and educational material for patient and family) (Strader et al., 1997). This combined approach does not address the incidence of treatment-resistant cases, though the 93% response rate after 8 weeks of treatment suggests that the combined model is highly efficacious in PPD.

## Impact of the illness

The adverse impact of untreated or partially treated maternal mental illness during pregnancy on long-term infant outcome is not well documented, and investigations provide some discordant results. One group, using the General Health Questionnaire, concludes that symptoms of depression and anxiety do not adversely affect the rate of obstetric complications (Perkin et al., 1993). In contrast, Steer and colleagues (1992) find a risk of 3.97 for lower birth weight ( $< 2500 \, gm$), a risk of 3.39 for preterm delivery ( $< 37$ weeks' gestation), and a risk of 3.02 for small for gestational age ( $< 10th$ percentile) in a group of adult women, derived from an inner city population, with Beck Depression Inventory (BDI) scores of 21 or higher. A second study by Hedegaard et al. (1993) confirms the risk for preterm delivery in women reporting psychological distress in the 30th week of gestation. Similarly, Wadhwa and colleagues (1993), in a prospective study, demonstrate a significant relationship between maternal stress and early delivery. The results from these studies are not conclusive, but do suggest a potential for lower birth weight and an enhanced risk for preterm delivery in women with increased psychological distress. The clinician should consider the data on the negative impact of maternal depression on obstetric outcome while making a risk–benefit assessment with the patient.

Unlike the scarcity of data existing for pregnancy, the adverse impact of untreated maternal mental illness and maternal separation on infant well-being is clearly documented. The potential deleterious effects of an emotionally unresponsive maternal figure on an infant are also well documented. There are over four decades of data on the adverse impact of maternal separation from human infants (Bowlby, 1951). Laboratory studies, starting in the early sixties, demonstrate adverse effects on socialization in maternally deprived offspring of primates (Harlow & Harlow, 1962). Various animal models of maternal separation show long lasting and persistent alterations in numerous neuroendocrine axes (Plotsky

& Meaney, 1993), in neurotransmitter systems (Matthew et al., 1996), in behavior (for review, see Statham, 1998), in CNS cytoarchitecture and receptors (McEwen et al., 1992; Sutanto et al., 1996), and in neuronal firing patterns (Stowe et al., 1998). Human postpartum studies on maternal mental illness demonstrate negative effects on maternal–infant attachment, cognitive competence, and child development (Avant, 1981; Brazelton, 1975; Campbell et al., 1995; Cogill et al., 1986; Cradon, 1979; Cutrona et al., 1986; Murray & Cooper, 1996; Teti et al., 1995; Whiffen & Gotlib, 1989; Zahn-Waxler et al., 1984). Another series of studies with depressed mothers demonstrates a decrease in mother–infant behavioral and EKG synchrony (Field, 1989, 1990) as well as depressed infant behavior (Field et al., 1988). The entry criteria of these depressed subjects was a BDI > 12. The population of these studies was made up of a community-based sample which most likely represented the 'walking wounded' (e.g. mild to moderate depression). This underscores the need to identify and treat maternal mental illness in order to minimize the negative impact of this illness on both mother and infant.

The incidence and potential impact of untreated or partially treated depression provides the basis from which the clinician can begin the risk–benefit assessment. The other salient factors to consider in the risk–benefit assessment are: the data on obstetrical outcome, the physiology of pregnancy and lactation, and the available data on somatic therapies.

## Obstetrical outcome

Of documented pregnancies past 12 weeks' gestation, 84.5% result in the birth of a viable infant (Kiely, 1991; McBride, 1972), 2–4% of infants have malformations that impair function and/or require surgical correction, and up to 12% have minor malformations (Riccardi, 1977). The Collaborative Perinatal Project followed a cohort of 50 282 mother–infant pairs from 12 medical centers, and found an overall infant malformation rate of 6.5% (Heinonen et al., 1977). The etiology of these malformations is unknown in greater than 65% of the cases, and environmental factors which include medication exposure account only for approximately 3% of them. There may also be a bias in associating birth defects with psychotropic medications. For example, the association of 'in utero' lithium exposure with Ebstein's anomaly of the heart is still a widely held view, yet comprehensive reviews of the available data (Cohen et al., 1994) place the risk for this malformation at less than 0.1%.

Several factors confound the interpretation of reproductive safety data on medication. First, greater than 40% of pregnancies are inadvertent conceptions, with most women learning of their pregnancy at approximately 6 weeks' gestation, or some even later. Therefore, vitamins are often not taken during critical developmental periods. Developmental studies demonstrate that the majority of major malformations occur during the embryonic period (i.e. the 3rd through 8th week of gestation), before many women know they are pregnant. After the 11th week of gestation, most of the organ systems (except for the central nervous system [CNS], teeth, ears, eyes, and external genitalia) are developed (Sadler, 1985). Secondly, 90% of women take medications, other than prenatal vitamins (PNV), during pregnancy (Rayburn & Andresen, 1982). Greater than 30% of women take a sedative, tranquilizer, or antidepressant (Heinonen et al., 1977; Doering & Stewart, 1978) at some point in a pregnancy. Finally, the majority of the reproductive safety reports do not control for maternal age, tobacco use, alcohol and drug abuse, potential exposure to environmental toxins, and the extent of prenatal care received. Considering this information, a controlled definitive study on psychotropic medications is unlikely.

# Physiology

## Pregnancy

The physiologic changes that occur during pregnancy, which affect the metabolism and disposition of psychotropic medications in the body, complicate the pharmacologic treatment of the depressed pregnant woman. The majority of relevant data concerning the physiologic changes associated with pregnancy are derived from therapeutic plasma drug monitoring with non-psychotropic medications (Boobis & Lewis, 1983). Physiologic changes that occur during pregnancy which may alter maternal serum concentrations of psychotropic medications include: (i) delayed gastric emptying, which results in increased maternal and fetal exposure to an acidic environment and degradative enzymes; (ii) decreased gastrointestinal motility, presumably related to increased progesterone, which potentially enhances complete absorption of medication; (iii) increased volume of distribution (increased body fat, plasma volume, total body water), producing a decreased serum concentration for a given dose; (iv) decreased protein binding capacity, thus increasing serum-free medication concentrations (Wood & Hytten, 1981); and (v) increased hepatic metabolism, resulting in more rapid degradation of certain medications. These factors may alter the medication concentration to which the fetus is exposed and the maternal dose needed to maintain therapeutic concentrations. Wisner and colleagues (1993) found that, to maintain therapeutic serum concentrations and response of TCAs in pregnant patients, maternal medication dose was increased, on average, to 1.6 times the original dose by the time of patient's delivery. This is consistent with such physiological alterations of pregnancy. Similar alterations have been described with lithium. A clear relationship between therapeutic response and serum concentrations does not exist for most of the newer antidepressants. Studies with sertraline, fluoxetine, paroxetine, fluvoxamine, venlafaxine, nefazadone, and mirtazapine reveal no relationship between plasma medication concentrations and clinical response.

Although there is no evidence of placental filtering of psychotropic medications, a formal study is lacking. All psychotropics studied cross the blood–placental barrier. The mechanism of placental transport is thought to be simple diffusion that is dependent on several properties of the individual medication: molecular size, percentage of protein binding, polarity, lipid solubility, and duration of exposure (Rayburn & Andresen, 1982). The fetus is exposed to maternal medication, but it is noteworthy that the fetal exposure is based on the maternal serum concentration and not the maternal dose (Stowe et al., 1997a).

## Lactation

Lactation is another special circumstance in which the treatment of a depressed woman, especially by pharmacologic intervention, warrants careful consideration and a risk–benefit assessment involving several factors. The neonate continues to exhibit physiological characteristics different than an adult for several months after birth. The neonate has decreased activity of certain hepatic metabolic enzyme systems, making him/her susceptible to slower elimination of some chemicals (Warner, 1986). Both glucuronidation and oxidation systems can be as low as 20% of adult levels (Atkinson et al., 1988); the maturation of both systems will be even more delayed in premature infants. In addition, rates of glomerular filtration and tubular secretion are relatively low in neonates – 30–40% and 20–30% lower than adult levels, respectively (Welch & Findlay, 1981). Therefore, the potential for the infant to be exposed to higher serum concentrations of parent compounds and metabolites of any medication needs to be considered.

The excretion of medications into breast milk is a complex system (Pons et al., 1994), and there is no evidence of a breast milk–blood barrier for psychotropic medications. The number of women who breast-feed is on the rise, with recent estimates indicating that more than 50% of new mothers who leave the hospital after delivery plan to nurse (Briggs et al., 1996). The excretion of psychotropic medications in breast milk has been reviewed (Buist et al., 1990; Llewellyn & Stowe, 1998; Wisner et al., 1996). The literature is difficult to interpret secondary to differences in the methodology of drug concentration assays. Additionally, there is an identified gradient in breast milk with respect to lipophilic characteristics, and protein content (Kauffman et al., 1994; Vorherr, 1974). Our group found such a gradient and time course for sertraline excretion into breast milk (Stowe et al., 1997b). Time course determinations may become important in creating feeding recommendations for women to reduce infant exposure to medications.

The American Academy of Pediatrics (1994) published a committee report on the excretion of drugs and other chemicals into human breast milk. Although they admit it is not complete, the report's list of psychotropic medications underscores a need to encourage further collaboration between psychiatrists and pediatricians. The Academy's classification of individual psychotropic medications include: (i) medications that are contraindicated during breast-feeding; (ii) drugs whose effect on nursing infants is unknown but may be of concern (i.e. no adverse events have been reported, but the medications are present in human milk and thus conceivably alter CNS development); and (iii) maternal medications usually compatible with breast-feeding. The bulk of antidepressants are listed as unknown, and only lithium is considered contraindicated.

In summary, the physiologic alterations of pregnancy may affect both maternal and fetal serum medication concentrations. The complex nature of excretion into breast milk renders clinical decisions based on milk/plasma ratios speculative (Llewellyn & Stowe, 1998). The clinician should consider monitoring of infant serum concentrations as well as other indices affected by medications (e.g. TSH, electrolytes) and parents should be educated about potential side effects.

## Somatic therapies in pregnancy and lactation

As noted previously, this topic has been extensively reviewed. To date, the Food and Drug Administration (FDA) has not approved any psychotropic medication for use during pregnancy or lactation. The decision of whether or not to use psychotropic medications during pregnancy and/or lactation is not only a difficult clinical decision, but it also carries ethical and potential legal consequences regardless of what decision is made. It is suggested that non-pharmacologic interventions be used prior to psychotropic agents or electroconvulsive therapy (ECT) (Cohen, 1989; Miller, 1991). There are studies by O'Hara (1994) which demonstrate efficacy of interpersonal psychotherapy in the treatment of PPD. In many cases, however, it becomes necessary to try psychopharmacologic treatment intervention. The following is brief overview of the most salient information on the antidepressants, mood stabilizers, benzodiazepines, and ECT.

### Antidepressants

Tricyclic antidepressants have been available in the United States since 1963, and the addition of non-TCA antidepressants has broadened the scope of their use well beyond the treatment of depression. Despite the widespread use of TCAs during pregnancy, no clear association with congenital malformations has been demonstrated (for review, see Elia et al., 1987). Altshuler and colleagues (1996) review 14 studies of in utero exposure to TCAs, both prospective and retrospective in design, representing over 300 000 total live births. Only 13 malformations are noted in 414 first-trimester exposures, an incidence of 3.14%. Similar rates are noted by McElhatton and colleagues (1996) in a review of data from the European Network of Teratology Information Services. This is within the baseline incidence of 2% to 4%. There have been several reports of neonatal withdrawal syndromes associated with in utero exposure to TCAs (Misri & Sivertz, 1991; Prentice & Brown, 1989). Withdrawal symptoms can include: tachypnea, tachycardia, cyanosis, irritability, hypertonia, clonus, and spasm (for review, see Eggermont, 1973; Miller, 1991; for review, see Webster, 1973). The issue of neonatal withdrawal is complicated by the lack of data about maternal dosing during labor. As mentioned previously, Wisner et al. (1993) reported that the TCA dosage requirement for women with depression during pregnancy may increase over the course of pregnancy to maintain adequate therapeutic serum concentrations and response. In contrast to the TCAs, animal studies demonstrate teratogenic effects associated with the MAOIs (Poulson & Robson, 1964). The dietary constraints and potential for hypertensive crisis are relative contraindications to the use of MAOIs during pregnancy (Wisner & Perel, 1988).

The literature on the use of the SSRIs during pregnancy is steadily accumulating, and as a class rivals that of most medications. In one of the first investigations of first-trimester exposure to fluoxetine (mean dose 25.8 mg/day), no demonstrable increase in fetal anomalies is noted among 128 women participants (Pastuszak et al., 1993). The manufacturer's index currently lists over 1700 first-trimester exposures to fluoxetine, with no evidence of an increased incidence of congenital malformations nor a clustering of any particular anomaly (personal communication, Eli Lilly, Inc., 1997). More recently McElhatton et al. (1996) report that, among 92 women treated with SSRI monotherapy during pregnancy, only two cases of major infant malformations were noted. An initial study of paroxetine found no congenital malformations in 63 pregnancies with known first-trimester exposure (Inman et al., 1993). The postmarketing data on fluvoxamine from its use in Europe and the data from clinical trials with sertraline do not demonstrate teratogenic effects but these data have not been published in peer reviewed journals. Extending this data set, a recent publication on 267 women taking SSRIs (sertraline, paroxetine, fluvoxamine) during pregnancy demonstrates no adverse impact on obstetric outcome (Kulin et al., 1998). In contrast, one report indicates that third-trimester fluoxetine exposure is associated with decreased birth weight and an increase in minor anomalies (Chambers et al., 1996). The numerous confounds present in this study, however, make it difficult to render definitive conclusions.

The interpretation of obstetric outcomes is not limited to physical malformations. Pastuszak et al. (1993) note that the rate of spontaneous abortion is higher among SSRI- and TCA-treated women than in controls (14.8%, 12.2%, and 7.8%, respectively). Two groups have found a slight decrease in birth weight among neonates exposed to fluoxetine during pregnancy, but these differences do not achieve statistical significance (Chambers et al., 1993; Nulman et al., 1997). It is possible that this trend towards lower birth weight may be a correlate of maternal mental illness rather than medication exposure. In a landmark study, Nulman and colleagues (1997) conducted extensive neurodevelopmental assessment of children exposed in utero to antidepressant medications (TCA $n = 80$; fluoxetine $n = 55$, no exposure $n = 84$). Children were assessed between 16 and 86 months of age for such factors as global IQ, language development, temperament, mood, activity level, and behavior using numerous study measures and diagnostic tools. The children whose mothers received antidepressants during pregnancy – either fluoxetine or a TCA – did not differ from the no exposure control children on any measure of neurodevelopment. Further, global IQ and language development scores were nearly identical among all groups. In conclusion, 'in utero' exposure to fluoxetine or TCAs did not affect either neurodevelopment or behavior in preschool-aged children.

The use of TCAs in breast-feeding is reviewed (Wisner et al., 1996). This group concludes that TCAs readily enter breast milk, although most parent compounds and metabolites are undetectable in infant serum by 10 weeks of age, and there is no evidence of drug or metabolite accumulation in the neonate. The only exception to this is doxepin, which is present in concentrations of 3 ng/ml in infant serum. Doxepin is also the only TCA associated with an adverse effect on the nursing infant (respiratory depression) (Matheson et al., 1975). Wisner et al. communicates that most TCAs (amitriptyline, nortriptyline, desipramine, clomipramine, and dothiepin) are relatively safe for use during breast-feeding with a preference for the secondary amines.

The SSRI data in breast-feeding now exceeds the data for all other psychotropic medications. Earlier case reports suggested that fluoxetine concentration is disproportionately elevated in infant serum compared to maternal dose (Lester et al., 1993). It is noteworthy that this may not represent accumulation, but rather a higher steady state as repeat infant serum measures are not complete. In contrast, several groups (Kim et al., 1997; Kumar & Robson, 1984; Birnbaum and colleagues – personal communication) do not find evidence of accumulation for fluoxetine in breast-feeding infants. Only a single case report is available for fluvoxamine, in which no adverse effects were shown (Wright et al., 1991). An expanding experience with sertraline (Altshuler et al., 1995; Birnbaum et al., 1999; DeVane, 1992; Epperson et al., 1997; Stowe et al., 1997b; Wisner et al., 1998) demonstrates predominantly undetectable infant serum concentrations. A detailed study of sertraline excretion into breast milk demonstrates both a concentration gradient from 'fore' milk to 'hind' milk and a time course of excretion that parallels the gastrointestinal absorptive phase (Stowe et al., 1997b). Peak concentrations occur 7 to 10 hours following maternal dose and by discarding one feeding (at 7 to 8 hours postmaternal dose), the total daily dose to which an infant is exposed could be cut by nearly 25%. The ability to accurately estimate levels of medication in breast milk would allow the development of individually tailored therapeutic regimens that maximize maternal care while minimizing infant exposure. The follow-up data on infants exposed during breast feeding are sparse. Llewellyn and colleagues (1997) found no adverse effects on growth and milestone achievement in 13 infants exposed to sertraline at 12-month follow up.

In summary, there is currently no evidence that TCAs and SSRIs cause birth defects. The burgeoning data on their use in breast-feeding exceed most other classes of medication, and the infant (while exposed) typically has very low serum concentrations of medications. However, in both in utero and breast-feeding exposures additional long-term follow-up data are needed.

## Mood-stabilizing medications

The primary mood stabilizer utilized in the treatment of refractory depression is lithium carbonate. The Registry of Lithium Babies was established in 1969 for Danish women after cases of congenital malformations following in utero exposure to lithium were reported (Schou, 1976). Registries are now established in Canada and the United States, culminating in the International Register of Lithium Babies. Initial studies suggest a marked increase in cardiovascular malformations, particularly Ebstein's anomaly (Nora et al., 1974; Weinstein & Goldfield, 1975). However, as noted previously, Cohen and colleagues (1994) document an extensive survey of the available information and note an increase in the relative risk ratio of cardiac malformations of 1.2–7.7 and an overall increase in the relative risk for congenital malformations of 1.5–3.0 for in utero lithium exposure. Similarly, Altshuler et al. (1996) find that the risk for Ebstein's anomaly following in utero lithium exposure rose from 1 in 20 000 to 1 in 1000. A 5-year follow-up study of infants exposed to lithium in utero failed to find any significant behavioral, teratogenetic sequele (Schou, 1976). The recent outcome studies on lithium discontinuation and relapse rates for patients with bipolar disorder (Tohen et al., 1990) underscore the need to carefully assess the severity of illness (Cohen et al., 1994) before abrupt discontinuation of lithium. While lithium clearly is a teratogen, the window of risk for cardiac malformation is typically between 4 and 9 weeks' gestation. For women taking lithium during this period, it is recommended that the clinician obtain a level II ultrasound between the 16th and 18th week of gestation to assess cardiac development. In addition to the cardiac risk, the neonate may experience symptoms of toxicity including: flaccidity, lethargy, and poor suck reflexes possibly persisting for over 7 days (Woody et al., 1971). Lithium can also produce reversible changes in thyroid function (Karlsson et al., 1975), cardiac arrhythmia (Wilson et al., 1983), hypoglycemia, and diabetes insipidus (Mizrahi et al., 1979). The previously noted physiological alterations during pregnancy are of importance in the management of lithium. The changes in glomerular filtration rate during and at parturition, along with the associated rapid fluid status changes, and the potential for dehydration warrant close monitoring of lithium levels throughout pregnancy and at delivery.

The utility of anticonvulsants in refractory depression has not been demonstrated, though their widespread use in psychiatry warrants their inclusion. The bulk of the literature on the teratogenic risk of these compounds is derived from studies on the treatment of epilepsy during pregnancy. In utero exposure to both carbamazepine and valproic acid increases the congenital malformation rate in infants of epileptic mothers (Jones et al., 1989; Lindhout & Schimdt, 1986). Fetal serum concentrations of carbamazepine are approximately 50–80% of the maternal concentrations (Nau et al., 1982). The risk for spina bifida associated with fetal exposure to carbamazepine is 1% (relative risk is about 13.7) (Rosa, 1991). Similarly, valproic acid is a known human teratogen with a 1–2% risk of neural tube defects. As noted by Janz (1982), almost all major and minor malformations associated with anticonvulsants are reported from infants of epileptic mothers, confounding direct extrapolation to mood disorders. Intrauterine growth retardation is one of the most commonly cited potential complications of in utero exposure to valproic acid (for review, see Briggs et al., 1996). In contrast to the lithium follow-up data, Gaily and colleagues (1988) compare the IQ of 148 children born to epileptic mothers (both treated and untreated) and 105 control subjects at $5\frac{1}{2}$ years of age. Four of the children of epileptic mothers are mentally deficient or of borderline intelligence, whereas none of the control children has mental deficiencies.

Similar to other psychotropic medications, mood-stabilizing medications are present in breast milk. Nursing infants can achieve serum lithium concentrations that are 40–50% of maternal levels (Schou & Amdisen, 1973; Kirksey & Groziak, 1984). Although there are the reports of infant side effects associated with lithium and nursing, these are confounded by in utero exposure and failure to document infant health status (e.g. hydration exposure to NSAIDs) . The potential for such toxicity warrants close observation of the infant's hydration status and avoidance of NSAIDs. In comparison, both carbamazepine and valproic acid appear in low concentrations in human milk and are both considered compatible with breast-feeding (American Academy of Pediatrics, 1994).

## Anxiolytics

Benzodiazepines (BZD) are among the most commonly used medications for the treatment of anxiety disorders, mixed depression states, and as adjuncts in symptom relief in refractory cases. A recent retrospective survey of the Medicaid records (1980–1983) of 104 339 pregnant women finds that at least 2% receive one or more prescriptions for a benzodiazepine (Bergman et al., 1992). As a class, benzodiazepines readily traverse the placenta, and the presence of benzodiazepines in umbilical cord plasma demonstrates that these drugs show higher fetal circulation concentrations after prolonged administration (Mandelli at al., 1975; Shannon et al., 1971). Early studies report an increased risk of oral clefts following in utero exposure to diazepam (Aarkog, 1975; Saxen, 1975; Saxen & Saxen, 1974); later studies fail to demonstrate this association (Entman & Vaughn, 1984; Rosenberg et al., 1984; Shiono & Mills, 1984). Altshuler and colleagues (1996) pool data from several studies investigating the association of oral cleft with in utero benzodiazepine exposure. They find that, while exposure does confer an increase in risk of oral cleft, the absolute risk increases only 0.01%, from 6 in 10 000 to 7 in 10 000. Like lithium, the clinician should consider the gestational timing of exposure, as the lip and palate develop during weeks 8–14. Outside this window of risk, the utility of benzodiazepines for symptom relief may be relatively safer than other alternatives.

One group describes a 'benzodiazepine exposure syndrome' which includes: growth retardation, dysmorphism, and both mental and psychomotor retardation for infants exposed to these medications in utero (Laegreid et al., 1987). The same group later reported that predominant symptoms are neonatal sedation and withdrawal (Laegreid et al., 1987). A second group that looks at children exposed to chlordiazepoxide finds no increase in incidence of behavioral abnormalities at 8 months of age, and no difference in IQ scores at 4 years of age (Hartz et al., 1975). Lorazepam (Ativan) and oxazepam (Serax) bypass hepatic metabolism, and may therefore have less potential for metabolic accumulation in the neonate. Clonazepam (Klonopin, FDA category C) appears to have minimal teratogenic risks (Sullivan & McElhatton, 1977).

Finally, Buist and colleagues (1990) conclude that benzodiazepines at relatively low doses present no contraindications to nursing. However, long-term follow-up data are lacking.

## Electroconvulsive therapy (ECT)

The use of electroconvulsive therapy in pregnancy has not been associated with an increase in adverse obstetric outcome (Impastato et al., 1964; for review, see Miller

1994b). The majority of the reports predate the rigor and monitoring with which ECT is now conducted. Miller points out that, without proper preparation, the primary complications included: aspiration, aortocaval compression, and respiratory alkalosis. In addition, transient fetal bradycardia (Varan et al., 1985) has been described. A total of 28 complications from 300 cases of ECT in pregnancy have been reported (Miller 1994b); the number of treatments ranged from 2 to 35, and many women had additional risk factors such as prior treatments including insulin coma therapy. Infant follow-up data on 16 infants exposed to ECT in the first or second trimester did not demonstrate developmental or physical abnormalities (Forssman, 1955). Our group recently completed maintenance ECT during the second and third trimester for a woman with refractory depression (Z.N. Stowe, unpublished observation). Guidelines for minimizing complications (for review, see Miller, 1994b) include: limitation of anticholinergic agents, adequate pretreatment hydration, elevation of right hip to avoid compression of abdominal vasculature, and post-treatment monitoring of uterine contractions.

## Augmentation options during pregnancy and lactation

Pharmacological augmentation strategies have not been well documented in pregnancy. It is reasonable to assume that some of the women in the Lithium Registry and in the SSRI and stimulant data bases were taking other medications, though formal documentation, dose, and duration are unknown. Considering the variety of augmentation strategies available (Nemeroff, 1997) and lack of information for use in pregnancy, any recommendations are speculative and empirically derived. Reasonable guidelines include:

(i) Maximize monotherapy – monitor serum concentrations if appropriate
(ii) Rule out medical conditions common in pregnancy (e.g. anemia, thyroid dysfunction)
(iii) Adjunctive psychotherapy
(iv) Diagnostic reconsideration
(v) Consider consultation with Center Specializing in Treatment during Pregnancy
(vi) Electroconvulsive therapy, particularly if first trimester
(vii) Choose augmentation strategies with documented rate of response
(viii) Avoid windows of high teratogenic risk
    Anticonvulsants – Neural tube defects (0–4 weeks' gestation)
    Lithium Carbonate – Cardiac malformations (4–9 weeks' gestation)
    Benzodiazepines – Cleft lip and palate (8–14 weeks' gestation)
(ix) Adding vs. switching medications
    Fetal clearance of psychotropic medications is unknown, therefore chang-

ing medications results in exposure to both. If a partial response has been obtained on one medication, adding is preferable to switching.

(x) Known risk is better than unknown

Newer agents with no reproductive safety data should be avoided.

The clinician enters the realm of unknown when dealing with the majority of pharmacological augmentation strategies. The following general guidelines for completing a risk–benefit assessment and developing management strategies provide the basis for clinical decision-making in the absence of definitive data.

## The risk–benefit assessment

A thorough risk–benefit analysis, taking into account such factors as maternal psychiatric history, potential deleterious effects of untreated illness on both the mother and fetus, and what is known with regard to somatic, perinatal, and long-term neurobehavioral teratogenicity of the different classes of psychotropic medications should be completed for each woman presenting with psychiatric illness during pregnancy and lactation. Table 16.1(a) and 16.1(b) summarizes the basic risk–benefit assessment; these should be individualized, based on prior history and the patient's treatment goals.

Central to the risk–benefit assessment is that the clinician must 'choose a path.' If the decision is to provide somatic therapy in the treatment of affective disorders during pregnancy and lactation, the treatment should be the most efficacious possible, reasonably aggressive, and continuous during the postpartum period. Partial treatment, or symptom reduction approaches leave the patient with both the risks of the illness and of the medication. No decision is risk free, and pregnancy and the postpartum period are not the time to experiment with novel treatment modalities or medications with limited data.

## Clinical guidelines

### General

Because the clinician seldom knows when a patient will conceive, the following steps should be taken in the treatment of affective disorders in women during their reproductive years (e.g. treatment for pregnancy begins prior to conception).

(i) Document method of birth control – this reduces medical–legal liability

(ii) Encourage healthy lifestyle – no tobacco, no alcohol or illicit drugs, weight should be within ±15% of ideal body weight, taking a daily vitamin supplement

(iii) Discourage daily exposure to substances with no reproductive safety data, e.g. herbal, 'natural remedies,' or other chemicals, and, if present, document their use.

**Table 16.1(a).** General risk–benefit assessment – pregnancy

*Known – Pregnancy*

85% of all pregnancies result in live births.

7–14% of deliveries are premature.

2–4% of infants have significant malformations and up to 12% have minor anomalies.

< 3% of malformations are related to environmental or medication factors.

Relatively few medications are known teratogens.

> 80% of all women take at least one prescription medication during pregnancy.

The ideal pregnancy, as defined by the Centers for Disease Control, is ± 15% of the Ideal Body Weight and on Prenatal Vitamins with folic acid for 6 weeks prior to conception.

Most women learn of pregnancy at 5–8 weeks' gestation, therefore may be past window of highest risk.

*Increasing data*

Pregnancy is not protective from psychiatric illness.

Major Depressive Episodes (MDE) demonstrate similar incidence during pregnancy compared to non-gravid periods.

Untreated maternal depression is associated with lower birth weight and preterm delivery.

The teratogenic risk of psychotropic medications has been historically overestimated.

Increasing obstetric outcome and infant follow-up data on psychotropic medications that is comparable in sample size to most other classes of medication.

*Unknown*

The potential long-term impact of untreated maternal psychiatric illness during pregnancy on infant development.

The long-term neurobehavioral effects of in utero exposure to psychotropic medications, though initial studies do not demonstrate adverse impact for several medications.

(iv) Assume patient will conceive soon after psychiatric treatment is initiated. Choose a medicine based on the available data for pregnancy and postpartum. For patients being treated with anticonvulsants, recommend folic acid supplementation.

(v) If pharmacotherapy is indicated, choose a medication based on the following:

- greatest documentation of prior use in pregnancy and lactation – use medications with some published data on relative safety. It is preferable to prescribe medications with a known risk over those with no data; being the first to use a particular medication in pregnancy or lactation is not recommended.

- concordant data – avoid medications with conflicting data; use a clinically comparable alternative if available. This recommendation should also reduce any potential legal liability.

**Table 16.1(*b*).** General risk-benefit assessment – lactation

*Known – postpartum*

> 60% of women plan to breast-feed during the puerperium.

5–17% of all nursing women take a prescription medication during breast-feeding.

12–20% of nursing women smoke cigarettes.

Benefits of breast-feeding to infant.

Supported by all professional organizations as ideal form of nutrition.

The postnatal period is a high-risk time for onset/relapse of psychiatric illness.

All psychotropic medications studied to date are excreted in breast-milk.

*Increasing data*

Untreated maternal mental illness has an adverse impact on mother–infant attachment, and later infant development.

Laboratory data demonstrates long-lasting adverse impact on multiple neuroendocrine and neurotransmitter systems of maternal separation on offspring.

Adverse effects of psychotropic agents on infants are limited to case reports.

Nursing infant daily dose of psychotropic agents is less than maternal daily dose.

Psychotropic medications are excreted into breast-milk with specific individual time course allowing for minimizing infant exposure while continuation of breast-feeding.

*Unknown*

The long-term neurobehavioral effects of breast-feeding exposure to psychotropic medications.

- fewer side effects – medications with fewer hypotensive and anticholinergic side effects are preferable. Additionally, medications that affect seizure threshold and potentially interact with commonly used obstetric anesthetic and analgesic agents should be minimized.
- maximize monotherapy – considerable data exists on single medications. However, when two or more medications are used, reproductive outcome data are essentially unknown. The bulk of clinical data on medication dose were not obtained in women of reproductive years.

(vi) Provide the patient and significant other(s) with educational materials. Educational materials from peer-reviewed journals and review-type articles can often be of benefit to patients and foster questions. Support group literature can also be of benefit (e.g. Depression After Delivery, Postpartum Support International, the American Association of Breastfeeding Medicine, and the Marce Society).

(vii) Document the patient's perception of elective termination. Considering the high rate of inadvertent conceptions and the potential impact of mood state on decision processes – knowing this information prior to conception provides the clinician with a framework for obstetric or mental status assessments if, for instance, a patient relapses and her views on termination dramatically change (e.g. patient does not view termination as option based on religious and or personal convictions; then she inadvertently conceives and medications are discontinued or tapered. Later, she relapses and while severely depressed requests an elective abortion – what is the clinician's role?).

## Inadvertent conception

Inadvertent conception is probably the most common clinical situation encountered. The primary rule is 'don't panic' – the bulk of exposure during the high risk period for organ teratogenesis has already occurred and the clinician should be mindful not to change treatment secondary to his/her anxiety, but rather base the clinical decision on patient's history and desire.

(i) Do not abruptly discontinue medications – lithium and BZD are the only psychotropics with a known gestational window of risk where the clinician has the opportunity to intervene. Abrupt discontinuation increases the risk for clinical confusion of psychiatric disorder with withdrawal syndrome and relapse of illness.

(ii) Discuss and document a comprehensive risk–benefit assessment.

(iii) Retrospectively document all environmental exposures (e.g. medications, toxins), starting at approximately 6 weeks before knowledge of pregnancy and continued through entire pregnancy.

(iv) If medication discontinuation is indicated or desired – develop treatment plan while patient is euthymic for possibility of relapse and/or postpartum prevention. The clinician should also discuss criteria (number of symptoms, functional impairment) for intervention at this time.

(v) Minimize all other exposures (e.g. tobacco, alcohol).

(vi) Start Prenatal Vitamins (PNV). Often patients do not start PNV until first obstetric visit, and their initial communication may be with a psychiatrist.

(vii) If history of drug abuse or any suspicion – obtain urine drug screen. While not cost effective, we encourage obtaining a urine toxicology screen at the slightest indication, and documenting the rationale when one is not obtained.

(viii) A reduction in number of medications may be warranted, though substitution to an agent with more reproductive data is not. Once conception has occurred, to change medications to one with greater data (hence the general recommendations above) actually increases the fetal exposure to the total number of medications. The safety data was not derived from populations where such changes were made. A similar approach would apply to breast-feeding. For example, if a woman takes a particular medication during pregnancy, changing to an agent with greater breast-feeding data at delivery is actually increasing neonatal exposure by adding exposure to a second medication. Again, starting a new medication during the high risk postpartum period is not recommended.

## Planned conception

Should a patient want to stay on medication until pregnancy is confirmed and then attempt a taper, the following procedures are recommended:

(i) Confirm ovulation. Attempt to confirm ovulation time by using basal body temperature records or ovulation test kits.

(ii) Assess for seasonal variation of illness. If the patient's history demonstrates a seasonal component, attempt to plan conception to occur so that first trimester is timed with season of best affect. This can offer a window in which successful medication taper is possible.

(iii) Monitor current treatment strategies prior to conception. Measure serum concentrations of medications several times if possible before conception. In case of unsuccessful or undesired medication taper, knowing prepregnancy concentrations can aid in clinical decisions to increase medication dosage. These levels will change in pregnancy.

(iv) Treat with the minimum effective dose for every medication in each patient.

(v) Discuss and document treatment plan. Before the pregnancy occurs, discuss and document with the patient, the treatment plan for preconception and each trimester of the pregnancy Discuss what severity of symptoms and which symptoms will indicate reinstitution of pharmacologic treatment or increase in dose. Document what obstetric assessments you recommend and when (maternal AFP, level II USG, amniocentesis).

## Management in pregnancy

For women whose history or choice indicates no or minimal exposure:

(i) Taper medications. Taper medications (ones of greatest concern, e.g. lithium, anticonvulsants, stimulants) over 3–5 days following completion of the menses and hope they get pregnant quickly. Uterine/placental blood does not establish for 10–12 days and this method will minimize fetal exposure.

(ii) Conduct weekly home pregnancy tests. Begin tests 2 weeks after ovulation and intercourse so that gestational timing will be known for remainder of pregnancy with respect to specific windows of teratogenic risk. This can provide a method for minimizing exposure to medications during their greatest windows of risk (4–9 weeks' gestation for lithium, and 8–14 weeks' gestation for BZD).

(iii) History of illness, impairment, duration to stabilize, and risk of harm should guide the decision about medication discontinuation.

(iv) Avoid additional medications. Some medications place an increased metabolic load on the fetal system (e.g. NSAIDs and lithium, or acetominophen and anticonvulsants). Avoid multiple medications to treat symptoms of the mental illness; it may be preferable to increase dose than to expose the fetus to more than one medication for the same illness.

(v) Monitor serum concentrations. Monitor concentrations throughout pregnancy and adjust medication to maintain therapeutic levels. The majority of dose increases in previous studies occurred in the late second trimester.

(vi) Obstetric monitoring is recommended. Obstetric tests recommended include: Level II USG at 16 weeks gestation for lithium and anticonvulsants to evaluate fetal heart and vertebral body formation.

(vii) Prepare for labor and delivery. During labor and delivery anticipate rapid alterations in serum concentrations changes of psychotropic medications due to stress and rapid volume change. One must also anticipate a high likelihood of exposure to other medications.

(viii) Monitor neonate for signs of toxicity and/or withdrawal.

## Management during postpartum period and lactation

The high risk of relapse for women with affective disorders in the postpartum period and the documented adverse impact of maternal depression on infant well-being warrants continuation of treatment. The benefits of breast-feeding are well documented and all professional organizations support breast-feeding. Guidelines concerning the use of psychotropic medications during lactation are sparse. A reasonable set of general guidelines includes:

(i) Do not change to a novel treatment modality during the postpartum period.

(ii) Discuss rationale for breast-feeding. The impact on maternal sleep and continued neonatal exposure to medications may not warrant a trial of breast-feeding.

(iii) Infant serum monitoring should be routine and should include other indices affected by medications (lithium – TSH, chemistry; anticonvulsants – liver enzymes, platelets, etc.). The frequency of such monitoring should exceed adult monitoring and be repeated if any suspected clinical alterations occur in the infant.

(iv) Caution patient about inadvertent conception while breast-feeding.

## Conclusions

The lack of large-scale epidemological studies regarding the adverse effects of untreated major psychiatric illness on the fetus or infant vs. the potential adverse effect of psychopharmacological treatment prevents the development of widely applicable treatment algorithms for managing the treatment of pregnant or postpartum women with existing and/or new-onset psychiatric illness. Pregnant and nursing women are generally excluded in clinical studies of novel pharmacological agents, and routine postmarketing registries are not maintained by most pharmaceutical companies; thereby limiting the available data. It is doubtful that well-controlled studies will ever be conducted. It has been suggested that conducting such studies in pregnant and nursing women is unethical (Kerns, 1986). An opposing view is that failure to conduct such studies increases the overall risk to women and infants over time and may deprive some women of adequate treatment.

The lack of data concerning the frequency of conception in women with treatment-resistant illness, and of the incidence of treatment-resistant illness in pregnancy and the postpartum period precludes an appreciation of how often these situations are encountered. The guidelines and risk–benefit assessment presented in this chapter are consistent with those at our center and can be applied to other categories of psychiatric illnesses. In summary, pregnancy and lactation may complicate psychiatric treatment but do not preclude it.

## REFERENCES

Aarkog, D. (1975). Association between maternal intake of diazepam and oral clefts (letter). *Lancet*, **ii**, 921.

Affonson, D.D., Lovett, S., Paul S.M. et al. (1990). A standardized interview that differentiates pregnancy and postpartum symptoms from perinatal clinical depression. *Birth*, **17**, 121–30.

Altshuler, L.L., Burt, V.K., McMullen, M., & Hendrick, V. (1995). Breastfeeding and sertraline: a 24-hour analysis. *Journal of Clinical Psychiatry*, **56**, 243–5.

Altshuler, L.L., Cohen, L., Szuba, M.P. et al. (1996). Pharmacologic management of psychiatric illness during pregnancy: dilemmas and guidelines. *American Journal of Psychiatry*, **153**, 592–606.

American Academy of Pediatrics, Committee on Drugs (1994). The transfer of drugs and other chemicals into human breast milk. *Pediatrics*, **93**, 137–50.

American Psychiatric Association. *Diagnostic and Statistical Manual of Mental Disorders.*(1994). 4th edn, Washington, DC.

Appleby, L. (1991). Suicide during pregnancy and in the first postnatal year. *British Medical Journal*, **302**, 137–40.

Appleby, L., Warner, R., Whitton A. et al. (1997). A controlled study of fluoxetine and cognitive-behavioral counseling in the treatment of postnatal depression. *British Medical Journal*, **314**, 932–6.

Atkinson, H.C., Begg, E.J., & Darlow, B.A. (1988). Drugs in human milk: clinical pharamacokinetic considerations. *Clinical Pharmacokinetics*, **14**, 217–40.

Avant, K. (1981). Anxiety as a potential factor affecting maternal attachment. *Journal of Obstetrics, Gynecology and Neonatal Nursing*, **10**, 416–19.

Beck, C.T. (1995). Screening methods for postpartum depression. *Journal of Obstetrics, Gynecology and Neonatal Nursing*, **24**, 308–12.

Bergman, U., Rosa, F.W., Baum, C. et al. (1992). Effects of exposure to benzodiazapine during fetal life. *Lancet*, 694–6.

Birnbaum, Cohen, L.S., Bailey, J.W., Grush, L.R., Robertson, L.M., & Stowe, Z.N. (1999). Serum concentrations of antidepressants and benzodiazapines in nursing infants: a case series. *Pediatrics*, **104**, e11.

Boobis, A.R. & Lewis, P.J. (1983). Pharmacokinetics in pregnancy. In *Clinical Pharmacology in Obstetrics*, ed. P. Lewis, pp. 6–54. Boston, MA: Wright-PSG.

Bowlby, J. (1951). Maternal care and mental health. *WHO Monograph Series*, **2**, Geneva: World Health Organization.

Brazelton, T.B. (1975). Mother infant reciprocity. In *Maternal Attachment and Mothering Disorders: A Roundtable*, ed. M.H. Klaus, T. Leger, & M.A. Trause, pp. 49–54. North Bruswick, NJ: Johnson and Johnson.

Briggs, G.G., Freeman, R.K., & Yaffe, S.J. (1996). *Drugs in Pregnancy and Lactation*, 4th edn, vol. 9, No. 1, Williams & Wilkins, Baltimore, MD.

Buist, A., Norman, T.R., & Dennerstein, L. (1990). Breastfeeding and the use of psychotropic medication: a review. *Journal of Affective Disorders*, **19**, 197–206.

Campbell, S.B., Cohn, J.F., & Meyers, T. (1995) Depression in first-time mothers: mother–infant interaction and depression chronicity. *Developmental Psychology*, **31**, 349–57.

Chambers, C.D., Johnson, K.A., & Jones, K.L. (1993). Pregnancy outcome in women exposed to fluoxetine. *Reproductive Toxicology*, **7**, 155–6.

Chambers, C.D., Johnson, K.A., Dick, L.M. et al. (1996). Birth outcomes in pregnant women taking fluoxetine. *New England Journal of Medicine*, **335**, 1010–15.

Cogill, S.R., Caplan, H.L., & Alexandra, H. (1986). Impact of maternal postnatal depression on cognitive development of young children. *British Medical Journal*, **292**, 1165–6.

Cohen, L.S. (1989). Psychotropic drug use in pregnancy. *Hospital and Community Psychiatry*, **40**, 566–7.

Cohen, L.S., Friedman, J.M., Jefferson, J.W. et al. (1994). A reevaluation of risk of in utero exposures to lithium. *Journal of the American Medical Association*, **2**, 146–50.

Cooper, P.J. & Murray, L. (1995). Course and recurrence of postnatal depression: evidence for the specificity of the diagnostic concept. *British Journal of Psychiatry*, **166**, 191–5.

Cradon, A.J. (1979). Maternal anxiety and neonatal wellbeing. *Journal of Psychosomatical Research*, **23**, 113–15.

Cutrona, C.E. & Troutman, B.R. (1986). Social support, infant temperament, and parenting self-efficacy: a mediational model of postpartum depression. *Child Development*, **57**, 1507–18.

DeVane, C.L. (1992). Pharmacokinetics of the selective serotonin reuptake inhibitors. *Journal of Clinical Psychiatry*, **53** (Feb Suppl), 13–20.

Doering, J.C. & Stewart, R.B. (1978). The extent and character of drug consumption during pregnancy. *Journal of the American Medical Association*, **239**, 843–6.

Duffy, C.L. (1983). Postpartum depression: identifying women at risk. *Genesis*. June/July 11 & 21.

Eggermont, E. (1973). Withdrawal symptoms in neonates associated with maternal imipramine therapy. *Lancet*, **ii**, 680.

Elia, J., Katz, I.R., & Simpson, G.M. (1987). Teratogenicity of psychotherapeutic medications. *Psychopharmacol Bulletin*, **23**, 531–86.

Entman, S.S. & Vaughn, W.K. (1984) Lack of relation of oral clefts to diazepam use in pregnancy. *New England Journal of Medicine*, **310**, 1121–2.

Epperson, C.N., Anderson, G.M., & McDougle, C.J. (1997) Sertraline and breast-feeding (letter to the editor). *New England Journal of Medicine*, **336**, 1189–90.

Field, T., Healy, B., Goldstein, S. et al. (1988). Infants of depressed mothers show 'depressed' behavior even with nondepressed adults. *Child Development*, **59**, 1569–79.

Field, T., Healy, B., & LeBlanc, W.G. (1989). Sharing and synchrony of behavior states and heart rate in non-depressed versus depressed mother–infant interactions. *Infant Behavior and Development*, **12**, 357–76.

Field, T., Healy, B., Goldstein, S., & Guthertz, M. (1990). Behavior-state matching and synchrony in mother–infant interactions of nondepressed versus depressed dyads. *Developmental Psychology*, **26**, 7–14.

Forssman, H. (1955). Follow-up study of sixteen children whose mothers sere given electric convulsive therapy during gestation. *Acta Psychiatrica et Neurologica Scandinavica*, **30**, 437–41.

Gaily, E., Kantola-Sorsa, E., & Granstrom, M. L. (1988). Intelligence of children of epileptic mothers. *Journal of Pediatrics*, **113**, 677–84.

Harlow, H.F., & Harlow, H.F. (1962). Social deprivation of monkeys. *Scientific American*, **207**, 136–46.

Harris, B. (1993). A hormonal component to postnatal depression. *British Journal of Psychiatry*, **163**, 403–5.

Harris, B., Lovett, L., Roberts, S. et al. (1993). Cardiff puerperal mood and hormone study. *Hormone Research*, **39**, 138–45.

Hartz, S.C., Heinonen, O.P., Shapiro, S. et al. (1975). Antenatal exposure to meprobamate and chlordiazepoxide in relation to malformations, mental development, and childhood mortality. *New England Journal of Medicine*, **292**, 726–8.

Hedegaard, M., Henriksen, T.B., Sabroe, S. et al. (1993). Psychological distress in pregnancy and preterm delivery. *British Medical Journal*, **307**, 234–9.

Heinonen, O.P., Stone, D., & Shapiro, S. (1977). *Birth Defects and Drugs In Pregnancy*. Littleton MA: Publishing Sciences Group.

Impastato, D.J., Gabriel, A.R., & Lardaro, H.H. (1964). Electric and insulin shock therapy during pregnancy. *Diseases of the Nervous System*, **25**, 542–6.

Inman, W., Kubotu, K., & Pearce, G. (1993). Prescription event monitoring of paroxetine.

*Prescription Event Monitoring Reports*, 1–44.

Janz, D. (1982). Antiepileptic drugs and pregnancy: altered utilization patterns and teratogenesis. *Epilepsia*, **23**(Suppl 1), S53–S63.

Jones, K.L., Larco, R.V., Johnson, K.A. et al. (1989). Pattern of malformations in the children of women treated with carbamazepine during pregnancy. *New England Journal of Medicine*, **320**, 1661–9.

Karlsson, K., Lindstedy, G., & Lundberg, P.A. (1975). Transplacental lithium poisoning: reversible inhibition of fetal thyroid (letter). *Lancet*, **i**, 1295.

Kauffman, R.E., Banner, W. Jr, & Berline, C.M. Jr (1994). The transfer of drugs and other chemicals into human milk. *Pediatrics*, **93**, 137–50.

Kendall, R.E., Chalmers, J.C., & Platz, C. (1987). Epidemiology of puerperal psychosis. *British Journal of Psychiatry*, **150**, 662–73.

Kerns, L.L. (1986). Treatment of mental disorders in pregnancy: a review of psychotrophic drug risks and benefits. **174**, 652–9.

Kiely, M. (1991). *Reproductive and Perinatal Epidemiology*. Boca Raton, FL: CRC Press.

Kim, J., Misri, S., Riggs, K.W. et al. (1997). Stereoselective excretion of fluoxetine and norfluoxetine in breast milk and neonatal exposures. American Psychiatric Association Annual Meeting. San Diego, CA.

Kirksey, A. & Groziak, S.M. (1984). Maternal drug use: evaluation of risks to breast-fed infants. *World Review of Nutrition and Dietetics*, **43**, 60–79.

Kitamura, T., Shima, S., Sugawara, M. et al. (1993). Psychological and social correlates of the onset of affective disorders among pregnant women. *Psychological Medicine*, **23**, 967–75.

Klein, M.H., & Essex, M.J. (1995). Pregnant or depressed? The effect of overlap between symptoms of depression and somatic complaints of pregnancy on rates of major depression in the second trimester. *Depression*, **2**, 308–14.

Koren, G., Pastuszak, A., & Ito, S. (1998). Drugs in pregnancy. *New England Journal of Medicine*, **338**, 1128–37.

Kulin, N.A., Pastuszak, A., Sage, S.R. et al. (1998). Pregnancy outcome following maternal use of the new selective serotonin reuptake inhibitors. *Journal of the American Medical Association*, **279**, 609–10.

Kumar, R. & Robson, K.M. (1984). A prospective study of emotional disorders in childbearing women. *British Journal of Psychiatry*, **144**, 35–47.

Laegreid, L., Olegard, R., Walstrom, J. et al. (1987). Teratogenic effects of benzodiazepine use during pregnancy. *Journal of Pediatrics*, **114**, 126–31.

Lester, B.M., Cucca, J., Andreozzi, L. et al. (1993). Possible assocation between fluoxetine hydrochloride and colic in an infant. *Journal of the American Academy of Child and Adolescent Psychiatry*, **32**, 1253–5.

Lindhout, D. & Schimdt, D. (1986). In utero exposure to valproate and neural tube defects. *Lancet*, **i**, 329–33.

Llewellyn, A. & Stowe, Z.N. (1998). Psychotropic medications in lactation. *Journal of Clinical Psychiatry*, **59**(Suppl. 2).

Llewellyn, A.M., Stowe, Z.N., & Nemeroff, C.B. (1997). Infant outcome after sertraline exposure. American Psychiatric Association Annual Meeting.

Llewellyn, A., Stowe, Z.N., Hostetter, A., & Strader, J.R. (1998). Suicidal Ideation in Pregnancy. Poster Session. American Psychiatric Association Annual Meeting. Toronto, Canada.

McBride, W.G. (1972). Limb deformities associated with iminodibenzyl hydrochloride. *Medical Journal of Australia*, **1**, 175–8.

McElhatton, P.R., Garbis, H.M., Elefant, E. et al. (1996). The outcome of pregnancy in 689 women exposed to therapuetic doses of antidepressants. A collaborative study of the European Network of Teratology Information Services (ENTIS). *Reproductive Toxicology*, **10**, 285–94.

McEwen, B.S., Gould, E.A., & Sakai, R.R. (1992). The vulnerability of the hippocampus to protective and destructive effects of glucocorticoids in relation to stress. *British Journal of Psychiatry*, **15**, 18–23.

McGorry, P. & Conell, S. (1990). The nosology and prognosis of puerperal psychosis: a review. *Comprehensive Psychiatry*, **31**, 519–34.

McNeil, T.F., Kaij, L., & Malmquist-Larsson, A. (1984a). Women with nonorganic psychosis: mental disturbance during pregnancy. *Acta Psychiatrica Scandinavica*, **70**, 127–39.

McNeil, T.F., Kaij, L., & Malmquist-Larsson, A. (1984b). Women with nonorganic psychosis: pregnancy's effect on mental health during pregnancy. *Acta Psychiatrica Scandinavica*, **70**, 140–8.

Mandelli, M., Morselli, P.L., Nordio, S. et al. (1975). Placental transfer of diazepam and its disposition in the newborn. *Clinical Pharmacology and Therapeutics*, **17**, 564–72.

Matheson, I., Pande, H., & Alertsen, A.R. (1985). Respiratory depression caused by N-desmethyldoxepin in breast milk. *Lancet*, **16**, 1124.

Matthew, K., Scott H.F., Wilkinson, L.S. et al. (1996). Retarded acquisition and reduced expression of conditional locomotor activity in adult rats following repeated early maternal separation: effects of prefeeding, D-amphetamine, dopamine antagonists, and clonidine. *Psychopharmacology*, **26**, 75–84.

Miller, L.J. (1991). Clinical strategies for the use of psychotropic drugs during pregnancy. *Psychiatric Medicine*, **9**, 275–99.

Miller, L.J. (1994a). Psychiatric medication during pregnancy: understanding and minimizing the risks. *Psychiatric Annals*, **24**, 69–75.

Miller, L.J. (1994b). Use of electroconvulsive therapy during pregnancy. *Hospital and Community Psychiatry*, **45**, 1994.

Misri, S. & Sivertz, K. (1991). Tricyclic drugs in pregnancy and lactation: a preliminary report. *International Journal of Psychiatry in Medicine*, **21**, 157–71.

Mizrahi, E.M., Hobbs, J.F., & Goldsmith, D.I. (1979). Nephrogenic diabetes insipidus in transplacental lithium intoxication. *Journal of Pediatrics*, **94**, 493–5.

Murray, L. & Cooper, P.J. (1996). The impact of postpartum depression on child development. *International Review Psychiatry*, **8**, 55–63.

Nau, H., Kuhnz, W., Egger, H.J. et al. (1982). Anticonvulsants during pregnancy and lactation: transplacental maternal and neonatal pharmacokinetcs. *Clinical Pharmacokinetics*, **7**, 508–43.

Nemeroff, C.B. (1997). Augmentation strategies in patients with refractory depression. *Depression and Anxiety*, **4**, 169–81.

Neziroglu, F., Anemone, R., & Yaryura, T.J.A. (1992). Onset of obsessive compulsive disorder in pregnancy. *American Journal of Psychiatry*, **149**, 947–50.

Nora, J.J., Nora, A.H., & Toews, W.H. (1974). Lithium, Ebstein's anomaly, and other congenital heart defects. *Lancet*, **ii**, 594–5.

Nulman, I., Rovet, J., Stewart, D.E. et al. (1997). Neurodevelopment of children exposed in utero to antidepressant drugs. *New England Journal of Medicine*, **336**, 258–62.

O'Hara, M.W. (1986). Social support, life events and depression during pregnancy and the puerperium. *Archives of General Psychiatry*, **43**, 569–73.

O'Hara M.W. (1991). Postpartum mental disorders. In *Gynecology and Obstetrics*, ed. W. Droegemeuller & J. Sciarra. PA: J.B. Lippincott Company.

O'Hara, M.W. (1994). Psychosocial Therapies in the Peripartum Period (paper presentation) Washington DC: Workshop on mental disorders during pregnancy.

O'Hara, M.W., Rehm, L.P., & Campbell, S.B. (1982). Predicting depressive symptomology: cognitive-behavioural models and postpartum depression. *Journal of Abnormal Psychology*, **91**, 457–61.

O'Hara, M.W., Neunaber, D.J., & Zekoski, E.M. (1984). Prospective study of postpartum depression: prevalence, course, and predictive factors. *Journal of Abnormal Psychology* , **93**, 158–71.

O'Hara, M.W., Zekoski, E.M., Phillips, L.H. et al. (1990). Controlled prospective study of postpartum mood disorders: comparison of childbearing and non-childbearing women. *Journal of Abnormal Psychology*, **99**, 3–15.

Pastuszak, A., Schick-Boschetto, B., Zuber, C. et al. (1993). Pregnancy outcome following first trimester exposure to fluoxetine (Prozac). *Journal of the American Medical Association*, **269**, 2246–8.

Pedersen, C.A., Stern, R.A., Pate, J. et al. (1993). Thyroid and adrenal measures during late pregnancy and the puerperium in women who have been mafor depressed of who become dysphoric postpartum. *Journal of Affective Disorders*, **29**, 201–11.

Perkin, R., Bland, J.M., Peacock, J.L., & Anderson, R. (1993). The effect of anxiety and depression during pregnancy on obstetrical complications. *Journal of Obstetrics and Gynecology*, **100**, 629–34.

Playfair, H.R., & Gowers, J.I. (1981). Depression following childbirth: a search for predictive signs. *Journal of the Royal College of General Practitioners*, **31**, 201–8.

Plotsky, P.M. & Meaney, M.J. (1993). Early, postnatal experience alters hypothalamic corticotropin-releasing factor (CRF) mRNA, median eminence Crf content and stress-induced release in adult rats. *Molecular Brain Research*, **18**, 195–200.

Polster, D.S. & Wisner, K. L. (1999). ECT-induced premature labor: a case report [letter]. *Journal of Clinical Psychiatry*, **60**, 53–4.

Pons, G., Rey, W., & Matheson, I. (1994). Excretion of psychoactive drugs into breast milk. *Clinical Pharmacokinetics in Special Populations*, **27**, 270–89.

Poulson, E. & Robson, J.M. (1964). Effect of phenelzine and some related compounds in pregnancy. *Journal of Endocrinology*, **30**, 205–15.

Prentice, A. & Brown, R. (1989). Fetal tachyarrhythmia and maternal antidepressant treatment. *British Medical Journal*, **298**, 190.

Pugh, T.F., Jerath, B.K., Schmidt, W.M. et al. (1963). Rates of mental disease related to childbearing. (1963). *New England Journal of Medicine*, **268**, 1224–8.

Rayburn, W.F. & Andresen, B.D. (1982). Principles of perinatal pharmacology. In Drug *Therapy in Obstetrics and Gynecology*, ed. W.F. Rayburn & F. Zuspan, pp. 1–8. Norwalk, CT: Appleton-Century-Crofts.

Riccardi, V.M. (1977). *The Genetic Approach to Human Disease.* New York, NY: Oxford University Press.

Richards, J.P. (1990). Postnatal depression: a review of recent literature. *British Journal of General Practice*, **40**, 472–6.

Robinson, H.E., Stewart, D.E., & Flak, E. (1986). The rational use of psychotrophic drugs in pregnancy and postpartum. *Canadian Journal of Psychiatry*, **31**, 183–90.

Rosa, F.W. (1991). Spina bifida in infants of women treated with carbamazepine during pregnancy. *New England Journal of Medicine*, **324**, 674–7.

Rosenberg, A.J. & Silver, E. (1965). Suicide, psychiatrists, and therapeutic abortion. *California Medicine*, **102**, 407–11.

Rosenberg, L., Mitchell, A.A., Parsells, J.L. et al. (1984). Lack of relation of oral clefts to diazepam use during pregnancy. *New England Journal of Medicine*, **309**, 1281–5.

Sadler, T.W. (ed) (1985). *Langman's Medical Embryology*, 5th edn, Baltimore, MD: Williams & Wilkens.

Saxen, I. (1975). Association between oral clefts and drugs taken during pregnancy. *International Journal of Epidemiology*, **4**, 37–44.

Saxen, I. & Saxen, L. (1974) Association between maternal intake of diazepam and oral clefts (letter). *Lancet*, **2**, 498.

Schou, M. (1976). What happened later to the lithium babies?: follow-up study of children born without malformations. *Acta Psychiatrica Scandinavica*, **54**, 193–7.

Schou, M. & Amdisen, A. (1973). Lithium and pregnancy, III: lithium ingestion by children breast-fed by women on lithium treatment. *British Medical Journal*, **2**, 138.

Shannon, R.W., Fraser, G.P., & Aitken, R.G. et al. (1971). Diazepam in preeclamptic toxaemia with special reference to its effect on the newborn infant. *British Journal of Clinical Practice*, **26**, 271–5.

Shiono, P.H. & Mills, J.L. (1984). Oral clefts and diazepam use during pregnancy (letter). *New England Journal of Medicine*, **311**, 919–20.

Sibert, T.E. (1993). Recognizing and treating postpartum depression. Greenwich. (Report #11).

Sichel, D.A., Cohen, L.S., Rosenbaum, J.F. et al. (1993). Postpartum onset of obsessive-compulsive disorder. *Psychosomatics*, **34**, 277–9.

Sim, M. (1963). Abortion and the psychiatrist. *British Medical Journal*, **5350**, 145–8.

Statham, A. (1998). Current evidence from animal investigations of a role for early mother–infant relationships in the aetiology of major depressive illness. *Neurosciences in Psychiatry*, **1**, 40–4.

Steer, R.A., Scholl, T.O., Hediger, M.L., & Fisher, R.L. (1992). Self-reported depression and negative pregnancy outcomes. *Epidemiology*, **45**, 1093–9.

Stowe, Z.N. & Nemeroff, C.B. (1995a). Psychopharmacology during pregnancy and lactation. In *APA Textbook of Psychopharmacology*, ed. Schatzberg & C.B. Nemeroff, pp. 823–37. Washington, DC: APA Press.

Stowe, Z.N. & Nemeroff, C.B. (1995b). Women at risk for postpartum-onset major depression. *American Journal of Obstetrics and Gynecology*, **173**, 639–45.

Stowe, Z.N., Landry, J.C., Porter, M.F., & Nemeroff, C.B. (1995). The Use of Depression Rating Scales in Women with Postpartum Depression. *American Psychiatric Association*. Abstract.

Stowe, Z.N., Llewellyn, A.M., Strader, J.R. et al. (1997a). Placental passage of antidepressants. American Psychiatric Association Annual Meeting. Abstract.

Stowe, Z.N., Owens, M., Landry, J.C. et al. (1997b). Sertraline and desmethylsertraline in human breast milk and nursing infants. *American Journal of Psychiatry*, **154**, 1255–60.

Stowe, Z.N., Hostetter, A., Cox, M., Ritchie, J.C., & Owens, M.J. (1998). SSRIs In Breastmilk and Nursing Infants. *American Psychiatric Association*. (submitted)

Strader, R., Baugh, C.L., Llewellyn, A.M., & Stowe, Z.N. (1997). Predictors of treatment response in postpartum depression. American Psychiatric Association Annual Meeting. Abstract.

Stuart, S. & O'Hara, M.W. (1995). Interpersonal psychotherapy for postpartum depression: a treatment program. *Journal of Psychotherapy Practice and Research*, **4**, 18–29.

Sullivan, F.M. & McElhatton, P.R. (1977). A comparison of the teratogenic activity of the antiepileptic drugs carbamazepine, clonazepam, ethosuximide, phenobarbital, phenytoin, and pyrimidone in mice. *Toxicology and Applied Pharmacology*, **40**, 365–78.

Sutanto, W., Rosenfeld, P., de Kloet, E.R. et al. (1996). Long-term effects of neonatal maternal deprivation and ACTH on hippocampal mineralocorticoid and glucocorticoid receptors. *Developmental Brain Research*, **92**, 156–63.

Teti, D.M., Messinger, D.S, Gelfand, D.M. et al. (1995). Maternal depression and the quality of early attachment: an examination of infants, preschoolers, and their mothers. *Developmental Psychology*, **31**, 364–76.

Tohen, M., Waternaux, C.M., & Tsuang MT. (1990). Outcome in mania: a 4-year prospective follow-up of 75 patients utilizing survival analysis. *Archives of General Psychiatry*, **47**, 1106–11.

Troutman, B. & Cutrona, C. (1990). Nonpsychotic postpartum depression among adolescent mothers. *Journal of Abnormal Psychology*, **99**, 69.

Varan, L.R., Gillieson M.S., Skene D.S. et al. (1985). ECT in an acutely psychotic pregnant woman with actively aggressive (homicidal) impulses. *Canadian Journal of Psychiatry*, **30**, 363–7.

Vorherr, H. (1974). Drug excretion in breast milk. *Postgraduate Medicine*, **56**, 97–104.

Warner, A. (1986). Drug use in the neonate: inter-relationships of pharmacokinetics, toxicity and biochemical maturity. *Clinical Chemistry*, **32**, 721–7.

Watson, J.P., Elliot, S.A., Rugg, A.J. et al. (1984). Psychiatric disorder in pregnancy and the first postnatal year. *British Journal of Psychiatry*, **147**, 453–62.

Webster P.A.C. (1973). Withdrawal symptoms in neonates associated with maternal antidepressant therapy. *Lancet*, **ii**, 318–19.

Weinstein, M.R. & Goldfield, M.D. (1975). Cardiovascular malformations with lithium use during pregnancy. *American Journal of Psychiatry*, **132**, 529–31.

Weissman, N.M. & Olfson, M. (1995). Depression in women: implications for health care research. *Science*, **269**, 799–801.

Welch, R. & Findlay, J. (1981). Excretion of drugs in human breast milk. *Drug Metabolism Review*, **12**, 261–77.

Whiffen, V.E. & Gotlib, I.H. (1989). Infants of postpartum depressed mothers: temperament and cognitive status. *Journal of Abnormal Psychology*, **98**, 274–9.

Wilson, N., Forfar, J.C., & Godman, M.J. (1983). Atrial flutter in the newborn resulting from maternal lithium ingestion. *Archives of Disease in Childhood*, **58**, 538–49.

Wisner, K.L. & Perel, J.M. (1988). Psychopharmacologic agents and electroconvulsive therapy during pregnancy and the puerperium. In *Psychiatric Consultation in Childbirth Settings: Parent- and Child-Oriented Approaches*, ed. R.L. Cohen, pp. 165–206. New York: Plenum Medical Book Company.

Wisner, K.L., Perel, J.M., & Wheeler, S.B. (1993). Tricyclic dosage requirements across pregnancy, *Amererican Journal of Psychiatry*, **150**, 1541–2.

Wisner, K.L., Perel, J.M., & Findling, R.L. (1996). Antidepressant treatment during breast-feeding. *American Journal of Psychiatry*, **159**, 1132–7.

Wisner, K.L., Perel, J.M., & Blumer, J. (1998). Serum sertraline and n-desmethylsertraline levels in breast-feeding mother–infant pairs. *American Journal of Psychiatry*, **155**, 690–2.

Wood, S.M. & Hytten, F.E. (1981). The fate of drugs in pregnancy. *Clinical Obstetrics and Gynecology*, **8**, 255–9.

Woody, J. et al. (1971). Lithium toxicity in a newborn. *Pediatrics*, **47**, 94–6.

Wright, S., Dawling, S., & Ashford, J.J. (1991). Excretion of fluvoxamine in breast milk. *British Journal of Clinical Pharmacology*, **31**, 209.

Yoshida, K., Smith, B., Craggs, M., & Kumar, R.C. (1998). Fluoxetine in breast-milk and developmental outcome of breast-fed infants. *British Journal of Psychiatry*, **172**, 175–9.

Zahn-Waxler, C., Cummings, E.M., Ianoff, R.J. et al. (1984). Young offspring of depressed patients: a population of risk for affective problems and childhood depression. In *Childhood Depression*, ed. D. Cichette & Schneider-Rosen, pp. 81–105. San Francisco: Jossey-Bass.

Zajick, E. (1981). Psychiatric problems during pregnancy, In *Pregnancy: A Psychological and Social Study*, ed. S. Wolkind & E. Zajicek, pp. 57–73. London: Academic Press.

## 17

# Preliminary algorithms for treatment-resistant bipolar depression

Robert M. Post, Mark A. Frye, Kirk D. Denicoff, Andrew M. Speer, Susan R. B. Weiss, and Gabriele S. Leverich

## Introduction

In this chapter a series of treatment algorithms are presented which may be used as a general guide in sequencing treatment so that patients who fail to respond to first-line conventional treatment may still very likely achieve a substantial amelioration, if not complete remission, of depressive syndromes or recurrences. Caution should be noted that most of the conclusions and recommendations presented are highly provisional, often based on databases from uncontrolled studies, and as such reflect the authors' clinical experiences and biases. However, as there are relatively few randomized, controlled trials that address the necessary treatment decisions often required for the treatment-resistant bipolar patient, the clinician as well as the clinical research investigator is often faced with making the best possible judgment based on direct inferences from other illnesses and controlled case series. Despite these major caveats, depression in most treatment-resistant bipolar patients can usually be adequately treated. The optimal sequencing of these treatments in the general bipolar patient population, and how to most rapidly achieve this optimal sequencing in the individual patient with defined clinical or biochemical characteristics, is less clear.

A series of principles are emphasized in attempting to arrive at optimal pharmacotherapeutics. These principles involve: (i) carefully mapping the prior illness to ascertain patterns of (a) partial responsiveness to treatment agents alone or in combination, (b) non-responsiveness, and (c) illness exacerbation; (ii) developing an even more detailed, prospective, graphic chart of the illness course to delineate alterations in manic and depressive episode severity, frequency, duration, and patterning; (iii) using agents with different and novel mechanisms of action (Table 17.1) applied sequentially and often in combination; (iv) carefully titrating medication doses against side effects to maximize therapeutic outcome, even with complex combinations; (v) using drugs with broader symptom target profiles and more acceptable side effects profiles in relation to a patient's presenting problems and potential side effects liabilities; (vi) carefully incorporating any family history of both bipolar illness and treatment response into treatment algorithms; (vii) initiating pharmacoprophylaxis early in the illness course to prevent malignant progression; (viii) engaging the patient and family in an active, ongoing psycho-educational approach to the illness; (ix) treating the potential for episode recurrence, comorbidity, and catastrophic outcome as seriously as the initial acute episode; and finally, (x) engaging all of the patients' and families' resources to recruit them as collaborators in the treatment of the illness (often requiring a combination of pharmacotherapy and psychotherapy) and to help insure adequate compliance.

## Mapping the illness course using the life chart method (LCM)

Detailed retrospective charting of the illness course and potential responsiveness to prior treatments (Figs. 17.1–17.2(a)) is recommended at the first consultation, along with continuing this charting on a prospective basis (Fig. 17.2(b)) using patient's daily ratings of sleep, mood, and illness-driven functional incapacitation (Leverich & Post, 1998). This longitudinal approach to the illness from the outset emphasizes the potential for illness recurrence (Fig. 17.3) and the need to approach bipolar illness with care equal to that given to other chronic, recurrent, potentially life-threatening medical illnesses such as epilepsy, diabetes, and congestive heart failure. In many instances, the graphic depiction of the illness and its prior responsivity to treatment may provide almost instantaneous guidelines on new ways to approach the illness. Should initial treatment efforts prove inadequate, life charting nonetheless provides a basis for rational decision-making and reconsultation if needed.

Involving the family in the consultation often greatly assists in making a bipolar II diagnosis in which, in some instances, clearly manic behavior is recognized as abnormal or bizarre by family members, but denied or minimized as part of the usual behavior by the patient. The retrospective life chart can be constructed (Fig. 17.2(a)) with an initial description of the patient's typical depressive symptomatology, worst episode, or most recent episode, and then proceeding to other episodes that share these characteristics (and have a minimal, substantial, or major impact on functional incapacity) and chart accordingly. Similarly, one can chart mania as mild, moderate, or severe, and elicit hypomanic symptoms in a positive manner; hypomanic symptoms such as decreased need for sleep or increased energy may be associated with improved functioning, rather than functional impairment, in the context of either a euphoric or dysphoric mood. As best one can, medications should be charted along with the episode course so that partial

**Table 17.1.** Positive and negative selection factors for choice of mood stabilizer

| | Lithium (Li) | | Carbamazepine (CBZ) | | Valproic acid (VPA) | |
|---|---|---|---|---|---|---|
| Target symptoms and auxiliary responsive syndromes | Euphoric ++++ <br> Family history positive +++ <br> MDI pattern +++ <br> Steroid-induced ++ <br> Suicidal +++ | | Euphoric ++++ <br> Schizoaffective ++ <br> Organic-affective +++ <br> Aggressive +++ <br> Dysphoric + <br> Alcohol ++ <br> Cocaine ± <br> PTSD + <br> Steroid-induced ± <br> Pain syndromes ++++ | | Dysphoric +++ <br> Rapid cycling +++ <br> Organic-affective +++ <br> Panic + <br> Migraine ++++ <br> Alcohol ± <br> Cocaine ± <br> PTSD + <br> Pain syndromes ++ | |

| | Choose – Li | Avoid – Li | Choose – CBZ | Avoid – CBZ | Choose – VPA | Avoid – VPA |
|---|---|---|---|---|---|---|
| Side effects profiles: | ↑WBC (c) | Wt gain (c) | Minimal cognitive changes | Many drug interactions! (c) | Few drug interactions | Wt gain (c) |
| (c) = common | ↑Ca++ (c) | Tremor (c) – DR | Little Wt Gain | ↓Potency of birth control pills (c) | Tolerated in O.D. | GI distress (c) |
| (r) = rare | | | | | | Tremor (c) – DR |
| (vr) = very rare | Renal excretion | Subjective (c) – DR cog. Slowing | Tolerated in O.D. | | Minimal cognitive changes | Alopecia (r) – I |
| | | | | | | Pancreatitis (vr) – I |
| DR = Dose-related | Non-sedating | ↓ Thyroid (c) | | Rash (10–15%) (c) | | Polycystic ovaries (?) |
| I = Idiosyncratic | | ↓ Renal | | Ataxia/sedation (c) | | ↓ platelets (c) |
| | | – ↑ DI (c) | | Hyponatremia (c) | | Liver failure |
| | | – ↓ GFR (r) | | Agranulocytosis (r) – I | | – (Child < 2) (vr) |
| | | Toxic in O.D. | | Aplastic anemia (vr) – I | | Pregnancy |
| | | – Cardiac (c) | | Allergy – I | | – Spina bifida (2–6%) (r) |
| | | – Cerebellar (r) | | Pregnancy | | |
| | | Poor in MS and neurological illness | | – Spina bifida (1–3%) (r) | | |
| | | Pregnancy? | | | | |
| | | – Ebstein's anomaly (vr) | | | | |

response to prior drug regimens can be ascertained. Important psychosocial events can be charted with this mood line, as they often assist in recollecting periods of symptomatic dysfunction. If regular seasonal components to episodes or anniversary reactions become evident, they can be incorporated into more rigorous psychotherapeutic and pharmacotherapeutic interventions at the appropriate time in the future. Moreover, this life charting exercise should be used to set up a prospective early warning system, so that if patients begin to develop early precursors of an episode, they can be instructed to increase medication or contact the physician accordingly in an attempt to prevent a renewed episode.

**Table 17.1** (*cont.*)

| Target symptoms and auxiliary responsive syndromes | Lamotrigine (LTG) Rapid cycling ++ Treatment resistant ++ Pain syndromes ++ | | Gabapentin (GPN) Parkinsonian symptoms ++ Insomnia ++ Anxiety + | | Topiramate (TOP) Bulemia ++ | |
|---|---|---|---|---|---|---|
| | Choose – LTG | Avoid – LTG | Choose – GPN | Avoid – GPN | Choose – TOP | Avoid – TOP |
| Side effects profiles: | Non-sedating | Rash (c): 5–10% | Renal excretion | Inhibits own uptake – requires T.I.D., Q.I.D. dosing May exacerbate mania | Weight loss (c) (sometimes sustained) | 1% incidence renal calculi |
| (c) = common (r) = rare (vr) = very rare | Weight neutral to weight loss | Risk of severe rash: 1/500 (r) | Few interactions Helps essential tremor | | | Psychomotor slowing (c) |
| DR = Dose-related I = Idiosyncratic | Antidepressant; Mood not set below baseline | Slow titration required | | | | Difficulty with word finding (c) |
| | | ↑ levels (× 2) with VPA | | | | Possible insomnia |
| | | ↓ levels (× 2) with CBZ | | | | |

Abbreviations: MDI = Mania-Depression-Well Interval; DI = diabetes insipidus; GFR = glomular filtration rate; PTSD = posttraumatic stress disorder; WBC = white blood cells; O.D. = overdose; GI = gastro-intestinal; T.I.D. = three times/day; Q.I.D. = four times/day; MS = multiple sclerosis.

Key: (±)–(++++)=strength of evidence

## Persistent treatment-resistant depression

### Lessons from unipolar illness

Faced with an extended treatment-resistant depression, one may approach bipolar illness similarly to unipolar illness, except that cotreatment with one or more mood stabilizers is required (Fig. 17.5). One can then progress through a sequence of antidepressant treatment algorithms attempting to terminate the extended episode. The author's bias is to use bupropion as the first-line antidepressant because of its positive side effects profile, including lack of sexual dysfunction and lack of weight gain, the latter of which is often problematic in patients on mood

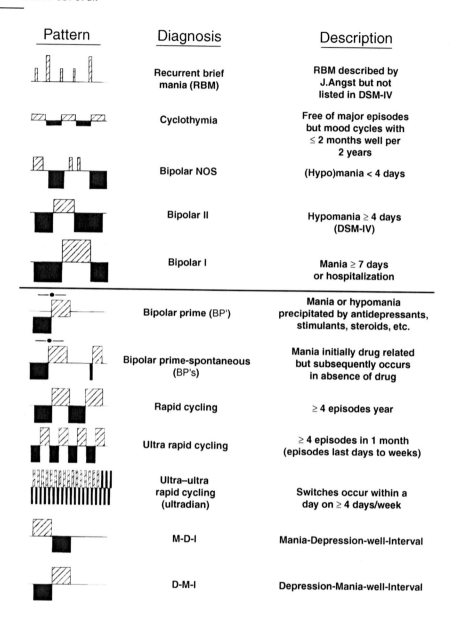

| Pattern | Diagnosis | Description |
|---|---|---|
| | Recurrent brief mania (RBM) | RBM described by J.Angst but not listed in DSM-IV |
| | Cyclothymia | Free of major episodes but mood cycles with ≤ 2 months well per 2 years |
| | Bipolar NOS | (Hypo)mania < 4 days |
| | Bipolar II | Hypomania ≥ 4 days (DSM-IV) |
| | Bipolar I | Mania ≥ 7 days or hospitalization |
| | Bipolar prime (BP') | Mania or hypomania precipitated by antidepressants, stimulants, steroids, etc. |
| | Bipolar prime-spontaneous (BP's) | Mania initially drug related but subsequently occurs in absence of drug |
| | Rapid cycling | ≥ 4 episodes year |
| | Ultra rapid cycling | ≥ 4 episodes in 1 month (episodes last days to weeks) |
| | Ultra–ultra rapid cycling (ultradian) | Switches occur within a day on ≥ 4 days/week |
| | M-D-I | Mania-Depression-well-Interval |
| | D-M-I | Depression-Mania-well-Interval |

Fig. 17.1.    Life chart patterns (*left*), corresponding with diagnoses and their descriptions.

stabilizers (particularly lithium or valproate), neuroleptics (especially the atypicals) and some antidepressants (especially many of the older tricyclics). Moreover, if a patient is taking one of the mood stabilizing anticonvulsants, there is less concern about reaching or even exceeding bupropion's traditional 450 mg/day maximum because of the liability of seizures. Carbamazepine markedly diminishes the levels of the parent compound of bupropion with a marked increase in

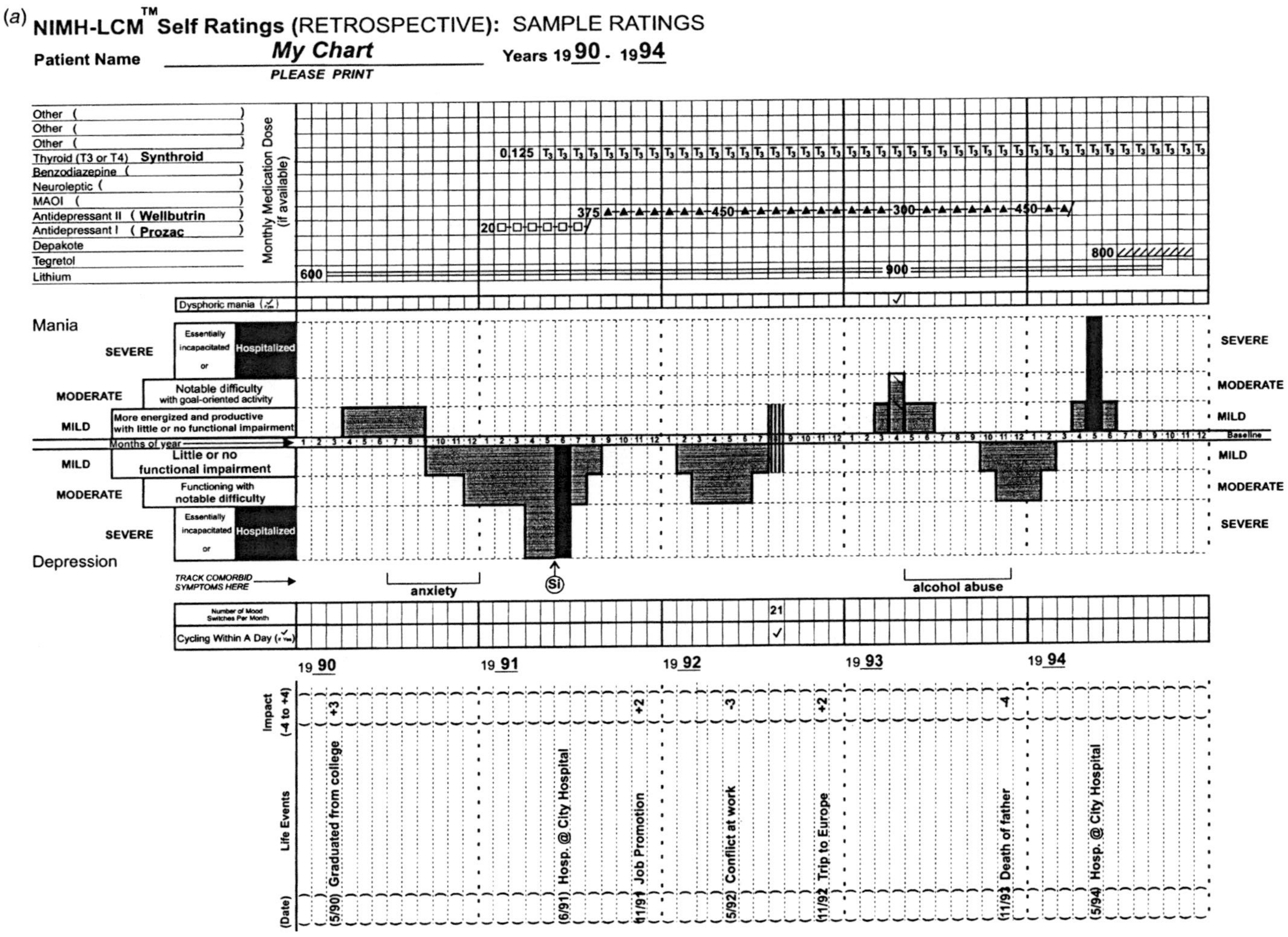

Fig. 17.2(a). An example of a completed retrospective life chart template.

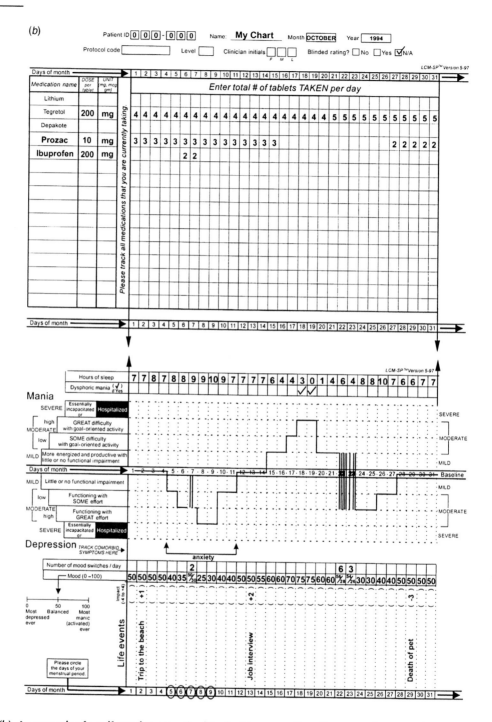

Fig. 17.2(b). An example of a self-rated prospective life chart incorporating all aspects of prospective daily charting.

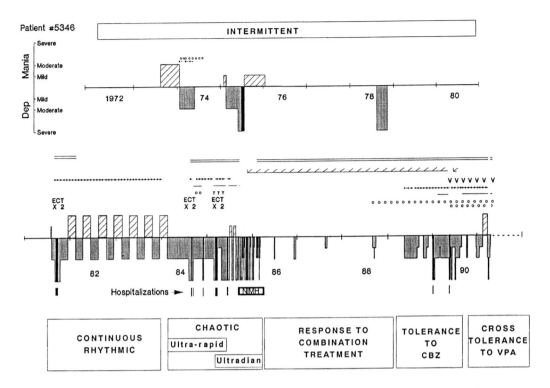

Fig. 17.3.  Life chart showing phases in evolution and treatment response in a bipolar II female. Key: lithium carbonate ══ ; carbamazepine (CBZ): ⤺⤺⤺; valproate (VPA): v v v v ·; tricyclics: ·········· ; benzodiazepines: ── ; Other: °°°°° ; ECT = electroconvulsive therapy.

dihydroxybupropion, a metabolite also thought to be active. In contrast, there are lesser effects with valproate on the ratio of bupropion to its hydroxy metabolite, and it is unclear which is preferable for optimal pharmacodynamic antidepressant effects. However, it is clear that there is no need to measure bupropion blood levels during concomitant treatment with carbamazepine, since they are likely to be negligible in relationship to the active hydroxy metabolite.

With partial but inadequate antidepressant response, one might consider augmentation with triiodothyronine ($T_3$) even in the absence of baseline thyroid abnormalities (Joffe & Singer, 1990), particularly in female patients in whom several studies have suggested a higher antidepressant potentiation rate as a function of female gender (Extein & Gold, 1988). After 2 to 3 weeks of $T_3$ administration, if the patient is not already on concomitant lithium treatment, one might consider switching to lithium potentiation for the treatment-resistant bipolar patient (Joffe et al., 1993). Lithium is a highly effective adjunctive modality, and across multiple studies has highly suggestive antisuicide effects, even when its acute or long-term prophylactic antidepressant effects are less obvious (Müller-

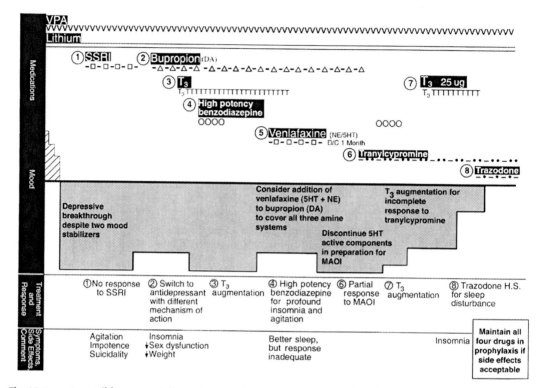

Fig. 17.4.    A possible sequential algorithm for the treatment-resistant bipolar depressed patient.
VPA=valproate; SSRI=serotonin-selective reuptake inhibitor; DA=dopamine;
T₃=triiodothyronine; NE=norepinephrine; 5HT=serotonin; D/C=discontinue;
MAOI=monoamine oxidase inhibitor; H.S.=at night (hours of sleep).

Oerlinghausen et al., 1992a,b; Baldessarini et al., 1999).

If response is inadequate to one or more mood stabilizers in combination with bupropion, one might consider the addition of venlafaxine, given its combined and potent actions on noradrenergic and serotonin reuptake. In this way with bupropion increasing dopamine levels in the striatum and nucleus accumbens, all three amine systems would be potentiated at the reuptake mechanism in an apparent parallel to the monoamine oxidase inhibitors (MAOIs), which have an equally broad spectrum in inhibiting the breakdown of all three amine systems.

In cases of lack of efficacy to this broad spectrum, second-generation antidepressant treatment, one might then be more than justified in switching to a classical MAOI with its 60–80% response rate in treatment-resistant unipolar or bipolar depression, which is significantly higher than more traditional tricyclic antidepressants (Himmelhoch et al., 1991). This switch could be accomplished by discontinuing venlafaxine or any other serotonin-selective reuptake inhibitor (SSRI) and maintaining bupropion until the transition to the MAOI. In this way,

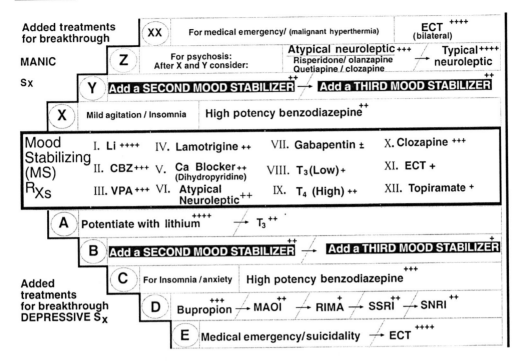

Fig. 17.5.    Treatment options for rapid and ultra-rapid cyclers. ECT = electroconvulsive therapy; Li = lithium; CBZ = carbamazepine; VPA = valproate; Ca = calcium; $T_3$ = triiodothyronine; $T_4$ = thyroxine; MAOI = monoamine oxidase inhibitor; RIMA = reversible inhibitor of monoamine oxidase; SSRI = serotonin-selective reuptake inhibitor; SNRI = serotonin–norepinephrine reuptake inhibitor; Sx = symptoms. Key: (+)–(++++)=strength of evidence.

antidepressant coverage would be maintained, while the serotonin-selective agents were discontinued for 3 to 6 weeks in order to avoid the potential of a catastrophic serotonergic syndrome with the MAOI addition.

In light of the recent controlled data on the efficacy of lamotrigine in bipolar and unipolar depression (Frye et al., 2000a; Calabrese et al., 1999; Bowden et al., 1999), one might consider the use of this agent (discussed in more detail below) in the treatment sequence either before or after an MAOI. As more data become available, lamotrigine may be used even earlier in the treatment algorithm of bipolar patients because of its potential antidepressant and mood-stabilizing properties.

If a patient has failed these approaches, it would perhaps be advisable to change the mood stabilizer regimen to find an agent or combination with more effective acute antidepressant properties (Fig. 17.5). In this regard, carbamazepine has been used as an acute antidepressant with some success in approximately one-third of bipolar patients (Fig. 17.6) (Post et al., 1986) and its properties as an adjunctive antidepressant have also been noted (Post, 1991; Otani et al., 1996). The

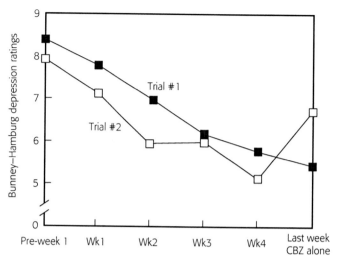

Fig. 17.6.   Repeated antidepressant response to carbamazepine (double-blind; N = 10; off–on–off–on design). This subgroup of responsive patients (Post et al., 1986) was treated a second time with active drug to confirm individual responsiveness.

antidepressant effects of gabapentin are not well documented, but because of its significant effects on gamma-aminobutyric (GABA)-ergic transmission (increasing GABA levels in cerebrospinal fluid [CSF]), it may have antianxiety and antidepressant effects in some patients (Dimond et al., 1996; McLean, 1995; Altshuler et al., 1999), particularly those who are younger, lower in weight, and have a shorter duration of illness (Frye et al., 2000a; Obrocea et al., unpublished data).

If this series of options fails, one might wish to consider the addition of high dose $T_4$ treatment (150–400 µg/day) (Bauer & Whybrow, 1990; Baumgartner et al., 1994), as this strategy, which has been used to improve mood in both phases of rapid cycling bipolar illness (Whybrow, 1994), also appears to be effective in some patients with treatment-resistant depression (Bauer et al., 1998).

When confronted with acute suicidality or another medical emergency, considering electroconvulsive therapy (ECT) becomes a high priority given its rapid onset of action. However, in the bipolar patient, one is then still faced with the problem of what regimen to use for long-term prophylaxis if a good acute response to ECT is achieved. Although a few case reports have suggested the long-term utility of prophylactic ECT on a once-every-2-weeks or once-a-month basis (Abrams, 1990; Bonds et al., 1998), this has not been systematically studied in the literature, and the ability to sustain the response, particularly in bipolar patients, is not at all certain. Moreover, the cost and inconvenience of a major procedure which requires general anesthesia on a regular basis, would not appear optimal for any but those with the most intractable depressions.

## Symptom targeting

A sequence of drug treatments may also be based on a drug's relative assets to liability profile (Table 17.1) or on type of manic and cyclic presentation (Table 17.2). For the patient with extreme motor retardation and/or lack of response to a variety of approaches noted previously, one might consider augmentation with the psychomotor stimulants as an acute transition while waiting for a better long-term antidepressant response. For the low-energy, psychomotor-slowed depressed patient, this augmentation may provide enough of a mood and energy stimulant to allow patients to function better at work and in their usual social roles. Again, acute controlled studies and the benefits of long-term follow-up for bipolar patients have not been adequately reported. J. Fawcett and associates (1994, personal communication) have indicated that most previously treatment-resistant patients will become tolerant to stimulant augmentation, although they report that this is less likely to occur if patients are on the combination of a psychomotor stimulant with an MAOI. A number of investigators in the field (Fawcett et al., 1991; Feighner et al., 1985) have suggested that, despite the *Physicians Desk Reference* contraindications for using stimulants with an MAOI, they can be carefully titrated into the regimen (White & Simpson, 1981) and, under these circumstances, are not apparently associated with loss of efficacy via tolerance (J. Fawcett, 1994, personal communication).

For significant comorbid symptoms of anxiety and insomnia, gabapentin or the high potency benzodiazepines lorazepam and clonazepam might be considered adjunctively, particularly if the patient is struggling with acute suicidality. Fawcett et al. (1990) have indicated that extreme and panicky anxious agitation is sometimes a precursor of a completed suicide attempt, and while attempting to treat a patient's depression with other modalities, appropriate support and acute pharmacological assistance in anxiety reduction should also be considered. The degree of anxiety may also play a role in the choice of a mood stabilizer, since valproate has been reported to have antianxiety and antipanic effects in some patient populations (Keck et al., 1993), and carbamazepine is reportedly highly effective for anxiety in patients with treatment-resistant epilepsy (Trimble, 1988). Gabapentin has been reported to be effective in the treatment of social phobia (Pande et al., 1999).

## Unconventional approaches

The use of precursor strategies, such as choline (Stoll et al., 1996) or the amino acids tyrosine or tryptophan, have received some attention in treatment-resistant bipolar depression, but are not widely used in most clinicians' algorithms.

Another experimental approach is to use high doses of inositol (12–16 g/day), which has also been reported as a useful antianxiety and antidepressant modality,

**Table 17.2.** Preliminary clinical impressions of comparative clinical and side effects profiles of lithium, nimodipine, and the putative mood-stabilizing anticonvulsants in adults

| | Lithium[b] (0.5–1.2 meq/l) | Carbamazepine (4–12 μg/ml) | Valproate (50–120 μg/ml) | Nimodipine | Lamotrigine[a] | Gabapentin | Topiramate |
|---|---|---|---|---|---|---|---|
| *Clinical profiles* | | | | | | | |
| Acute episodes | | | | | | | |
| Mania (M) | ++ | ++ | ++ | + | (±) | — | (±) |
| Dysphoric mania | + | (++) | ++ | (+) | ? | (±) | (±) |
| Depression (D) | + | + | ± | (+) | ++ | (±) | (±) |
| Prophylaxis | | | | | | | |
| Mania | ++ | ++ | ++ | (+) | (+) | — | (±) |
| Depression | + | + | + | (+) | + | (+) | (±) |
| Rapid cycling | + | + | ++ | (+) | (+) | (±) | (+) |
| Seizures | | | | | | | |
| Generalized (and complex partial) | — | ++ | ++ | ± | ++ | ++ | ++ |
| Absence | — | — — | ++ | ? | ++ | ? | ? |
| Paroxysmal pain syndromes | — | ++ | + | — | (+) | ++ | ? |
| Migraine | + | ± | ++ | + | ? | (±) | ? |
| *Side effects profiles* | | | | | | | |
| White blood cell count | ↑↑[b] | ↓↓ | (↓) | — | — | — | — |
| Diabetes insipidus | ↑↑[b] | → | — | — | — | — | — |
| Thyroid hormones: T3, T4 | ↓↓ | ↓↓ | → | — | ? | (↑)? | ? |
| Thyroid stimulating hormone | ↑↑[b] | — | ? | — | — | — | ? |
| Serum calcium | ↑ | → | ? | ? | ? | ? | ? |
| Weight | ↑↑ | (↑) | ↑↑ | — | → | ↑ | ↓↓ |
| Tremor | ↑↑ | — | ↑↑ | — | ← | ↓,↑ | ↑↑ |
| Memory disturbances | ↑ | ↑ | ← | → | (↑) | ← | (↑) |
| Diarrhea, gastrointestinal distress | ↑↑ | ↑ | ↑↑ | (↓) | — | (↑) | (↑) |

| | | | | | | |
|---|---|---|---|---|---|---|
| Teratogenesis | (↑) | ↑ | ↑↑ | — | — | ? |
| Psoriasis | ↑ | — | (↑) | — | — | — |
| Rash | ↑ | ↑↑ | (↑) | ↑↑ᵃ | (↑) | ? |
| Alopecia | (↑) | — | ↑ | — | — | — |
| Agranulocytosis, aplastic anemia | — | (↑) | — | — | — | — |
| Thrombocytopenia | — | (↑) | ↑ | — | — | — |
| Hepatitis | — | ↑ | ↑ | ? | — | (↑)? |
| Hyponatremia, water intoxication | — | ↑ | — | — | — | — |
| Dizziness, ataxia, diploplia | (↑) | ↑↑ | ↑ | ↑ | ↑ | ↑ |

*Clinical efficacy:* — = none; ± = equivocal; + = effective; ++ = very effective; ( ) = weak or questionable data; ? = unknown; — — = exacerbation

*Side effects:* ↑ = increase; ↓ = decrease; ( ) = inconsistent or rare; — = absent

ᵃ Lamotrigine rash is common in approximately 10% of patients; severe, life-threatening rash occurs in about 1 out of every 100 children and is thus not recommended for children under the age of 16.

ᵇ Effect of lithium predominates over that of carbamazepine when used in combination.

including a few patients with bipolar illness in a recent report (Benjamin et al., 1995; Levine, 1997). Excellent success with high dose omega-3 fatty acids has been reported in one small controlled study (Stoll et al., 1999).

The vitamin supplements ascorbate (Naylor & Smith, 1981; Kay et al., 1984) and folate (Coppen et al., 1986; Coppen & Bailey, 2000) have also been reported in some studies to augment other mood-stabilizing regimens and, in light of their benign side effects profile, might be considered in an overall strategy for patients with treatment-resistant bipolar illness.

## Cyclic treatment-resistant depressions in the context of bipolar illness

The authors' experience is that the majority of patients with treatment-resistant bipolar depression present with recurrent episodes of depression interspersed with a dysthymic baseline or hypomanic or manic episodes, rather than an intractable single episode (Fig. 17.3). These intercurrent hypomanias and full-blown manias are often more readily treatable with mood stabilizers than the recurrent depressions. Moreover, it appears that some antidepressant modalities may actually lead to a cycle acceleration, either by shortening each depressive episode, or the 'well' or hypomanic/manic interval between episodes (Fig. 17.3).

Although not clearly established, it is the authors' impression that patients with initially rapid cycling presentations are at a particularly high risk for this phenomenon (Post, 1992a; Kramlinger & Post, 1996; Post et al., 1997; Altshuler et al., 1995), as well as those patients with continuous cycling without a well interval. Those with a non-cyclic course may be much less prone to switching (Kupfer et al., 1988; Peet, 1994; Young et al., 2000). Thus, in patients with continuous or rapidly recurring cycling patterns, the authors' approach is to make greater use of primary mood-stabilizing regimens prior to the use of adjunctive antidepressants.

Lithium and carbamazepine have been used in combination with some success in approximately 50% of rapid cycling bipolar patients (Fig. 17.7) in the study of Denicoff et al. (1997), wherein both agents in monotherapy may only be effective in 25% of rapid cycling patients. Similarly, the adjunctive use of valproate in the lithium-treatment-resistant bipolar patient is often associated with clinical improvement in both phases of the illness (Lambert, 1984; Lambert & Venaud, 1987; McElroy et al., 1988b; Pope et al., 1991; Calabrese et al., 1992) (Figs. 17.8, 17.9). In illness which has not responded to lithium and carbamazepine with or without adjunctive treatment with antidepressants or MAOIs, some patients might respond to valproate combination or monotherapy (Fig. 17.8). In the National Institute of Mental Health (NIMH) group of highly treatment-resistant affectively ill patients, lamotrigine appeared most effective for bipolar males with fewer numbers of hospitalizations for depression and fewer numbers of prior medication trials, and showed a trend for those who had not had a prior trial of carbamazepine (Frye et al., 2000a; Obrocea et al., unpublished data).

### Rationale for combination treatment rather than sequential monotherapies

Despite the occasional monotherapy responder (Fig. 17.8), it would appear prudent in most individuals to add rather than substitute valproate to the lithium regimen (Fig. 17.9). This recommendation is based on a series of indirect logistical issues that are pertinent to the time frame of clinical response and, potentially, to the overall safety of the patient. The same principle would apply for the addition of other mood-stabilizing anticonvulsants such as carbamazepine, lamotrigine, or nimodipine.

(i) If one uses the second agent (such as lithium, carbamazepine, or valproate) adjunctively, one is applying a maximum therapeutic modality to the patient's recurrent clinical course, which might have the advantage of using two drugs with different mechanisms of action to combat the illness.

(ii) To the extent that combination therapy is found to be required (Fig. 17.10), it will be implemented and achieved more quickly, rather than having an extra trial of monotherapy inserted into the sequence. The same argument would apply even more strongly if the patient is eventually found to not respond to this combination therapy; again, the time of an entire extra monotherapy trial will have been saved.

(iii) In addition, if one discontinues lithium or another mood stabilizer, one is asking the new agent to treat both the treatment-resistant illness as well as any potential illness exacerbation induced by the discontinuation phase. This could further confound interpreting the potential efficacy of the new drug, which might be helpful as an adjunctive agent, but might not be sufficient to induce a remission in the context of a further illness exacerbation or during a withdrawal reaction.

(iv) Lithium maintenance treatment may be an antisuicide measure, even if lithium is not sufficient to reduce episodes. Müller-Oerlinghausen et al. (1992a,b) and Tondo et al. (1998) have observed some patients who were showing inadequate mood response to lithium who committed suicide after discontinuation, apparently because of the loss of the separate antisuicide effect of lithium independent of its clinical effect on the affective episode. In a meta-analysis, Baldessarini et al. (1999) have found a 20-fold increased incidence of suicide in those who stop lithium in year 1 vs. those who continue lithium prophylaxis.

(v) If a patient shows an excellent response to the combination, one can later decide whether or not to taper the initial agent slowly to assess whether it is

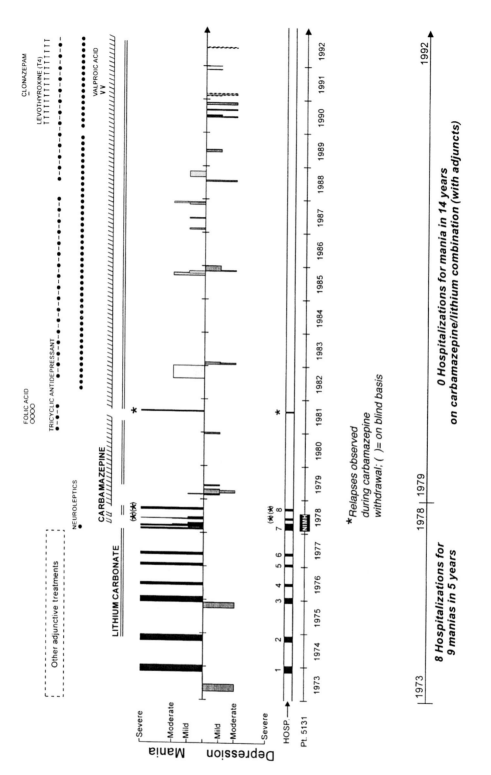

Fig. 17.7. Life chart showing confirmed* acute and prophylactic response to carbamazepine in a lithium non-responder.

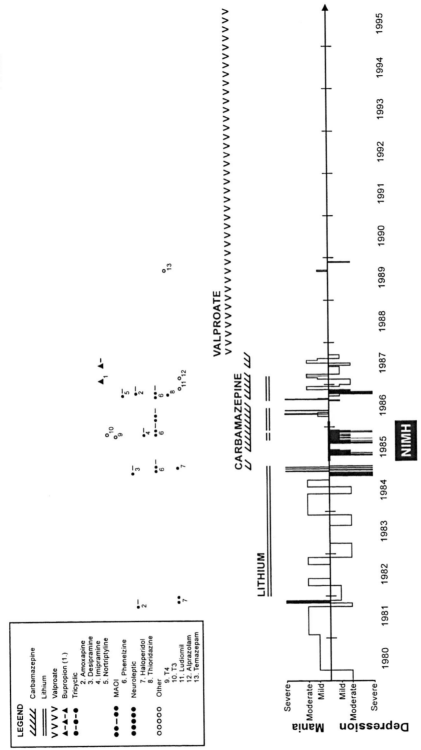

Fig. 17.8.    Life chart showing prophylactic response to valproate in a non-responder to lithium/carbamazepine plus antidepressant augmentation.

PT. 244

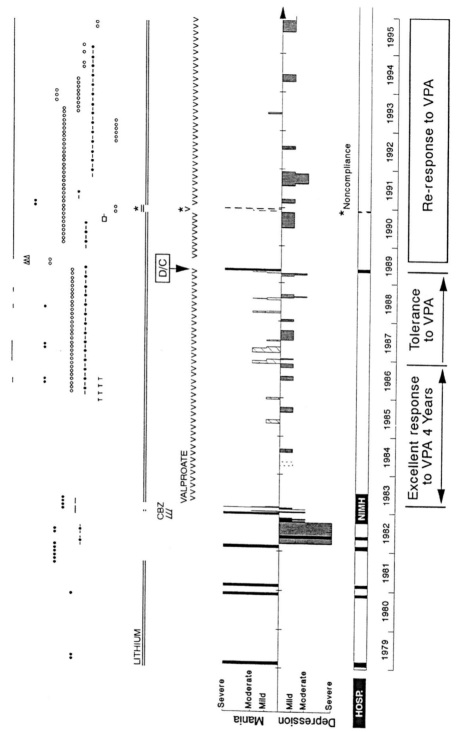

Fig. 17.9. Life chart showing tolerance and re-response to the prophylactic effects of valproate as an adjunct to lithium.

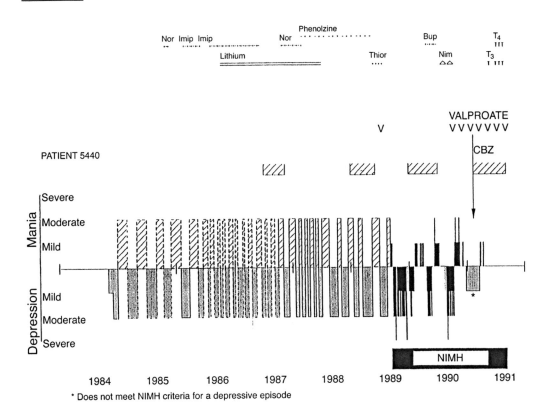

Fig. 17.10.  Life chart showing response to valproate–carbamazepine combination. Nor=nortriptyline; Imip=imipramine; Thior=thioridazine; Bup=bupropion; Nim=nimodipine; T₄=thyroxine; T₃=triiodothyronine.

needed in the regimen. This taper should be done extremely slowly and cautiously, if at all, especially if the patient is euthymic and has no side effects.

(vi) We take an extremely conservative view and recommend that, in the relative absence of side effects, many patients should consider continuation therapy with their combined mood stabilizer treatment for several different reasons: (a) the possibility that patients may develop tolerance to the mood stabilizer in monotherapy at a higher incidence than in combination, as discussed subsequently; thus, with a dual mood stabilizer approach one would be providing more protection than in monotherapy; (b) moreover, if one were to find that the illness was showing progressive evidence of breaking through a previously effective treatment (i.e. a minor episode or 'flurries' preceding more major ones in a pattern suggestive of tolerance), then it might be more difficult to reassert control over the illness than if one maintained the patient in a state of complete remission. Keller et al. (1992) have reported that 'flurries' herald more major episode breakthroughs, and we have seen repeatedly in our studies of tolerance development that minor episodes herald more major ones (Post & Weiss, 1995; see Fig. 17.9, 1984–1989). Thus, it may be preferable to be conservative from the outset, since one does not know the predictors of which patients are going to develop tolerance to the mood-stabilizing anticonvulsants; and finally, (c) discontinuation of effective lithium treatment, for example, may be associated with the occurrence of a new episode. This phenomenon, in turn, has a series of additional liabilities, some of which are not obvious or well understood.

### Liabilities of lithium discontinuation

The first liability of lithium discontinuation is that the new episode may be extremely problematic in terms of the renewal of symptoms and their associated morbidity and loss of social or employment opportunities. It is also possible that the patient may require rehospitalization. A manic or depressive exacerbation could be a severe stressor in an already shaky marriage; a marital breakup could be associated with further deterioration or the resumption of drug or alcohol abuse. Finally, it is possible for the new episode to engender a different neurobiological process that renders a patient more difficult to treat and no longer responsive to lithium alone or in conjunction with another previously effective agent (Post, 1992b; Post & Weiss, 1995). In the worst case scenario, new episodes may be associated with a completed suicide to which patients who discontinue lithium are at much higher risk (Baldessarini et al., 1999).

My colleagues and I have described the phenomenon of lithium discontinuation-induced treatment resistance in a series of patients (Post et al., 1992, 1993), and other clinicians have noted it as well (Koukopoulos et al., 1995; Bauer, 1994; Maj et al., 1995; Tondo et al., 1997). Even Coryell et al. (1998) who reported no overall evidence of a lithium discontinuation effect in their small series, indicated that one patient did fail to rerespond. No amount of time 'well' on a regimen including lithium appears to preclude the liability of such a phenomenon. We have observed patients who have been well for 18 years who have discontinued lithium, experienced a relapse, and then had extreme difficulty in reacquiring an adequate response. In some instances, this has been associated with a complete failure to renew responsivity despite a whole host of new pharmacotherapeutic measures, many of which have been discussed in this chapter. This failure to renew responsivity is viewed from the potential theoretical context of a new episode engendering a further neurobiological process which then renders the illness less amenable to the previously effective treatment (Post, 1992b). This could be conceptualized as similar to a metastasis in cancer, wherein the primary tumor might be highly responsive to a drug, but once the tumor reaches a new stage, it is no longer responsive to the original regimen.

The incidence of lithium discontinuation-induced treatment-resistance is unknown in the general population, but after reviewing life chart records of 66 patients referred to the NIMH for treatment-resistance, it appeared that 14% of such patients arrived at the clinical research unit via this route. Another 35% who appeared to have had good initial responses to lithium then lost response despite continued treatment at adequate doses, through a process that appeared to be the development of tolerance. The incidence of lithium discontinuation-induced treatment resistance and tolerance in a population not selected for treatment resistance remains to be ascertained in the general population, but is likely to be small, perhaps about 10%. Nonetheless, it appears worth advising patients that an additional potential risk of lithium discontinuation is the lack of a guarantee of as complete a response as originally experienced.

### Choosing mood stabilizers over antidepressants

Additional support for the use of two mood stabilizers in combination (Figs. 17.7, 17.9, 17.10), rather than immediately after an antidepressant adjunct, is the data concerning the liability of antidepressants to precipitate manic episodes or cycle acceleration, as described previously. This liability appears to be a problem in approximately one-third of treatment-resistant bipolar patients in whom the switch appears attributable to the antidepressant agent, in that it either occurs earlier than expected or with a greater magnitude of mania than the prior course of illness would suggest (Altshuler et al., 1995; Post et al., 1997). However, a switch into mania may occur during prophylaxis with a regimen including an antidepressant in 60–70% of treatment-resistant rapid cycling patients (Altshuler et al., 1995), although the majority of these switches are attributable to the expected prior course of illness rather than antidepressant related. Nonetheless, it is this potential liability that leads one, in many instances, to consider a second mood stabilizer in preference to an antidepressant. This clinical preference may or may not stand the test of time since Young et al. (2000) found paroxetine preferable to the second mood stabilizer (either lithium or valproate) in non-rapid cycling patients. Moreover, we have observed a low switch rate (about 12%) in 100 patients treated for 10 weeks with either bupropion, sertraline, or venlafaxine in a randomized fashion for a depression breaking through a mood stabilizer (R.M. Post et al., 2000, unpublished data).

Another factor influencing our preference is the clinical data analyzed from the NIMH unit in treating treatment-resistant patients over the past three decades. We have observed increasingly fewer of our patients (preselected for prior unresponsiveness) who are able to be discharged on monotherapy (even with the advent of a series of newer agents). In the assessment of their discharge medicines, only in the minority (10–20%) have adjunctive antidepressants or neuroleptics been necessary to their therapeutic regimens. In most cases, patients are discharged on one or more mood stabilizers, and this is often sufficient to decrease cycling, if not end it completely (Frye et al., 2000b).

A third potential rationale for choosing mood stabilizers over unimodal antidepressants has been alluded to previously; that is, patients may be prone to tolerance development with monotherapy and, in many instances, even with several drugs used in combination (Figs. 17.3, 17.9). In patients successfully discharged from the NIMH on a regimen involving carbamazepine (usually in conjunction with lithium and other agents), a loss of efficacy has been found in 40.7% of patients followed for an average of 8.5 years. The loss of efficacy appeared in the second or third year of treatment, after an average of 3.6 years (G.S. Leverich et al., 1998, unpublished data). With a slightly lower incidence rate but in a parallel fashion, 27% of patients on valproate followed on long-term prophylaxis showed loss of efficacy, after an average of 5.8 years on valproate (R.M. Post et al., 1998, unpublished data).

One must raise the caveat that these patients were highly treatment-resistant to begin with, and were referred to a tertiary clinical research evaluation center (the NIMH), and thus might represent a patient group over-represented with rapid cycling and more inclined to malignant progression of the illness and tolerance development than the general population. Nonetheless, tolerance has been reported by others in other populations (Koukopoulos et al., 1995), including a high incidence of loss of efficacy to carbamazepine for a variety of reasons (Frankenburg et al., 1988), and reports of the loss of efficacy to carbamazepine and valproate as well via an apparent tolerance mechanism (S.L. McElroy and P.E. Keck, personal communication).

## A preclinical model for loss of efficacy to the anticonvulsants and potential clinical implications

The authors have been able to model the loss of efficacy via tolerance to the anticonvulsants carbamazepine, lamotrigine, diazepam, and valproate in the model of amygdala-kindled seizures (Weiss et al., 1995; Post & Weiss, 1996). In these instances, initially successful doses of drug become inadequate in preventing breakthroughs of amygdala-kindled seizure episodes. This happens more readily with carbamazepine, lamotrigine, and the anticonvulsant benzodiazepines than with valproate. Nonetheless, when tolerance does occur, it manifests in an episodic fashion with an occasional seizure breaking through the anticonvulsant, and then more rapid and consistent seizure episodes progressing to complete loss of efficacy. The tolerance is contingent on the association between drug and kindling stimulation; if the drug is given after (rather than before) kindled seizures occur, tolerance does not develop.

With loss of efficacy to carbamazepine and diazepam, Weiss and colleagues (1995) found that seizures fail to induce the same range of endogenous adaptive alterations in gene expression as they usually do in the absence of tolerance; that is, seizures induce a variety of transient changes in gene expression that may represent endogenous anticonvulsant mechanisms. These include increases in $GABA_A$ and benzodiazepine receptors as well as increases in peptides that are putatively anticonvulsant such as thyrotropin-releasing hormone (TRH), neuropeptide Y (NPY), and cholecystokinin (CCK) (Rosen et al., 1993, 1994a,b; Zhang et al., 1996; Clark et al., 1994). If seizures occur in the context of tolerance to the anticonvulsant effects of carbamazepine and diazepam, it is of some interest that the $GABA_A$ receptors (specifically its $\alpha$-4 subunit) fail to increase as they ordinarily would in the non-tolerant condition. Similarly, the neuropeptide TRH mRNAs are not induced by the seizure in the context of tolerance development. Since seizures and their downstream consequences are helpful to the anticonvulsant effects of carbamazepine and diazepam, it is possible that the failure of these putative anticonvulsant adaptations during tolerance could be mechanistically important in the loss of anticonvulsant efficacy. TRH administered directly into the hippocampus has been shown to be anticonvulsant (Wan et al., 1998).

In a parallel manner, we have postulated that some of the abnormal neurochemistry of the affective disorders is related to its primary pathology and some to its secondary adaptations, potentially representing endogenous antidepressant principles (Post & Weiss, 1992, 1996). We have reached this postulate from the preclinical data in the kindling model and have preliminarily tested and confirmed it in patients, with the observation that TRH administered intrathecally is an acute antidepressant modality in patients with treatment-resistant bipolar illness (Marangell et al., 1997; Callahan et al., 1997). These observations suggest that the evidence of increased TRH in depression (as revealed by increases in CSF TRH and blunted thyrotropin-stimulating hormone [TSH] responses to TRH) may represent attempts at endogenous antidepressant adaptation that need to be enhanced, rather than part of the primary pathology that needs to be suppressed.

## Predictions from the model

To the extent that this preclinical seizure model has predictive validity for other types of tolerance that develop in affectively ill individuals, it would suggest a variety of potential treatment approaches, each of which requires prospective clinical studies for validation:

(i) moving to drugs with different mechanisms of action that do not show cross-tolerance;

(ii) using more potent rather than less potent drugs such as valproate instead of benzodiazepines (with their high tolerance proclivity);

(iii) using higher, tolerated doses, rather than lower, minimally-effective doses;

(iv) treating patients earlier rather than later in the course of the illness. In the kindling model tolerance occurs more rapidly to similar doses of drug after animals have experienced a large number of seizures as opposed to only a limited number;

(v) potentially using combination therapy in preventing tolerance development; if one uses carbamazepine and valproate in combination (at doses that in monotherapy are associated with the early development of tolerance), tolerance is substantially delayed. The same may be true for the addition of gabapentin to animals already tolerant to lamotrigine (even though gabapentin itself is not effective in this model). It remains to be explicitly tested clinically as to whether mood-stabilizing anticonvulsant combination therapy would also be useful in warding off the development of tolerance in the mood disorders, as observed in the seizure disorders.

(vi) giving patients who have developed loss of efficacy via tolerance a period of time off that drug (associated with the putative renewal of endogenous adaptive mechanisms), which may enable patients to rerespond to the initial treatment regimen.

It is noteworthy that this suggestion for a period of time off drug in the face of tolerance development is contrary to what would be recommended with a period of extended wellness. In instances of long-term therapeutic efficacy, discontinuing the effective agent might lead to episode renewal and be a negative factor in illness progression, as described previously. In contrast, in instances of loss of efficacy via tolerance, a period of time off drug may be associated with the later renewal of a drug's efficacy.

Thus, the preclinical model would suggest a different approach to drug discontinuation depending on the interaction of the course of illness with pharmacotherapy. In addition, the biochemical changes that accompany tolerance also appear to be contingent on the interaction of the drug and the episode being treated, i.e. animals that are treated with the same doses of drug *after* a seizure has been induced do not become tolerant and continue to show the usual seizure-induced biochemical adaptations previously mentioned. Thus, the failure of TRH mRNA and of the GABA$_A$ receptors (at the level of the $\alpha$-4 subunit) to increase occurs only in tolerant animals that experience seizures in the context of concurrent drug treatment. In animals that experience the same number of seizures and receive the same amount of drug (but given after the seizure has occurred), the usual seizure-induced adaptations continue to be observed.

Taken together, the emerging clinical evidence and its preclinical supporting principles suggest that treatment with the most effective regimens from the outset may have the best chance at lessening illness progression. In this regard, Kalynchuk et al. (1994) have suggested that the slow increases in drug in order to prevent potential seizures from breaking through is the regimen that leads to the fastest rate of tolerance development and eventual inefficacy. In contrast, maintenance of high doses or even lower doses appears more effective than 'chasing' the episodes with dose increases, as one is more likely to do clinically. These data are convergent with those of Kupfer et al. (1992) concerning the prophylaxis of recurring unipolar depression, wherein recommendations for full doses appears to have considerable merit. When patients who were well maintained for 3 to 5 years on full doses of imipramine (200 mg/day) were then blindly given a dose reduction to 100 mg/day, a high relapse rate was observed approximately equivalent to that of placebo substitution. These data, taken with those of Gelenberg et al. (1989), that higher doses of lithium are more effective than lower doses (even with reinterpretation of the data (Keller et al., 1992)), suggest that full effective doses, rather than marginal doses or dose reductions, are more likely to be useful in maintaining long-term efficacy.

Some support is also provided for this strategy by the indirect data of Fava et al. (1995) with full dose treatment in recurrent unipolar depression. In patients who became well on fluoxetine (20 mg/day), a modest relapse rate was observed in patients on follow-up over the next six months to one year. In another cohort of patients at even higher risk for early relapses, who had also responded to 20 mg/day acutely, the dose of fluoxetine was increased to 40 mg for prophylaxis, which was accompanied by a substantially reduced relapse rate compared with the first group or compared with that predicted for this high risk group of patients.

Thus, although formal prospective clinical trials remain to be assessed in non-treatment-resistant and treatment-resistant bipolar patients, it appears that the postulate that doses that are sufficient to stabilize the illness are best for long-term prophylaxis may be as good a principle as any to follow until other data are shown to be relevant. However, this theory should be balanced with the caveat that patients who do not consistently take higher doses of their medicine because of side effects may be at an even greater risk of sustained non-compliance and associated relapse from medication discontinuation. An optimal regimen of keeping each drug below its side effects threshold may be in the patient's long-

**Table 17.3.** Steps in the treatment algorithm of the bipolar patient

A    *Diagnostic clarification*

    1. Retrospective course (BPI, BPII, BP-NOS, RBM, Rapidity of cycling)

    2. Medication history (Antidepressant-induced; tolerance; or seasonal pattern)

    3. Family history of bipolar disorder and medication response

    4. Principle: Treatment 1st; blood levels, chemistries later

B    *Maximize current treatment regimen*

    1. Increase dose if side effects allow

    2. Change timing of dose (especially at night – for sleep/side effects/compliance)

    3. Treat dose limiting side effects:

        (a) Use another antimanic agent is possible (i.e. one with two-for-one return)

            (i) Propranolol (for Lithium tremor)

            (ii) $Ca^{2+}$ blocker (for Lithium diarrhea)

            (iii) *Li* (for CBZ→↓ WBC)

            (iv) Thyroid (for Li →↓ thyroid)

        (b) Decrease dose (if response allows)

        (c) Discontinuation (for intolerable side effects)

C    *Augment:* especially with partial efficacy, occasionally with little or no efficacy (i.e. do not discontinue ineffective Li without careful reconsideration of risk–benefit ratio, including its antisuicide effects)

    1. PRN High potency benzodiazepine (Clonazepam or Lorazepam)

    2. With second mood stabilizer (especially acute efficacy)

    3. Use third mood stabilizer if needed

    4. PRN Neuroleptic (low dose)

        Atypical: Olanzapine/Quetiapine/Risperidone/Clozapine

        Typical: Haloperidol/Thiothixene/Molindone

    Use drug with new mechanism of action (i.e. with profile of effects in different cycle frequencies or illness patterns)

        (a) Dihydropyridine $Ca^{2+}$ blocker (for ultradian cycling)

        (b) VPA (for migraine)

        (c) CBZ (as atypical antidepressant/mood stabilizer) active at peripheral-type benzodiazepine receptor

        (d) Clonidine (for panic and opiate withdrawal)

        (e) Consider Trimipramine as atypical antidepressant with $D_2$ blocking and antipsychotic effects

D    *Discontinuation of potential mania-inducing or cycle-inducing agents, such as:*

    1. Antidepressant and Alprazolam

    2. Cocaine and related stimulants

    3. Steroids (if possible)

E    *Substitution* (if side effects present and drug is ineffective)

    1. Drug with different side effects profile

    2. Use drugs with different mechanisms of action

F    *Refocus on Early Warning System (EWS) and Prophylaxis*

    1. Mood chart and contract of mediation changes and contact M.D. for given degrees of symptom emergence

    2. Education and compliance

    3. Principle: Maintain Effective Prophylaxis

        (a) Be conservative when good medication responses are achieved

        (b) Be more radical and make changes when adequate response not achieved

RBM = recurrent brief mania; Ca=calcium; Li=lithium; CBZ=carbamazepine; WBC=white blood cells; PRN=as needed; VPA=valproic acid.

term interests rather than pushing to the theoretically maximum doses that might lead to greater numbers of missed doses or non-compliance altogether.

Another caveat is that dosing strategies that are optimal for maintaining prophylactic efficacy for lamotrigine are not known. In the kindling seizure model, tolerance develops rapidly to lamotrigine and higher doses are paradoxically less effective than lower or intermittent high and low doses. The incidence of clinical tolerance development to lamotrigine in the affective disorders and dose regimens most likely to prevent this occurrence require further observation and study.

## Sequencing of mood stabilizers

### Accepted mood stabilizers: lithium, valproate, carbamazepine

What is the appropriate sequencing of mood stabilizers (Tables 17.3, 17.4)? Conventional wisdom suggests that one would add carbamazepine or valproate to lithium as the major second-line strategy. The literature from adjunctive studies suggests an approximate 50% improvement rate with either agent. There are relatively few markers of response, so one may rely largely on side effects profiles (Tables 17.1, 17.2). In a patient with major weight gain, lithium tremor, or gastrointestinal distress, one might choose carbamazepine before valproate in light of the potential added liability of valproate on these target symptoms.

However, valproate is easier to use than carbamazepine in terms of fewer pharmacokinetic interactions (Tables 17.5, 17.6). Valproate is also safer in conjunction with birth control pills, as carbamazepine's enzyme induction properties render many low-dose birth control devices ineffective. Moreover, a variety of drugs can induce carbamazepine toxicity, including erythromycin and its congeners, the calcium channel blockers verapamil and diltiazem (but not nifedipine or nimodipine), and a variety of other agents. In this regard, valproate will subtly increase carbamazepine's efficacy by increasing the free fraction of carbamazepine (displaced from protein binding) and preventing the breakdown of carbamazepine-10,11-epoxide, a metabolite active both for therapeutic efficacy and side effects, but its presence is not obviously detected in the routine measures of carbamazepine levels. The treatment principle in the use of carbamazepine and valproate in combination is to decrease carbamazepine dose with the addition of valproate, particularly if the patient is already at or near their side-effects threshold. Adding carbamazepine to valproate is readily accomplished with slow upward titration avoiding side effects.

Valproate also appears particularly useful in bipolar patients with dysphoric mania and rapid-cycling (Table 17.1) (Calabrese et al., 1992, 1993). Carbamazepine appears somewhat less effective in rapid cycling compared with non-rapid cycling patients, although in conjunction with lithium, a 50% response

**Table 17.4.** Drugs in the prevention of manic depressive episodes and cycling (strength of supporting evidence + to ++++)

| Primary drug (Putative Mood Stabilizer MS) | Adjunctive drugs | Bipolar-depression (D) |
|---|---|---|
| MS # First line for Mania (M) or Cycling (C) | First line – Mania (M) | |
| | | |
| MS I. Lithium ++++ | M – 1. Benzodiazepines (high potency) | D-1 Bupropion ++ |
| | (a) Clonazepam (Klon) +++ | D-2 SSRI |
| MS II. VPA ++ | (b) Lorazepam (Lor) ++ | (a) Fluoxetine ++ |
| | | (b) Sertraline ++ |
| MS III. CBZ +++ | | (c) Paroxetine ++ |
| | M – 2. Typical neuroleptics ++++ | (d) Fluvoxamine ± |
| Second line | (a) Butyrophenone (Haloperidol) | (e) Citalopram ± |
| | (b) Phenothiazine (Chlorpromazine) | |
| MS IV. Lamotrigine ++ | (c) Thiothixene (Navane) | D-3 SNRI |
| | (d) Molindone (Moban) | Venlafaxine ++ |
| | | |
| MS V. Ca²⁺ blocker ++ | | D-4 MAOI +++ |
| A. Dihydropyridine | M –3. Atypical neuroleptics (M and C) | (a) Typical |
| 1. Amlodipine (Norvasc) ± | (a) Olanzapine (Zyprexia) | 1. Tranylcypromine |
| 2. Isradipine (Dynacirc) ++ | (b) Risperidone (Risperdal) | (Parnate) ++ |
| 3. Nimodipine (Nimotop) +++ | (c) Quetiapine (Seroquel) | 2. Phenelzine |
| B. Phenylalkylamine | (d) Clozapine (Clozaril) | (Nardil) + |
| 1. Verapamil (Calan) ++ | | (b) RIMA – maclobemide |
| C. Diltiazam | Second line (M, D, & C) | D-5 Nefazodone (Serzone) ± |
| | | D-6 NeRI |
| MS VI. Atypical | MS VIII. T₃ (replacement) 25–37.5 μg ++ | (a) DMI ± |
| Risperidone + | T₃ (replacement) 75–150 μg + | (b) nortirptyline |
| Olanzapine + | | (c) maprotiline (Ludiomil) ± |
| Quetiapine ± | MS IX. T₄ (hypermetabolic) + | D-7 Clomipramine ± |
| | free thyroxine index > 150% | D-8 α2 antagonist mirtazapine (Remeron) ± |
| | (T₄ 150–400 μg) | D-9 Da Active |
| MS X. Clozapine ++ | | (a) pramipexole |
| | Third line | (b) Bromocriptine + |
| | | (c) Amoxapine ± |

Third line

MS IX.  Topiramate

MS VII.  Gabapentin +

MS XI.  ECT ++++

MS XII.  Trimipramine (±)

Fourth line

Omega-3 fatty acids (9 gms) +
Calcitonin +
Clonidine ±
Propranolol (High dose)
Mysoline ±
Phenytoin ±
Spironolactone

M – 4. Choline ±
     Acetazolamide ±

Fourth line

M – 5. Folate ± [a]
M – 6. Ascorbate + [a]
M – 7. Methylene blue +
M – 8. Smoking cessation ( ) [a]

D-10 rTMS ±
D-11 Precursors
    (a) Inositol ++
    (b) Tyrosine ±
    (c) Tryptophan ±
D-12 Psychomotor stimulants
    (a) methylphenidate (Ritalin) ±
    (b) Amphetamine (Dexedrine) ±
    (c) Pemoline (cylert) ±
D-13 High-intensity light ± 10 000 lux esp. in
     a.m.
D-14 Sleep deprivation ++
D-15 TRH ±
D-16 Anti-glucocorticoid
    (a) Ketoconazole ++
    (b) aminoglutethimide
D-17 Glucocorticoids
    (a) Prednisone ±
    (b) Dexamethazone ±
D-18 Inositol, 12–14 grams

| | | | | | |
|---|---|---|---|---|---|
| Established | ++++ | Multiple Controlled Trials | Equivocal | ± | Cases Only |
| Solid | +++ | Some Controlled Trials | No Data | () | Speculative |
| Substantial | ++ | Multiple Studies or One Controlled Study | | [a] | Relatively benign side effects |
| Weak | + | Few Studies | | | dictates greater use |

VPA=valproic acid; CBZ=carbamazepine; SSRI=serotonin-selective reuptake inhibitor; SNRI=serotonin–norepinephrine reuptake inhibitor; MAOI=monoamine oxidase inhibitor; RIMA=reversible inhibitor of monoamine oxidase; NeRI=norepinephrine reuptake inhibitor; rTMS=repetitive transcranial magnetic stimulation.

Note: Mood Stabilizer roman numerals (eg, MS I, MS IV, etc.) are from Fig. 17.5.

**Table 17.5.** Carbamazepine (CBZ) properties relevant to pharmacokinetics and drug interactions

| Property | Relevance |
|---|---|
| A.   Induces catabolic enzymes | ↓ Levels of CBZ and other drugs |
| | ↓ Thyroid hormones,[a] ↓ androgens[a] |
| | ↓ Effects of mild inducers on CBZ (induction ceiling?) |
| | ↑ 6-$\beta$-hydroxycortisol excretion |
| | ↑ Pseudocholinesterase |
| B.   Exclusively hepatic metabolism | ↑ CBZ levels with certain enzyme inhibitors |
| CYP3A3/4 | ↓ CBZ levels with certain robust inducers |
| | (phenytoin, phenobarbital, primidone) |
| | No kinetic interactions with lithium |
| C.   Active (CBZ-E) metabolite | Occult ↑ therapeutic and side effects with inducers of |
| | CBZ metabolism and inhibitors of CBZ-E metabolism |
| D.   Induces anabolic enzymes | ↑ HDL and total cholesterol, ↑ cortisol[a] |
| | ↑ Sex hormone binding globulin |
| | ↑ $\alpha_1$-acid glycoprotein |
| E.   Antidiuretic hormone agonist | Hyponatremia (↑ with diuretics)[a] |
| | ↑ Antidiuretic drug effects[a] |
| | ↑ Diuretic drug effects[a] |
| F.   Plasma protein binding not extensive | Generally few binding interactions |
| G.   Primary albumin binding | ↑ Free CBZ with valproate (displaced) |
| H.   Secondary $\alpha_1$-acid glycoprotein binding | ↑ Bound CBZ and other drugs (CBZ induction and |
| | acute disease) |
| | Interindividual variations in free CBZ |

[a]Entirely or partially pharmacodynamic mechanism hypothesized.
*Source:* Adapted from Ketter et al., 1991.

rate is evident in the study of Denicoff et al. (1997). Other potential targets or relative liabilities of the mood stabilizers are listed in Table 17.1.

## Thyroid augmentation

It is not clear whether T$_3$ augmentation is a mood-stabilizing treatment, in addition to its role as an adjunct for depression. Although Bauer and Whybrow (1990) reported mood stabilization with high dose T$_4$, it is our clinical impression that T$_3$ may not only be a antidepressant augmenter but also help stabilize some patients with inadequate degrees of mood control. Delineating whether or not this is the case requires controlled, randomized, prospective studies. Nonetheless, T$_3$ augmentation appears useful to counter lithium's ability to induce mild hypothyroidism (in some instances associated with cognitive dysfunction). T$_3$ augmentation (25–50 µg/day), with its short half-life and benign side effects profile, might also be placed higher in the treatment algorithm compared with the high

**Table 17.6.** Carbamazepine drug interactions

| | |
|---|---|
| *CBZ→ ↓ drug* | B. *Drug→ ↑ CBZ* (*toxicity) |
| Alprazolam (?) | Acetazolamide* |
| Amitriptyline | Baclofen (?) |
| Azole antifungals (?) | Cimetidine |
| Bupropion | Clarithromycin |
| Clobazam | **Danazol*** |
| Clonazepam | **Dextropropoxyphene*** |
| Clozapine[a] | **Diltiazem*** |
| Cyclosporine (?) | **Erythromycin*** |
| Dexmethasone (false-positive DST) | **Fluoxetine*** |
| **Dicumarol (?)** | Flurithromycin |
| Doxacurium | **Fluvoxamine*** |
| Doxepin | Gemfibrozil |
| **Doxycycline** | **Isoniazid*** |
| Ethosuximide | Josamycin* |
| Felbamate | Lamotrigine (↑ CBZ-E ?) |
| Fentanyl | Nicotinamide |
| Fluphenazine (?) | Ponsinomycin |
| **Haloperidol** | **Propoxyphene** |
| **Hormonal contraceptives** | Tefenadine (↑ free CBZ ?) |
| Imipramine | **Triacetyloleandomycin*** |
| Lamotrigine | **Valproate** (↑ CBZ-E, ↑ free CBZ) |
| **Methadone** | **Verapamil*** |
| Methylprednisolone | **Viloxazine*** |
| Mianserin | |
| Nimodipine (?) | |
| Oxiracetam (?) | |
| **Pancuronium** | I. *Drug → ↓ CBZ* |
| Phenytoin (↑/↓/=) | |
| Prednisolone | Adriamycin and cisplatin (?) |
| Primidone | **CBZ (autoinduction)** |
| **Theophylline** | Felbamate |
| Thiothixene (?) | Isoretinoin (?) |
| Valproate | **Phenobarbital** |
| Vecuronium | **Primidone** |
| **Warfarin** | Valproate (↑/↓/= CBZ) |
| *CBZ→ ↑ drug* | |
| False negative pregnancy tests | |
| Phenytoin (↑/↓/=) | |

**Boldface indicates risk of important drug inefficacy or CBZ intoxication.**

[a]Combination with CBZ not advised due to risk of agranulocyctosis.

(?) Slight or contradictory evidence. ↑ Increased; ↓ Decreased; = unchanged

*Source:* Adapted from Ketter et al., 1991.

| | Phenylalkylamine (on outside of Ca$^{2+}$ channel) | Dihydropyridines (inside membrane and Ca$^{2+}$ channel) | | |
|---|---|---|---|---|
| | **Verapamil** | **Nimodipine** | **Isradipine** | **Amlodipine** |
| | Calan® | Nimotop® | DynaCirc® | Norvasc® |
| | Isoptin® | | | |
| Half-life | Short (5–12 hours) | Short (1–2 hours) | Short (8 hours) | Long (30–50 hours) |
| Starting dose | 30 mg T.I.D. | 30 mg T.I.D. | 2.5 mg B.I.D. | 5 mg H.S. |
| Peak daily dosage | 480 mg | 240-480 mg | 15 mg | 10-15 mg |
| Antimanic | ++ | ++ | (++) | ( )* |
| Antidepressant | ± | + | (+) | ( )* |
| Antiultradian | ± | ++ | (++) | ( )* |
| Anticocaine (Dopamine) | - | ++ | ++ | ( )* |

*No systematic studies; only case reports and clinical observation.

Fig. 17.11.    Half-lives, dosages and effectiveness of l-type calcium channel inhibitors in mood disorders. Ca = calcium; T.I.D. = three times/day; B.I.D. = two times/day; H.S. = at night.

dose T$_4$ strategy, which has medical liabilities and is additionally confounded by T$_4$'s extremely long half-life.

## Calcium Channel Blockers (CCBs)

Nimodipine represents a class of dihydropyridine L-type CCBs that may have antidepressant and mood-stabilizing properties beyond those observed with the phenylalkylamine L-type CCB verapamil (Fig. 17.11). A number of controlled studies suggest the potential antimanic utility of verapamil (Dubovsky, 1995); its prospects in depression are dubious, particularly considering the controlled studies showing no more effectiveness than placebo, and substantially less effective-

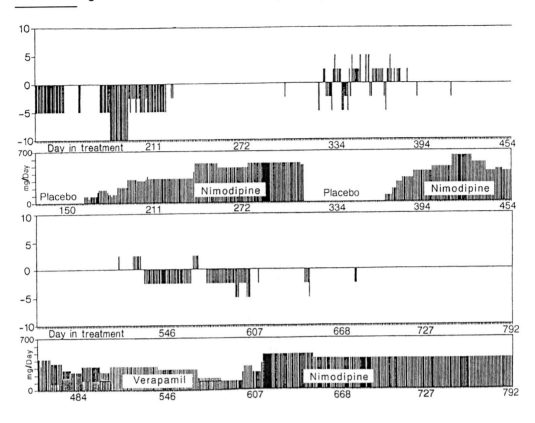

**Fig. 17.12.**   Prospective daily life chart ratings of mood (above) by nurses blind to medication status (below). Boxes above the horizontal line (euthymia) represent mild, moderate, or severe mania. Boxes below the line represent mild, moderate, or severe depression. A complete record of all her medications for each day of the study is depicted below each life chart line. Numbers indicating the day of the patient's hospitalization are in 2-month intervals.

ness than tricyclic antidepressants (Hoschl & Kozeny, 1989; Hoschl et al., 1990).

In an attempt to study a new CCB with a different profile that might be more effective, nimodipine was chosen because of its greater penetration in the brain, its lack of tolerance development in the treatment of migraine, and a differential anticonvulsant and biochemical profile, including the ability to block cocaine-mediated hyperactivity and the associated dopamine overflow (Pazzaglia et al., 1993). Nimodipine was shown to have clinically relevant mood-stabilizing properties in ten of the first 30 treatment-resistant depression cases studied at the NIMH on a double-blind basis (Pazzaglia et al., 1998). In some instances full or partial responses were confirmed in a B–A–B–A (off–on–off–on) placebo substitution design (Fig. 17.12). However, in the majority of cases, improvement was incomplete on nimodipine monotherapy and further augmentation with other agents was required. In one-third of the patients augmented with carbamazepine,

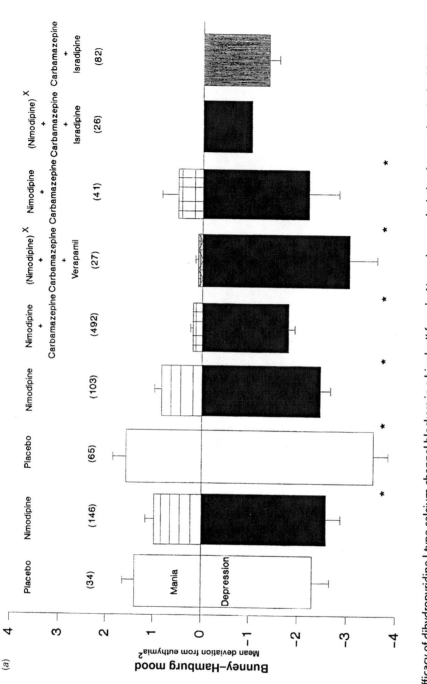

Fig. 17.13(a). Efficacy of dihydropyridine l-type calcium channel blockers in a bipolar II female. Nurses' mean deviation from euthymia double-blind ratings (number of days in parentheses) in a BP II ultra–ultra-rapid cycling patient showing the following: efficacy of nimodipine monotherapy; efficacy of nimodipine–carbamazepine combination therapy; unsuccessful transition from nimodipine to verapamil; successful reinstitution of nimodipine–carbamazepine combination therapy; and finally, successful transition to isradipine–carbamazepine combination therapy. *$P < 0.05$; × nimodipine slowly tapered to zero. [2] Mean using days depressed or manic only.

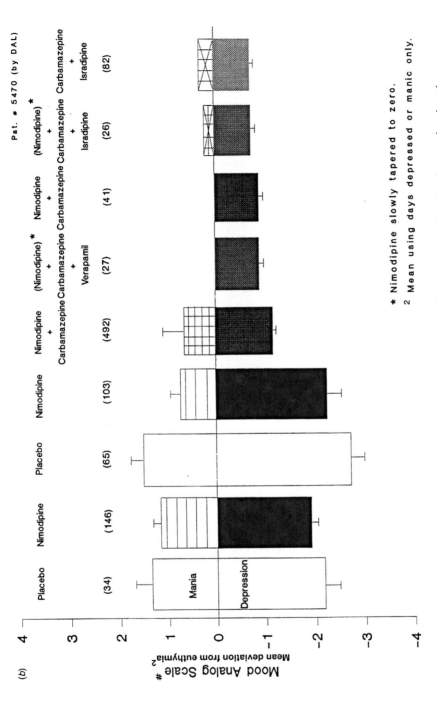

Pat. # 5470 (by DAL)

* Nimodipine slowly tapered to zero.
2 Mean using days depressed or manic only.

Fig. 17.13(b). Efficacy of dihydropyridine l-type calcium channel blockers in a bipolar II female: self-ratings. Mean deviation from euthymia ratings (number of days in parentheses) on the Mood Analog Scale in a BP II ultra-rapid cycling patient. In contrast to Fig. 13(A), the patient's ratings failed to identify significant depression exacerbation on the carbamazepine–verapamil trial.

**Table 17.7.** Lamotrigine in affective illness

| Investigator(s) | Subjects | Design | Duration | Dosage (mg/day) | Adjunctive meds | Results | Responders/ Non-responders |
|---|---|---|---|---|---|---|---|
| Weisler et al. (1994) | 1 BP | Open | 9 months | 200 | Yes | – Patient greatly improved; CGI values dropped from 7 to 3 | 2/2 |
| | 1 RC | | 8 months | 400 | | – Patient improved, relapsed after running out of lamotrigine, and again improved after restarting; CGI dropped from 5 to 1 | |
| Walden et al. (1996) | 1 BP | Open | 1 year | 150 | Valproate | Patient much improved; CGI values between 1 and 2 | 1/1 |
| Calabrese et al. (1997) | 64 BP: 25 manic phase | Open | 6 months | ? | Yes | 19/25 moderate to marked improvement in manic phase; SADS-C dropped from 21 $\pm$ 8.0 to 8.0 $\pm$ 9.9 | 46/64 |
| | 39 depressed phase | | | | | 27/39 moderate to marked improvement in depressed phase; CGI dropped from 4.7 to 3.6 | |
| Ferrier et al. (1997) | 7 BP RC | Open | 2–3 years | 150–200 | Yes | 3/7 marked reduction in frequency and severity of episodes | 3/7 |
| Fogelson & Sternbach (1997) | 6 BP (4 RC) 1 SA | Open | 8–65 weeks | 200–400 | Yes | 4/7 moderate to marked improvement | 4/7 |
| Hoopes & Snow (1997) | 47 (31 BP, 2 Cyclo., 10 MDD, 2 MD, 1 Conduct Dis.) | Open | 25–400 | | | 20/28 showed significant improvement, with lamotrigine alone or in combination with other medications, particularly younger females with rapid cycling BP II | 20/28 |
| Sporn & Sachs (1997) | 16 BP (8 RC) | Open | 5 weeks | 50–250 | Yes | 8/16 rated as responders (CGI $\leqslant$ 2) | 8/16 |
| Kusumakar & Yatham (1997a) | 7 BP RC | Open | 4 weeks | 50–150 | Valproate | 5/7 responded by end of week 4 (1 pt. developed rash, discontinued, and then restarted on lamotrigine) | 5/7 |

| Study | Design | Duration | Dose (mg) | Concurrent medication | Results | Response ratio |
|---|---|---|---|---|---|---|
| Kusumakar & Yatham (1997b) | Open | 4 weeks | 50–100 | Valproate | 16/22 (72%) responded by end of week 4 (≥ 50% reduction in HAM-D score compared to baseline) | 16/22 |
| Mandoki (1997) | Open | ? | 50–200 | Valproate + Lamotrigine | 10/10 children and adolescents improved CGI score | 10/10 |
| Kotler & Matar (1998) | Open | 6 months / 4 months | 25–100 / 25–100 | Yes / Yes | LTG added to Li stabilized patient / LTG added to Li, perphenazine and fluoxetine stabilized patient | 2/2 |
| Fatemi et al. (1997) | Open | 226 days ± 28 days | 185.0 ± 33.5 | Yes | 5/5 treatment-resistant rapid cycling patients showed significant improvement on mean BDI score after treatment with lamotrigine | 5/5 |
| Calabrese et al. (1999) | Double-blind | 7 weeks | 50 or 200 | No | 51% of patients on 200 mg/day, and 41% on 50 mg/day, showed ≥ 50% reduction on HAM-D or MADRS scales, or much to very much improved on CGI-I | 26/64 50 mg; 32/63 200 mg |
| Bowden et al. (1999) | Open | 48 weeks | 50–700 | Yes (N = 60) | 58% RC/manic markedly improved on MRS vs. 91% NRC; 48% RC/depressed and 48% NRC/depressed markedly improved on HAM-D; 49% RC markedly improved on GAS vs. 69% NRC | |
| Frye et al. (2000) Obrocea et al., unpublished data | Double-blind crossover | 6 weeks each phase | 50–500 | None | 20/39 (51%) responded to LTG; 11/40 (28%) responded to GPN; 8/38 (21%) responded to placebo; P<0.05 Cochran's Q for depression and overall illness | |
| | | | | | Overall response rate: | 200/337 (59%) |

BP, bipolar; CGI, Clinical Global Impressions scale; RC, rapid cycling; SA, schizoaffective; Cyclo, Cyclothymic; MDD, major depressive disorder; MD, mood disorder; SADS-C, Schedule for Affective Disorders and Schizophrenia: Change Version; DEP, depressed; HAM-D, Hamilton Rating Scale for Depression; LTG, lamotrigine; BDI, Beck Depression Inventory; Li, lithium; MADRS, Montgomery-Asberg Depression Rating Scale; MRS, Mania Rating Scale; NRC, non-rapid cycling; GAS, Global Assessment Scale.

**Table 17.8.** Topiramate in mood disorders

Open case series experience:

| Target symptoms | Dose | Trial duration | Response (%) | Investigator(s) |
|---|---|---|---|---|
| Mania | 614 mg/day (mean) | 28 days | 5/11 (45%) | Calabrese et al. (1998) |
| Treatment-resistant mood disorders | 200 mg/day | 16 wks | 23/44 (52%) | Marcotte et al. (1998) |
| Rapid cycling | 105.2 mg/day (mean) | 16 wks | 10/15 (67%) | Kusumakar et al. (1999) |
| Treatment-resistant mood disorders | 100–300 mg/day | 5 wks | 12/20 (60%) | Roy Chengappa et al. (1999) |
| 30 Manic | 193 ± 122 mg/day | 10 wks | 19/30 (63%) | McElroy et al. (2000) |
| 11 Depressed | | | 3/11 (27%) | |
| Mania | 50 mg/day | 15 days/16 days | 1/1 (100%) | Normann et al. (1999) |
| Rapid cycling ($n = 1$) | 200 mg/day | 3 months | 1/1 (100%) | Gordon & Price (1999) |
| Major depression ($n = 1$) | 300 mg/day | 2 months | 0/1 (0%) | |
| Total: | | | 74/134 (55%) | |

a substantial degree of added clinical benefit was observed. Among those responsive to nimodipine monotherapy or in combination with carbamazepine were patients with extremely rapid or ultradian cycling patterns of mood fluctuation (multiple mood switches in a single day) (Fig. 17.13(a),(b)).

It is unclear whether the L-type calcium channel blocking action of nimodipine is supplemented by carbamazepine's ability to block calcium influx through the NMDA receptor or through some other mechanism of action of carbamazepine unrelated to calcium (Post et al., 2000). Nonetheless, the ability to block calcium influx through two different mechanisms with carbamazepine and nimodipine, respectively, is of interest in relation to the large database suggesting that unipolar and bipolar depressed patients have increased intracellular calcium (as measured in their blood elements, perhaps reflective of neuronal accumulations as well) (Dubovsky et al., 1992; Post et al., 2000). It is also likely that calcium entering cells by voltage-dependent ion channels (blocked by the dihydropyridines) and ligand-gated, NMDA-mediated channels (blocked by lithium, carbamazepine, valproate, and lamotrigine) maintain separate signal transduction pathways in the cell and have a differential impact on the expression of immediate early genes. In this manner, one could conceptualize a dual approach to increased intracellular calcium with better long-term regulatory effects when a dihydropyridine is used in combination with carbamazepine or another calcium-active agent working through the NMDA receptor or some other different site of action.

Response to nimodipine may show cross-responsivity to other agents in the dihydropyridine class but not necessarily to verapamil (Fig. 17.13(a)). Several patients were successfully transferred to isradipine or, in uncontrolled observations, amlodipine, but did not maintain their clinical improvement on maximally tolerated doses of the phenylalkylamine verapamil (Pazzaglia et al., 1993, 1998). Amlodipine may be particularly convenient because of its long half-life, especially compared with nimodipine or isradipine, which require multiple daily dosing. Thus, we would suggest considering use of the dihydropyridine L-type CCBs as an adjunct to lithium in light of the data of Manna (1991), or as a substitute for lithium in those patients unable to tolerate its side effects profile.

### Lamotrigine, gabapentin, and topiramate

Lamotrigine and gabapentin are two newly approved agents for adjunctive treatment in epilepsy. Lamotrigine is thought to exert its actions through a blockade of sodium channels and associated decrease and release of excitatory amino acids, i.e. mechanisms related to those of carbamazepine and phenytoin (Fitton & Goa, 1995; Taylor et al., 1998). However, it would appear to have other, as yet undefined actions in light of its much broader spectrum in the treatment of a variety of epilepsies, including not only complex partial and major motor seizures as with carbamazepine, but also absence and atonic seizures (that carbamazepine may not only inadequately treat but may even exacerbate).

Calabrese et al. (1999) reported that lamotrigine was highly effective (50 mg or 200 mg/day) in monotherapy in treatment-resistant bipolar depression. The response rate was 51% on the Clinical Global Impressions scale (CGI) for lamotrigine 200 mg/day, and 41% on the CGI for lamotrigine 50 mg/day. In addition, there did not appear to be switch induction, and therefore lamotrigine appears to be a potential mood-stabilizing drug. In double-blind clinical trials on our unit (Frye et al., 2000a; Obrocea et al., 2000, unpublished observations) we have observed positive effects of lamotrigine in 20 of the first 39 patients studied in monotherapy. Slightly better antidepressant than antimanic effects were suggested; average doses in our study were 274 mg/day ± 128 mg (Table 17.7).

When used in combination with valproate, levels of lamotrigine should be markedly reduced, as valproate increases lamotrigine levels by a factor of about two (Ketter et al., 1999). In this regard, it is important to start very slowly when using lamotrigine as an adjunct to valproate, as the rate of increase in lamotrigine appears somewhat proportional to the incidence of rash, which is already at a high level (approximately 10%) in the absence of combination therapy. Since the rash can lead to severe Stevens–Johnson or Lyells syndromes in rare instances, the appearance of a rash should lead to drug discontinuation (Matsuo, 1999).

A number of open studies suggest the efficacy of topiramate in adjunctive mood stabilization (Table 17.8). In 54 patients studied by the Stanley Foundation Bipolar Network (SFBN), antimanic and anticycling, but not acute antidepressant

**Table 17.9.** Gabapentin in affective illness

| Investigator(s) | Subjects | Design | Duration | Dosage range (mg/day) | Other meds | Results | Responders/ non-responders |
|---|---|---|---|---|---|---|---|
| Bennett et al. (1997) | 5 BP | Open | Unknown | 600–2400 | Yes | 4 of 5 (80%) had moderate to marked response to adjunctive gabapentin | 4/5 |
| Marcotte et al. (1997) | 47 BP | Open | 6 months | 600–4800 | Yes | Majority of patients improved | |
| McElroy et al. (1997) | 9 BP (6 RC) | Open, used as adjunct | 1–10 months | 300–4800 | Yes | 8 patients (89%) showed moderate or marked improvement 1 to 3 months after adjunctive gabapentin; 6 of these 8 (75%) showed sustained antimanic response for 1–7 months | 6/8 |
| Ryback et al. (1997) | 73 BP (41 RC) | Open | | 200–3500 | No? | 67 of 73 (92%) responded positively to gabapentin, with the resumption of normal activities, mood, and behavior | 67/73 |
| Schaffer & Schaffer (1997) | 28 BP | Open | 1–9 months | 33–2700 | Yes | 18 of 28 (64%) positive response as judged by both treating psychiatrist and patient. Treatment discontinued in 10 patients, 2 because of greater rapid cycling | 18/28 |
| Stanton et al. (1997) | 1 BP | Open | 10 days | 900–3600 | None | Young Mania Rating Scale score decreased from 34 (at baseline) to 17 | 1/1 |
| Young et al. (1997) | 15 BP (10 RC) | Open | 6 weeks | 300–2400 | Yes | 8 of 15 patients (53%) responded (3 marked, 5 partial; Young Mania Rating Scale, Hamilton Depression Rating Scale) | 8/15 |
| Knoll et al. (1998) | 12 BP | Open | 2–60 weeks | 300–3300 | Yes | 8 of 12 (67%) had moderate to marked response on CGI | 8/12 |

| Study | Sample | Design | Duration | Dose | Concurrent medication | Outcome | Response |
|---|---|---|---|---|---|---|---|
| Erfurth et al. (1998) | 14 BP | Open | 21 days | 1200–4800 | Antimanic medication in six patients | 10/14 (71%) significant reduction in BRMAS score (6/6 in add-on group, 4/8 monotherapy group) | 10/14 |
| Ghaemi et al. (1998) | 40 BP | Open | 12.8 weeks (mean) | 100–5600 | Yes | 13/40 (33%) moderate to marked response on CGI-I | 13/40 |
| Altshuler et al. (1999) | 28 BP (5 RC) | Open | Varied with response | 300–3600 | Yes | 20/28 (71%) much or very much improved on CG-BP | 20/28 |
| Frye et al. (2000a) | 31 BP/UP (23 RC) | Double-blind | 6 weeks | 3987 ± 856 | | 8 of 31 (26%) responded on CGI 7 of 31 (23%) responded to placebo Both inferior to LTG | 8/31 |
| Pande et al. (2000) | BP | Double-blind | 10 weeks | 900–3600 | Yes | No significant differences between gabapentin and placebo in mania | |
| | | | | | | Overall response rate: | 163/255(64%) |

effects, were observed, however (McElroy et al., 2000). Its potentially positive side effect of appetite suppression and weight loss make it a potentially highly useful adjunctive or alternative to other mood stabilizers and atypical neuroleptics, which often are associated with mild to substantial weight gain. It also has a 1% incidence of kidney stones because it is a carbonic anhydrase inhibitor as well as a blocker of AMPA glutamate receptors. Too rapid dose increases may also be associated with speech or word finding difficulties.

The response to gabapentin was 8 of 31 patients (27%) in our double-blind study, a rate that did not exceed placebo (23%) and was significantly inferior to that of lamotrigine (52%) (Frye et al., 2000a). Possible antianxiety or antidepressant effects were observed at high doses averaging 3987 mg/day ± 856 mg, which was much higher than that used in most open add-on studies (Table 17.9). The controlled study of Pande et al. (2000) in mania was also negative.

Gabapentin is thought to block the L-amino acid transporter and increase GABA levels in brain and CSF (Beydoun et al., 1995). It is not a reuptake blocker, and whether the presumptive effect on the GABA transporter is related to its anticonvulsant and psychotropic actions remains to be determined (Kocsis & Mattson, 1996). In light of its potential antianxiety effects and positive effects in social phobia, one should consider using this agent in mood disordered patients with anxiety target symptoms (Pollack et al., 1998). It also may be useful in patients with insomnia and somatic pain syndromes. The addition of this agent to other combination therapies in some instances (but not in monotherapy) has resulted in important degrees of clinical improvement in some instances. Moreover, this agent does not appear to have pharmacokinetic interactions with most other agents and is excreted almost exclusively by the kidney and not metabolized in the liver. Thus, it has the advantage of having a relatively simple profile when used in complex combination regimens (Ketter et al., 1999) and titration can readily be achieved against side effects and therapeutic efficacy without concern about effects on either lithium level (Frye et al., 1998b) or, theoretically, other enzyme-inducing or blocking agents.

## Neuroleptics

The algorithms for using neuroleptics (Table 17.10) have dramatically changed in the last several years with the availability of clozapine and its unique profile of action in bipolar illness and schizophrenia, and even more recently with the availability of a number of other atypical antipsychotic agents. Whereas clozapine requires weekly blood counts because of a several percentage incidence of agranulocytosis, the newer atypical agents do not share this liability (Tamminga & Lahti, 1996). Low doses of risperidone have been reported to be an effective mood stabilizer in some patients (Tohen et al., 1996), although, somewhat surprisingly, higher doses in the 6–8 mg range have been reported to facilitate the induction of mania (Barkin et al., 1997; Lane et al., 1998). The overall utility of risperidone in treatment-resistant bipolar and dysphoric manic patients remains to be better delineated, particularly in relation to its dose/efficacy profile. Equally promising is the availability of olanzapine, another atypical that has a minimum proclivity for parkinsonian side effects, even with higher doses (McElroy et al., 1998a) and quetiapine.

Since these drugs have also been reported to be effective against the negative symptoms of schizophrenia, they provide the possibility of an augmentation treatment for treatment-resistant bipolar mania without the possibility of exacerbating the next depressive phase or extending its duration, as has been reported with typical neuroleptics (Koukopoulos et al., 1980; Ahlfors et al., 1981). To the extent that these atypical agents do not have the proclivity to induce tardive dyskinesia with either long-term or intermittent use (based on their relative lack of dopamine $D_2$ receptor blockade in the neostriatum), they would also have considerable merit and preference over the typical neuroleptics which potently block $D_2$ receptors in the striatum and are particularly prone to causing tardive dyskinesia in bipolar patients (Hunt & Silverstone, 1991).

The incidence of tardive dyskinesia in patients with bipolar illness has been estimated to be between 20% and 40%, and using only intermittent dosing strategies for intercurrent psychotic manias or depressions may actually be a risk factor for, rather than a protection against, the emergence of tardive dyskinesia (Jeste & Wyatt, 1982). Clozapine has been reported to be effective in both dysphoric manic and rapid cycling patients (Calabrese et al., 1996; Kimmel et al., 1994; Suppes et al., 1992; Zarate et al., 1995; Frye et al., 1996). To the extent that olanzapine and some of the other atypical antipsychotics more closely approximate its profile effects (Tamminga & Lahti, 1996; Frye et al., 1998a), one can hope that these agents will provide a new range of mood-stabilizing augmentation treatment for treatment-resistant cycling patients as well as those with schizoaffective illness and the need for long-term neuroleptics. The use of the atypical or the typical neuroleptics is to be highly encouraged in the acute treatment of bipolar illness, even in the absence of current controlled studies of their long-term efficacy. However, other more classical non-neuroleptic mood stabilizers may be preferable based on either efficacy or side effects profiles. Since atypical neuroleptics are clearly effective in the schizophrenic psychoses, including schizoaffective illness, and the negative syndrome of schizophrenia, one hopes they will be better antidepressants than the typical neuroleptics for bipolar illness. Ziprasidone may have a more positive side-effects profile than other atypicals with lesser degrees of weight gain and cognitive impairment (Daniel et al., 1999).

Parenthetically, an interesting potential atypical neuroleptic masquerading as

**Table 17.10.** Neuroleptic use in mania

| Drug (database) (Trade name) (Dose range in mg) | Mechanism | Assets ( + ) | Liabilities ( − ) | Comment | Relative CPZ equiv. |
|---|---|---|---|---|---|
| Clozapine ( + + + ) (Clozaril) (300–900) | ↓ $D_1$ ( + + ) <br> ↓ $D_2$ ( + + ) <br> ↓ $D_4$, 5-$HT_2$ <br> ↓ $\alpha_1,\alpha_2$ <br> ↓ $H_1$, $M_1$ | + No risk of tardive dyskinesia <br> + Well studied and effective in dysphoric mania and rapid cycling | − Weekly blood monitoring <br> − Sedation <br> − Hypotension <br> − Sialorrhea <br> − Weight gain <br> − Seizures | Blood monitoring for agranulocytosis inconvenient and expensive <br> Do not exceed ↑ 50 mg every 2 days <br> Can ↑ OCD <br> 5-HT block 10 times > D2 block | 100 |
| Risperidone ( + ) (Risperdal) (2–10) | ↓ $D_1$ ( + + ) <br> ↓ $D_2$ ( + + + + ) <br> ↓ $5HT_2$, $\alpha_1,\alpha_2$ | + Few EPS in low doses | − EPS in ↑ doses <br> − ?Antimanic <br> − Hypotension <br> − ↑ Prolactin <br> − Tachycardia <br> − Sexual dysfunction | Reports of exacerbation of mania with doses over 6–8 mg/day | 1.5 |
| Trimipramine ( ± )?? (Surmontil) (50–300) | ↓ $D_2$, $D_4$ <br> ↓ $M_1$ | + Proven antidepressant | − Sedating <br> − Unproven antipsychotic properties | Can ↑ OCD <br> $D_2$, $D_4$ blocker and antidepressant <br> ?Mood stabilizer | |
| Olanzapine ( + ) (Zyprexa) (7.5–20) | ↓ $D_1$ ( + + + ) <br> ↓ $D_2$ ( + + + ) <br> ↓ $D_3$, $D_4$, 5-$HT_2$ <br> ↓ $\alpha_1,\alpha_2$ <br> ↓ $H_1$, $M_1$ | + No blood monitoring <br> + Proven antimanic <br> + Less EPS | − Sedation <br> − Weight gain <br> − Nausea/dyspepsia <br> − Orthostatic hypotension | Most similar biochemical profile to clozapine <br> Most widely used atypical | 4 |

| Quetiapine (Seroquel) | $\downarrow D_1$ (+)<br>$\downarrow D_2$ (++)<br>$\downarrow \alpha_1$<br>$\downarrow H_1, M_1$ | + No ↑ prolactin | – Somnolence<br>– Alopecia<br>– Constipation<br>– Weight gain<br>– Hypotension | Limbic selective<br>Few anticholinergic side effects | 100 |
| Ziprasidone (Zeldox) | $\downarrow D_1$ (+)<br>$\downarrow D_2$ (++++)<br>$\downarrow 5HT_2, \alpha_1,$ | + No weight gain | – Somnolence<br>– Dizziness<br>– Nausea<br>– Hypotension | | 50 |

---

$D_1, D_2, D_3, D_4$=dopamine receptors; 5-HT=serotonin; $\alpha_1, \alpha_2$=alpha receptors; $H_1$=histamine receptors; $M_1$=muscarinergic receptors; EPS=extrapyramidal side effects; CLZ=clozapine; OCD=obsessive–compulsive disorder.

Key: (+)–(++++)=strength of evidence.

**Table 17.11.** *Principles in the treatment of bipolar illness*

| | |
|---|---|
| Dual treatment: Focus acute prophylaxis. | Develop Early Warning System (E.W.S.). |
| Mania: Treat first, chemistries later. | Develop specific clinical contracts. |
| Load valproate and lithium; start slow lamotrigine. | Regular visits; monitor course and side effects. |
| Second mood stabilizers (M.S.) over neuroleptics. | Encourage PRN phone contact. |
| Benzodiazepines instead of neuroleptics. | |
| Combination treatment; ↓ side effects. | Develop 'fire drill'. |
| Chart illness. | Prevent comorbid alcohol and drug abuse. |
| Augmentation rather than substitution. | Psychotherapy and medicalization of illness. |
| | Give statistics: 50% relapse in first five months off lithium |
| Simplify regimen (for side effects). | Patient as a co-P.I. |
| Slow taper of lithium, if at all. | Conservative T$_x$, if successful. |
| Educate family. | Radical T$_x$, if inadequate response. |
| Assess compliance and suicidality. | |

an antidepressant may be the tricyclic trimipramine. Trimipramine is approved for the treatment of depression, but has recently been shown to be a weak blocker of amine reuptake in contrast to other tricyclics, and yet is a relatively potent blocker of D$_2$ and D$_4$ receptors in vitro (Gross et al., 1991). This is consistent with the recent open study of its potential utility in the treatment of acute schizophrenia (Eikmeier et al., 1991). Whether it could have a positive role in the treatment of bipolar patients, as suggested by M. Berger et al. (1994, personal communication) remains to be determined.

## Conclusions

With the availability of a large number of putative treatment agents within each class of drug for bipolar illness (mood stabilizers, antidepressants, and antimanics) appropriate sequencing and management of complex drug combinations may be fraught with difficulty, but at the same time potentially life-saving. It is hoped that some of the principles outlined here will prove to be of value (Tables 17.3, 17.11), even if many of the provisional algorithms are radically altered by the availability of new data from comparative and controlled clinical trials and the emergence of additional treatment approaches.

## REFERENCES

Abrams, R. (1990). ECT as prophylactic treatment for bipolar disorder. *American Journal of Psychiatry*, **147**, 373–4.

Ahlfors, U.G., Baastrup, P.C., Dencker, S.J. et al. (1981). Flupenthixol decanoate in recurrent manic depressive illness. A comparison with lithium. *Acta Psychiatrica Scandinavica* **64**, 226–37.

Altshuler, L.L., Post, R.M., Leverich, G.S., Mikalauskas, K., Rosoff, A. & Ackerman, L. (1995). Antidepressant-induced mania and cycle acceleration: a controversy revisited. *American Journal of Psychiatry*, **152**, 1130–8.

Altshuler, L.L., Keck, P.E. Jr, McElroy, S.L. et al. (1999). Gabapentin in the acute treatment of refractory bipolar disorder. *Bipolar Disorders*, **1**, 61–5.

Baldessarini, R.J., Tondo, L., & Hennen, J. (1999). Effects of lithium treatment and its discontinuation on suicidal behavior in bipolar manic-depressive disorders. *Journal of Clinical Psychiatry*, **60** [suppl 2], 77–84.

Barkin, J.S., Pais, V.M.J., & Gaffney, M.F. (1997). Induction of mania by risperidone resistant to mood stabilizers [letter]. *Journal of Clinical Psychopharmacology*, **17**, 57–8.

Bauer, M. (1994). Refractoriness induced by lithium discontinuation despite adequate serum lithium levels [letter]. *American Journal of Psychiatry*, **151**, 1522.

Bauer, M.S. & Whybrow, P.C. (1990). Rapid cycling bipolar affective disorder. II. Treatment of refractory rapid cycling with high-dose levothyroxine: a preliminary study. *Archives of General Psychiatry*, **47**, 435–40.

Bauer, M., Hellweg, R., Graf, K.J., & Baumgartner, A. (1998). Treatment of refractory depression with high-dose thyroxine. *Neuropsychopharmacology*, **18**, 444–55.

Baumgartner, A., Bauer, M., & Hellweg, R. (1994). Treatment of intractable non-rapid cycling bipolar affective disorder with high-dose thyroxine: an open clinical trial. *Neuropsychopharmacology*, **10**, 183–9.

Benjamin, J., Agam, G., Levine, J., Bersudsky, Y., Kofman, O., & Belmaker, R.H. (1995). Inositol treatment in psychiatry. *Psychopharmacology Bulletin*, **31**, 167–75.

Bennett, J., Goldman, W.T., & Suppes, T. (1997). Gabapentin for treatment of bipolar and schizoaffective disorders. *Journal of Clinical Psychopharmacology*, **17**, 141–2.

Beydoun, A., Uthman, B.M., & Sackellares, J.C. (1995). Gabapentin: pharmacokinetics, efficacy, and safety. *Clinical Neuropharmacology*, **18**, 469–81.

Bonds, C., Frye, M.A., Coudreaut, M.F. et al. (1998). Cost reduction with maintenance ECT in refractory bipolar disorder. *Journal of Electroconvulsive Therapy*, **14**, 36–41.

Bowden, C.L., Calabrese, J.R., McElroy, S.L. et al. (1999). The efficacy of lamotrigine in rapid cycling and non-rapid cycling patients with bipolar disorder. *Biological Psychiatry*, **45**, 953–8.

Calabrese, J.R., Markovitz, P.J., Kimmel, S.E., & Wagner, S.C. (1992). Spectrum of efficacy of valproate in 78 rapid-cycling bipolar patients. *Journal of Clinical Psychopharmacology*, **12**, 53S–6S.

Calabrese, J.R., Woyshville, M.J., Kimmel, S.E., & Rapport, D.J. (1993). Predictors of valproate response in bipolar rapid cycling. *Journal of Clinical Psychopharmacology*, **13**, 280–3.

Calabrese, J.R., Kimmel, S.E., Woyshville, M.J. et al. (1996). Clozapine for treatment-refractory mania. *American Journal of Psychiatry*, **153**, 759–64.

Calabrese, J.R., Bowden, C.L., McElroy, S.L. et al. (1997). Lamotrigine in bipolar disorder: preliminary data. Syllabus and Proceedings Summary of the 150th American Psychiatric Association Meeting, May 17–22, 1997 Abstract No. 33B.

Calabrese, J.R., Shelton, M.D. III, Keck, P.E. Jr, McElroy, S.L., & Werkner, J.E. (1998). Topiramate in severe treatment-refractory mania. *American Psychiatric Association New Research Program and Abstracts Abstract NR202*, 121.

Calabrese, J.R., Bowden, C.L., Sachs, G.S., Ascher, J.A., Monaghan, E., & Rudd, G.D. (1999). A double-blind placebo-controlled study of lamotrigine monotherapy in outpatients with bipolar I depression. Lamictal 602 Study Group. *Journal of Clinical Psychiatry*, **60**, 79–88.

Callahan, A.M., Frye, M.A., Marangell, L.B. et al. (1997). Comparative antidepressant effects of intravenous and intrathecal thyrotropin-releasing hormone: Confounding effects of tolerance and implications for therapeutics. *Biological Psychiatry*, **41**, 264–72.

Clark, M., Massenburg, G.S., Weiss, S.R.B., & Post, R.M. (1994). Analysis of the hippocampal GABA$_A$ receptor system in kindled rats by autoradiographic and in situ hybridization techniques: Contingent tolerance to carbamazepine. *Molecular Brain Research*, **26**, 309–19.

Coppen, A., Chaudhry, S., & Swade, C. (1986). Folic acid enhances lithium prophylaxis. *Journal of Affective Disorders*, **10**, 9–13.

Coppen, A. & Bailey, J. (2000). Enhancement of the antidepressant action of fluoxerine by folic acid: a randomised placebo controlled trial. *Journal of Affective Disorders*, **60**, 121–30.

Coryell, W., Solomon, D., Leon, A.C. et al. (1998). Lithium discontinuation and subsequent effectiveness. *American Journal of Psychiatry*, **155**, 895–8.

Daniel, D.G., Zimbroff, D.L., Potkin, S.G., Reeves, K.R., Harrigan, E.P., & Lakshminarayanan, M. (1999). Ziprasidone 80 mg/day and 160 mg/day in the acute exacerbation of schizophrenia and schizoaffective disorder: a 6-week placebo-controlled trial. Ziprasidone Study Group. *Neuropsychopharmacology*, **20**, 491–505.

Denicoff, K.D., Smith-Jackson, E.E., Disney, E.R., Ali, S.O., Leverich, G.S., & Post, R.M. (1997). Comparative prophylactic efficacy of lithium, carbamazepine, and the combination in bipolar disorder. *Journal of Clinical Psychiatry*, **58**, 470–8.

Dimond, K.R., Pande, A.C., Lamoreaux, L., & Pierce, M.W. (1996). Effect of gabapentin (Neurotonin) on mood and well-being in patients with epilepsy. *Progress in Neuropsychopharmacology and Biological Psychiatry*, **20**, 407–17.

Dubovsky, S.L. (1995). Calcium channel antagonists as novel agents for manic-depressive disorder. In *Textbook of Psychopharmacology*, ed. A.F. Schatzberg & C.B. Nemeroff, pp. 377–88. Washington DC: American Psychiatric Press.

Dubovsky, S.L., Murphy, J., Thomas, M., & Rademacher, J. (1992). Abnormal intracellular calcium ion concentration in platelets and lymphocytes of bipolar patients. *American Journal of Psychiatry*, **149**, 118–20.

Eikmeier, G., Berger, M., Lodemann, E., Muszynski, K., Kaumeier, S., & Gastpar, M. (1991). Trimipramine – an atypical neuroleptic? *International Clinical Psychopharmacology*, **6**, 147–53.

Erfurth, A., Kammerer, C., Grunze, H., Normann, C., & Walden, J. (1998). An open label study of gabapentin in the treatment of acute mania. *Journal of Psychiatric Research*, **32**, 261–4.

Extein, I.L. & Gold, M.S. (1988). Thyroid hormone potentiation of tricyclics. *Psychosomatics*, **29**, 166–74.

Fatemi, S.H., Rapport, D.J., Calabrese, J.R., & Thuras, P. (1997). Lamotrigine in rapid-cycling bipolar disorder. *Journal of Clinical Psychiatry*, **58**, 522–7.

Fava, M., Rappe, S.M., Pava, J.A., Nierenberg, A.A., Alpert, J.E., & Rosenbaum, J.F. (1995).

Relapse in patients on long-term fluoxetine treatment: response to increased fluoxetine dose. *Journal of Clinical Psychiatry*, **56**, 52–5.

Fawcett, J., Scheftner, W.A., Fogg, L. et al. (1990). Time-related predictors of suicide in major affective disorder. *American Journal of Psychiatry*, **147**, 1189–98.

Fawcett, J., Kravitz, H.M., Zajecka, J.M., & Schaff, M.R. (1991). CNS stimulant potentiation of monoamine oxidase inhibitors in treatment-refractory depression. *Journal of Clinical Psychopharmacology*, **11**, 127–32.

Feighner, J.P., Herbstein, J., & Damlouji, N. (1985). Combined MAOI, TCA, and direct stimulant therapy of treatment-resistant depression. *Journal of Clinical Psychiatry*, **46**, 206–9.

Ferrier, I.N., Potkins, D., & Eccleston, D. (1997). Lamotrigine treatment in rapid cycling bipolar disorder (BPD): clinical and biological correlates. Proceedings of the Second International Conference on Bipolar Disorder, 15.

Fitton, A. & Goa, K.L. (1995). Lamotrigine. An update of its pharmacology and therapeutic use in epilepsy. *Drugs*, **50**, 691–713.

Fogelson, D.L. & Sternbach, H. (1997). Lamotrigine treatment of refractory bipolar disorder. *Journal of Clinical Psychiatry*, **58**, 271–3.

Frankenburg, F.R., Tohen, M., Cohen, B.M., & Lipinski, J.F. Jr (1988). Long-term response to carbamazepine: a retrospective study. *Journal of Clinical Psychopharmacology*, **8**, 130–2.

Frye, M.A., Altshuler, L.L., & Bitran, J.A. (1996). Clozapine in rapid cycling bipolar disorder [letter]. *Journal of Clinical Psychopharmacology*, **16**, 87–90.

Frye, M.A., Ketter, T.A., Altshuler, L.L. et al. (1998a). Clozapine in bipolar disorder: treatment implications for other atypical antipsychotics. *Journal of Affective Disorders*, **48**, 91–104.

Frye, M.A., Kimbrell, T.A., Dunn, R.T. et al. (1998b). Gabapentin does not alter single-dose lithium pharmaco- kinetics. *Journal of Clinical Psychopharmacology*, **18**, 461–4.

Frye, M.A., Ketter, T.A., Kimbrell, T.A. et al. (2000a). A placebo controlled study of lamotrigine and gabapentin monotherapy in refractory mood disorders. *Journal of Clinical Psychopharmacology*, **20**, 607–14.

Frye, M.A., Ketter, T.A., Leverich, G.S. et al. (2000b). The increasing use of polypharmacotherapy for refractory mood disorders: twenty-two years of study. *Journal of Clinical Psychiatry*, **61**, 9–15.

Gelenberg, A.J., Kane, J.M., Keller, M.B. et al. (1989). Comparison of standard and low serum levels of lithium for maintenance treatment of bipolar disorder. *New England Journal of Medicine*, **321**, 1489–93.

Ghaemi, S.N., Katzow, J.J., Desai, S.P., & Goodwin, F.K. (1998). Gabapentin treatment of mood disorders: a preliminary study. *Journal of Clinical Psychiatry*, **59**, 426–9.

Gordon, A. & Price, L.H. (1999). Mood stabilization and weight loss with topiramate [letter]. *American Journal of Psychiatry*, **156**, 968–9.

Gross, G., Xin, X., & Gastpar, M. (1991). Trimipramine: pharmacological reevaluation and comparison with clozapine. *Neuropharmacology*, **30**, 1159–66.

Himmelhoch, J.M., Thase, M.E., Mallinger, A.G., & Houck, P. (1991). Tranylcypromine versus imipramine in anergic bipolar depression. *American Journal of Psychiatry*, **148**, 910–16.

Hoopes, S. & Snow, M. (1997). Clinical effectiveness of lamotrigine in affective disorders. Proceedings of the Second International Conference on Bipolar Disorder, 26.

Hoschl, C. & Kozeny, J. (1989). Verapamil in affective disorders: a controlled, double-blind study. *Biological Psychiatry*, **25**, 128–40.

Hoschl, C., Vackova, J., & Janda, B. (1990). Mood stabilizing effect of verapamil. *Bratislavske Lekarske Listy*, **93**, 208–9.

Hunt, N. & Silverstone, T. (1991). Tardive dyskinesia in bipolar affective disorder: a catchment area study. *International Clinical Psychopharmacology*, **6**, 45–50.

Jeste, D.V. & Wyatt, R.J. (1982). *Understanding and Treating Tardive Dyskinesia*. New York: Guilford Press.

Joffe, R.T. & Singer, W. (1990). A comparison of triiodothyronine and thyroxine in the potentiation of tricyclic antidepressants. *Psychiatry Research*, **32**, 241–51.

Joffe, R.T., Singer, W., Levitt, A.J., & MacDonald, C. (1993). A placebo-controlled comparison of lithium and triiodothyronine augmentation of tricyclic antidepressants in unipolar refractory depression. *Archives of General Psychiatry*, **50**, 387–93.

Kalynchuk, L.E., Kim, C.K., Pinel, J.P.J., & Kippin, T.E. (1994). Effect of an ascending dose regimen on the development of tolerance to the anticonvulsant effect of diazepam. *Behavioral Neuroscience*, **108**, 213–16.

Kay, D.S., Naylor, G.J., Smith, A.H., & Greenwood, C. (1984). The therapeutic effect of ascorbic acid and EDTA in manic-depressive psychosis: double-blind comparisons with standard treatments. *Psychological Medicine*, **14**, 533–9.

Keck, P.E., McElroy, S.L., Tugrul, K.C., Bennett, J.A., & Smith, J.M.R. (1993). Antiepileptic drugs for the treatment of panic disorder. *Neuropsychobiology*, **27**, 150–3.

Keller, M.B., Lavori, P.W., Kane, J.M. et al. (1992). Subsyndromal symptoms in bipolar disorder. A comparison of standard and low serum levels of lithium. *Archives of General Psychiatry*, **49**, 371–6.

Ketter, T.A., Post, R.M., & Worthington, K. (1991). Principles of clinically important drug interactions with carbamazepine. Part I. *Journal of Clinical Psychopharmacology*, **11**, 198–203.

Ketter, T.A., Frye, M.A., Cora-Locatelli, G., Kimbrell, T.A., & Post, R.M. (1999). Metabolism and excretion of mood stabilizers and new anticonvulsants. *Cellular and Molecular Neurobiology*, **19**, 511–32.

Kimmel, S.E., Calabrese, J.R., Woyshville, M.J., & Meltzer, H.Y. (1994). Clozapine in treatment-refractory mania. *Journal of Clinical Psychiatry*, **55**, 91–3.

Knoll, J., Stegman, K., & Suppes, T. (1998). Clinical experience using gabapentin adjunctively in patients with a history of mania or hypomania. *Journal of Affective Disorders*, **49**, 229–33.

Kocsis, J.D. & Mattson, R.H. (1996). GABA levels in the brain: a target for new antiepileptic drugs. *The Neuroscientist*, **2** (6), 326–34.

Kotler, M. & Matar, M.A. (1998). Lamotrigine in the treatment of resistant bipolar disorder. *Clinical Neuropharmacology*, **21**, 65–7.

Koukopoulos, A., Reginaldi, D., Laddomada, P., Floris, G., Serra, G., & Tondo, L. (1980). Course of the manic-depressive cycle and changes caused by treatment. *Pharmacopsychiatry and Neuropsychopharmacology*, **13**, 156–67.

Koukopoulos, A., Reginaldi, D., Minnai, G., Serra, G., Pani, L., & Johnson, F.N. (1995). The long term prophylaxis of affective disorders. *Advances in Biochemical Psychopharmacology*, **49**, 127–47.

Kramlinger, K.G. & Post, R.M. (1996). Ultra-rapid and ultradian cycling in bipolar affective illness. *British Journal of Psychiatry*, **168**, 314–23.

Kupfer, D.J., Carpenter, L.L., & Frank, E. (1988). Possible role of antidepressants in precipitating mania and hypomania in recurrent depression. *American Journal of Psychiatry*, **145**, 804–8.

Kupfer, D.J., Frank, E., Perel, J.M. et al. (1992). Five-year outcome for maintenance therapies in recurrent depression. *Archives of General Psychiatry*, **49**, 769–73.

Kusumakar, V. & Yatham, L.N. (1997a). Lamotrigine treatment of rapid cycling bipolar disorder [letter]. *American Journal of Psychiatry*, **154**, 1171–2.

Kusumakar, V. & Yatham, L.N. (1997b). An open study of lamotrigine in refractory bipolar depression. *Psychiatry Research*, **72**, 145–8.

Kusumakar, V., Yatham, L.N., O'Donovan, C., & Kutcher, S.P. (1999). Topiramate augmentation in women with refractory rapid cycling bipolar disorder and significant weight gain from previous treatment. *Bipolar Disorders*, **1**[Suppl. 1], 38–9.

Lambert, P.A. (1984). Acute and prophylactic therapies of patients with affective disorders using valpromide (dipropylacetamide). In *Anticonvulsants in Affective Disorders*, ed. H.M. Emrich, T. Olcuma, & A.A. Muller, pp. 33–44. Amsterdam: Excerpta Medica.

Lambert, P.A. & Venaud, G. (1987). [Use of valpromide in psychiatric therapeutics]. *Encephale*, **13**, 367–73.

Lane, H.Y., Lin, Y.C., & Chang, W.H. (1998). Mania induced by risperidone: dose related? [letter]. *Journal of Clinical Psychiatry*, **59**, 85–6.

Leverich, G.S. & Post, R.M. (1998). Life charting of affective disorders. *CNS Spectrums*, **3**, 21–37.

Levine, J. (1997). Controlled trials of inositol in psychiatry. *European Neuropsychopharmacology*, **7**, 147–55.

McElroy, S.L., Pope, H.G. Jr, Keck, P.E. Jr, & Hudson, J.I. (1988). Treatment of psychiatric disorders with valproate: a series of 73 cases. *Psychiatrie and Psychobiologie*, **3**, 81–5.

McElroy, S.L., Soutullo, C.A., Keck, P.E. Jr, & Kmetz, G.F. (1997). A pilot trial of adjunctive gabapentin in the treatment of bipolar disorder. *Annals of Clinical Psychiatry*, **9**, 99–103.

McElroy, S.L., Frye, M., Denicoff, K. et al. (1998). Olanzapine in treatment-resistant bipolar disorder. *Journal of Affective Disorders*, **49**, 119–22.

McElroy, S.L., Suppes, T., Keck, P.E. Jr et al. (2000). Open-label adjunctive topiramate in the treatment of bipolar disorders: a clinical case series. *Biological Psychiatry*, **47**, 1025–33.

McLean, M.J. (1995). Gabapentin. *Epilepsia*, **36**, S73–86.

Maj, M., Pirozzi, R., & Magliano, L. (1995). Nonresponse to reinstituted lithium prophylaxis in previously responsive bipolar patients: prevalence and predictors. *American Journal of Psychiatry*, **152**, 1810–11.

Mandoki, M. (1997). Lamotrigine/valproate in treatment resistant bipolar disorder in children and adolescents. *Biological Psychiatry*, **41**, 93S–4S.

Manna, V. (1991). [Bipolar affective disorders and role of intraneuronal calcium. Therapeutic effects of the treatment with lithium salts and/or calcium antagonist in patients with rapid polar inversion]. *Minerva Medica*, **82**, 757–63.

Marangell, L.B., George, M.S., Callahan, A.M. et al. (1997). Effects of intrathecal protirelin (thyrotropin-releasing hormone) in refractory depressed patients. *Archives of General Psychiatry*, **54**, 214–22.

Marcotte, D. (1998). Use of topiramate, a new anti-epileptic as a mood stabilizer. *Journal of Affective Disorders*, **50**, 245–51.

Marcotte, D.B., Fogleman, L., Wolfe, N., & Nemire, R. (1997). Gabapentin: an effective therapy for patients with bipolar affective disorder. APA New Research Program and Abstracts (Abstract NR261), 138.

Matsuo, F. (1999). Lamotrigine. *Epilepsia*, **40** Suppl 5, S30–6.

Müller-Oerlinghausen, B., Ahrens, B., Grof, E. et al. (1992a). The effect of long-term lithium treatment on the mortality of patients with manic-depressive and schizoaffective illness. *Acta Psychiatrica Scandinavica*, **86**, 218–22.

Müller-Oerlinghausen, B., Muser-Causemann, B., & Volk, J. (1992b). Suicides and parasuicides in a high-risk patient group on and off lithium long-term medication. *Journal of Affective Disorders*, **25**, 261–9.

Naylor, G.J. & Smith, A.H. (1981). Vanadium: a possible aetiological factor in manic depressive illness. *Psychological Medicine*, **11**, 249–56.

Normann, C., Langosch, J., Schaerer, L.O., Grunze, H., & Walden, J. (1999). Treatment of acute mania with topiramate [letter]. *American Journal of Psychiatry*, **156**, 2014.

Otani, K., Yasui, N., Kaneko, S., Ohkubo, T., Osanai, T., & Sugawara, K. (1996). Carbamazepine augmentation therapy in three patients with trazodone-resistant unipolar depression. *International Clinical Psychopharmacology*, **11**, 55–7.

Pande, A., Crockatt, J.G., Janney, C.A., Werth, J.L., Tsaroucha, G. (2000). Gabapentin in bipolar disorder. A placebo-controlled trial of adjunctive therapy. *Bipolar Disorders*, **2**, 249–55.

Pande, A.C., Davidson, J.R., Jefferson, J.W. et al. (1999). Treatment of social phobia with gabapentin: a placebo-controlled study. *Journal of Clinical Psychopharmacology*, **19**, 341–8.

Pazzaglia, P.J., Post, R.M., Ketter, T.A., George, M.S., & Marangell, L.B. (1993). Preliminary controlled trial of nimodipine in ultra-rapid cycling affective dysregulation. *Psychiatry Research*, **49**, 257–72.

Pazzaglia, P.J., Post, R.M., Ketter, T.A. et al. (1998). Nimodipine monotherapy and carbamazepine augmentation in patients with refractory recurrent affective illness. *Journal of Clinical Psychopharmacology*, **18**, 404–13.

Peet, M. (1994). Induction of mania with selective serotonin reuptake inhibitors and tricyclic antidepressants. *British Journal of Psychiatry*, **164**, 549–50.

Pollack, M.H., Matthews, J., & Scott, E.L. (1998). Gabapentin as a potential treatment for anxiety disorders [letter]. *American Journal of Psychiatry*, **155**, 992–3.

Pope, H.G., McElroy, S.L., Keck, P.E. Jr, & Hudson, J.I. (1991). Valproate in the treatment of acute mania. *Archives of General Psychiatry*, **48**, 62–8.

Post, R.M. (1991). Anticonvulsants as adjuncts or alternatives to lithium in refractory bipolar illness. In *Advances in Neuropsychiatry and Psychopharmacology*, volume 2, *Refractory Depression*, ed. J. Amsterdam, pp. 155–65. New York: Raven Press.

Post, R.M. (1992a). Rapid cycling and depression. In *Long-term Treatment of Depression*, ed. S.A. Montgomery & F. Rouillon, pp. 41–195. London: John Wiley.

Post, R.M. (1992b). Transduction of psychosocial stress into the neurobiology of recurrent affective disorder. *American Journal of Psychiatry*, **149**, 999–1010.

Post, R.M. & Weiss, S.R.B. (1992). Endogenous biochemical abnormalities in affective illness: therapeutic vs. pathogenic. *Biological Psychiatry*, **32**, 469–84.

Post, R.M. & Weiss, S.R.B. (1995). The neurobiology of treatment-resistant mood disorders. In *Psychopharmacology: The Fourth Generation of Progress*, ed. F.E. Bloom & D.J. Kupfer, pp. 1155–70. New York: Raven Press.

Post, R.M. & Weiss, S.R.B. (1996). A speculative model of affective illness cyclicity based on patterns of drug tolerance observed in amygdala-kindled seizures. *Molecular Neurobiology*, **13**, 33–60.

Post, R.M., Uhde, T.W., Roy-Byrne, P.P., & Joffe, R.T. (1986). Antidepressant effects of carbamazepine. *American Journal of Psychiatry*, **143**, 29–34.

Post, R.M., Leverich, G.S., Altshuler, L., & Mikalauskas, K. (1992). Lithium discontinuation-induced refractoriness: preliminary observations. *American Journal of Psychiatry*, **149**, 1727–9.

Post, R.M., Leverich, G.S., Pazzaglia, P.J., Mikalauskas, K., & Denicoff, K. (1993). Lithium tolerance and discontinuation as pathways to refractoriness. In *Lithium in Medicine and Biology*, ed. N.J. Birch, C. Padgham, & M.S. Hughes, pp. 71–84. Lancashire, UK: Marius Press.

Post, R.M., Denicoff, K.D., Leverich, G.S., & Frye, M.A. (1997). Drug-induced switching in bipolar disorder: epidemiology and therapeutic implications. *CNS Drugs*, **8**, 352–65.

Post, R.M., Pazzaglia, P.J., Ketter, T.A. et al. (2000). Carbamazepine and nimodipine in refractory affective illness: efficacy and mechanisms. In *Pharmacotherapy for Mood, Anxiety, and Cognitive Disorders*, ed. U. Halbreich & S. Montgomery, pp. 77–110. Washington DC: American Psychiatric Press.

Rosen, J.B., Abramowitz, J., & Post, R.M. (1993). Co-localization of TRH mRNA and Fos-like immunoreactivity in limbic structures following amygdala kindling. *Molecular and Cellular Neurosciences*, **4**, 335–42.

Rosen, J.B., Kin, S., & Post, R.M. (1994a). Differential regional and time course increases in thyrotropin-releasing hormone, neuropeptide Y and enkephalin mRNAs following an amygdala kindled seizure. *Molecular Brain Research*, **27**, 71–80.

Rosen, J.B., Weiss, S.R., & Post, R.M. (1994b). Contingent tolerance to carbamazepine: alterations in TRH mRNA and TRH receptor binding in limbic structures. *Brain Research*, **651**, 252–60.

Roy Chengappa, K.N., Rathore, D., Levine, J. et al. (1999). Topiramate as add-on adjunctive treatment for patients with bipolar I or schizoaffective disorder–bipolar type disorder experiencing manic or mixed episodes. *Bipolar Disorders*, **1**[Suppl. 1], 27.

Ryback, R.S., Brodsky, L., & Munasifi, F. (1997). Gabapentin in bipolar disorder. [letter]. *Journal of Neuropsychiatry and Clinical Neurosciences*, **9**, 301.

Schaffer, C.B. & Schaffer, L.C. (1997). Gabapentin in the treatment of bipolar disorder [letter]. *American Journal of Psychiatry*, **154**, 291–2.

Sporn, J. & Sachs, G. (1997). The anticonvulsant lamotrigine in treatment-resistant manic-depressive illness. *Journal of Clinical Psychopharmacology*, **17**, 185–9.

Stanton, S.P., Keck, P.E. Jr, & McElroy, S.L. (1997). Treatment of acute mania with gabapentin [letter]. *American Journal of Psychiatry*, **154**, 287–7.

Stoll, A.L., Sachs, G.S., Cohen, B.M. et al. (1996). Choline in the treatment of rapid-cycling bipolar disorder: clinical and neurochemical findings in lithium-treated patients. *Biological Psychiatry*, **40**, 382–8.

Stoll, A.L., Severus, W.E., Freeman, M.P. et al. (1999). Omega 3 fatty acids in bipolar disorder: a preliminary double-blind, placebo-controlled trial. *Archives of General Psychiatry*, **56**, 407–12.

Suppes, T., McElroy, S.L., Gilbert, J., Dessain, E.C., & Cole, J.O. (1992). Clozapine in the treatment of dysphoric mania. *Biological Psychiatry*, **32**, 270–80.

Tamminga, C.A. & Lahti, A.C. (1996). The new generation of antipsychotic drugs. *International Clinical Psychopharmacology*, **11**, 73–6.

Taylor, C.P., Gee, N.S., Su, T.Z. et al. (1998). A summary of mechanistic hypotheses of gabapentin pharmacology. *Epilepsy Research*, **29**, 233–49.

Tohen, M., Zarate, C.A. Jr, Centorrino, F., Hegarty, J.I., Froeschl, M., & Zarate, S.B. (1996). Risperidone in the treatment of mania. *Journal of Clinical Psychiatry*, **57**, 249–53.

Tondo, L., Baldessarini, R.J., Floris, G., & Rudas, N. (1997). Effectiveness of restarting lithium treatment after its discontinuation in bipolar I and bipolar II disorders. *American Journal of Psychiatry*, **154**, 548–50.

Tondo, L., Baldessarini, R.J., Hennen, J., Floris, G., Silvetti, F., & Tohen, M. (1998). Lithium treatment and risk of suicidal behavior in bipolar disorder patients. *Journal of Clinical Psychiatry*, **59**, 405–14.

Trimble, M.R. (1988). Carbamazepine and mood: evidence from patients with seizure disorders. *Journal of Clinical Psychiatry*, **49**, (Suppl) 7–12.

Walden, J., Hesslinger, B., Van Calker, D., & Berger, M. (1996). Addition of lamotrigine to valproate may enhance efficacy in the treatment of bipolar affective disorder. *Pharmaco-psychiatry*, **29**, 193–5.

Wan, R.Q., Noguera, E.C., & Weiss, S.R. (1998). Anticonvulsant effects of intra-hippocampal injection of TRH in amygdala kindled rats. *Neuroreport*, **9**, 677–82.

Weisler, R.H., Risner, M.E., Ascher, J.A., & Houser, T.L. (1994). Use of lamotrigine in the treatment of bipolar disorder. APA New Research Program and Abstracts Abstract NR611, 216.

Weiss, S.R.B., Clark, M., Rosen, J.B., Smith, M.A., & Post, R.M. (1995). Contingent tolerance to the anticonvulsant effects of carbamazepine: relationship to loss of endogenous adaptive mechanisms. *Brain Research Reviews*, **20**, 305–25.

White, K. & Simpson, G. (1981). Combined MAOI-tricyclic antidepressant treatment: a reevaluation. *Journal of Clinical Psychopharmacology*, **1**, 264–82.

Whybrow, P.C. (1994). The therapeutic use of triiodothyronine and high dose thyroxine in psychiatric disorder. *Acta Medica Austriaca*, **21**, 47–52.

Young, L.T., Robb, J.C., Patelis-Siotis, I., MacDonald, C., & Joffe, R.J. (1997). Acute treatment of bipolar depression with gabapentin. *Biological Psychiatry*, **42**, 851–3.

Young, L.T., Joffe, R.T., Robb, J.C., MacQueen, G.M., Marriott, M., & Patelis-Siotis, I. (2000). Double-blind comparison of addition of a second mood stabilizer versus an antidepressant to an initial mood stabilizer for treatment of patients with bipolar depression. *American Journal of Psychiatry*, **157**, 124–6.

Zarate, C.A. Jr, Tohen, M., Banov, M.D., Weiss, M.K., & Cole, J.O. (1995). Is clozapine a mood stabilizer? *Journal of Clinical Psychiatry*, **56**, 108–12.

Zhang, L-X., Smith, M.A., Kim, S-Y., Rosen, J.B., Weiss, S.R.B., & Post, R.M. (1996). Changes in cholecystokinin mRNA expression after amygdala kindled seizures: an in situ hybridization study. *Molecular Brain Research*, **35**, 278–84.

# 18

# Medical disorders and treatment-resistant depression

John P. O'Reardon and Jay D. Amsterdam

## Definition of treatment-resistant depression

To date, there is no established consensus as to the definition of treatment-resistant depression (TRD). Nevertheless, a useful pragmatic approach is to define TRD broadly, as the failure of an episode of major depression to respond fully to a treatment known to be effective in major depression. This implies that TRD exists along a continuum rather than as an all-or-none phenomenon with varying degrees of treatment resistance. It ranges from a minimal or zero response to adequate antidepressant treatment (what has been termed treatment-refractory depression by Fawcett, 1994), to the more general problem of partial but incomplete response, where clinically there is some improvement in the patients condition but insufficient to achieve remission. In the literature remission in clinical studies is usually defined as an endpoint score on the Hamilton Rating Scale for Depression (HDRS) of $\leqslant 7$, and possibly in addition, a physician rated Clinical Global Impression-Improvement (CGI-I) score $= 1$ (i.e. very much improved). When this more rigorous benchmark is applied, only about 30% of patients in clinical trials will actually achieve remission of symptoms at the end of a 6- or 8-week trial of an antidepressant, so the problem of TRD, to one extent or another, is a very substantial one.

## Categories of TRD

Given the fact that the population of TRD patients is a heterogeneous one, some stratification is important in both conceptualization and development of treatment approaches. Patients with TRD fall into four major groups:

- Patients who have failed at least a single adequate trial of antidepressant treatment (either a complete failure of minimal to zero response, or a partial but clinically inadequate response falling short of remission).
- Some antidepressant treatment was administered but is judged retrospectively

to be inadequate in dose, duration, or both and so the patient was labeled, either prematurely or falsely, as treatment resistant (a form of pseudo-TRD).

- Misidentification or misdiagnosis of the disorder as treatment-resistant major depression, when, in reality, it is an underlying medical condition masquerading as major depression. Examples might include hypothyroidism, Cushing's syndrome or an intra-abdominal neoplasm presenting as major depression, which then fails to respond to antidepressant treatment.
- Concurrent presence of major depression in the setting of chronic medical illness such as poststroke, ischemic heart disease or cancer. In such situations major depression may be persistent and disabling and yet adequate treatment is inhibited by either a failure to recognize its presence, or else to adequately pursue appropriate antidepressant treatment. In this situation, the true bedrock level of TRD cannot be determined until adequate treatment is administered, though it is probable that it is, at a minimum, no less of a problem than situations where such comorbidity does not exist.

The difficulties posed by the first two situations, true-TRD and pseudo-TRD (due to inadequacy of treatment), are already the subject of a previous chapter. In this chapter specific consideration will be given to the problem of a second form of pseudo-TRD, where a medical condition is misdiagnosed as major depression and so does not respond to antidepressant treatment. In addition TRD will be reviewed in the general medical setting, where major depression is frequently overlooked or inadequately treated, such that it persists unresolved in consequence of what might be termed an approach of not so benign neglect.

## Relationship between medical disorders and major depression

Given that medical issues are an important consideration in patients putatively designated as TRD, each case assessed needs a thorough clinical evaluation. Failure to do so will result in misidentification of underlying medical disorders as TRD, and persistence of the TRD condition unresolved. With recognition of the medical disorder and appropriate treatment the syndrome of depression should resolve.

In addition to directly causing or precipitating major depression, many medical conditions such as stroke, cancer and myocardial infarction are important contributors to TRD. In such situations the biggest problem is not misidentifying the medical condition as major depression, but rather the failure either to recognize or treat adequately the comorbid major depression. When identified, the major depression is often dismissed as a normal psychological reaction to the burden of chronic physical illness, and as such, not requiring treatment in its own right. Such

**Table 18.1.** Some common medical contributors to TRD

*Endocrinopathies*
Thyroid disease
Hypercortisolism (Cushing's syndrome)
Hyperparathyroidism
Addison's disease

*Neurologic*
Poststroke
Parkinson's disease
Huntington's disease
Epilepsy
Autoimmune diseases (SLE, MS)

*Neoplastic syndromes*
Pancreatic carcinoma
Lymphoma
Bronchogenic carcinoma

*Sleep disorders*

under-recognition and lack of treatment is very common, for instance, in patients poststroke and postmyocardial infarction, where less than 10% of these patients comorbid with major depression receive an antidepressant (Robinson & Price 1982; Frasure-Smith et al., 1993), when treatment as usual is administered. This category of patients may well form the bulk of patients with persistent unresolved major depression in the medical setting. However, since systematic antidepressant treatment is only occasionally undertaken or evaluated, the level of true-TRD (failure to respond fully to treatment known to be effective in major depression), is unknown. A list of important causes and contributors to TRD is provided in Table 18.1 and will provide a framework for this chapter.

The coexistence of a medical disorder and major depression raises the question of the relationship between the two and what conclusions might be drawn, based on the evidence. The possibilities are:

- It is merely the co-ocurrence of two common conditions, a coincidence, and there is no significant interaction between the two.
- The presence of the medical condition has indirectly caused the major depression through its non-specific effect of increasing the burden of coping on an individual who is dealing with an incapacitating, chronic illness. At some point, when coping resources are exhausted, a 'reactive' major depression results.
- The medical condition has directly brought about specific biological changes, which then cause or precipitate a major depression.

- The presence of major depression has either directly or indirectly induced the medical illness.

In this chapter evidence will be presented, indicating that in many medical disorders biological changes ensue in important mood-regulating systems within the brain, and so may directly cause depression rather than through an indirect stress-reactive model. However, it should be borne in mind that, from a treatment standpoint, whether the cause of the major depression was direct or indirect with respect to the medical illness is irrelevant as far as the decision to treat. As per the atheoretical stance of the *Diagnostic and Statistical Manuals* as developed by the American Psychiatric Association, a strong case can be made that, if the patient meets criteria for major depression, and there is either significant impairment in functioning or moderate to severe distress, then treatment may well be warranted, either of a pharmacotherapy or psychotherapeutic kind. Whether the reverse can happen, i.e. major depression causing physical disease, has long been a topic of interest in psychosomatic medicine and, while there is evidence for depression lowering immunity, the evidence for major depression causing specific disease states remains limited. In any event, it is important for the clinician to recognize that, whenever major depression and a medical disorder coexist, there is a dynamic two-way relationship between the two, and one can only be ignored at the expense of the other. Both must be recognized and treated appropriately.

## Screening for medical illness in the setting of treatment-resistant depression

Each case of putative TRD needs a physical examination (whether by the primary care physician or the psychiatrist) and a targeted, focused work-up to ensure identification of possible underlying medical disorders presenting as major depression. In Table 18.2 a basic outline of the medical evaluation of all patients with some degree of treatment-resistant major depression is described. This will need to be adapted for the individual patient in light of age and risk factors, and further additional tests ordered as guided by preliminary clinical and laboratory findings.

In the physical examination, the vigilant clinician will be alert for any specific indicators of likely underlying clinical disease linked to depression. Severe weight loss in the middle-aged to older patient may suggest the wasting of malignancy. Finger clubbing can be an important pointer to bronchogenic neoplasia. Enlarged lymph nodes, especially if hard in texture, may suggest lymphoma and its subtypes. Neck examination for thyroid disease will reveal the presence or absence of a goiter. In neurological examination, the presence of tremor at rest, hypokinesia,

**Table 18.2.** Standard work-up in patients with treatment-resistant depression

Physical, including neurological examination

CBC + Differential, Electrolytes BUN, Creatinine, Thyroid function tests including TSH, LFT, Calcium, Phosphate, Albumin, Total Protein, Sedimentation rate, Urinalysis

> 40 years

The above plus

      EKG

      CXR

Presence of neurological signs or symptoms

All of the above plus

      CT scan or MRI

and increased tone, forms the classical triad of Parkinson's disease. In earlier cases, only tremor or mild loss of manual dexterity may be evident. Fundoscopy to examine for papilledema as a sign of raised intracranial pressure produced by a cerebral tumor is useful. The presence of specific neurologic deficit patterns will suggest conditions such as stroke or MS.

## Endocrine causes of TRD

Amongst medical causes of depression the most frequent appear to be endocrine, in particular thyroid (Gold et al., 1981; Prange et al., 1990). A number of findings point to a significant relationship between major depression and thyroid function. Hypothyroid patients exhibit many of the signs and symptoms of depression (Hall et al., 1981). Viewed from the opposite vantage point, approximately 25% of all patients with major depression exhibit blunted thyrotropin (TSH) responses to exogenously administered thyrotropin-releasing hormone (TRH) in the TRH stimulation test (Loosen & Prange, 1982). Furthermore, the addition of a thyroid hormone (triiodothyronine, T3) has been shown to both reduce the latency of onset and potentiate the therapeutic effects of tricyclic antidepressants (Thase & Rush 1995).

In considering further the relationship between hypothyroidism and major depression, it is useful to see hypothyroidism along a continuum rather than all or none, with varying degrees of thyroid failure from mild to severe. Accordingly, there is a gradual progression whereby all the baseline thyroid function tests become abnormal in a stepwise fashion over time. The grading stages of hypothyroidism from Grade I to IV, as proposed by Prange et al. (1990), are outlined in Table 18.3.

In the setting of major depression there is now good evidence for varying degrees of thyroid failure in a significant proportion of cases, perhaps as much as

**Table 18.3.** Grades of primary hypothyroidism

| Grade | Free T4 | Basal TSH | Response to TRH | Antibodies |
|---|---|---|---|---|
| I (overt) | Low | Elevated | Elevated | Usually + |
| II (subclinical) | Normal | Elevated | Elevated | Usually + |
| III (subclinical) | Normal | Normal | Elevated | Usually + |
| IV (subclinical) | Normal | Normal | Normal | + |

20%. The frequency of thyroid autoantibodies (Grade IV) has been investigated by Nemeroff et al. (1985) in a series of 45 psychiatric inpatients with depressive symptoms. Nine patients (20%) were found to have detectable titers of antithyroid antibodies, about double the rate reported in the general population of 5–10%. All nine had normal baseline TFTs (TRH testing was not performed), and none had a goiter. The presence of antithyroid antibodies by itself cannot be taken as normal since there is evidence such individuals will over time go on to develop symptomatic autoimmune thyroiditis (Amino et al., 1976).

In a larger series of 250 consecutive patients with major depression, thyroid status was examined by Gold et al. (1981). An overall frequency of thyroid dysfunction of 16% was found (20/250). Only 1% had clinically overt hypothyroidism (two patients), whilst 3.2% had Grade II (eight patients), and 10% (ten patients) had Grade III hypothyroidism. Thus in this study, even though patients were not screened for the mildest form of hypothyroidism, Grade IV, a strikingly high frequency of subclinical hypothyroidism was found. Furthermore, half of the total cases would not have been identified without performing a TRH stimulation test (which, in this instance, provides the opposite result from what is ordinarily found in most patients with depression – namely a rise in TSH above what occurs in normal controls, i.e. a rise of $\geqslant 25$ mIU/ml – vs. the blunted response found in 25% of patients with major depression). Of the ten patients with Grade III hypothyroidism (with the only thyroid abnormality detected being the abnormal TRH test), in half of these cases, it was judged clinically that the hypothyroidism was the likely etiology of major depression. Two of these five cases had in fact manifested a TRD type course of illness, with several failed medication trials, and these cases now responded successfully to an open trial of thyroid hormone administration. In the other five cases, the abnormal TRH response was considered to be either an early indicator of thyroid failure most likely co-occurring with the major depression, or else of uncertain significance as far as the causation of major depression.

In summary, taking the results of these two studies together, there appears to be a high prevalence of thyroid dysfunction in depressed patients, ranging from the mildest degree, Grade IV (with a frequency of 20%) to clinically overt hypothyroidism, Grade I (1%). This, in turn, raises the question of whether TRH stimulation testing should be performed as a routine in patients with documented TRD. To maximize yield from testing, it would perhaps be useful first to screen for Grade IV hypothyroidism, the presence of antithyroid antibodies, since, if these are absent, then thyroid failure is unlikely. In our practice we recommend TRH testing in the setting of TRD, if antithyroid antibodies are present and standard thyroid function tests (Free T4, TSH) are normal.

In terms of treatment there is good evidence from the work of Targum et al. (1984) that supplementation with T3 may be the most effective augmentation strategy in TRD patients with subclinical hypothyroidism, even in cases where it may appear uncertain that there is an etiological link. Even where subclinical hypothyroidism is not the direct cause of a case of TRD, it may still be making a significant contribution to the syndrome, such that thyroid treatment may be a necessary even if not sufficient intervention to restore euthymia.

Looking at the thyroid–depression relationship from the opposite perspective, the presence of hypothyroidism itself will produce a clinical picture similar but not identical to depression. The mood state is more frequently described as apathetic or irritable rather than depressed. Complaints of cold intolerance, sluggishness, and memory difficulty are prominent. An early classic paper by Asher (1949) on 'myxedematous madness' described the relationship between advanced hypo-thyroidism and psychosis. In each of the 14 cases described there was a paranoid flavoring to the symptoms. The most common subtype of psychosis was a delirium with psychotic features (five cases), two patients presented with dementia, five with what was felt to be a schizophrenic picture. Only two cases had a clinical picture of depression with psychosis, the least common subtype in this series. A generally favorable response to thyroid replacement is reported (Jellinek, 1962), unless the psychosis had persisted untreated for more than 2 years (Tonks, 1964).

The association between major depression and hyperthyroidism is less clearcut. Rather, these patients more typically have features of generalized anxiety disorder. In Kathol et al.'s (1986) series of 29 consecutive patients with hyperthyroidism, 80% met criteria for generalized anxiety disorder, with a strong correlation between its presence and the degree of elevation in the free thyroxine index. However, major depression was also common, with one-third of the series meeting criteria. In the great majority of cases symptoms of both anxiety and depression resolved with antithyroid treatment alone, implying that the psychiatric syndromes were secondary to the thyrotoxicosis. In converse, viewed from the opposite vantage point, the presence of hyperthyroidism amongst psychiatric patients is low. In a survey of over 1200 hospitalized psychiatric patients the frequency of hyperthyroidism was less than 1% (McLarty et al., 1978). Thus hyperthyroidism is an infrequent consideration in the setting of TRD.

## Hypercortisolism and major depression

The presence of major depression is associated with the presence of sustained hypercortisolemia in about 50% of cases. In turn, patients with Cushing's syndrome often have the syndrome of major depression. In this regard it is of interest that, in a relatively large prospective series of 29 patients with Cushing's syndrome examined by Cohen (1980), about half had a family history of depression or suicide, and six patients had a significant loss shortly preceding the onset of the endocrine condition, implying some overlap between the two conditions. In Cohen's series, a very large majority of the patients (86%) were significantly depressed. This was particularly so in the patient's with a pituitary origin for the Cushing's syndrome (i.e. Cushing's disease), where all but one of the 21 patients were depressed. Of the remaining eight patients four had adenomas of the adrenal gland, and four had carcinomas. The majority of these (five out of eight) were also depressed. However the uneven distribution between the two groups of major depression implies that, if there is an absence of major depression in a patient with Cushing's syndrome it is much more likely that the syndrome is a consequence of a peripheral tumor rather than being of pituitary origin. About 15% of the series had severe depression and one patient was psychotic. Successful treatment of the cause of the syndrome resulted in remission of the depression. In those with Cushing's disease who were treated surgically with bilateral adrenalectomy, improvement was rapid in onset in most cases with symptoms improving as early as a few days post surgery. A few cases did require up to a year to resolve completely.

An important clinical implication of the overlap between Cushing's Syndrome and major depression for the psychiatrist is that it may be impossible to distinguish the obese patient with major depression from early Cushing's. Thus the underlying endocrine condition and cause of the major depression may easily be overlooked. Such major depression may persist labeled as refractory to treatment until the proper diagnosis is made. Cortisol measurements are helpful in this instance. In a study by Gold et al. (1986), normal controls had a mean evening basal cortisol level (drawn at 8 p.m. in the evening when the hypothalamic–pituitary–adrenal axis is quiescent), of 3.5 $\mu$g/dl compared to a mean level of 7.5 $\mu$g/dl for patients with major depression ($P < 0.001$). In Cushing's Syndrome the degree of hypercortisolemia is significantly greater with a mean evening basal level of 20 $\mu$g/dl ($P < 0.001$). However, these mean figures can mislead as they fail to reveal the considerable overlap between the two groups of patients. In this study 11 out 30 (more than a third) of the depressed patients had levels of basal evening cortisol overlapping with the values of those with Cushing's Disease. The use of a corticotrophin releasing hormone (CRH) stimulation test may help to distinguish the two conditions as the plasma ACTH response to CRH injection move in opposite directions compared to the response of normal controls. In the study by Gold et al. (1986) patients with major depression had attenuated rises in ACTH levels in response to CRH injection compared to normal controls ($P < 0.001$). However, patients with Cushing's disease had quite exaggerated responses compared to normal controls ($P < 0.001$). Thus where the level of hypercortisolemia falls in uncertain territory in a patient with TRD, the use of a CRH stimulation test should allow patients with the hypercortisolemia of major depression to be distinguished from patients with hypercortisolemia secondary to Cushing's syndrome.

Finally, there may one other important area of overlap between Cushing's syndrome and major depression. It is noteworthy that the hippocampus contains the highest concentration of glucocorticoid receptors in the brain. A neuroimaging study by Starkman et al. (1992) found evidence of hippocampal volume loss in 3 out 11 patients with Cushing's disease with the degree of volume loss correlating positively with memory impairment and negatively with cortisol level. Memory complaints are also quite common in patients with major depression, and in the elderly may be so prominent as to initially suggest a diagnosis of dementia, the so-called 'pseudodementia' of depression. It is tempting to speculate that the loss of modulation of cortisol levels may be the shared pathophysiologic mechanism in both disorders leading to these symptoms in both groups of patients.

## Other endocrine causes

In contrast to Cushing's syndrome, Addison's disease is characterized by very low levels of all adrenal steroids, consequent to autoimmune destruction of the adrenal gland. Common presenting symptoms are weight loss and fatigue. Symptoms of depression occur in about 50% of cases and paranoia with delusions in 5% (Cleghorn, 1965). However, other clinical features help to distinguish Addison's from major depression. These include pigmentation on exposed skin surfaces, hypotension and abnormal electrolytes with hyponatremia and hyperkalemia (present in 90% and 65% of cases, respectively; Edwards, 1966). Thus the routine work up of a patient with TRD as outlined in Table 18.2 should permit recognition of the condition.

In hyperparathyroidism the commonest mental change is depression with anergia (Lishman, 1998). Again, routine screening of patients with putative TRD with routine laboratory tests will allow the hypercalcemia to be detected and so the diagnosis considered. Of particular interest regarding the mental disturbances observed in hyperparathyroidism is the close correlation with serum calcium levels. In Petersen's case series (1968) affective disorders were found in patients with a serum calcium in the range of 12–16 mg/dl. Above 16 mg/dl, range delirium was much in evidence, and at levels above 19 mg/dl somnolence and coma supervened. Consistent with this observation, psychiatric symptoms are rapidly and wholly reversed by lowering of serum calcium by peritoneal dialysis or by removal of the causative parathyroid adenoma. Therefore, TRD in this instance is really more an artifact of the correct diagnosis not being considered or identified. Once made, affective symptoms respond rapidly to the appropriate treatment. Hypoparathyroidism is not linked particularly with major depression and the commonest psychiatric syndrome secondary to the hypocalcemia is delirium.

## Neurological causes of TRD

Major depression frequently coexists with neurological conditions but often goes untreated because it is either overlooked or the major depression is dismissed as an understandable reaction to chronic disability resulting from the neurological condition. In this section evidence will be presented supporting a more direct link between many neurological disorders and major depression.

### Stroke

A pertinent example of this is the link between stroke and major depression. At one point it was felt by most clinicians that the development of depression poststroke was an understandable, non-pathological response of the patient to the resulting loss of function and chronic disability. Accordingly, it was rare for any of these patients to be prescribed antidepressants. In the series of 113 poststroke patients examined by Feibel et al. (1979), although fully one-third of the group were diagnosed as depressed, only a single patient was receiving an antidepressant. However, stroke patients do seem to have a high vulnerability to major depression, in excess of what can be expected on the basis of the burden of disability alone. This has been examined for by comparing stroke patients with matched groups of patients with equivalent or greater levels of physical disability (as measured by objective rating scales of disability) from other causes, such as motor neuron disease, traumatic spinal injury and patients with amputations consequent to peripheral vascular disease. Consistently, a higher incidence of major depression is found in stroke patients compared to controls (Folstein et al., 1977; Robinson & Szetela, 1981).

An important paper by Robinson and Price (1982) has explored further the link between stroke and onset of depression. A series of 103 outpatients attending a stroke clinic was evaluated for poststroke depression. As in the earlier series they found 30% of the group to be significantly depressed. However, there was no correlation between the degree of cognitive or physical disability and the severity of depression. They further classified the stroke patients into three groups; those with left hemisphere vs. right hemisphere lesions and those with brainstem lesions.

Patients with left hemisphere lesions were significantly more depressed than patients with either right hemisphere or brainstem lesions. Specifically, 49% of those with a left hemisphere lesion were diagnosed as depressed at initial interview, compared to 36% of those with brainstem lesions and only 7% of those with a right hemisphere injury. The peak period of onset of depression was in the 6-month to 2-year period poststroke. Of notable concern was the finding that none of the cases of depression were currently receiving any treatment for depression.

A possible neurobiological explanation for the propensity of left hemisphere lesions to result in major depression is suggested by a recent PET study in rats by Mayberg et al. (1988) using radiolabeled methylpiperone to detect serotonin-2 receptor binding. It was found that right but not left hemisphere strokes were associated with an increase in serotonin receptor binding in the uninjured parts of the hemisphere. This response within the right hemisphere may be a compensatory one that serves to prevent or attenuate depression. Therefore, in summary, it is important for the clinician to be alert to the development of major depression in poststroke patients. Otherwise, it will persist untreated undermining efforts at rehabilitation and lowering further the quality of life for these patients.

## Parkinson's disease

Analogous to the situation with poststroke patients, sufferers from Parkinson's disease also seem particularly vulnerable to major depression. Current evidence indicates that about half of patients with Parkinson's disease (PD) become depressed (Celesia & Wanamaker, 1972; Mindham, 1970). In a study by Robins (1976), 45 patients with Parkinson's disease were compared with an age and sex matched control group of 45 physically disabled patients. The control group was selected such that they had a significantly more physical disability (as measured on objective rating scales) than the group with Parkinson's disease. The control group included patients with severe chronic disability resulting from hemiplegia (almost half the cases), paraplegia, orthopedic conditions such as rheumatoid arthritis, and amputations consequent to severe peripheral vascular disease. Despite this it was found that the parkinsonian group was significantly more depressed ($P < 0.0001$). Even when scores for retardation were excluded from the Hamilton Depression Rating Scale (HDRS) scores, the mean HDRS score for the patients with PD remained significantly greater (HDRS score = 33.97 in PD group compared to HDRS score = 24.18 in the control group, $P < 0.001$). Thus, while both groups have high levels of depressive symptoms as indicated by the group mean HDRS scores, the level of depressive symptoms is substantially greater again in the group with PD. Patients with PD seem to have an added vulnerability to depression beyond the burden of physical handicap. Therefore some other mechanism must be in operation.

In this regard, attempts to relate major depression to changes in dopamine metabolism have been unsuccessful (Granerus et al., 1974; Hoehn et al., 1976, Vanderheyden et al., 1981). A study by Mayeux et al. (1984) has, however, demonstrated a link with serotonin depletion in the CSF of patients with PD. Lumbar puncture and CSF analysis for biogenic amine metabolites were performed in patients with PD, with or without depression and compared to 15 age-matched patient controls (with either stroke or neuromuscular disorders). The concentration of 5HIAA was significantly lower in PD patients with depression compared to either PD patients without depression ($P < 0.03$) or controls ($P < 0.0001$). In addition, within the depressed group the greatest reduction in CSF levels of 5HIAA was in those with major depression with a less marked reduction in those with dysthymia. However, CSF levels of either HVA or MHPG did not relate to depression. Thus the loss of serotonin function in PD which parallels loss of dopamine function may be a direct etiological link to the very high incidence of depression in this condition. This may have treatment implications in terms of managing either major depression or TRD in patients with PD. It appears that serotonin reuptake inhibitor antidepressants are effective in patients with major depression and PD. These findings would support their first-line use in PD patients who develop major depression. However, as of yet, there is no evidence to indicate that the specific serotonergic properties confer an additional advantage in antidepressive effect over other antidepressant classes in PD patients with major depression. In the setting of TRD in patients with PD, serious consideration should also be given to ECT as there is evidence that it reduces the hypokinesia of PD, at least in the short term as well as effectively treating major depression.

## Epilepsy

A close relationship between epilepsy and affective disorder has been surmised since the time of Hippocrates, who wrote 'melancholics ordinarily become epileptics, and epileptics become melancholics: of these two states, what determines the preference is the direction the malady takes; if it bears upon the body, epilepsy, if upon the intelligence, melancholy' (Lewis, 1934). There is good evidence for a significant vulnerability to major depression amongst patients with epilepsy. In a study of epileptic patients requiring psychiatric admission by Betts (1974), depression was the commonest psychiatric diagnosis, occurring in 31% of the sample of 74 patients. A larger series by Currie et al. (1971) of 666 patients with temporal lobe epilepsy, found rates of 19% for depression, and 11% for anxiety during the follow-up period. Whether there is a connection between the development of major depression and particular subtypes of epilepsy remains unclear. In one series, evidence was found for a connection between frequency of depressive episodes and the presence of temporal lobe epilepsy (Donigier, 1959), while another case series was negative in this regard (Trimble & Perez, 1980).

However, irrespective whether one subtype of epilepsy is more liable to cause or precipitate major depression than another clinicians need to be aware of the high frequency of suicide in patients comorbid with major depression and epilepsy. In the study by Henriksen et al. (1970), a representative sample of all neurological patients with epilepsy discharged from four clinics in Denmark were followed up long term, and the cause of death ascertained from death certificates. The number of deaths by suicide was three times the number that would have been predicted. Similarly, a follow-up study by White et al. (1979) of 2000 patients with epilepsy over a 60-year period, found a total of 21 deaths by suicide compared to an expected value of 4. Barraclough (1981), in a review of 11 articles in this area, concluded that overall the mortality rate by suicide for patients with epilepsy was elevated five-fold. Furthermore, the risk for patients with temporal lobe epilepsy was elevated even further, with a 25-fold increase in mortality by suicide. Viewed in totality, this evidence suggests a high prevalence of severe major depression in the setting of epilepsy, and either a failure to deliver adequate treatment or relative resistance to adequate treatment (TRD) or, most likely a combination of the two. Given such findings, clinicians, in particular neurologists, need to be alert for the presence of major depression in patients with epilepsy and to be prepared to utilize the services of psychiatrists freely in managing TRD in this setting.

A couple of additional links between epilepsy and major depression are also of interest. Some patients with epilepsy manifest only ictally related mood changes (perictal) and do not suffer from persistent major depression in the interictal periods. In these situations the mood episodes are closely linked in time with seizures and resolve spontaneously. They are distinguished from an aura or post-ictal automatism by lasting longer. In one case series (Mulder & Daly, 1952) of epileptics, 15% were found to manifest periictal mood changes, mostly dysphoria (in two-thirds of cases). Occasionally, such mood changes can be severe, as evinced in the case report by Betts (1982) of a patient cutting his throat during an ictal depressed state. An interaction in the opposite direction may also occur, as indicated by the frequent observation that fit frequency declines either prior to, or with the onset of a major depressive episode (Betts, 1974). Thus, as well as the full syndromal and treatment-resistant major depressive episodes, a more subtle interplay may also occur between mood and seizure disorders. In either event, the careful clinician needs to be attentive to mood changes in epileptic patients, and be prepared to manage TRD aggressively, in light of the high lethality of such episodes in this patient population.

## Multiple sclerosis

Affective disturbances are common in patients with multiple sclerosis (MS). They range from major depression and bipolar illness to disorders which are more unique to MS, namely euphoria and pathological laughing and crying. The latter two seem to be more clearly neurologically based, occurring late in the course of the disease and appear to be related to lesions in the frontal lobes, basal ganglia and temporal lobes (O'Malley, 1966).

Euphoria needs to be distinguished from bipolar hypomanic episodes. Euphoria in this setting may be defined as 'a persistent mental state of happiness, and optimism as to the future and prospects for ultimate recovery which is out of place and incongruous' (Cottrell & Wilson, 1926). Unlike hypomania, there is not the associated hyperactivity, racing thoughts or pressure of speech. Contrary to what one might predict, the development of euphoria in the course of MS is associated with severe disability and chronic progressive type MS. It is also strongly associated with the onset of cognitive impairment, and enlargement of ventricles on computed tomographic scans. It is not associated with MS confined to the spinal cord (Surridge, 1969; Rabins et al., 1986). The euphoric state is best construed as a neurologically based inability to appreciate the severity of the deficits present, rather than psychodynamically driven denial. Rabins (1990) has suggested the disconnection of cognition and emotion seen in the euphoria of MS reflects a frontal lobe disconnection syndrome consequent to periventricular demyelination of frontal pathways. Similarly, the syndrome of pathological laughing and crying may also be a type of disconnection syndrome, in this instance a disconnection between neuronal centers involved in perceived emotion and those involved in the displayed emotion. Reported prevalence rates for these complications of MS vary widely in the literature ranging from 5% (Kahana et al., 1971) to 63% (Cottrell & Wilson, 1926).

Similar to other neurological disorders reviewed, MS also is associated with a high prevalence of major depression. A variety of studies have suggested a point prevalence range of 27 to 52% (Whitlock & Siskind, 1980; Schiffer et al., 1983; Joffe, 1987). Furthermore there is an elevated suicide rate, in one study a 14-fold elevation above the rate of the general population (Kahana et al., 1971). This suggests that many of these depressive episodes are severe and likely to fall within the TRD category, albeit there are no systematic studies of TRD in MS patients with major depression. There is emerging evidence that there may be a direct biological link between MS and the elevated rates of major depression and suicide, as well as the more indirect factor of a chronic disabling illness like MS increasing the psychosocial burden on the patient. For instance, patients with MS exhibit higher levels of depression compared with patient controls with equivalent levels of disability from other neurological disorders such as spinal cord injury or ALS (Whitlock & Siskind, 1980). Within the MS group itself, patients with primarily cerebral involvement have a significantly higher propensity to major depression than those with predominantly cerebellar or spinal cord disease (Schiffer et al., 1983; Rabins et al., 1986).

A recent study by Honer et al. (1987) suggests that MS lesions in the temporal lobes may underlie this propensity. Magnetic resonance imaging results from eight MS patients with psychiatric disturbance (with onset after the diagnosis of MS was made), were compared to results from another group of eight MS patients matched for age, sex, severity and duration of illness. The psychiatric group was a heterogeneous group, not confined to cases of major depression. Three patients were diagnosed with major depression, two with bipolar disorder and the remainder with organic psychiatric syndromes. Whilst both groups had similar areas of total cerebral involvement when plaque area was measured, the psychiatric group had a significantly greater burden of temporal lobe involvement (a mean area of 488 mm vs. 280 mm; $P < 0.05$). This is preliminary evidence that temporal lobe involvement by MS lesions may underlie a significant portion of the pathophysiology of affective illness in MS patients.

## Huntington's disease (HD)

Affective symptoms, particularly depressed mood are found commonly in this hereditary neurological disorder. A survey of 88 patients with HD from a defined geographical area in Maryland has been conducted by Folstein et al. (1983). Multiple case-finding methods were used in order to ascertain all cases in the defined area. Following patient evaluation with a structured clinical instrument (NIMH Diagnostic Interview Schedule), the commonest psychiatric disorder was major depression with a frequency of 32%. The rate of bipolar disorder was also elevated at 9%. Dysthmic disorder was diagnosed in about 4% giving a total prevalence of 45% for affective disorders. In addition, it was found that affective disorder cases clustered within certain families. In most of the 34 patients with both affective disorder and HD, the affective disorder preceded the onset of chorea and dementia (23 out of 34 cases), on average by about 5 years. Taken as a whole, these findings suggest that it is unlikely that the occurrence of major depression in patients with HD is simply and exclusively a psychological reaction to having a fatal disabling illness. This would fail to explain both the markedly increased rate of bipolar disorder also seen (9%) and the fact that two-thirds of the cases of affective disorder preceded the diagnosis of HD rather than following in its wake, in some cases by as much as 20 years. The familial clustering of affective disorder and HD together suggest that genetic heterogeneity may be a more persuasive explanation.

Similar to both MS and epilepsy, suicide is a significant concern in HD. Huntington himself remarked on this in 1872 writing that, 'the tendency to insanity, and sometimes to that form of insanity that leads to suicide is marked'. In the Folstein case series most of the patients, with an affective disorder in addition to HD, had a history of suicide thought or attempts (55%). As with major depression, completed suicides also tend to cluster in families. The overall suicide rate amongst patients with HD who are non-institutionalized has been reported at 7% (Reed & Chandler, 1958). The relative contributions to this clinical course made by under-recognition, inadequate treatment of major depression vs. treatment-resistant major depression is unknown. Nevertheless, this patient group similarly to patients with MS and epilepsy, seem to have heightened vulnerability to both major depression and death by suicide, and therefore should command from the clinician a heightened vigilance for the detection of major depression and delivery of systematic antidepressant strategies.

## Cerebral tumors

Albeit rare, it is important that consideration be given to the possibility of an underlying brain tumor in the setting of TRD. Tumors that give rise to psychiatric rather than to neurological symptoms as an early manifestation tend to be slow growing such as meningiomas, or else located in a brain region such as the frontal lobes where space permits considerable 'silent' growth in the absence of neurological signs or symptoms. Thus the diagnosis is easily missed. Anderson (1970) reported an autopsy series from state mental hospitals in Denmark in which a tumor frequency of 3% was detected at autopsy, two-thirds of which had gone undetected during life. Most of these patients had been hospitalized for less than 6 months, so it is likely in that at least a portion of cases the tumor was causally related to the psychiatric presentation and admission. Similarly, a series of 88 cases from the Boston State Hospital by Raskin (1956) reported a tumor frequency of 3.5% with meningiomas making up the largest single group (30% compared to general frequency of 15% amongst all neurological patients with brain tumors).

Whilst brain tumors may initially present with a wide variety of possible psychiatric syndromes, including classically, dementia or isolated memory difficulties or delirium, on occasion the presentation is with a syndrome of TRD. This applies particularly to frontal and temporal lobe tumors, as in the series reported by Hecaen and Ajuraguerra (1956) where affective symptoms were found to be twice as common in tumors in these locations compared to all other brain tumors. Frontal lobe tumors are particularly likely to mislead as to diagnosis. Disturbances of affect such as irritability, depressed mood, euphoria and apathy are common with frontal tumors. In Direkze's series of 25 patients with frontal tumors, some had initially been admitted to psychiatric inpatient units with clinical depression and treated unsuccessfully with ECT before the correct diagnosis was made (Direkze et al., 1971). In Lishman's classic text *Organic Psychiatry: The Psychological Consequences of Cere-bral Disorder* (1998) he cites a case report initially reported by Maurice-Williams and Sinar (1984), illustrating the presence of TRD may blind the clinician to other possibilities even in the face of evidence to the contrary:

An intractable depressive illness in a female patient responded to bilateral leukotomy 23 years before her left frontal meningioma was diagnosed. It seemed probable, moreover, that the tumor had caused or precipitated the depression since its onset coincided with the development of focal seizures involving the right arm and face. An EEG carried out prior to the leukotomy had shown a left frontotemporal focus, but inexplicably was ignored. The depression remained in abeyance following the leukotomy, though the seizures had continued. At the time of her depression the patient had been obsessed that her fits were due to a brain tumor!

Two approaches will assist the clinician immensely dealing with a case of TRD in avoiding these unsatisfactory outcomes. The first is to have an awareness and knowledge of other coexisting signs or symptoms that may suggest the possibility of a brain tumor, and the second is a readiness to utilize neuroimaging tools of CT scanning and magnetic resonance imaging when in doubt. With frontal tumors, the commonest initial symptoms are memory impairment suggestive of dementia. In addition to depressed mood, apathy is a frequent finding often accompanied by psychomotor slowing. The latter is sometimes so severe that the patient is rendered mute and immobile, the syndrome of akinetic mutism. Personality changes, in particular irritability and disinhibition are common usually developing without accompanying insight. Finally, incontinence is often an early feature and should be a suggestive symptom for the alert clinician.

In temporal lobe tumors, as with frontal tumors, affective symptoms of depressed mood, irritability and anxiety are common, possibly more frequent with tumors on the dominant hemisphere (Keschner et al., 1936). Like frontal tumors, early progressive dementia is also common. However, in other respects the clinical picture is different. Temporal lobe epilepsy occurs in 50% (Strobos, 1953). In addition, dysphasia with dominant lesions is an early feature. With respect to pituitary tumors, a presenting syndrome of TRD is not uncommon in this instance as concomitant with the endocrinopathy, as with Cushing's disease and prolactinomas. An awareness of the clinical stigmata of the endocrine effects of these tumors should permit their diagnosis in the setting of TRD, as discussed earlier in this chapter. Finally, in dealing with TRD as a possible presentation of an insidiously growing brain tumor, it is useful to bear in mind that the absence of signs or symptoms of raised intracranial pressure such as headache, vomiting or papilledema on fundoscopic examination by no means excludes the possibility, as it is in the nature of these lesions that raised intracranial pressure is a late manifestation. Therefore, if any doubt exists, the definitive reassurance rests with negative neuroimaging, specifically an MRI when available.

## Coronary artery disease

The frequency of major depression in patients with coronary artery disease (CAD) is in the 15–20% range across a number of studies (Carney et al., 1987; Lloyd & Cawley, 1983; Schleifer et al., 1989). Point prevalence rates in the aftermath of a myocardial infarction (MI) are even higher, ranging from 20 to 30% (Frasure-Smith et al., 1993), yet major depression very frequently goes unrecognized and untreated. In a recent prospective study by Frasure-Smith et al. (1993) of treatment as usual in 222 patients hospitalized post-MI, a total of 35 cases of major depression were diagnosed (a prevalence of 18%) following screening of all cases utilizing a diagnostic interview schedule instrument administered by trained research assistants. The screening process operated concurrently with, but independent of, treatment as usual, so the treating cardiologists were blind to diagnoses made and were free to consult psychiatric services as they saw fit. However, per treatment as usual, in only half of the group diagnosed as depressed was a psychiatric consultation requested, and in only a few of these was any antidepressant treatment initiated by the consulting psychiatrist. When patients were followed prospectively, however, the cardiac mortality rate in the group diagnosed with major depression was markedly higher than in the non-depressed group (17% vs. 3%; $P < 0.0$), even after controlling for other prognostic risk factors, such as history of previous MI, Killip class of heart failure, and presence of PVCs. These important findings have now been extended out to 18 months post-MI with the same results (adjusted odds ratio for Beck Depression Inventory Score $\geqslant 10$ in 2-week period following an MI = 6.64, 95% confidence interval: 1.76, 25.09; $P = 0.026$) (Frasure-Smith et al., 1995). Other studies have produced similar findings. For instance, Carney et al. (1988) found that major coronary events were twice as common in depressed patients compared with non-depressed patients (78% vs. 35%; $P < 0.02$). Given that major depression has such an unfavorable impact on the course of CAD, it makes recognition and treatment in this setting vital.

Regarding treatment, a recent comparative study (Roose et al., 1998) found equivalent response rates between a serotonin reuptake inhibitor (paroxetine) and a tricyclic antidepressant (nortriptyline) in depressed patients with ischemic heart disease. With response defined rigorously as both a reduction in initial HDRS score of at least 50%, and an end-point score of $\leqslant 8$ (in effect remission criteria), on an intent to treat analysis the response rate for paroxetine was 61% and for nortriptyline 55%. There was no placebo control group in the study. In terms of tolerability though, paroxetine was much better tolerated with adverse cardiac events occurring in only 1 out of 41 patients (2%), compared to 8 of 41 patients treated with nortriptyline (18%). As of yet there are no formal studies reported in depressed patients in the post-MI period. A multicenter, double blind, randomized trial of sertraline vs. placebo in patients with major depression post-MI is currently ongoing. In summary therefore, it appears at this juncture that, in this large group of patients, analogous to patients poststroke, recognition and adequate treatment of major depression is a more pressing problem, than treatment resistance *per se*.

## Cancer

Prevalence rates of major depression in cancer in general are also high, on average 24% across a range of tumors (Evans et al., 1996/97). As before, undertreatment is the norm, with only 3% of the patients hospitalized at Sloane-Kettering Cancer Center in 1987 receiving an antidepressant (Steifel et al., 1990). A particularly high rate (50%) has been reported in association with carcinoma of the pancreas suggesting a special connection (McDaniel et al., 1995). An early study by Fras et al. (1967) compared 46 patients presenting with pancreatic carcinoma to a control group of patients with carcinoma of the colon. Patients were evaluated psychiatrically when first referred to the medical or surgical clinic, and prior to the diagnosis being established. About half of the patients with pancreatic cancer reported only psychiatric symptoms as the first symptoms noticed, which preceded physical symptoms on average by 6 months. Overall, prior to any surgery and so definite confirmation of the diagnosis, 76% of the pancreatic cancer group reported psychiatric symptoms, most often depressed mood and loss of drive, compared to only 17% of the group with colon cancer. Similarly, other neoplasms such as lymphoma, leukemia and lung cancer may first present with major depression. Thus in patients, with progressive weight loss in the setting of TRD, an underlying tumor manifesting as a case of pseudo-TRD should be considered, even in the absence of specific physical symptoms.

## HIV and AIDS

The background prevalence rate of major depression is already high in two groups of patients at risk for HIV infection, namely homosexual men and intravenous drug users. HIV infection appears to increase the high base rate even further

(Perkins et al., 1994). On occasion a new episode of major depression can be the first manifestation of a complication of HIV infection such as AIDS encephalitis (Beresford et al., 1986) or rarer complications, namely bacillary angiomatosis (Baker et al., 1995), or destruction of the thyroid gland secondary to invasion by Kaposi's sarcoma (Mollison et al., 1991). Whether the development of major depression, by affecting underlying immunity, alters for the worse the prognosis with HIV infection is still an open question. One study found no relationship between psychological variables and CD4 + cell counts (Rabkin et al., 1991), while another study (Evans et al., 1995) did find a decline in CD8 + and NK cell counts in association with stress in HIV + men compared to no association for HIV− women.

   With regard to treatment resistance in this setting, there is as of yet no evidence of a heightened level of resistance. In a placebo-controlled trial with imipramine the response rate at 6 weeks, in 96 HIV-infected patients with either major depression or dysthymia, was significantly greater at 76% compared to a placebo response of just 26% (Rabkin et al., 1994a). Open trials of both fluoxetine and sertraline in smaller patients groups have also been positive with better tolerability compared to imipramine (Rabkin et al., 1994b; Markowitz et al., 1994). In each of these studies antidepressant treatment had no effect on CD4 + counts. It also appears that psychosocial interventions can be effective. In one study of HIV + homosexual men group therapy alone was as effective at 12 weeks as the combination of group therapy and fluoxetine. Both were significantly superior to placebo (Targ et al., 1994). Therefore, a reasonable approach to a case of TRD in this setting would be to pursue treatment in a logical stepwise fashion as with any other case of TRD, whilst, at the same time, being alert to the possibility that treatment resistance might be an indicator of a medical complication of HIV or AIDS, as of yet not detected.

## Conclusions

In this chapter a selective review of treatment-resistant depression in the medical setting has been conducted. Generally speaking, the presence of documented treatment resistance in any patient with major depression should prompt a consideration of possible underlying medical illness that might be causing, or at a minimum, contributing to the state of failure to respond to antidepressant treatment. To proceed blindly with treatment without a basic medical work-up is to invite misdiagnosis and therefore mismanagement of the case. This responsibility in practice will often fall to the psychiatrist to whom the patient has been referred to ensure that such an approach is adopted. In addition, psychiatrists and other mental health professionals can make an indispensable contribution by raising awareness amongst their colleagues of the importance and frequent neglect of major depression in many common medical disorders ranging from stroke to coronary artery disease. In these situations better recognition and treatment of major depression can only but make a very valuable contribution to enhancing patient care.

## REFERENCES

Andersson, P.G. (1970). Intracranial tumors in a psychiatric autopsy material. *Acta Psychiatrica Scandinavica*, **46**, 213–24.

Asher, R. (1949). Myxoedematous madness. *British Medical Journal*, 555–62.

Baker, J., Ruiz-Rodriguez, R., Whitfield, M. et al. (1995). Bacillary angiomatosis: a treatable cause of acute psychiatric symptoms in human immunodeficiency virus infection. *Journal of Clinical Psychiatry*, **56**, 161–6.

Barraclough, B. (1981). Suicide and epilepsy. In *Epilepsy and Psychiatry*, ed. E.H. Reynolds & M.R. Trumble, pp. 72–6. Edinburgh: Churchill Livingstone.

Beresford, T.P., Blow, F.C., & Hall, R.C.W. (1986). AIDS encephalitis mimicking alcohol dementia and depression. *Biological Psychiatry*, **21**, 934–7.

Betts, T.A. (1974). A follow-up study of a cohort of patients with epilepsy admitted to psychiatric care in an English city. In *Epilepsy: Proceedings of the Hans Berger Centenary Symposium*, ed. P. Harris & C. Mawdsley, pp. 326–38. Edinburgh: Churchill Livingstone.

Betts, T.A. (1982). Psychiatry and epilepsy: Part 1. In *A Textbook of Epilepsy*, 2nd edn, ed. J. Laidlaw & A. Richens, pp. 227–70. Edinburgh: Churchill Livingstone.

Carney, R.M., Rich, M.W., teVelde, A. et al. (1987). Major depressive disorder in coronary artery disease. *American Journal of Cardiology*, **60**, 1273–5.

Carney, R.M., Rich, M.W., teVelde, A. et al. (1988). Major depressive disorder predicts cardiac events in patients with coronary artery disease. *Psychosomatic Medicine*, **50**, 627–33.

Celesia, G.G. & Wanamaker, W.M. (1972). Psychiatric disturbances in Parkinson's disease, **33**, 577–83.

Cleghorn, R.A. (1965). Hormones and humors. In *Hormonal Steroids: Biochemistry, Pharmacology and Therapeutics*. Vol. 2. ed. L. Martini & A. Pecile. New York: Academic Press.

Cohen, S.I. (1980). Cushing's syndrome: a psychiatric study of 29 patients. *British Journal of Psychiatry*, **136**, 120–4.

Cottrell, S.S. & Wilson, S.A.K. (1926). The affective symptomatology of disseminated sclerosis. *Journal of Neurology and Psychopathology*, **7**, 1–30.

Currie, S., Heathfield, K.W.G., Henson, R.A. et al. (1971). Clinical causes and prognosis of temporal lobe epilepsy: a survey of 666 patients. *Brain*, **94**, 173–90.

Direkze, M., Bayliss, S.G., & Cutting, J.C. (1971). Primary tumors of the frontal lobe. *British Journal of Clinical Practice*, **25**, 207–13.

Dongier, S. (1959). Statistical study of clinical and electroencephalographic manifestations of 536 psychotic episodes occurring in 516 epileptics between clinical seizures. *Epilepsia*, **1**, 117–42.

Edwards, C.R.W. (1966). Adrenocortical diseases: section 12.7.1. In *Oxford Textbook of Medicine*, 3rd edn, ed. D.J. Weatherall, J.G.G. Ledingham, & D.A. Warrell. Oxford: Oxford University Press.

Evans, D.L., Leserman, J., Perkins, D.O. et al. (1995). Stress associated reductions of cytotoxic T lymphocytes and natural killer cells in asymptomatic HIV infection. *American Journal of Psychiatry*, **152**, 543–50.

Evans, D.L., Staab, J., Ward, H. et al. (1996/97). Depression in the medically ill: management considerations. *Depression and Anxiety*, **4**, 199–208.

Fawcett, J. (1994). Progress in treatment-resistant and treatment-refractory depression: we still have a long way to go. *Journal of Clinical Psychiatry*, **24**, 214–16.

Feibel, J.H., Berk, S., & Joynt, R.J. (1979). The unmet needs of stroke survivors. *Neurology*, **29**, 592.

Folstein, M.F., Maiberger, R., & McHugh, R. (1977). Mood disorder as a specific complication of stroke. *Journal of Neurology, Neurosurgery, and Psychiatry*, **40**, 1018–20.

Folstein, S.E., Abbott, M.H., Chase, G.A. et al. (1983). The association of affective disorder with Huntington's Disease in a case series and in families. *Psychological Medicine*, **13**, 537–42.

Fras, I., Litin, E.M., & Pearson, J.S. (1967). Comparison of psychiatric symptoms in carcinoma of the pancreas with those in some other intra-abdominal neoplasms. *American Journal of Psychiatry*, **123**, 1553–62.

Frasure-Smith, N., Lesperance, F., & Talajiic, M. (1993). Depression following myocardial infarction: impact on 6-month survival. *Journal of the American Medical Association*, **270**, 1819–61.

Frasure-Smith, N., Lesperance, F., & Talajiic, M. (1995). Depression and 18 month prognosis after myocardial infarction. *Circulation*, **91**, 999–1005.

Gold, M.S., Pottash, A.L.C., & Extein, I. (1981). Hypothyroidism in depression: evidence from complete thyroid function evaluation. *Journal of the American Medical Association*, **245**, 1919–22.

Gold, P.W., Loriaux, D.L., Roy et al. (1986). Responses to corticotropin releasing hormone in the hypercortisolism of depression and Cushing's disease: pathophysiologic and diagnosis implications. *New England Journal of Medicine*, **314**, 1329–35.

Granerus, A.K., Magnusson, T., Roos, B.E. et al. (1974). Relationship of age and mood to monoamine metabolites in cerebrospinal fluid in parkinsonism. *European Journal of Clinical Pharmacology*, **7**, 105–9.

Hall, R.C., Gardner, E.R., Popkin et al. (1981). Unrecognized physical illness prompting psychiatric admission: a prospective study. *American Journal of Psychiatry*, **138**, 629–35.

Hecaen, H. & Ajuriaguerra, J.D.E. (1956). *Troubles Mentaux au Cours des Tumeurs Intracraniennes*. Masson: Paris.

Huntington, G. (1972). On chorea. *Medical and Surgical Reporter*, **26**, 317.

Henriksen, B., Juul-Jensen, P., & Lund, M. (1970). The mortality of epileptics. In *Life Assurance Medicine: Proceedings of the 10th International Conference of Life Assurance Medicine*, ed. Brackenridge. London: Pitman.

Hoehn, M.M., Crowley, T.J., & Rutledge, C.O. (1976). Dopamine correlates of neurological and psychological status in untreated parkinsonism. *Journal of Neurology, Neurosurgery and Psychiatry*, **39**, 941–51.

Honer, W.G., Hurwitz, T., Li, D.K.B. et al. (1987). Temporal lobe involvement in multiple sclerosis patients with psychiatric disorders. *Archives of Neurology*, **44**, 187–90.

Jellinek, E.H. (1962). Fits, faints, coma and dementia in myxoedema. *Lancet*, **ii**, 1010–12.

Joffe, R.T., Lippert, G.P., Gray, T.A. et al. (1987). Mood disorder and multiple sclerosis. *Archives of Neurology*, **44**, 376–8.

Kahana, E., Leibowitz, U., & Alter, M. (1971). Cerebral multiple sclerosis. *Neurology*, **21**, 1179–85.

Kathol, R.G., Turner, & Delahunt, J. (1986). Depression and anxiety associated with hyperthyroidism: response to antithyroid therapy. *Psychosomatics*, **27**, 501–5.

Keschner, M., Bender, M.B., & Strauss, I. (1936). Mental symptoms in cases of tumor of the temporal lobe. *Archives of Neurology and Psychiatry*, **35**, 572–96.

Lewis, A.J. (1934). Melancholia: a historical review. *Journal of Mental Science*, **80**, 1–42.

Lishman, W.A. (1998). *Organic Psychiatry: The Psychological Consequences of Cerebral Disorder*, 3rd edn, p. 235. Oxford: Blackwell Science.

Lloyd, G.G. & Cawley, R.H. (1983). Distress or illness? A study of psychological symptoms after myocardial infarction. *British Journal of Psychiatry*, **142**, 120–5.

Loosen, P.T. & Prange, A.J. Jr (1982). The serum thyrotropin (TSH) response to thyrotropin releasing hormone (TRH) in depression: a review. *American Journal of Psychiatry*, **139**, 405–6.

McDaniel, J.S., Musselman, D.J., Porter, M.R. et al. (1995). Depression in patients with cancer: Diagnosis, biology, and treatment. *Archives of General Psychiatry*, **52**, 89–99.

McLarty, D.G., Ratcliffe, W.A., Ratcliffe, J.G. et al. (1978). A study of thyroid function in psychiatric inpatients. *British Journal of Psychiatry*, **133**, 211–18.

Markowitz, J.C., Rabkin, J.G., & Perry, S.W. (1994). Treating depression in HIV-posiitve patients. *AIDS*, **8**, 403–12.

Maurice-Williams, R.S. & Sinar, E.J. (1984). Depression caused by an intracranial meningioma relieved by leucotomy prior to diagnosis of the tumor. *Journal of Neurology, Neurosurgery and Psychiatry*, **47**, 844–85.

Mayberg, H.S., Robinson, R.G., Wong, D.F. et al. (1988). Pet imaging of cortical S2 serotonin receptors after stroke: lateralized changes and relationship to depression. *American Journal of Psychiatry*, **14S**, 937–43.

Mayeux, R., Yaakov, S., Cote, L. et al. (1984). Altered serotonin metabolism in depressed patients with Parkinson's disease. *Neurology*, **34**, 642–6.

Mindham, R.H.S. (1970). Psychiatric syndromes in parkinsonism. *Journal of Neurology, Neurosurgery and Psychiatry*, **30**, 188–91.

Mollison, L.C., Miijch, A., McBride, G. et al. (1991). Hypothyroidism due to destruction of the thyroid gland by Kaposi's sarcoma. *Review of Infections Diseases*, **13**, 826–7.

Mulder, D.W. & Daly, D. (1952). Psychiatric symptoms associated with lesion of the temporal lobe. *Journal of the American Medical Association*, **150**, 173–6.

Nemeroff, C.B., Simon, J.S., Haggerty, J.J. et al. (1985). Antithyroid antibodies in depressed patients. *American Journal of Psychiatry*, **142**(7), 840–3.

O'Malley, P.P. (1966). Severe mental symptoms in disseminated sclerosis: a neuropathological study. *Journal of the Irish Medical Association*, **58**, 115–27.

Perkins, D.O., Stern, R.A., Golden, R.N. et al. (1994). Mood disorders in HIV infection: prevalence and risk factors in a nonepicenter of the AIDS epidemic. *American Journal of Psychiatry*, **151**, 233–6.

Petersen, P. (1968). Psychiatric disorders in primary hyperparathyroidism. *Journal of Clinical Endocrinology and Metabolism*, **28**, 1491–5.

Prange, A.J., Mason, G.A., & Garbutt, J.C. (1990). Thyroid axis syndromes in depression: definitions and interpetations. In *Pharmacotherapy of Depression: Applications for the Outpatient Practitioner*, ed. J.D. Amsterdam, pp. 35–55. New York: Marcel Dekker, Inc.

Rabins, P.V. (1990). Euphoria in mutiple sclerosis. In *Neurobehavioral Aspects of Multiple Sclerosis*, ed. S.M. Rao Chap. 11. Oxford: Oxford University Press.

Rabins, P.V., Brooks, B.R., O'Donnell, P. et al. (1986). Structural brain correlates of emotional disorder in multiple sclerosis. *Brain*, **109**, 585–97.

Rabkin, J.G., Williams, J.B.W., Remien, R.H. et al. (1991). Depression, distress, lymphocyte subsets, and human immunodeficiency virus symptoms on two occasions in HIV-positive homosexual men. *Archives of General Psychiatry*, **48**, 111–19.

Rabkin, J.G., Rabkin, R., Harrison, W. et al. (1994a). Effect of imipramine on mood and enumerative measures of immune status in depressed patients with HIV illness. *American Journal of Psychiatry*, **151**, 516–23.

Rabkin, J.G., Rabkin, R., Harrison, W. et al. (1994b). Effects of fluoxetine on mood and immune status in depressed patients with HIV illness. *Journal of Clinical Psychiatry*, **55**, 92–7.

Raskin, N. (1956). Intracranial neoplasms in psychotic patients. *American Journal of Psychiatry*, **112**, 481–4.

Reed, T.E. & Chandler, J.H. (1958). Huntington's chorea in Michigan.1, Demographics and genetics. *American Journal of Human Genetics*, **10**, 201–25.

Robins, A.H. (1976). Depression in patients with Parkinsonism. *British Journal of Psychiatry*, **128**, 141–5.

Robinson, R.G. & Price, T.R. (1982). Post-stroke depressive disorders: a follow-up study of 103 patients. *Stroke*, **13**, 635–41.

Robinson, R.G. & Szetala, B. (1981). Mood change following left hemisphere brain injury. *Annals of Neurology*, **9**, 447–53.

Roose, S.P., Laghrissi-Thode, F., Kennedy, J.S. et al. (1998). Comparison of paroxetine and nortriptyline in depressed patients with ischemic heart disease. *Journal of the American Medical Association*, **279**, 287–91.

Schiffer, R.B., Caine, E.D., Bamford, K.A. et al. (1983). Depressive episodes in patients with multiple sclerosis. *American Journal of Psychiatry*, **140**, 1498–500.

Schleifer, S.J., Macari-Hinson, M.M., Coyle, D.A. et al. (1989). The nature and course of depression following myocardial infarction. *Archives of Internal Medicine*, **149**, 1785–9.

Starkman, M.N., Gebarski, S.S., Berent, S. et al. (1992). Hippocampal formation volume, memory dysfunction, and cortisone levels in patients with Cushing's Syndrome. *Biological Psychiatry*, **32**, 756–65.

Steifel, F.C., Kornblith, A.B., & Holland, J.C. (1990). Changes in the prescription patterns of psychotropic drugs for cancer patients during a 10-year period. *Cancer*, **65**, 1048–53.

Strobos, R.R.J. (1953). Tumors of temporal lobe. *Neurology*, **3**, 752–60.

Surridge, D. (1969). An investigation into some psychiatric aspects of multiple sclerosis. *British Journal of Psychiatry*, **115**, 749–64.

Targ, E.F., Karasic, D.H., Diefenbach, P.N. et al. (1994). Structured group therapy and fluoxetine to treat depression in HIV-positive persons.

Targum, S.D., Greenberg, R.D., Harmon, R.L. et al. (1984). Thyroid hormone and the TRH stimulation test in refractory depression. *Journal of Clinical Psychiatry*, **45**, 345–6.

Thase, M.E. & Rush, A.J. (1995). Treatment-resistant depression. In *Pharmacology: The Fourth Generation of Progress*, ed. F.E. Bloom & D.J. Kupfer. New York: Raven Press Ltd.

Tonks, C.M. (1964). Mental illness in hypothyroid patients. *British Journal of Psychiatry*, **110**, 706–10.

Trimble, M.R. & Perez, M.M. (1980). Quantification of psychopathology in adult patients with epilepsy. In *Epilepsy and Behavior 1979: Proceedings of Wopassey I*, ed. B.M. Kulig, H. Meinhardi, & G. Stores. Lisse: Swets and Zeitlingber.

Vanderheyden, J.E., Noel, G., & Mendlewicz, J. (1981). Biogenic amine disturbance in cerebrospinal fluid in parkinsonism and unipolar depression: use of the probenecid. *Neuropsychobiology*, **7**, 137–51.

White, S.J., McLean, A.E.M., & Howland, C. (1979). Anticonvulsant drugs and cancer: a cohort study in patients with sever epilepsy. *Lancet*, **ii**, 458–61.

Whitlock, F.A. & Siskind, M.M. (1980). Depression as a major symptom of multiple sclerosis. *Journal of Neurology, Neurosurgery and Psychiatry*, **43**, 861–5.

# 19

# Psychiatric comorbidity in treatment-resistant depression

Jonathan E. Alpert and Isabelle T. Lagomasino

## Introduction

Extensive co-occurrence of major depressive disorder (MDD) with other psychiatric disorders, particularly anxiety, personality, and alcohol and substance use disorders has been well documented within clinical and community samples (Blazer et al., 1994; Corruble et al., 1996; Markowitz et al., 1992; Rohde et al., 1991; Sanderson et al., 1990, 1992). Based on estimates from the National Institute of Mental Health Epidemiological Catchment Area Study (Robins et al., 1991) and the US National Comorbidity Survey (Kessler et al., 1996) as many as one-half to three-quarters of individuals in the community with MDD suffer from an additional one or more psychiatric disorders. Psychiatric comorbidity appears to be particularly high among juvenile depressed populations (Angold & Costello, 1993; Biederman et al., 1995; Birmaher et al., 1996) and among adults with an early age of onset of first depression (Alpert et al., 1994; Fava et al., 1996; Kasch & Klein, 1996). Moreover, results of the US National Comorbidity Survey suggest a disproportionate increase across recent birth cohorts in the prevalence of MDD with comorbidity, but not depression without comorbidity or 'pure' depression (Kessler et al., 1996). This trend was found to be largely accounted for by an increase in MDD secondary, in order of chronology, to other psychiatric disorders . In addition, individuals with lower educational attainment, lower income, and non-white ethnicity/race were reported to have an increased risk of comorbid compared with 'pure' depression (Blazer et al., 1994). While lifetime rates of MDD appear to vary as much as ten-fold across countries, the high prevalence of psychiatric comorbidity is characteristic of depression cross-nationally (Weissman et al., 1996). Epidemiological studies support the clinical impression that the co-occurrence of other psychiatric disorders with depression is associated with a greater likelihood of receiving treatment (Merikangas et al., 1996; Sartorius et al., 1996) but also with a more severe and protracted course of illness (Kessler et al., 1996) and greater risk of persistent disability (Kessler & Frank 1997).

There are few studies on treatment-resistant depression (TRD) that are methodologically sound and directly relevant to the issue of psychiatric comorbidity. In the absence of more rigorously established management guidelines for the treatment of TRD with comorbidity, thoughtful efforts to develop rational pharmacological and psychotherapeutic strategies for particular co-occurrent syndromes in TRD (Nunes et al., 1996; Thase, 1996) largely derive from the clinical and research literature on depressed patients with comorbid psychiatric illness (without reference to TRD) (Asnis & Faisal, 1997) and on patients with TRD (without reference to comorbidity) (Amsterdam & Hornig-Rohan, 1996; Nierenberg & McColl, 1996; Rosenbaum et al., 1995). Additional inferences about prognosis and treatment have been drawn from naturalistic and controlled studies evaluating potential predictors of treatment outcome – including psychiatric comorbidity – as they relate to acute response, longer-term function, and risk of relapse and recurrence among individuals with MDD (Akiskal, 1982; Joyce & Paykel, 1989; Katon et al., 1994; Keller et al., 1992; Nelson & Dunner, 1995; Thase & Howland, 1994).

## Clinical challenges

The clinician faces a series of challenges in the approach to a patient with TRD and psychiatric comorbidity, the first of which concerns establishing a valid diagnosis. Personality pathology and anxiety symptoms, in particular, are often amplified by and difficult to disentangle from unremitting depressive symptoms. The reporting of premorbid personality traits by depressed patients also appears to be influenced by their depressive state (Akiskal et al., 1983; Hirschfeld & Shea 1992; Loranger et al., 1991; Millon & Kotik-Harper, 1995; Stuart et al., 1992). Evaluation of depression during a period of active alcohol or substance use often presents similar challenges (Nunes et al., 1996; Schuckit et al., 1997). Furthermore, psychiatric comorbidity may potentially mask or alter the presentation, and thereby delay diagnosis, of conditions that might account for treatment resistance, including rapid cycling bipolar disorder and psychotic depression.

Psychiatric comorbidity may also interfere with treatment adherence and optimization. Thus, for example, anxiety disorders, particularly panic disorder, may be associated with heightened sensitivity to medication side effects which may compromise the adequacy of antidepressant dose and duration, reduce patient acceptance of adjunctive, combination, and high dose pharmacotherapy, and increase attrition from treatment (Brown et al., 1996; Cowley et al., 1997; Pohl et al., 1988), while patients with eating disorders may be severely intolerant of side effects such as weight gain, food cravings, or sensations of bloating thus greatly limiting the range of treatment options in available to target TRD. Significant personality and substance use disorders may strain a working alliance, jeopardize the safety of aggressive pharmacotherapy, and occur together with marked psychosocial disruption further impeding compliance with recommended treatment (Gastfriend, 1996; Nunes et al., 1996; Shea et al., 1992; Thase, 1996).

Expertise in the approach to TRD is not necessarily accompanied by equal familiarity with state-of-the-art treatment of other disorders. The shamed revelation by a patient with TRD that he or she has been binging and purging, compulsively hoarding, or abusing narcotics may be silently greeted by the clinician as an unwelcome diversion from the task at hand rather than as an additional avenue of treatment or consultation. Furthermore, the clinician and patient may be left with an impression of 'moving targets' and may have difficulty establishing which interventions have seemed to help or exacerbate the many symptoms under attack. Therapeutic nihilism on the part of clinician, patient, and family and other supports – a never distant problem in the treatment of TRD – is all the more easily fueled in the presence of comorbidity.

Finally, a frustrating lack of correspondence between the results of controlled clinical trials and clinical experience is often encountered when seeking insights from the literature on treatment or prognosis that might apply to the patient with TRD and comorbidity. In large part this relates to the under representation of patients with significant psychiatric (or medical) comorbidity in depression treatment trials, owing both to specific exclusion criteria (e.g., severe suicidality, current or recent alcohol or substance use, or an anxiety disorder judged to be a primary problem) and because of referral patterns which tend to divert complex patients away from studies toward more 'individualized' treatments. On the other hand, those studies that are more typically inclusive (e.g., naturalistic) are less well suited to testing particular treatment strategies and controlling for other sources of variability that may affect outcome. There continues to be much need for randomized, double-blind clinical trials focused on depressed populations with particular comorbid disorders of moderate or greater severity.

The intent of this chapter is to help clarify salient features of psychiatric comorbidity in MDD as well as limitations of current knowledge in this area, and to offer practical strategies for the management of TRD when complicated by co-occurrent psychiatric illness.

## Conceptual and methodological issues

Like many relatively young areas of clinical research, the literature on comorbidity in depression is still encumbered by a lack of standardized terms and methods. An appreciation of the heterogeneity of definitions and methods is crucial to evaluation of the diverse range of studies reported.

In its narrowest sense, comorbidity refers to the co-occurrence of two (or more) disorders only when the rate of co-occurrence exceeds that predicted by base rates of each disorder individually in the population under study. The finding of comorbidity in this strict sense of the term may be used to support the

**Table 19.1.** Models of psychiatric comorbidity in major depressive disorder

1. Coincidental co-occurrence of MDD and another psychiatric disorder ('A') as would be predicted by base rates of MDD and 'A' in the same population.

2. MDD and 'A' as phenotypic expressions of a single underlying disorder.

3. MDD and 'A' as distinct disorders sharing similar risk factors (e.g., social disruption, trauma).

4. MDD and 'A' as distinct disorders whose risk of occurrence is each increased by a third psychiatric (or other) disorder.

5. MDD + 'A' as a distinct disorder or subtype, differing from 'pure' MDD or 'A' along meaningful lines (e.g., etiology, familiality, course, treatment responses).

6. Co-occurrence as related, in whole or part, to overlapping diagnostic criteria (e.g., avoidant personality disorder and social phobia).

7. MDD as an exacerbating (or causal) factor in development of 'A' and/or,

8. 'A' as an exacerbating (or causal) factor in development of MDD.

hypothesis of some unique association among the co-occurring disorders. In most studies and reviews, however, comorbidity is defined more broadly as any co-occurrence of two (or more) disorders, whether or not that co-occurrence occurs at a rate higher than predicted by coincidence. Increasingly sophisticated models have been developed to test the nature of interrelationships among comorbid disorders. Nevertheless application of these models to comorbidity in depression is at an early stage (First et al., 1996; Neale & Kendler, 1995) and the basis for association between depression and other psychiatric disorders remains largely to be defined (Table 19.1).

When first introduced by Feinstein (1970), comorbidity referred to the co-occurrence of another disorder sometime during the course of the index disorder under study. In the subsequent psychiatric literature, the study of comorbidity was extended not only to *current* but often more broadly to lifetime co-occurrence of two or more disorders in the same individual, potentially separated in time by many years. Both definitions of comorbidity appear to be meaningful. Lifetime comorbidity is likely to be an important designation in family-genetic, imaging, and psychobiological studies of comorbidity where the underlying diathesis is the concern, while in clinical practice the greatest challenges appear to be posed by patients presenting with two or more unremitted disorders simultaneously complicating treatment.

In their simplest sense the terms 'primary' and 'secondary' applied to comorbid disorders refer only to temporal order, which may or may not be possible to establish depending on the patient, the disorders, and the quality of corroborating evidence. However, 'primary' has been used also to indicate assumptions about causality (e.g., depression as a 'complication' of persistent panic attacks), greater severity, family history, or a course apparently independent from (but not necessarily preceding the onset of) another disorder (Depression Guideline Panel, 1993; Moras & Barlow, 1992; Winokur et al., 1988). In the context of multiple connotations, the terms 'primary' and 'secondary' need to be defined in each context in which they are used.

'Pure' depression is typically compared with depression with comorbidity or 'combined' depression (Blazer et al., 1994). The purity of the depression in many clinical studies, however, refers only to the absence of the particular comorbid condition under scrutiny rather than to an absence of psychiatric comorbidity more generally. We therefore prefer the more specific designations, such as MDD with or without panic disorder, when describing study or clinical populations.

In addition, psychiatric disorders are by no means uniformly distributed among individuals with mental illness. Nearly half of the lifetime psychiatric disorders detected in the National Comorbidity Survey were concentrated in 14% of individuals with psychiatric illness who had three or more lifetime psychiatric disorders (Kessler et al., 1994). Individuals with anxiety disorders and MDD, for example, are also more likely to have a diagnosable personality disorder (Alnaes & Torgersen, 1990; Brown et al., 1996) and, within that triad, social phobia, avoidant personality disorder and atypical depression appear to cluster (Alpert et al., 1997). So too, the comorbidity of depression and anxiety disorders is also associated with an elevated risk of alcohol and drug abuse (Kamerow, 1988). When comparing two depressed populations with respect to the presence or absence of a particular comorbid disorder, therefore, it should be recognized that clinically important differences may exist between the populations with respect both to the overall burden of comorbidity (total number, duration, and severity of comorbid diagnoses) and the distribution of particular comorbid disorders which, though not necessarily assessed, may have a substantial influence on treatment outcome extending beyond the impact of the comorbid disorder under study.

In recent years there has been renewed attention devoted to subsyndromal presentations, such as mixed anxiety-depression (Boulenger et al., 1997), in which one or both comorbid conditions present with clinically significant symptoms which are, nevertheless, not of a severity, persistence or number to reach full DSM-IV diagnosis for a disorder (Angst et al., 1997). In much of the comorbidity literature, distinctions between subsyndromal presentations and categorical diagnoses are blurred so that 'anxious depression' has been used variously to refer to depression with anxiety symptoms, with panic disorder (lifetime or current), or with any anxiety disorder (lifetime or current) (Clayton et al., 1991; DiNardo & Barlow, 1990; Fava et al., 1997b; Fawcett & Kravitz, 1983; Joffe et al., 1993). So too, personality comorbidity has been used to refer to personality diagnoses made clinically, by structured interview, or by self-rating questionnaires as well as to personality dimensions, particularly neuroticism (Eysenck, 1967), which do not translate into a particular DSM-IV personality disorder or cluster (Shea et al., 1992; Thase, 1996). In so far as the relationship between symptoms, traits, and disorders among conditions comorbid with depression is far from clear, a degree of circumspection is called for when attempting to generalize findings from one domain to another.

These important caveats notwithstanding, ample evidence as reviewed below has shown that psychiatric comorbidity in MDD has important clinical and public health implications and the field is ripe for further research elucidating more precisely the role of comorbidity in TRD and providing guidelines for optimizing treatment.

## Anxiety disorders

Estimates of anxiety disorder comorbidity in MDD, ranging from 33–85%, indicate a high degree of co-occurrence, among both community and patient cohorts (Wetzler & Katz, 1989; Kessler et al., 1996; Lydiard, 1991: Zajecka & Ross, 1995) Depressed patients have been estimated to have 14 times the odds of having an anxiety disorder compared with non-depressed subjects (Boyd et al., 1984). Over 95% of patients with depression have at least one symptom of anxiety (Hamilton, 1988).

### Course and treatment outcome

In a large outpatient cohort ($n = 454$), over three-quarters of patients with depression had significantly elevated scores ($\geqslant 12$) on the Hamilton Rating Scale for Anxiety and the presence of anxiety was associated with greater severity of depression, work absenteeism, and social instability (Tollefson et al., 1993). Comorbidity of MDD with panic disorder, the most well-studied of the anxiety disorders among depressed individuals, has been associated with greater severity of anxiety and depressive symptoms, greater psychological and psychosocial impairment, and a higher rate of suicide than either disorder alone (Andrade et al., 1994; Bronish & Wittchen, 1994; Coryell et al., 1992; Fawcett, 1997; Gorman & Coplan, 1996; Johnson et al., 1990; King et al., 1995; Kessler et al., 1996; Lepola et al., 1996; Lesser et al., 1988; Reich et al., 1993).

Naturalistic and clinical studies have found a poorer prognosis and greater chronicity among patients suffering from MDD and panic disorder (Alnaes & Torgersen, 1990; Angst & Dobler-Mikola, 1985; Clayton et al., 1991; Cowley et al., 1997; Fawcett & Kravitz, 1983; Hecht et al., 1989; Lydiard, 1991; Kessler et al., 1996; Stavrakaki & Vargo, 1986). Coryell and colleagues reported that 50% of patients with MDD with panic disorder had recovered at two years compared to 74% of patients with MDD alone, while work impairment occurred in 66% of patients with both depression and panic compared to 28% of those with depression alone (Coryell et al., 1988).

In addition, patients with depression and anxiety may be at greater risk for depressive recurrence (Keller et al., 1992) and may be more likely to undergo psychiatric hospitalization (Kessler et al., 1996).

Sherbourne and Wells (1997) conducted a large study among primary care patients to examine the extent to which comorbid anxiety disorders influenced the clinical course of depression over a 2-year period. Among patients with subthreshold depression, those with comorbid anxiety disorders were significantly more likely to develop a full episode of MDD (e.g., 40% of those with comorbid generalized anxiety disorder (GAD) developed full depression compared to 14% of those without). Among those patients with MDD, those with comorbid anxiety disorders had a lower tendency to remit (e.g., 21% of patients with comorbid panic disorder remitted during the first year of the study compared to 44% of those without panic disorder) even when baseline rates of severity were controlled for. Patients with either subthreshold depressive symptoms or MDD and comorbid anxiety disorders had more severe symptoms for the entire length of the study.

Depressed patients who have comorbid anxiety disorders compared with depressed patients without comorbid anxiety have higher treatment rates, defined by any professional contact for mental health problems (Judd, 1994; Merikangas et al., 1996; Meredith et al., 1997). They independently seek treatment more often (Vollrath & Angst, 1989), and general practitioners more frequently recognize their need for services (Ormel et al., 1991). Unfortunately, anxious depressives also tend to terminate treatment more prematurely than those who suffer from depression alone (Brown et al., 1996).

With few exceptions (Joffe et al., 1993; Lesser et al., 1988), the presence of comorbid depression and anxiety has been associated with a decreased responsiveness to treatment (Albus & Sheibe 1993; Buller et al., 1986; Coryell et al., 1988; Liebowitz et al., 1990; Liebowitz, 1993; Noyes, 1990; Noyes et al., 1990; Van Valkenburg et al., 1984) and slower recoveries (Clayton et al., 1991; Stein & Uhde, 1988; Brown et al., 1996). Among psychiatrically hospitalized patients treated with tricyclic antidepressants (at least 150 mg of imipramine or desipramine daily) or a monoamine oxidase inhibitor (at least 60 mg of phenelzine) those with comorbid MDD and panic disorder did significantly less well than those with MDD alone (Grunhaus et al., 1986, 1988). Although both groups began with similar symptom severity, only 15% of those with comorbid conditions, compared to 53% of those with MDD without panic, experienced at least a 50% reduction in depression severity scores after three weeks of treatment; 50% and 71%, respectively, had a similar reduction in symptoms at discharge. If the criteria were set more stringently (Hamilton Depression Rating Scale (HDRS) score $\leqslant 5$), the two groups did not differ significantly at three weeks, but did at discharge, with 17% of the comorbid group and 57% of the depression alone group experiencing remission of depressive symptoms. Similarly, in another study, depressed non-responders to tricyclic antidepressants were found to have had higher anxiety scores at baseline (Roose et al., 1986). In one study patients with primary MDD and a secondary anxiety disorder were found to be more likely to recover completely than patients with secondary MDD (Nutzinger & Zapotoczky, 1985), although the effect of temporal order of comorbidity on treatment outcome is largely unknown.

Fava and colleagues (Fava et al., 1997b) enrolled 294 patients with MDD subtypes (melancholic, atypical, hostile, double [comorbid dysthymia], and panic, anxiety or personality disordered) in an eight-week trial with a fixed daily dose of fluoxetine (20 mg). Of those patients with comorbid anxiety disorders during their lifetime, a majority were diagnosed with social phobia (58%) and/or simple phobia (32%) and a smaller number with panic (14%), agoraphobia (9%), obsessive-compulsive disorder (8%) and/or generalized anxiety disorder (16%). These anxious depressives showed as a group significantly poorer response to the selective serotonin reuptake inhibitor (SSRI) than the other groups, even when response was adjusted for baseline depressive severity, which was highest for individuals with comorbid anxiety disorders, personality disorders, and melancholia. The rate of non-response for anxious depressives was 25.8% compared with 13.8% for depressives without comorbid anxiety suggesting a higher rate of treatment resistance or, at the least, a slower rate of recovery of MDD with comorbid anxiety as has been suggested by Clayton and colleagues (Clayton et al., 1991). A *post hoc* analysis prompted by the observation that social and simple phobias appeared to be more common among depressed adults with juvenile compared with later onset major depressive disorder (Alpert et al., 1999), revealed that the differences in treatment outcome between the anxious depressives and other depressed groups in this study may have been partly accounted for by their differences in age of depression onset in addition to the presence or absence of an anxiety disorder.

Brown and colleagues (Brown et al., 1996) recently completed the first randomized, controlled trial to investigate the clinical and treatment implications of comorbid depression and anxiety disorders, lifetime or current, in the primary care setting. A total of 276 depressed patients from four medical centers were randomized to receive care as usual, a structured interpersonal psychotherapy intervention, or a structured pharmacotherapy intervention using nortriptyline. Those patients with comorbid anxiety disorders were found to be characterized by older age, greater self-reported depressive and anxiety symptoms and suicidal thoughts, and poorer health-related and psychosocial functioning. They were also more likely to be diagnosed with a personality disorder. Higher proportions of patients with MDD and comorbid anxiety disorders than with MDD alone discontinued treatment before the completion of the study (55% vs. 44%, respectively, in the psychotherapy protocol, and 43% vs. 36%, respectively, in the pharmacotherapy protocol). Similar differences in attrition were seen in the acute and continuation phases of the protocols. Almost half of those who left treatment did so during the first month, with no differences in rates between those receiving psychotherapy and those receiving medication.

Among depressed primary care patients who received treatment, those with comorbid anxiety disorders, showed less improvement over the eight-month trial, regardless of whether they had psychotherapy or nortriptyline (Brown et al., 1996). Patients with comorbid anxiety took twice as long as those with MDD alone to demonstrate a similar magnitude of improvement, supporting previous impressions of a slower rate of recovery (Clayton et al., 1991). Of those receiving psychotherapy, 55–62% of those with MDD alone or with MDD and GAD were fully recovered at eight months, compared with only 38% of those with MDD and panic disorder. Similarly, of patients receiving pharmacotherapy, 57–62% with MDD alone or with MDD and GAD were fully recovered in eight months, compared to 33% of patients with MDD and panic. Therapy and medication thus appeared to be equally effective in the treatment of MDD with or without GAD in this primary care population while they were each less effective in MDD with panic disorder.

In a smaller cohort of older subjects (60 years or older) with recurrent MDD treated with both nortriptyline and interpersonal therapy, anxiety symptoms emerged as one of the significant predictors of lower likelihood of rapid, sustained response to antidepressants along with earlier age of first depressive episode, greater severity of depressive symptoms, higher levels of life stress, and greater sleep disturbance (Dew et al., 1997). Categorical anxiety diagnoses were not assessed among these individuals.

## Treatment approaches

Despite the prevalence and clinical implications of comorbidity, optimal treatments of MDD comorbid with anxiety have not been systematically studied in controlled trials (Asnis & Faisal, 1997; Nutt, 1997). In TRD complicated by anxiety, either psychic anxiety, or agitation may be a symptom not of an anxiety disorder but of depression, an adverse reaction to medication including akathisia, a consequence of persistent insomnia, a manifestation of alcohol, caffeine or other drug use or withdrawal, or expression of a previously undetected disorder such as partial complex seizures or hyperthyroidism which may have additional relevance for the depression. The accuracy of diagnosing an anxiety disorder is enhanced by evidence of the disorder prior to the onset of MDD or during previous periods of depressive remission, a family history, or a classic rather than atypical presentation of the anxiety symptoms.

Although antidepressants constitute the main treatment of comorbid depression and anxiety, an adjunctive anxiolytic agent may be helpful throughout the first several weeks, until the antidepressant reaches full efficacy, with an attempt to taper the anxiolytic thereafter. Reducing initial anxiety symptoms may help increase treatment compliance (Coplan & Gorman, 1990: Fawcett, 1990). Moreover, the early phases of treatment should be carefully monitored in an attempt to prevent dropouts (Brown et al., 1996), with ample attention to patient education about anticipated side effects, latency of response, and duration of treatment.

## Panic disorder

Tricyclic antidepressants (TCAs) have been used widely in the treatment of depression with comorbid panic disorder. Caution must be taken to start the medications more slowly than usual, perhaps at 25–50% of the usual initial dose (e.g., imipramine 10–25 mg daily), in order to avoid overstimulation or induction of a panic attack (Lydiard & Ballenger, 1987; Liebowitz, 1993). Recommendations for target dose levels of TCAs in the treatment of panic disorder have paralleled those for depression (i.e. 150–300 mg/day of imipramine or its equivalent) so that steady titration should be pursued, at least to approximately 2.25 mg/kg/day beyond which response rates for panic and treatment adherence may fall (Mavissakalian & Perel, 1994; Pollack & Smoller, 1996). Clomipramine, which is not uncommonly recruited in the approach to TRD, is also an effective antipanic agent (Modigh et al., 1992). SSRIs may similarly be initiated at low doses (e.g. 5–10 mg/day fluoxetine, 25 mg/day sertraline or fluvoxamine, and 10 mg/day paroxetine) and titrated up toward full antidepressant doses (Pollack & Smoller, 1996). Similarly venlafaxine may be initiated at 18.75 mg b.i.d. (Pollack et al., 1996) or nefazodone at 50 mg b.i.d. (DeMartinis et al., 1996) with gradual dose escalation . The combination of TCA and SSRI, as used for TRD, may represent an effective strategy for treatment-resistant panic as well (Tiffon et al., 1994). Monoamine oxidase inhibitors (MAOIs) are indicated in TRD with comorbid panic disorder, especially if features of an atypical depression are present (Liebowitz et al., 1985; Thase et al., 1995). In contrast, bupropion, trazodone and maprotiline have not been found to have much efficacy in the treatment of panic disorder (Coplan & Gorman, 1990). High-potency benzodiazepines may help control panic attacks during the first weeks of treatment, until the antidepressant effect is felt (Liebowitz, 1993). High-potency benzodiazepines, including alprazolam and particularly clonazepam, have been linked with worsening or emergence of depression and should be used with careful monitoring as a potential, if infrequent (Kravitz et al., 1993) impediment to antidepressant response (Lydiard et al., 1987; Pollack, 1987; Liebowitz, 1993). In some instances, adjunctive buspirone, which also may have weak antidepressant properties, may help reduce anticipatory anxiety in the patient with panic disorder (Gastfriend & Rosenbaum, 1989). A few investigators have reported some success with valproic acid for the treatment of panic (Keck et al., 1993; Primeau et al., 1990). The antipanic efficacy of other anticonvulsants used in the treatment of mood disorders, such as lamotrigene or gabapentin, remains to be explored.

### Generalized anxiety disorder

As in panic disorder, TCAs can produce a good response in patients with depression and GAD with potentially greater anxiolytic effect than benzodiazepines (Liebowitz, 1993; Rickels et al., 1993). However, since their effect may take up to 6 or 8 weeks, the temporary adjunctive use of a benzodiazepine such as clonazepam or lorazepam may be helpful (Liebowitz, 1993). MAOIs and SSRIs have also been found individually beneficial, although stimulating SSRIs such as fluoxetine may need to be started at low doses (Liebowitz, 1993). Unlike its apparent lack of efficacy in panic, trazodone achieved efficacy at least comparable to diazepam in a patient population with GAD without MDD (Rickels et al., 1993). Nefazodone, which is structurally related, has been similarly shown to reduce GAD symptoms (Hedges et al., 1996) and anxiety symptoms associated with depression (Zajecka, 1996). Buspirone, which has been shown to be effective in GAD and in the adjunctive treatment of MDD, may play a useful role in the treatment of the two disorders when they co-occur (Coplan & Gorman, 1990; Lydiard, 1991; Sramek et al., 1996; Zajecka & Ross, 1995). Beta-blockers, clonidine, guafacine, and antihistamines may also help alleviate anxiety symptoms (Zajecka & Ross, 1995) although, as with the benzodiazepines, close surveillance for worsening of depressive symptoms on these agents should be routine.

### Social phobia

MAOIs have been found to have greater efficacy than TCAs in the treatment of social phobia, and may have more effect in the treatment of MDD comorbid with social phobia (Liebowitz et al., 1990; Liebowitz, 1993). Initial trials of reversible, non-FDA approved MAOIs, which may entail fewer restrictions on diet, have shown promise including moclobemide (Versiani et al., 1992) and brofaromine (van Vliet et al., 1994). Fluoxetine and other SSRIs also appear to be effective (Lydiard, 1991; Tancer & Uhde, 1997; van Vliet et al., 1994; Zajecka & Ross, 1995). Potentially useful adjunctive agents include benzodiazepines (Coplan & Gorman, 1990; Davidson et al., 1993; Liebowitz, 1993; Zajecka & Ross, 1995) and buspirone

(Coplan & Gorman, 1990; Zajecka & Ross, 1995), as well as beta-blockers, though mainly for performance anxiety (Coplan & Gorman, 1990; Zajecka & Ross, 1995).

## Obsessive-compulsive disorder (OCD)

Clomipramine and SSRIs are indicated in the pharmacotherapy of depression comorbid with OCD (Liebowitz, 1993). Higher doses of SSRIs (e.g., 60–80 mg of fluoxetine) (Coplan & Gorman, 1990; den Boer, 1997; Zajecka & Ross, 1995) and longer duration of treatment (12 weeks rather than 4 to 6) (Zajecka & Ross, 1995) may be needed for full effect, which is generally a partial rather than complete remission of OCD symptoms. In contrast to other anxiety disorders, the implementation of SSRIs at usual rather than minute doses in OCD is often well tolerated. In studies of OCD and temporally secondary depressions, reviewed by den Boer (1997), OCD and depression improved significantly on SSRIs, although the improvement in OCD symptoms was generally independent of baseline severity of depression, with the exception of one study (Perse et al., 1987) in which there was a trend toward greater non-response of OCD symptoms to fluvoxamine among those individuals with more severe depression. In a comparative study of fluvoxamine and desipramine, the predominantly noradrenergic TCA, was unsuccessful as a treatment not only for the OCD but also for the secondary depression both of which improved on the SSRI (Goodman et al., 1990). Nevertheless, in the event that OCD symptoms improve but depressive symptoms do not, the addition of a noradrenergic agent such as desipramine, or a switch to another SSRI or clomipramine, may be worthwhile (Goodman et al., 1992). Anti-obsessional efficacy has been demonstrated with phenelzine as monotherapy, the MAOI comparable to clomipramine in one 12-week trial (Vallejo et al., 1992). Buspirone and clonazepam have also been studied with favorable results as has dextroamphetamine at least on acute administration (Rauch et al., 1996). Adjunctive agents which have been reported to be of some benefit include benzodiazepines, buspirone, fenfluramine, TCAs, trazodone, lithium, neuroleptics such as pimozide, haloperidol, or risperidone as well as clonidine (Goodman et al., 1992; Zetin & Kramer, 1992; Keller & Hanks, 1995; McDougle, 1997; Rauch et al., 1996).

## Post-traumatic stress disorder

The symptom clusters targeted in PTSD include intrusive re-experiencing, avoidant behavior, numbing, and hyperarousal. In a double-blind study of PTSD, fluoxetine was found to be significantly better than placebo, among the a civilian but not among a more chronically ill veteran group, particularly with respect to arousal and numbing symptoms (van der Kolk, 1994). An open trial of fluoxetine also demonstrated efficacy (Nagy et al., 1993). Davidson (1997) reported on a positive open label study of fluvoxamine in civilians with PTSD and a small open label study of sertraline by Brady and colleagues among individuals with PTSD and comorbid alcohol abuse in which the investigators are reported to have found a 50% reduction in PTSD scores and reduction in alcohol use across the 12-week trial. Sertraline was also reported to be effective in another open trial among veterans with comorbid PTSD and depression (Kline et al., 1994) and among rape victims (Rothbaum et al., 1996), Significant improvement was found with paroxetine among patients with non-combat-related PTSD (Marshall et al., 1998) including reduction in hyperarousal, re-experiencing and dissociative symptoms as well as anxiety and depression. Improvement in PTSD symptoms has also been reported in an open trial of trazodone (Hertzberg et al., 1996). Drug-placebo differences have been found for imipramine (Frank et al., 1987) and amitriptyline (Davidson et al., 1990), but not desipramine which nevertheless helped with symptoms of depression among those patients with PTSD and MDD (Reist et al., 1989). The largest drug–placebo difference was in a study of phenelzine (44% vs. 5%; Kosten et al., 1991), particularly on intrusive and avoidant symptoms among combat veterans without MDD. However an earlier study failed to show similar magnitude effects with this MAOI (Shestatsky et al., 1988). Controlled PTSD trials have not demonstrated efficacy with alprazolam (Braun et al., 1990) nor inositol (Kaplan et al., 1996). Limited study of anticonvulsants, including valproate and carbamazepine, have shown promise in combat veterans, particularly on hostility and intrusive symptoms (Fesler, 1991; Lipper et al., 1986; Wolf et al., 1988). Lithium was helpful in an open trial among combat veterans across a number of symptoms including anger, flashbacks, alcohol abuse and sleep disturbance (van der Kolk, 1983). Clonidine, guanfacine, beta-blockers, and atypical antipsychotics have been inadequately studied but may have a role, while benzodiazepines should be used with caution in the absence of proven efficacy because of risks of disinhibition, substance abuse, and depression (Davidson, 1997; Marshall et al., 1996).

## Psychotherapy

Particular forms of psychotherapy have been shown to have efficacy in the treatment of anxiety disorders, particularly behavioral and cognitive-behavioral therapies which have been shown to be equivalent and, in some cases, superior to pharmacological treatments (Beck, 1988; Clum et al., 1993; Gorman & Coplan 1996; Klosko et al., 1990; Otto & Gould, 1996; Gould & Otto, 1996; Rauch et al., 1996; Shear et al., 1994; Sherbourne & Wells, 1997). Some patients who refuse medications, cannot take them, cannot tolerate their side effects, or are medication treatment-resistant may need to rely on therapy as their sole source of treatment (Keller & Hanks, 1995). Many others will seek psychotherapy in combination with pharmacotherapy because of the limitations inherent in pharmacotherapy alone for their condition (e.g., OCD). The role of psychotherapy in the patient with TRD and comorbid anxiety remains to be defined as does the comparative efficacy of combined vs. single modality treatments. However, clinical experience suggests that the integration of pharmacological and psychotherapeutic interventions is an important avenue of treatment for patients with TRD and moderate to severe anxiety, particularly when the latter appears to be an additional source of psychosocial impairment, distress, and work disability and/or when anxiety disorder symptoms interfere with a patient's ability to adhere to pharmacotherapy and other treatments aimed at reducing depression.

## Alcohol and substance use

Although the association of MDD with alcohol and other substance use disorders is less strong than the association of depression with anxiety disorders (Regier et al., 1990; Sharma et al., 1995), the co-occurrence with MDD with alcohol and substance use disorders is still appreciable (Coryell et al., 1992; Helzer & Pryzbeck, 1988; Kessler et al., 1994, 1995; Grant & Hartford, 1995; MacEwan & Remick, 1988; Merikangas & Gelernter, 1990; Merikangas et al., 1996; Sherbourne et al., 1993; Weissman & Myers, 1980) and, when present, these disorders pose formidable challenges to antidepressant treatment.

An analysis of the Epidemiological Catchment Area Study data (Helzer & Pryzbeck, 1988) demonstrated that, among male alcoholics compared with the total male sample, the risk of depression was only modestly elevated (5% vs. 3%) while among female alcoholics the risk of depression was more than double that of the total female sample (19% vs. 7%). Moreover, while alcoholism preceded the development of depression in the majority of men with both lifetime disorders (78%), depression appeared to be the antecedent disorder in the majority of women (66%). This finding suggests that there may be significant gender differences with respect to the nature of the relationship between the two disorders.

### Impact on treatment outcome

In the management of TRD, alcohol and other substance intoxication (and withdrawal) may wreak havoc in myriad ways (Gastfriend, 1996; Nunes et al., 1996) including their physiological consequences both acute and subacute (e.g., sleep disturbance, irritability, dysphoria, heightened risk of drug interactions) and chronic (e.g., dementia, liver disease, HIV), their psychosocial ramifications (e.g., marital disruption, unemployment), and their association with other comorbid disorders (e.g., antisocial personality disorder, attention deficit hyperactivity disorder, anxiety disorders) that may themselves further complicate recovery from depression. Although it is widely agreed that alcohol and substance abuse/

dependence in MDD should be vigorously addressed, often starting with respectful but tenacious confrontation of denial and recruitment of formally structured substance abuse treatment, acceptable lower limits of use, if any, among non-abusing patients, are by no means agreed upon. In support of abstinence as an ideal, a study by Worthington and colleagues (Worthington et al., 1996) found that, among an outpatient sample of 94 non-drug or alcohol abusing adults with MDD who were enrolled in an 8-week open trial of fluoxetine, alcohol consumption at baseline was a significant predictor of poorer depression outcome even though mean self-reported alcohol consumption was unexceptional at just under 1 fl oz per day.

Among depressed patients with alcohol or substance abuse/dependence disorders, it is frequently difficult to exclude the possibility of a DSM-IV defined substance induced mood disorder (American Psychiatric Association: *Diagnostic and Statistical Manual of Mental Disorders*, 1994) rather than MDD unless there has been a month of more of documented abstinence. Under those circumstances, Nunes and colleagues (Nunes et al., 1996) advise evaluation of features of the clinical presentation that may count in favor of the latter diagnosis, namely: (i) depression antedates the onset of regular substance use; (ii) depression has persisted in the past during periods of abstinence; (iii) symptoms of depression are chronic across fluctuating patterns of substance use; (iv) depression emerges during a period of stable rather than escalating (or diminishing) use; (v) positive family history of mood or anxiety disorders is elicited; (vi) mood and anxiety symptoms are symptoms not typically associated with drug toxicity or withdrawal (e.g., severe sustained suicidal ideation, social phobia); and (vii) the type of drug involved is not as frequently associated with induction of mood disorder symptoms during use or withdrawal (e.g., opiates and benzodiazepines less commonly than alcohol and stimulants).

In a comparison of alcohol induced vs. independent MDD among 2945 alcoholic subjects in the Collaborative Study on the Genetics of Alcoholism of whom 41.6% had depressive symptoms serious enough to qualify for a diagnosis of MDD at some time during their alcoholic course, independent MDD was defined as depression that occurred either before the onset of alcohol dependence or during a period of 3 or more months of abstinence, whereas an induced depression was one that occurred during a period of active alcohol dependence (Schuckit et al., 1997). Clinical variables associated with independent vs. substance-induced depression included being female, married, and Caucasian, having a first degree relative with a major mood disorder, having made a suicide attempt, and having had less treatment for alcoholism and experience with fewer drugs than those individuals with an alcohol induced mood disorder (Schuckit et al., 1997). Although the distinction between independent and substance-induced – or 'primary' and 'secondary' – depression in alcohol and substance use disorders appears to be clinically meaningful, its relevance to predicting antidepressant responsiveness is not established.

There are abundant clinical and naturalistic data to suggest that comorbidity of alcohol and substance use with depression carries a poor prognosis including persistence of depression and drug use, and an elevated risk of suicide (Akiskal, 1982; Carroll et al., 1993; Coulehan et al., 1987; Grant, 1997; Helzer & Pryzbeck, 1988; Madden, 1991; Murphy et al., 1992; Rousanville et al., 1986, 1987). There is also ample clinical experience to suggest that sobriety should be the goal in the ongoing treatment of established TRD, in which eradication of all factors potentially confounding treatment takes on particular significance. Nevertheless, abstinence sustained over one or more months may be difficult to achieve despite multiple hospitalizations and an unremitting depression may in some cases, reciprocally, perpetuate alcohol and substance use (Khantzian, 1985; Nunes et al., 1996). Hence interest has focused upon the development of treatment strategies in the approach to the dually diagnosed depressed individual in whom reduction of alcohol or other substance use as well as remission of depression are concurrent goals.

## Alcohol abuse/dependence

Although alcohol is likely to hinder response to antidepressants, an evolving literature has suggested antidepressant efficacy and some degree of reduction of alcohol use among recently abstinent or currently drinking outpatients with mild to moderate alcohol dependence and MDD who are treated with SSRI or TCA antidepressants.

Among the most encouraging of these studies was a double-blind, placebo-controlled trial conducted by Cornelius and colleagues (Cornelius et al., 1997) involving 51 adults with comorbid MDD and alcohol dependence who were started on fluoxetine 20–40 mg daily following inpatient detoxification and then were discharged two weeks later for outpatient treatment consisting of weekly supportive psychotherapy sessions, weekly meetings with a psychiatrist expert in dual-diagnosis, and encouragement of attendance of Alcoholics Anonymous. Not surprisingly, both the placebo and fluoxetine assigned groups showed marked drops in HDRS depression scores following detoxification. However, on follow-up, only the fluoxetine treated group showed significant, if only moderate, further improvement in depression during the 12-week trial. In addition, fluoxetine treated outpatients showed a two-thirds reduction in total alcohol consumption when compared with the placebo group and fewer days of heavy drinking. The rates of complete abstinence during the 12 weeks, however, were under 30% in both treatment groups and did not differ significantly between them.

In contrast, Kranzler and colleagues (Kranzler et al., 1995) were unable to demonstrate notable effects of fluoxetine on alcohol consumption among a group of alcoholics of whom only a subset (14%) had comorbid depression, although they found a reduction in HDRS scores. This result supports the hypothesis that comorbidity with MDD may be a positive predictor of response when fluoxetine is used in the treatment of alcoholism.

Similarly designed trials with the TCAs include the double-blind, placebo-controlled outpatient trial of imipramine by McGrath and colleagues (McGrath et al., 1996) in which 69 actively drinking alcoholics were enrolled who suffered from a current depressive disorder judged to be either antecedent to alcoholism or present during previous periods. Individuals were excluded if they were felt to be in need of inpatient detoxification. Imipramine dosing was aggressive (mean dose 262 mg/day; mean plasma level 322 ng/ml). Post-treatment HDRS scores were significantly, if modestly, lower for imipramine compared with placebo treated subjects and response rates, measured globally as much or very much improved, with respect to depression and alcoholism were significantly greater. Tempering these findings are the observations that antidepressant efficacy was not demonstrable using other criteria for response (including an HDRS score $\leqslant 6$ and/or 50% reduction in the HDRS) and that effects on drinking were limited to those subjects who also experienced mood improvement. In addition, despite provision of weekly relapse prevention counseling and weekly meetings with a psychologist along with pharmacotherapy, the completion rate of this 12-week trial was only 51%. Nevertheless the study supported the safety and partial efficacy of full dose imipramine in this population of moderate alcoholics with depression for whom TCAs have traditionally been discouraged.

Mason and colleagues (Mason et al., 1996) have reported generally comparable results with desipramine showing moderate efficacy for depression and for alcohol relapse among individuals with MDD and antecedent alcohol dependence. Since MDD followed alcoholism in these patients, these results underscore the question of whether the distinction between independent and induced (or 'primary' and 'secondary') depression is relevant to predicting antidepressant efficacy in this population. Further studies of antidepressants among depressed alcoholics are warranted, even for those depressions which appear to be one of the consequences of alcohol dependence. In general, however, depressive symptoms which are truly the result of alcoholism typically remit with abstinence over 3–4 weeks and therefore do not usually require antidepressant treatment (Brown et al., 1995).

As yet there have been no systematic studies of adjunctive treatments for comorbid alcohol dependence and depression. In particular, naltrexone (50 mg daily) has been shown to be safe and effective monotherapy for relapse prevention (O'Malley et al., 1996), at least among compliant patients (Volpicelli et al., 1997), putatively by blocking reinforcing effects of alcohol and possibly influencing conditioned neuroendocrine responses to environmental cues paired with drinking. A promising extension of this work will be trials combining the opiate receptor antagonist, antidepressants, and dual diagnosis counseling among patients with MDD and alcohol dependence.

## Substance abuse/dependence

Early placebo controlled studies showed antidepressant efficacy of TCAs in depressed methadone maintenance or detoxification patients receiving doxepin (Titievsky et al., 1982; Woody et al., 1975), a finding supported by more recent studies with imipramine among methadone patients with better characterized primary or chronic depressions (Nunes et al., 1991, 1996) Self-reported concurrent use of other substances was less clearly improved by antidepressant treatment in these trials. Promising results in a similar patient cohort were found in a pilot study of fluoxetine (Petrakis et al., 1994). Among cocaine abusers, imipramine or desipramine alone or in combination with dopamine agonists, as well as fluoxetine, have also shown antidepressant efficacy in subgroups of abusers who were also depressed and may reduce postwithdrawal cocaine craving (Arndt et al., 1992; Carroll & Billet, 1994; Gawin et al., 1989; Gianni et al., 1987; Kosten et al., 1992a; Nunes et al., 1995), although there have been some contradictory reports (Kosten et al., 1992b) and TCA related jitteriness has been reported to be associated with cocaine relapse in a small series (Weiss, 1988). Fluoxetine appears to have limited use in cocaine dependence based on preliminary studies (Covi et al., 1995; Grabowsky et al., 1995). The partial $\mu$ opiate receptor agonist, $\kappa$ antagonist, buprenorphine, has been shown to be comparable on sublingual administration (12 mg) to oral methadone (65 mg) for reduction of illicit opioid use and more modest attenuation of concurrent cocaine abuse/dependence, a frequently comorbid disorder among opioid abusers (Schottenfeld et al., 1997). In the treatment of antidepressant-treatment-resistant unipolar depression, among a small sample of non-substance-abusing adults with TRD, intranasal or sublingual administration of buprenorphine, at much lower doses, has been observed to produce rapid-onset reduction of depressive symptoms, although in several subjects initial benefit did not persist into continuation treatment (Bodkin et al., 1995). The potential antidepressant efficacy of this agent among substance abusing populations with MDD remains to be clarified.

Inpatient treatment is a priority for those patients with severe substance dependence and, in this context, temporary cessation or delay in antidepressant pharmacotherapy is appropriate at least until the patient has undergone detoxification and is medically stable (Nunes et al., 1996). For those patients with more moderate substance abuse/dependence outpatient substance abuse treatment programs have been shown to be effective, particularly if they include flexibility to target additional, if inter-related, problems (e.g., psychiatric, employment related) with which patients inevitably present (McLellan et al., 1997; Woody et al., 1984). It is especially important for the TRD patient that treatment takes place in a setting in which the pressing need for depression reassessment and treatment, including pharmacotherapy, can be recognized and facilitated.

Implementation or continuation of antidepressants in a depressed patient found to have substance abuse/dependence may include a 'pharmacotherapy contract' (Gastfriend, 1993) including the stipulation that pharmacological treatments are contingent upon active participation in substance abuse treatment and, perhaps, also self-help groups including Alcoholic or Narcotics, Cocaine Anonymous; that urine or blood testing may be required at any time to provide an independent source of data about the course of chemical dependence; and that unilateral changes in medication by the patient are to be considered unacceptable and may be an early sign of relapse. When family or other significant persons are in a position to serve as additional observers of the patient's moods, behavior and substance use and as advocates for compliance with treatment, their involvement can also be a crucial asset.

## Dysthymia

As many as one-quarter of adults presenting with MDD are thought to have a 'double depression' in which dysthymia is conceptualized as a comorbid disorder upon which MDD is superimposed (Keller & Shapiro, 1982; Sanderson et al., 1990). In naturalistic studies, comorbidity with dysthymia appears to be related to greater functional impairment than MDD alone (Klein 1996; Wells et al., 1992) and a higher risk of relapse or recurrence of MDD (Steffens et al., 1996, Keller et al., 1983, 1992). The degree to which dysthymia and MDD are truly distinct disorders, however, remains a question, particularly because dysthymia, double depression, and MDD have been difficult to distinguish in family-genetic studies (Remick et al., 1996) and pharmacological trials.

Dysthymia has been shown to respond in double-blind, placebo controlled studies to sertraline (Thase et al., 1996); fluoxetine (Hellerstein et al., 1993; Vanelle et al., 1997); imipramine (Lecrubier et al., 1997; Thase et al., 1996; Vallejo et al., 1987); phenelzine (Vallejo et al., 1987); and amisulpride, a D2 and D3 dopamine receptor antagonist (Lecrubier et al., 1997). An open trial of fluoxetine was effective among elderly patients with dysthymia (Nobler et al., 1996). 'Double depression' has been shown to respond to imipramine (Kocsis et al., 1988), desipramine (Marin et al., 1994); fluoxetine (Hellerstein et al., 1993; Lapierre, 1994; Fava et al., 1997b), MAOIs including moclobemide (Duarte et al., 1996,

Versiani, 1994) and the 5-HT$_2$ serotonin receptor antagonist, ritanserin (Bakish et al., 1993; Bersani et al., 1991; Reyntjens et al., 1986). Similarly, in an acute and long-term treatment study of dysthymics, double depressives, and chronic major depressives, the three groups did not differ in their response to initial open-label treatment with desipramine nor with respect to prophylactic benefit against recurrence derived from desipramine vs. placebo during a subsequent randomized, double-blind maintenance phase of up to 2 years (Kocsis et al., 1996). An early trial of continuation treatment with phenelzine also showed a significant drug–placebo difference among a small sample of patients with dysthymia and double depression (Harrison et al., 1986).

Thus, naturalistic studies have suggested that comorbidity with dysthymia implies a poorer prognosis but evidence from controlled clinical trials in which treatment is optimized have suggested that dysthymia and double depression may respond initially in much the same way as MDD alone. Nevertheless, while evidence is lacking to suggest that comorbid dysthymia accounts for non-response of MDD to standard treatment, there have been two studies suggesting greater persistence of at least minor depressive symptoms (i.e. less complete remission) following treatment of double depression compared with MDD without dysthymia. Keller and colleagues (Keller et al., 1983) reported on patients with double depression who recovered quickly from their MDD episode but then recovered slowly from residual depressive symptoms. Moreover, the more persistent the minor depressive symptoms, the greater the probability of a recurrence of MDD over a two year follow-up. The NIMH Treatment of Depression Collaborative Research Program study also found that double depression was associated with greater depressive symptomatology at end point across all treatment conditions including interpersonal psychotherapy, cognitive-behavioral therapy, imipramine with clinical management, and placebo with clinical management (Sotsky et al., 1991). Further study of continuation and maintenance pharmacotherapy, psychotherapy (Markowitz, 1994) and combined treatment of double depression will be of much interest in further clarifying the relevance of this form of depressive comorbidity to the acute and long-term management of major depression.

## Personality disorders

Estimated rates of coexisting personality disorders among individuals with MDD range widely from approximately 20–80% among patient samples reflecting the heterogeneity of populations studied, varied time points of assessment with respect to depression severity and treatment, and the diversity of instruments and methodologies used to assess Axis II pathology (Corruble et al., 1996). Inpatient depressed samples have been characterized by higher rates of so-called Cluster B (dramatic, emotional, or erratic) personality disorders, particularly borderline and histrionic (Black et al., 1988; Charney et al., 1981; Pfohl et al., 1984), while outpatient samples have been associated with higher proportion of Cluster C (anxious or fearful) personality disorders, including avoidant, dependent and obsessive-compulsive (Pilkonis & Frank, 1988; Shea et al., 1987; Tyrer et al., 1983). Cluster B personality disorders as well as avoidant personality disorder were found to be significantly more common among depressed adult outpatients with a history of juvenile rather than adult onset MDD (Fava et al., 1996). Although the prevalence of personality disorders is likely to be elevated among clinical populations, nearly half of individuals with a history of MDD within one non-treatment sample were reported to meet criteria for one or more personality disorders (Zimmerman & Coryell, 1989). Some studies have suggested a greater preponderance of personality disorders among individuals with chronic depressive disorders, including dysthymia, double depressions, and chronic major depressions (Howland, 1993; Klein et al., 1988; Markowitz et al., 1992; Miller et al., 1986; Pepper et al., 1995; Sanderson et al., 1992). However in the DSM-IV field trials the rates of Axis II comorbidity among chronic and episodic MDD were not significantly different (Kaye et al., 1994).

As with other forms of comorbidity, the relationship between personality pathology and MDD is likely to be complex. The most influential hypotheses concerning this form of comorbidity have included the proposals that personality disorders predispose to depression directly or by virtue of their consequences; that personality disorders modify the symptom expression of depression; that depression, particularly when severe and unremitting, may have an enduring impact on features of personality; and that personality disorders are an attenuated expression of affective disorders (Akiskal et al., 1983; Gunderson & Phillips, 1991; Hirschfeld & Shea 1992; Thase, 1996).

Testing of these and related hypotheses regarding personality disorders in MDD has been hampered by the significant potential impact the depressive state has on assessment of and reporting of personality traits (Coppen & Metcalfe, 1965; Hirschfeld et al., 1983; Joffe & Regan, 1988; Reich et al., 1987; Stuart et al., 1992), only modest correlations between patient and informant reports of personality pathology (Zimmerman et al., 1988), and the differing levels of sensitivity and specificty and generally poor agreement among research instruments available to diagnose Axis II disorders (Fava et al., 1996; Perry, 1992) and between research and clinical approaches to personality assessment (Westen, 1997). Among TRD patients, the usual reasonable practice of deferring evaluation of personality until the depression is remitted is often not a foreseeable option and, in addition, there may be concerned parties, including family, other clinicians, and even the patient, who interpret antidepressant treatment resistance as confirmation of characterological problems, further amplifying the risk that Axis II pathology will be overdiagnosed in this population.

## Impact on treatment outcome

Summarizing contemporary views on the relevance of personality traits and disorders to treatment-resistance in depression, Thase (1996) has commented: 'At one extreme is the view that depressive phenomenology colors personality to such an extent that valid assessment is impossible. At the other extreme is the view that antidepressant resistance is uncommon among people with "healthy" personalities' (p. 287).

While fraught with methodological difficulties, studies on personality and treatment outcome have largely but certainly not uniformly (Davidson et al., 1985; Fava et al., 1994; Joffe & Regan, 1988; Sullivan et al., 1994) supported the widely espoused clinical impression that Axis II disorders are associated with a poorer response rate to antidepressants (Black et al., 1988; Reich & Vasile 1993; Shea et al., 1992; Nelson et al., 1994; Thase, 1996), slower recovery of social functioning (Shea et al., 1990, Patience et al., 1995; Quinton et al., 1995), chronicity (Andreoli et al., 1993; Vine & Steingart, 1994) and a higher rate of relapse (Alnaes & Torgersen, 1997) and hospital readmission (Labbate & Doyle, 1997). Within a statistical model developed to predict recovery among 1471 depressed inpatients, personality disorder was one of six predictive variables identified by stepwise multiple logistic regression along with anxiety, dysthymia, organic mental disorder, chronicity, and ECT (Black et al., 1991). Some investigators have suggested that particular personality clusters are associated with different patterns of antidepressant response, including relatively poorer outcome for depressed individuals with comorbid Cluster A (odd or eccentric) personality disorders especially schizoid PD (Sato et al., 1994) and a relatively better outcome for individuals with borderline personality disorder (Cluster B) (Fava et al., 1994). Other studies have not detected differential outcomes according to personality cluster (Shea et al., 1990). Conclusions drawn from studies regarding particular personality disorders must be made with caution in so far as different research methodologies for diagnosing personality disorders show much less agreement when used to reach specific personality disorder diagnoses than when used to determine simple presence or absence of a personality disorder *per se* (Westen, 1997).

It should be emphasized that available studies on antidepressant treatment of depressed patients with comorbid personality disorders generally speak more to effectiveness than efficacy in so far as a majority of studies were naturalistic and neither the adequacy nor aggressiveness of pharmacotherapy were standardized between personality and non-personality disordered patients. In addition, most studies were conducted before the widespread use of the SSRIs and may not generalize well to current practice.

Studies generally support the effectiveness of ECT as acute treatment in MDD with personality Axis II comorbidity but suggest a less favorable long-term prognosis. In a cohort of 40 depressed inpatients who received ECT and were followed over one year, personality disorders did not influence the speed of symptom response to ECT nor of readmission, however personality was associated with slower recovery of social function following discharge (Casey et al., 1996). Among 25 inpatients with MDD, those with DSM-III personality disorders did not differ from those without personality disorders in the proportion of those responding acutely to ECT with a decrease of 50% or more on the HDRS, although fewer reached the criterion set for remission (HDRS score $\leqslant$ 6; 20% vs. 53%) and on 6-month follow-up they continued to show greater depressive symptomatology despite similar levels of antidepressant treatment and an eight-fold risk of rehospitalization (Zimmerman et al., 1986). In a sample of 76 inpatients with MDD and personality disorders compared with 176 inpatients with MDD without personality disorders, personality comorbidity was associated with lower likelihood of receiving ECT or antidepressants, but those depressed patients with personality disorder comorbidity who did receive ECT showed a similar response to those without personality disorders (Black et al., 1988) while those who received antidepressants at adequate doses showed a significantly poorer response than patients without personality disorder comorbidity (26% vs. 64%). A similar pattern was observed among a smaller sample of inpatients with MDD, in whom the coexistence of personality disorders was associated with poorer response to antidepressants but not to ECT (Pfohl et al., 1984). Despite a widely held view that individuals with MDD with personality disorder comorbidity are poor candidates for ECT, available data suggests the contrary, that selected individuals with TRD and personality disorders may sustain greater advantage with ECT relative to medications compared to their non-personality disordered counterparts, assuming the two groups are matched along other lines, such as baseline depression severity, chronicity, and subtype, and level of psychosocial stress.

Axis II comorbidity has been reported to exert a negative influence upon depression-related outcome of psychodynamic psychotherapy (Thompson et al., 1988; Diguer et al., 1993), interpersonal therapy (Shea et al., 1990), behavior therapy (Thompson et al., 1988), psychodynamic-interpersonal psychotherapy (Hardy et al., 1995) and interpersonal therapy combined with imipramine (Frank & Kupfer, 1990). Although co-existing personality disorders did not appear to reduce the response to cognitive-behavioral therapy (Hardy et al., 1995; Shea et al., 1990; Stuart et al., 1992).

Taken together these results suggest the co-occurrence of personality disorders in MDD is associated with poorer short-term response to antidepressants but not ECT, albeit often studied under naturalistic circumstances and involving non-

SSRI antidepressants. Personality disorders may also predict poorer response to psychotherapy, with the possible exception of cognitive-behavioral therapy, at least on short-term follow-up.

Spanning the Axis II disorders are dimensions of personality that have been assessed with a wide variety of instruments. Among the more consistent findings concern 'neuroticism,' a construct developed by Eysenck (1967) to encompass vulnerability to proneness to anxiety, emotional instability and somatic responses under stress and higher scores are associated with greater likelihood of a categorical personality disorder. High neuroticism scores in MDD have been reported to predict less complete recovery at 1 and 4 months follow-up after starting antidepressants in primary care (Katon et al., 1994), more prolonged and erratic patterns of recovery (Frank et al., 1987), and poorer long-term outcome (Kerr et al., 1970; Weissman et al., 1978) with follow-up as long as 18 years following an index depressive episode (Duggan et al., 1990). Not all studies have found an association between neuroticism and poorer acute antidepressant response (Zuckerman et al., 1980; Davidson et al., 1985), however, and in one study with 1-year follow-up only less adequate social adjustment was predicted by neuroticism (Zuckerman et al., 1980). Personality features on the Millon Clinical Multiaxial Inventory such as assertiveness, independence, and competitiveness distinguished responders from non-responders to TCAs better than categorical personality diagnoses which were not found to be predictive in that study (Joffe & Regan, 1988). A similar dimension, high 'autonomy' with low 'sociotropy', was associated among 217 depressed outpatients with both a greater response to antidepressants and a larger drug–placebo difference (Peselow et al., 1994). Attention has also focused upon constructs developed by Cloninger and colleagues, including high 'reward dependence' and low 'harm avoidance,' as assessed with the Tridimensional Personality Questionnaire or Temperament and Character Inventory (Cloninger et al., 1994). These 'temperaments' were reported to be predictive of response to desipramine and clomipramine (Joyce et al., 1994), nefazodone (Nelson & Cloninger, 1995) and paroxetine (Tome et al., 1997) while response to augmentation of paroxetine with the 5-HT1A receptor antagonist, pindolol, was associated with high 'novelty seeking' and low 'harm avoidance' (Tome et al., 1997). Further confirmation of these results are needed and the relationship of these dimensions of temperament to Axis II psychopathology remains to be clarified.

## Treatment strategies

Some of the most promising approaches to the development of rational pharmacotherapy of personality disorders have focused upon aggregations of symptoms which characterize particular personality disorders and clusters (Gitlin

1995). Thus, for example, Coccaro and Siever (1995) propose five principal targets of psychotropic drug treatment including psychotic-like, deficit symptoms, impulsive aggressive traits and behaviors, affective-related traits, and anxiety-related traits. A growing number of studies have looked at SSRIs in the treatment of samples of individuals with Axis II disorders, typically heterogeneous with respect to Axis I comorbidity including MDD, particularly targeting anger, irritability and aggressive behavior. Thus, in a double-blind, placebo-controlled trial of fluoxetine (20–60 mg) among 40 impulsively aggressive patients with DSM-III-R personality disorders (but not current MDD), there was a sustained superiority of drug over placebo during a 3-month period with reduction of aggressive behavior that appeared to be independent of comorbid mood, anxiety, or alcohol or other substance use disorders (Coccaro & Kavoussi, 1997). A 43% study attrition rate during the 12 weeks underscored the challenges of working with a severely personality disordered population.

Similarly a reduction in anger, which was independent of depression, was reported among a sample of 22 individuals with mild borderline personality disorder or traits treated in a double-blind, placebo-controlled protocol with fluoxetine (40 mg) (Salzman et al., 1995). So, too, a reduction in self-injurious behavior, as well as depression, anxiety and psychotic-like symptoms, was found among 18 patients with DSM-III-R borderline and borderline/schizotypal personality disorders following open-treatment with fluoxetine (80 mg) (Markovitz et al., 1991). A reduction in impulsivity and depression was also observed during open-label treatment with fluoxetine (20–40 mg) among five patients with borderline personality disorder (Cornelius et al., 1993b). An anti-aggressive effect of fluoxetine (5–40 mg) was observed as early as 1 week into treatment among 12 patients with borderline personality disorder (Norden, 1989). Sertraline (100–200 mg) was also associated with reduction in aggression and irritability among nine patients, predominantly with borderline personality disorder, during an 8-week trial (Kavoussi et al., 1994). Venlafaxine and sertraline were each associated with improvement in irritability and hostility among personality disordered patients (Markovitz & Wagner, 1995). These results parallel findings among outpatients with 'anger attacks' and MDD, with or without personality disorders, in whom fluoxetine has been associated with marked improvement in irritability (Fava et al., 1993).

Thus SSRIs appear to have intrinsic efficacy for impulsive/aggressive behavior that may cut across diverse clinical populations. The specificity of this effect, however, has not been well tested. Among borderline and borderline/schizotypal personality disordered patients double-blind treatment with amitriptyline was associated with exacerbation in paranoia, hostility, and impulsivity, despite improvements in depression (Soloff et al., 1986, 1989), thus contributing to the belief that TCAs are less effective and potentially dangerous among impulsive/aggressive personality disordered patients. Nevertheless, among individuals with anger attacks in MDD and dysthymia (with or without Axis II comorbidity) anger attacks were reduced (not increased) on imipramine and the magnitude of reduction was similar to that associated with sertraline (Fava et al., 1997a). Similar SSRI vs. TCA comparison studies among personality disordered patients are lacking.

Limited study of MAOIs suggests that both tranylcypromine (Cowdry & Gardner, 1988) and phenelzine (vs. imipramine) (Parsons et al., 1989) have positive effects on mood and rejection sensitivity in borderline personality disorder, particularly in the context of atypical depression, although one study showed more modest effects (Soloff et al., 1993). MAOIs are likely to be helpful, as are SSRIs, in avoidant personality disorder (Deltito and Stam, 1989) which is often found in association with social phobia and atypical depression among adults with MDD (Alpert et al., 1997). The potential use of benzodiazepines in this setting has not been well studied.

The anticonvulsant mood stabilizers, carbamazepine (Cowdry & Gardner, 1988) and valproate (Wilcox, 1995), have been shown to produce significant reduction in impulsivity/behavioral dyscontrol among patients with borderline personality disorder, although the degree to which they reduce depression severity appears to be less impressive.

Antipsychotic agents, including haloperidol (Soloff et al., 1993), thiothixene (Goldberg et al., 1986), thioridazine (Teicher et al., 1989), trifluoperazine (Cowdry & Gardner, 1988), loxapine and chlorpromazine (Leone, 1982) and clozapine (Frankenburg & Zarini, 1993), studied among borderline, borderline/schizotypal and schizotypal patient samples, have been associated with variable impact on mood with attenuation of impulsivity and ideas of reference and other psychotic-like symptoms. Although available studies do not suggest a first-line role for these agents in most patients with non-psychotic MDD with personality comorbidity, the increasingly available atypical antipsychotics including risperidone, olanzepine and quetiapine, which have a broader spectrum of action than conventional agents and may carry a lower risk of tardive dyskinesia, deserve evaluation in this setting (Gitlin, 1995).

A limited adjunctive role for opiate antagonists, such as naltrexone, may be indicated among some personality disordered individuals with self-injurious behavior such as cutting in view of reported benefit in reducing the incidence of self-harm (Buzan et al., 1995).

Clinical experience and case reports suggest that patients with TRD and personality disorders benefit in crucial ways from a variety of forms of psychotherapy in which a therapeutic alliance is established, maladaptive, inflexible, and potentially dangerous behaviors are addressed, strategies to cope with overwhelming, painful and unstable feelings are learned, normalizing behaviors are modeled, and hope is maintained (Thase, 1996). With respect to depression outcome, however, as reviewed earlier, only cognitive-behavioral therapy has been associated with documented antidepressant efficacy during acute treatment in this population. Dialectical behavior therapy (DBT) was developed by Linehan (Linehan, 1993) as an extension of CBT intended to address intense suicidal and self-injurious behaviors and urges, particularly among individuals with borderline personality disorder, and to provide psychoeducation and skills to promote both validation and acceptance as well as change. These techniques have been further extended to substance abuse among personality disordered patients (Linehan, 1995). Further study of the influence of DBT on depression outcome will be of much interest as it remains to be seen whether DBT is associated with any greater impact on depression than conventional psychotherapies (Linehan et al., 1991).

## Other psychiatric comorbidity

MDD is the most common form of Axis I psychiatric comorbidity among treatment-seeking individuals with anorexia nervosa and bulimia nervosa (Herzog, 1996), and, reciprocally, problems associated with eating disorders not infrequently complicate treatment of MDD. Dissatisfaction with body image and intolerance of weight gain often hinder progress in antidepressant pharmacotherapy by restricting the range of options available. In addition, bulimic patients may have variable drug levels by virtue of purging while anorexic patients may have unusual drug pharmacokinetics and drug–drug interactions by virtue of alterations in serum proteins and their proportion of adipose tissue. A higher incidence of seizures on bupropion (Horne et al., 1988) restricted its use in this population. Relatively little is known about the impact of eating disorders upon the course of depression, although they may be associated with greater risk of chronicity and of relapse (Keller et al., 1989). Although bulimia nervosa has been shown to respond to antidepressants of all classes (Walsh & Devlin, 1995), typically at usual doses for depression although potentially higher for fluoxetine (60 mg vs. 20 mg) (Fluoxetine Bulimia Nervosa Collaborative Study Group, 1992), and also to cognitive-behavioral therapy (Wilson et al., 1997), there exist contradictory findings concerning the relationship between changes in bulimic symptoms and changes in depression severity. In addition antidepressants seem to work equally well for bulimia whether or not there is a comorbid major depression (Walsh & Devlin, 1995). Anorexia nervosa may have a more direct impact on depression severity in so far as malnutrition itself appears to intensify depressive symptoms (as well as anxiety and obsessionality) and these symptoms are reported to improve, albeit incompletely, upon weight restoration (Pollice et al., 1997).

Attention-deficit hyperactivity disorder (ADHD) and major depression are often found co-occurring in children and adolescents presenting for treatment of depression (Biederman et al., 1995) and, 12% of adults evaluated for a major depressive episode met threshold or subthreshold DSM-III-R criteria for ADHD with symptoms persisting into adulthood (Alpert et al., 1996). The impact of comorbid ADHD on depression outcome has not been well-studied. In the latter study, depressed adults with and without ADHD were treated with fluoxetine 20 mg per day for 8 weeks and rates of depressive remission did not differ significantly between the two groups, suggesting that comorbid ADHD had minimal influence on antidepressant response. In addition, the two groups were similar with respect to duration of index major depressive episode, number of lifetime depressive episodes, age of first onset of depression, and baseline depression severity. Those depressed individuals with ADHD were distinguished from those without ADHD only by higher self-reported personality disorder traits. While psychostimulants and all classes of antidepressants have been shown to have some efficacy in the treatment of ADHD, less consistent results have been obtained with the SSRIs, which in some cases have caused behavioral worsening, than with TCAs, bupropion, MAOIs, and venlafaxine (Spencer et al., 1996; Popper, 1997). However SSRIs with adjunctive psychostimulants (Findling, 1996), TCAs, or bupropion appear to be reasonable combination therapy when ADHD is suspected in a patient with major depression.

## Conclusions

Psychiatric comorbidity is a ubiquitous feature of MDD which may contribute to poorer response to acute treatment, greater risk of relapse and recurrence, and less adequate social or occupational functioning. Despite its considerable clinical relevance, psychiatric comorbidity as a factor in the approach to management of depression has received little systematic attention and its true impact on treatment-resistance is unknown. Contemporary research in this area is limited by lack of standardized terms and methodologies and much of the evidence suggesting that coexisting psychiatric disorders contribute to treatment resistance among depressed patients comes from naturalistic studies in which such variables as compliance, adequacy of medication dose and duration, choice of treatments provided, and psychosocial disruption associated with particular forms of comorbidity are likely to play an important role. Nevertheless, studies in which the adequacy of treatment has been confirmed, have shown a probable impact of major psychiatric comorbidity, on the acute and longer-term outcome of pharmacology and psychotherapy treatments of depression although the implications of these findings for treatment remain to be defined.

A number of questions must be asked when comorbidity is suspected in the depressed patient: (i) What is the level of certainty surrounding the diagnosis of a comorbid disorder and MDD? A reasonable degree of assurance would come from a history indicating that there had been intervals during the course of one disorder when it existed independently of the other, or, if the two disorders were never separated temporally, that the severity or treatment responses of one has not followed entirely upon the severity or treatment responses of the other; that criteria for the two or more diagnoses are met without relying upon symptoms held in common (e.g., sleep disturbance in MDD and PTSD); that there exists a family history of one or more of the disorders in question; and that the presentation of each disorder is more classic than atypical. (ii) Which of the two (or more) disorders are posing greatest immediate risks or causing most severe disability or distress? (iii) What potential inter-relationships exist between the two (or more) disorders currently? Does one disorder (or its consequences) appear to aggravate or, indeed, produce symptoms of the other, do they have mutual effects, or do they appear not to interact? (iv) Are the symptoms or behaviors associated with one disorder hindering effective treatment of the other? (v) Is treatment prescribed for one disorder making the other worse (e.g., depressogenic effect of clonazepam in a patient with panic disorder and MDD)? (vi) Are there additional safety concerns in treating MDD by virtue of one or more of the comorbid disorders (e.g., tranylcypromine in an impulsive personality disordered patient with active substance use, bupropion in a patient with bulimia nervosa, high dose triidothyronine in an anorexic patient with advanced bone demineralization)? (vii) Are there treatments that would target both TRD and the comorbid disorder(s) (e.g., stimulant augmentation of SSRIs in ADHD; clomipramine for SSRI-resistant depression and OCD), serving both goals at once? (viii) Are there specific psychotherapeutic interventions available to target the comorbid disorders (e.g., behavioral therapy for OCD) and/or enhance compliance? (ix) Are there ancillary factors, physiological or psychosocial, that ought to be addressed for optimal overall outcome (e.g., folate replacement in alcoholism; vocational counseling following a period of unemployment precipitated by depression and substance abuse)? (x) With greater resolution of depressive symptoms, has the diagnostic picture changed with respect to apparent comorbid psychiatric disorders? or, alternatively, (xi) With failure of depression to remit, are there additional diagnostic complexities that were missed on first pass (e.g., previously undisclosed psychotic symptoms, substance use, dementia)?

In the approach to patients with TRD and psychiatric comorbidity it is likely that several important treatment goals will exist simultaneously. Efforts to prioritize these goals are essential in order to direct resources to problems in greatest need of resolution. A classification system of psychiatric comorbidity is offered to

**Table 19.2.** Proposed classification of psychiatric comorbidity in major depressive disorder

| | |
|---|---|
| Class I | Comorbid disorder poses imminent safety risks, requires stabilization |
| Class II | Comorbid disorder causes or exacerbates depressive disorder |
| Class III | Comorbid disorder impedes adequate or optimal treatment |
| Class IV | Comorbid disorder produces additional impairment, distress |

help guide decisions regarding optimal treatment (Table 19.2). Within Class I comorbidities are disorders that, because of their nature and severity, are judged to pose imminent threats to safety including severe alcohol dependence, anorexia nervosa, or borderline personality disorder with active suicidality and self-mutilation. In this context, the need to address the immediate danger posed by comorbid problems temporarily supersedes depression treatment, and often involves hospitalization and stabilization as well as enrolment in more comprehensive treatment before antidepressant treatment can proceed further. Within Class II comorbidities are disorders that do not pose safety concerns, at least in the short term, but are thought to cause or, at the very least, significantly aggravate depressive symptoms including moderate alcohol or substance abuse/dependence, moderate anorexia nervosa, moderate to severe obsessive-compulsive disorder symptoms, post-traumatic stress disorder, and recurrent panic attacks. These conditions may not preclude depression treatment but require directed treatment on their own terms concurrently, along lines described in previous sections. So too with Class III comorbidities which are composed of disorders that may not directly worsen MDD but rather present defined impediments to effective treatment, including moderate panic, generalized anxiety, or eating disorders that interfere with the tolerability of drug side effects or establishment of consistent drug levels, personality disorders that interfere with treatment compliance and therapeutic alliance, and agoraphobia that interferes with keeping appointments. Class III comorbidity also requires concurrent treatment, albeit after treatment is put in place for comorbid disorders associated with Classes I and II. Within Class IV comorbidities are disorders that may have little actual impact on the nature or treatment responsiveness of the depression or on the adequacy of treatment but may be additional sources of impairment, distress and demoralization. Thus, for example, attention deficit disorder, social phobia or avoidant personality disorder, all of mild to moderate severity, may not preclude antidepressant responsiveness of a major depression but may interfere more globally with a patient's quality of life and, perhaps, contribute to residual depressive symptoms and/or to risk of relapses and recurrences of MDD. Although the disorders within Class IV can be addressed while the depression is under active treatment, often their treatments may be deferred pending reassessment of their severity once resolution of the depression is achieved.

Psychiatric comorbidity presents abundant challenges to clinical practice but fortunately also serves as a guide to developing rational treatments and innovative strategies in the approach to treatment-resistant depression in the complicated patient.

# REFERENCES

Akiskal HS. (1982). Factors associated with incomplete recovery in primary depressive illness. *Journal of Clinical Psychiatry*, **43**, 266–71.

Akiskal, H.S., Hirschfeld, R.M.A., & Yerevanian, B.I. (1983). The relationship of personality to affective disorders – a critical review. *Archives of General Psychiatry*, **40**, 801–10.

Albus, M. & Sheibe, G. (1993). Outcome of panic disorder with and without concomitant depression: a 2-year prospective follow-up study. *American Journal of Psychiatry*, **150**, 1878–80.

Alnaes, R., Torgersen, S. (1990). DSM-III personality disorders among patients with major depression, anxiety disorders, and mixed conditions. *Journal of Nervous and Mental Diseases*, **178**, 693–8.

Alnaes, R. & Torgersen, S. (1997). Personality and personality disorders predict development and relapses of major depression. *Acta Psychiatrica Scandinavica*, **95**, 336–42.

Alpert, J.E., Maddocks, A., Rosenbaum, J.F., & Fava, M. (1994). Childhood psychopathology retrospectively assessed among adults with early onset major depression. *Journal of Affective Disorders*, **31**, 165–71.

Alpert, J.E., Fava, M., Uebelacker, L.A., Nierenberg, A.A., Pava, J.A., & Rosenbaum, J.F. (1995). Patterns of comorbidity in early-onset vs. late-onset major depressive disorder. Part I: Axis I disorders. 148th Annual Meeting of the American Psychiatric Association. Miami, FL.

Alpert, J.E., Maddocks, A., Nierenberg, A.A. et al. (1996). Attention deficit hyperactivity disorder in childhood among adults with major depression. *Psychiatry Research*, **62**, 213–19.

Alpert, J.E., Uebelacker, L.A., McLean, N.E. et al. (1997). Social phobia, avoidant personality disorder and atypical depression: co-occurrence and clinical implications. *Psychological Medicine*, **27**, 627–33.

American Psychiatric Association (1994). *Diagnostic and Statistical Manual of Mental Disorders*, 4th edn. Washington, DC: American Psychiatric Association.

Amsterdam, J.D. & Hornig-Rohan, M. (1996). Treatment algorithms in treatment-resistant depression. *Psychiatric Clinics of North America*, **19**(2), 371–86.

Andrade, L., Eaton, W.W., & Chilcoat, H. (1994). Lifetime comorbidity of panic attacks and major depression in a population-based study. Symptom profiles. *British Journal of Psychiatry*, **165**, 363–9.

Angold, A. & Costello, E.J. (1993). Depressive comorbidity in children and adolescents: empirical, theoretical, and methodological issues. *American Journal of Psychiatry*, **150**, 1779–91.

Angst, J. & Dobler-Mikola, A. (1985). The Zurich study, VI: a continuum from depression to anxiety disorders? *European Archives Psychiatry and Neurological Science*, **235**, 178–86.

Angst, J., Merikangas, K.R., & Preisig, M. (1997). Subthreshold syndromes of depression and anxiety in the community. *Journal of Clinical Psychiatry*, **58**[Suppl. 8], 6–10.

Arndt, I.O., Dorozynsky, L., Woody, G.E., McLellan, A.T., & O'Brien, C.P. (1992). Desipramine treatment of cocaine dependence in methadone-maintenance patients. *Archives of General Psychiatry*, **49**, 888–93.

Asnis, G.M. & Faisal, I. (1997). Pharmacotherapy of major depressive disorder with comorbidity. In *Treatment Strategies for Patients with Psychiatric Comorbidity*, ed. S. Wetzler & W.C. Sanderson, pp. 163–85. New York: John Wiley and Sons.

Bakish, D., Lapierre, Y.D., Weinstein, R. et al. (1993). Ritanserin, imipramine and placebo in the treatment of dysthymic disorder. *Journal of Clinical Psychopharmacology*, **6**, 409–15.

Beck, A.T. (1988). Cognitive approaches to panic disorder: theory and therapy In *Panic: Psychological Perspectives*, ed. S. Rachman & J. Maser, pp. 23–38. Hillsdale, NJ: Lawrence Erlbaum Associates.

Bersani, A., Pozzi, F., Marini, S., Grispini, A., Pasini, A., & Ciani, N. (1991). 5HT-2 receptor antagonism in dysthymic disorder: a double-blind, placebo-controlled study with ritanserin. *Acta Psychiatrica Scandinavica*, **83**, 244–8.

Biederman, J., Faraone, S., Mick, E., & Lelon, E. (1995). Psychiatric comorbidity among referred juveniles with major depression: fact or artifact? *Journal of the American Academy of Child and Adolescent Psychiatry*, **34**, 579–90.

Birmaher, B., Ryan, N.D., Williamson, D.E., Brent, D.A., & Kaufman, J. (1996). Childhood and adolescent depression: a review of the past 10 years. Part II. *Journal of the American Academy of Child and Adolescent Psychiatry*, **35**, 1575–83.

Black, D.W., Bells, S., Hubert, J., & Nasrallah, A. (1988). The importance of Axis II in patients with major depression: A controlled study. *Journal of Affective Disorders*, **14**, 115–22.

Black, D.W., Goldstein, R.B., Nasrallah, A., & Winokur, G. (1991). The prediction of recovery using a multivariate model in 1471 depressed inpatients. *European Archives of Psychiatry and Clinical Neuroscience*, **241**, 41–5.

Blazer, D.G., Kessler, R.C., McGonagle, K.A., & Swartz, M.S. (1994). The prevalence and distribution of major depression in a national community sample: The National Comorbidity Survey. *American Journal of Psychiatry*, **151**, 979–86.

Bodkin, J.A., Zornberg, G.L., Lukas, S.E. et al. (1995). Buprenorphine treatment of refractory depression. *Journal of Clinical Psychopharmacology*, **15**, 49–57.

Boyd, J.H., Burke, J.D., Gruenberg, E. et al. (1984). Exclusion criteria of DSM-III: a study of co-occurrence of hierarchy-free syndromes. *Archives of General Psychiatry*, **41**, 983–9.

Boulenger, J-P., Fournier, M., Rosales, D., & Lavallee, Y-J. (1997). Mixed anxiety and depression: from theory to practice. *Journal of Clinical Psychiatry*, **58**, [Suppl. 8], 27–34.

Braun, P., Greenberg, D., Dasberg, H., & Lerer, B. (1990). Core symptoms of posttraumatic stress disorder unimproved by alprazolam treatment. *Journal of Clinical Psychiatry*, **51**, 236–8.

Bronish, T. & Wittchen, H.U. (1994). Suicidal ideation and suicide attempts: comorbidity with depression, anxiety disorders, and substance abuse disorder. *European Archives of Psychiatry and Clinical Neuroscience*, **244**, 93–8.

Brown, C., Schulberg, H.C., Madonia, M.J., Shear, M.K., & Houck, P.R. (1996). Treatment outcomes for primary care patients with major depression and lifetime anxiety disorders. *American Journal of Psychiatry*, **153**, 1293–1300.

Brown, R.A., Inaba, R.K., Gillin, J.C., Schuckit, M.A., Stewart, M.A., & Irwin, M.R. (1995). Alcoholism and affective disorder: clinical course of depressive symptoms. *American Journal of Psychiatry*, **152**, 45–52.

Brown, R.A., Evans, D.M., Miller, I.W., Burgess, E.S., & Mueller, T.I. (1997). Cognitive-behavioral treatment for depression in alcoholism. *Journal of Consulting and Clinical Psychology*, **65**, 715–16.

Brown, R.A., Monti, P.M., Myers, M.G. et al. (1998). Depression among cocaine abusers in treatment: relation to cocaine and alcohol use and treatment outcome. *American Journal of Psychiatry*, **155**, 220–5.

Buller, R., Maier, W., & Benkert, O. (1986). Clinical subtypes in panic disorder: their descriptive and prospective validity. *Journal of Affective Disorders*, **11**, 105–14.

Buzan, R.D., Thomas, M., Dubovsky, S.L., & Treadway, J. (1995). The use of opiate antagonists for recurrent self-injurious behavior. *Journal of Neuropsychiatric and Clinical Neuroscience*, **7**, 437–44.

Carroll, K.M., Power, M.E., Bryant, K.J., & Rousanville, B.J. (1993). One-year follow-up status of treatment-seeking cocaine abusers: Psychopathology and dependence severity as predictors of outcome. *Journal of Nervous and Mental Diseases*, **181**, 71–9.

Carroll, K.M., Rounsaville, B.J., Gordon, L.T. et al. (1994). Psychotherapy and pharmacotherapy for ambulatory cocaine abusers. *Archives of General Psychiatry*, **51**, 177–87.

Casey, P., Meagher, D., & Butler, E. (1996). Personality, functioning, and recovery from major depression. *Journal of Nervous and Mental Diseases*, **184**, 240–5.

Charney, D.S., Nelson, J.C., & Quinlan, D.M. (1981). Personality traits and disorders in depression. *American Journal of Psychiatry*, **138**, 1601–4.

Clayton, P.J., Grove, W.M., Coryell, W., Keller, M., Hirschfeld, R., & Fawcett, J. (1991). Follow-up and family study of anxious depression. *American Journal of Psychiatry*, **148**, 1512–17.

Clum, G., Clum, G., & Surls, R. (1993). A meta-analysis of treatments for panic disorder. *Journal of Consulting and Clinical Psychology*, **61**, 317–26.

Coccaro, E.F., & Kavoussi, R.J. (1997). Fluoxetine and impulsvie aggressive behavior in personality-disordered subjects. *Archives of General Psychiatry*, **54**, 1081–8.

Coccaro, E.F. & Siever, L.J. (1995). The neuropsychopharmacology of personality disorders. In *Psychopharmacology: The Fourth Generation of Progress*, ed. F.E. Bloom & D.J. Kupfer, pp. 1567–79. New York: Raven Press.

Coplan, J.D. & Gorman, J.M. (1990). Treatment of anxiety disorder in patients with mood disorders. *Journal of Clinical Psychiatry*, **51**[Suppl.], 9–13.

Coppen, A. & Metcalfe, M. (1965). Effect of a depressive illness on MPI scores. *British Journal of Psychiatry*, **111**, 236–9.

Cornelius, J., Salloum, I.M., Cornelius, M.D. et al. (1993). Fluoxetine trial in suicidal depressed alcoholics. *Psychopharmacology Bulletin*, **29**, 195–9.

Cornelius, J., Salloum, I.M., Ehler, J.G. et al. (1997). Fluoxetine in depressed alcoholics: a double-blind, placebo-controlled trial. *Archives of General Psychiatry*, **54**, 700–5.

Cornelius, J.R., Soloff, P.H., Perel, J.M. et al. (1993). Continuation pharmacotherapy of borderline disorder with haloperidol and phenelzine. *American Journal of Psychiatry*, **150**, 1843–8.

Corruble, E., Ginestet, D., & Guelfi, J.D. (1996). Comorbidity of personality disorders and unipolar depression: a review. *Journal of Affective Disorders*, **37**, 157–70.

Coryell, W., Endicott, A., Andreason, N.C. et al. (1988). Depression and panic attacks: the significance of overlap as reflected in follow-up and family study data. *American Journal of Psychiatry*, **145**, 293–300.

Coryell, W., Endicott, J., & Winokur, G. (1992). Anxiety syndromes as epiphenomena of primary major depression: outcome and familial psychopathology. *American Journal of Psychiatry*, **149**, 100–7.

Coryell, W., Winokur, G., Keller, M., Scheftner, W., & Endicott, J. (1992). Alcoholism and primary major depression: a family study approach to co-existing disorders. *Journal of Affective Disorders*, **24**, 93–9.

Covi, L., Hess, J.M., Kreifer, N.A. et al. (1995). Effects of combined fluoxetine and counseling in the outpatient treatment of cocaine abusers. *American Journal of Drug and Alcohol Abuse*, **21**, 327–44.

Cowdry, R. & Gardner, D.L. (1988). Pharmacotherapy of borderline personality disorder: alprazolam, carbamazepine, trifluoperazine, and tranylcypromine. *Archives of General Psychiatry*, **45**, 111–19.

Cowley, D.S., Ha, E.H., & Roy-Byrne, R.P. (1997). Determinants of pharmacologic treatment failure in panic disorder. *Journal of Clinical Psychiatry*, **58**, 555–61.

Davidson, J. (1997). The pharmacological treatment of PTSD. *American Society Clinical Psychopharmacology Progress Notes*, **8**(5), 2–8.

Davidson, J., Miller, R., & Strickland, R. (1985). Neurotocism and personality disorder in depression. *Journal of Affective Disorders*, **8**, 177–82.

Davidson, J.R.T., Kudler, H., Smith, R. et al. (1990). Treatment of post-traumatic stress disorder with amitriptyline and placebo. *Archives of General Psychiatry*, **47**, 259–66.

Davidson, J.R.T., Potts, N., Richichi, E. et al. (1993). Treatment of social phobia with clonazepam and placebo. *Journal of Clinical Psychopharmacology*, **13**, 423–8.

Deltito, J.A. & Stam, M. (1989). Psychopharmacological treatment of avoidant personality disorder. *Comprehensive Psychiatry*, **30**, 498–504.

DeMartinis, N.A., Schweizer, E., & Rickels, K. (1996). An open-label trial of nefazodone in high comorbidity panic disorder. *Journal of Clinical Psychiatry*, **57**, 245–8.

den Boer, J.A. (1997). Psychopharmacology of comorbid obsessive-compulsive disorder and depression. *Journal of Clinical Psychiatry*, **58**[Suppl. 8], 17–19.

Depression Guideline Panel. *Depression in Primary Care, Vol 2: Treatment of Major Depression, Clinical Practice Guideline Number 5*. Rockville, MD: Agency for Health Care Policy and Research, 1993. Publication 93-0551.

Dew, M.A., Reynolds, C.F. III, Houck, P.R. et al. (1997). Temporal profiles of the course of depression during treatment: predictors of pathways toward recovery in the elderly. *Archives of General Psychiatry*, **54**, 1016–24.

Diguer, L., Barber, J.P., & Luborsky, L. (1993). Three concomitants: personality disorders, psychiatric severity, and outcome of dynamic psychotherapy of major depression. *American Journal of Psychiatry*, **150**, 1246–8.

DiNardo, P.A. & Barlow, D,H. (1990). Syndrome and symptom co-occurrence in the anxiety disorders. In *Comorbidity of Mood and Anxiety Disorders*, ed. J. Maser & R. Cloninger, pp. 205–30, Washington, DC: American Psychiatric Press.

Duarte, A., Mikkelsen, H., & Delini-Stula, A. (1996). Moclobemide versus fluoxetine for double depression: a randomized double-blind study. *Journal of Psychiatric Research*, **30**, 453–8.

Duggan, C.F., Lee, A.S., & Murray, R.M. (1990). Does personality predict long-term outcome in depression? *British Journal of Psychiatry*, **157**, 19–24.

Eysenck, H.J. (1967). *The Biological Basis of Personality*. Springfield, IL: Charles C. Thomas.

Fava, M., Rosenbaum, J.F., Pava, J., McCarthy, M., Steingard, R., & Bouffides, E. (1993). Anger attacks in unipolar depression. Part 1. Clinical correlates and response to fluoxetine. *American Journal of Psychiatry*, **150**, 1158–63.

Fava, M., Bouffides, E., Pava, J.A., McCarthy, M.K., Steingard, R.J., & Rosenbaum, J.F. (1994). Personality disorder comorbidity with major depression and response to fluoxetine treatment. *Psychotherapy and Psychosomatics*, **62**, 160–7.

Fava, M., Alpert, J.E., Borus, J.S., Nierenberg, A.A., Pava, J.A., & Rosenbaum, J.F. (1996). Patterns of personality disorder comorbidity in early-onset versus late-onset major depression. *American Journal of Psychiatry*, **153**, 1308–12.

Fava, M., Nierenberg, A.A., Quitkin, F.M. et al. (1997a). A preliminary study on the efficacy of sertraline and imipramine on anger attacks. *Psychopharmacology Bulletin*, **33**, 101–3.

Fava, M., Uebelacker, L.A., Alpert, J.E., Nierenberg, A.A., Pava, J.A., & Rosenbaum, J.F. (1997b). Major depressive subtypes and treatment response. *Biological Psychiatry*, **42**, 568–76.

Fawcett, J. (1990). Targeting treatment in patients with mixed symptoms of anxiety and depression. *Journal of Clinical Psychiatry*, **51**[Suppl.], 40–3.

Fawcett, J. (1997). The detection and consequences of anxiety in clinical depression. *Journal of Clinical Psychiatry*, **58**[Suppl. 8], 35–50.

Fawcett, J. & Kravitz, H.M. (1983). Anxiety syndromes and their relationship to depressive illness. *Journal of Clinical Psychiatry*, **44**, 8–11.

Feinstein, A.R. (1970). The pre-therapeutic classification of comorbidity in chronic disease. *Journal of Chronic Disease*, **23**, 455–68.

Fesler, F.A. (1991). Valproate in combat-related posttraumatic stress disorder. *Journal of Clinical Psychiatry*, **52**, 361–4.

Findling, R.L. (1996). Open-label treatment of comorbid depression and attentional disorders with co-administration of serotonin reuptake inhibitors and psychostimulants in children, adolescents, and adults: a case series. *Journal of Child and Adolescent Psychopharmacology*, **6**, 165–75.

Flick, S.N., Roy-Byrne, P.P., Cowley, D.S., Shores, M.M., & Dunner, D.L. (1993). DSM-III-R personality disorders in a mood and anxiety disorders clinic: prevalence, comorbidity and clinical correlates. *Journal of Affective Disorders*, **27**, 71–9.

Fluoxetine Bulimia Nervosa Collaborative Study Group (1992). Fluoxetine in the treatment of bulimia nervosa: a multicenter, placebo-controlled, double-blind trial. *Archives of General Psychiatry*, **49**, 139–47.

Frank, E. & Kupfer, D.J. (1990). Axis II personality disorders and personality features in treatment-resistant and refractory depression. In *Treatment Strategies for Refractory Depression*, ed. S.P. Roose & A.H. Glassman, pp. 207–21. Washington, DC: American Psychiatric Press.

Frank, E., Kupfer, D.J., Jacob, M., & Jarrett, D. (1987). Personality features and response to acute treatment in recurrent depression. *Journal of Personality Disorders*, **1**, 14–26.

Frankenburg, F. & Zarini, M.C. (1993). Clozapine treatment of borderline patients: a preliminary study. *Comprehensive Psychiatry*, **34**, 402–5.

Gastfriend, D.R. (1993). Pharmacotherapy of psychiatric syndromes with comorbid chemical dependency. *Journal of Addictive Disorders*, **12**, 155–70.

Gastfriend, D.R. (1996). When a substance use disorder is the cause of treatment resistance. In *Challenges in Clinical Practice: Pharmacological and Psychosocial Strategies*, ed. M.H. Pollack, M.W. Otto, & J.F. Rosenbaum, pp. 329–54. New York, NY: Guilford Press.

Gastfriend, D.R. & Rosenbaum, J.F. (1989). Adjunctive buspirone in benzodiazepine treatment of four patients with panic disorder. *American Journal of Psychiatry*, **146**, 914–16.

Gawin, F.H., Kleber, H.D., Byck, R. et al. (1989). Desipramine facilitation of initial cocaine abstinence. *Archives of General Psychiatry*, **46**, 117–21.

Gianni, A.J. & Billett, W. (1987). Bromocriptine-desipramine protocol in treatment of cocaine addiction. *Journal of Clinical Pharmacology*, **27**, 549–54.

Gitlin, M.J. (1995). Pharmacotherapy for personality disorders. *Psychiatric Clinics of North America*, **2**, 151–85.

Goldberg, S.C., Schulz, S.C., Schulz, P.M., Resnick, R.J., Hamer, R.M., & Friedel, R.O. (1986). Borderline and schizotypal personality disorders treated with low-dose thiothixine versus placebo. *Archives of General Psychiatry*, **43**, 680–6.

Goodman, W.K., Price, L.H., Delgado, P.L. et al. (1990). Specificity of serotonin reuptake inhibitors in the treatment of obsessive-compulsive disorder: comparison of fluvoxamine and desipramine. *Archives of General Psychiatry*, **47**, 577–85.

Goodman, W.K., McDougle, C.J., & Price, L.H. (1992). Pharmacotherapy of obsessive compulsive disorder. *Journal of Clinical Psychiatry*, **53** [Suppl. 4], 29–37.

Gorman, J.M. & Coplan, J.D. (1996). Comorbidity of depression and panic disorder. *Journal of Clinical Psychiatry*, **57** [Suppl. 10], 34–41.

Gould, R.A. & Otto, M.W. (1996). Cognitive-behavioral treatment of social phobia and generalized anxiety disorder. In *Challenges in Clinical Practice: Pharmacological and Psychosocial Strategies*, ed. M.H. Pollack, M.W. Otto, & J.F. Rosenbaum, pp. 171–200. New York, NY: Guilford Press.

Grabowsky, J., Rhoades, H., Elk, R. et al. (1995). Fluoxetine is ineffective for treatment of cocaine dependence or concurrent opiate and cocaine dependence: two placebo-controlled trials. *Journal of Clinical Psychopharmacology*, **15**, 163–74.

Grant, B.F. (1997). The influence of comorbid major depression and substance use disorders on alcohol and drug treatment: results of a national survey. *NIDA Research Monographs*, **172**, 4–15.

Grant, B.F. & Hartford, T.C. (1995). Comorbidity between DSM-IV alcohol use disorders and major depression: results of a national survey. *Drug and Alcohol Dependency*, **39**, 197–206.

Grunhaus, L., Rabin, D., & Greden, J.F. (1986). Simultaneous panic and depressive disorder: response to antidepressant treatment. *Journal of Clinical Psychiatry*, **47**, 4–7.

Grunhaus, L., Harel, Y., Krugler, T., Pande, A., & Haskett, R. (1988). Major depressive disorder and panic disorder: Effects of comorbidity on treatment outcome with antidepressant medications. *Clinical Neuropharmacology*, **11**, 454–61.

Grunhaus, L., Pande, A.C., Brown, M.B., & Greden, J.F. (1994). Clinical characteristics of patients with concurrent major depression and panic disorder. *American Journal of Psychiatry*, **151**, 541–6.

Gunderson, J.G. & Phillips, K.A. (1991). A current view of the interface between borderline personality disorder and depression. *American Journal of Psychiatry*, **148**, 967–75.

Hamilton, M. (1988). Distinguishing between anxiety and depressive disorders. In *Handbook of Anxiety Disorders*, ed. C.A. Last & M. Hersen, pp. 143–55. New York, NY: Pergamon Press.

Hardy, G.E., Barkham, M., Shapiro, D.A., Stiles, W.B., Rees, A., & Reynolds, S. (1995). Impact of cluster C personality disorders on outcomes of contrasting brief psychotherapies for depression. *Journal of Consulting and Clinical Psychology*, **63**, 997–1004.

Harrison, W., Rabkin, J., & Stewart, J.W. (1986). Phenelzine for chronic depression: a study of continuation treatment. *Journal of Clinical Psychiatry*, **47**, 346–9.

Hecht, H., von Zerssen, D., Krieg, C., Possl, J., & Wirtchen, H. (1989). Anxiety and depression: Comorbidity, psychopathology, and social functioning. *Comprehensive Psychiatry*, **30**, 420–33.

Hedges, D.W., Reimherr, F.W., Strong, R.E., Halls, C.H., & Rust, C. (1996). An open trial of nefazodone in adult patients with generalized anxiety disorder. *Psychopharmacology Bulletin*, **32**, 671–6.

Hellerstein, D.J., Yanowitch, P., Rosenthal, J. et al. (1993). A randomized double-blind study of fluoxetine versus placebo in the treatment of dysthymia. *American Journal of Psychiatry*, **150**, 1169–75.

Helzer, J.E. & Pryzbeck, T.R. (1988). The co-occurrence of alcoholism and other psychiatric disorders in the general population and its impact on treatment. *Journal for Study of Alcohol*, **49**, 219–24.

Hertzberg, M.A., Feldman, M.E., Beckham, J.C., & Davidson, J.R.T. (1996). Trial of trazodone for posttraumatic stress disorder using a multiple base-line group design. *Journal of Clinical Psychopharmacology*, **16**, 294–8.

Herzog, D.B., Nussbaum, K.M., & Marmor, A.K. (1996). Comorbidity and outcome in eating disorders. *Psychiatric Clinics of North America*, **19**, 843–59.

Hirschfeld, R.M.A. & Shea, M.S. (1992). Personality. In *Handbook of Affective Disorders*, 2nd edn, ed. E.S. Paykel, pp. 185–94. New York: Guilford Press.

Hirschfeld, R.M.A., Klerman, G.L., Clayton, P.F., Keller, M.B., McDonald-Scott, P., & Larkin, B.H. (1983). Assessing personality: effects of depressive state on trait measurement. *American Journal of Psychiatry*, **140**, 695–9.

Horne, R.L., Ferguson, J.M., Pope, H.G. et al. (1988). Treatment of bulimia with bupropion: a multicenter controlled trial. *Journal of Clinical Psychiatry*, **49**, 262–6.

Howland, R.H. (1993). Chronic depression. *Hospital Community Psychiatry*, **44**, 633–9.

Joffe, R.T. & Regan, J.J. (1988). Personality and depression. *Journal of Psychiatric Research*, **22**, 279–86.

Joffe, R.T., Bagby, M., & Levitt, A. (1993). Anxious and nonanxious depression. *American Journal of Psychiatry*, **150**, 1257–8.

Johnson, J., Weissman, M.M., & Klerman, G.L. (1990). Panic disorder, comorbidity and suicide attempts. *Archives of General Psychiatry*, **47**, 805–8.

Joyce, P.R., Mulder, R.T., & Cloninger, C.R. (1994). Temperament predicts clomipramine and desipramine response in major depression. *Journal of Affective Disorders*, **30**, 35–46.

Joyce, P.R. & Paykel, E.S. (1989). Predictors of drug response in depression. *Archives of General Psychiatry*, **46**, 89–99.

Judd, L. (1994). Comorbidity and health costs. *International Medical News*, **92**, 4–5.

Kamerow, D.B. (1988). Anxiety and depression in the medical setting: an overview. *Medical Clinics of North America*, **72**, 745–51.

Kaplan, Z., Amir, M., Swartz, M., & Levine, J. (1996). Inositol treatment of post-traumatic stress disorder. *Anxiety*, **2**, 51–2.

Kasch, K.L. & Klein, D.N. (1996). The relationship between age at onset and comorbidity in psychiatric disorders. *Journal of Nervous Mental Diseases*, **184**, 703–7.

Katon, W., Lin, E., von Korff, M. et al. (1994). The predictors of persistence of depression in primary care. *Journal of Affective Disorders*, **31**, 81–90.

Kaye, A.L., McCullough, J.P., Roberts, W.C. et al. (1994). Differentiating affective and characterologic DSM-III-R psychopathology in non-treatment, community unipolar depressives. *Depression*, **2**, 80–8.

Keck, P.E., McElroy, S.L., Tugrul, K.C., Bennett, J.A., & Smith, J.M.R. (1993). Antiepileptic drugs for the treatment of panic disorder. *Neuropsychiatry*, **27**, 150–3.

Keller, M.B. & Hanks, D.L. (1993). Course and outcome in panic disorder. *Progress in Neuropsychopharmacology Biology and Psychiatry*, **17**, 551–70.

Keller, M.B. & Hanks, D.L. (1995). Anxiety symptom relief in depression treatment outcomes. *Journal of Clinical Psychiatry*, **56**[Suppl. 6], 22–9.

Keller, M.B. & Shapiro, R.W. (1982). 'Double depression': superimposition of acute depressive episodes on chronic depressive disorders. *American Journal of Psychiatry*, **139**, 438–42.

Keller, M.B., Lavori, P.W., Endicott, J., Coryell, W., & Klerman, G.L. (1983). 'Double depression': two year follow-up. *American Journal of Psychiatry*, **140**, 689–94.

Keller, M.B., Herzog, D.B., Lavori, P.W. et al. (1989). High rates of chronicity and rapidity of relapse in patients with bulimia and depression [letter]. *Archives of General Psychiatry*, **46**, 480–1.

Keller, M.B., Lavori, P.W., Mueller, T.I. et al. (1992). Time to recovery, chronicity, and levels of psychopathology in major depression: a 5-year prospective follow-up of 431 subjects. *Archives of General Psychiatry*, **49**, 809–16.

Kerr, T.A., Shapira, K., Roth, M., & Garside, R.F. (1970). The relationship between the Maudsley personality inventory and the course of affective disorder. *British Journal of Psychiatry*, **116**, 11–19.

Kessler, R.C. & Frank, R.G. (1997). The impact of psychiatric disorders on work loss days. *Psychological Medicine*, **27**, 861–73.

Kessler, R.C., McGonagle, K.A., Zhao, S. et al. (1994). Lifetime and 12-month prevalence of DSM-III-R psychiatric disorders in the United States: results from the National Comorbidity Survey. *Archives of General Psychiatry*, **51**, 8–19.

Kessler, R.C., Nelson, C.B., McGonagle, K.A., Edlund, M.J., Frank, R.G., & Leaf, P.J. (1995). The epidemiology of co-occurring addictive and mental disorders: implications for prevention and service utilization. *American Journal of Psychiatry*, **152**, 1026–32.

Kessler, R.C., Nelson, C.B., McGonagle, K.A., Liu, J., Swartz, M., & Blazer, G. (1996). Comorbidity of DSM-III-R major depressive disorder in the general population: results from the US National Comorbidity Survey. *British Journal of Psychiatry Suppl.* Jun(30), 17–30.

Kessler, R.C., Crum, R.M., Warner, L.A., Nelson, C.B., Schulanhang, J., & Anthony, J.C. (1997). Lifetime co-occurence of DSM-III-R alcohol abuse and dependence with other psychiatric disorders in the National Comorbidity Survey. *Archives of General Psychiatry*, **54**, 313–21.

Khantzian, E.J. (1985). The self-medication hypothesis of addictive disorders: focus on heroin and cocaine dependence. *American Journal of Psychiatry*, **142**, 1259–64.

King, M.K., Schmaling, K.B., Cowley, D.S. et al. (1995). Suicide attempt history in depressed patients with and without a history of panic attacks. *Comprehensive Psychiatry*, **36**, 25–30.

Klein, D.N. (1996). Social adjustment in dysthymia, double depression and episodic major depression. *Journal of Affective Disorders*, **37**, 91–101.

Klein, D.N., Taylor, B., Harding, K., & Dickstein, S. (1988). Double depression and episodic major depression: demographic, clinical, familial, personality, and socioenvironmental characteristics and short-term outcome. *American Journal of Psychiatry*, **145**, 1226–31.

Kline, N.A., Dow, B.M., Brown, S.A., & Matloff, J.L. (1994). Sertraline efficacy in depressed combat veterans with posttraumatic stress disorder. *American Journal of Psychiatry*, **151**, 621.

Klosko, J.S., Barlow, D.H., Tassinari, R. et al. (1990). A comparison of alprazolam and behavior therapy in treatment of panic disorder. *Journal of Consulting and Clinical Psychology*, **58**, 77–84.

Kocsis, J.H., Frances, A.J., Voss, C., Mann, J.J., Mason, B.J., & Sweeney, J. (1988). Imipramine treatment for chronic depression. *Archives of General Psychiatry*, **45**, 253–7.

Kocsis, J.H., Friedman, R.A., Markowitz, J.C. et al. (1996). Maintenance therapy for chronic depression. A controlled clinical trial of desipramine. *Archives of General Psychiatry*, **53**, 769–74.

Kosten, T.R., Frank, J.B., Dan, E., McDougle, C.J., & Giller, E.L. (1991). Pharmacotherapy for posttraumatic stress disorder using phenelzine or imipramine. *Journal of Nervous and Mental Diseases*, **179**, 366–70.

Kosten, T.R., Gawin, F.H., Kosten, T. et al. (1992a). Six-month follow-up of short-term pharmacotherapy for cocaine dependence. *American Journal of Addictions*, **1**, 40–9.

Kosten, T.R., Morgan, C.M., Falcione, J., & Schottenfeld, R. (1992b). Pharmacotherapy for cocaine-abusing methonadone-maintained patients using amantadine or desipramine. *Archives of General Psychiatry*, **49**, 894–8.

Kranzler, H.R., Burelson, J.A., Korner, P. et al. (1995). Placebo-controlled trial of fluoxetine as an adjunct to relapse prevention in alcoholics. *American Journal of Psychiatry*, **152**, 391–7.

Kravitz, H.M., Fawcett, J., & Newman, A.J. (1997). Alprazolam and depression: a review of risks and benefits. *Journal of Clinical Psychiatry*, **54** [Suppl.], 78–84.

Labbate, L.A. & Doyle, M.E. (1997). Recidivism in major depressive disorder. *Psychotherapy and Psychosomatics*, **66**, 145–9.

Lapierre, U.D. (1994). Pharmacological therapy of dysthymia. *Acta Psychiatrica Scandinavica*, **89**[Suppl. 383], 42–8.

LaPorte, D.J., McLellan, A.T., O'Brien, C.P., & Marshall, J.P. (1981). Treatment response in psychiatrically impaired drug abusers. *Comprehensive Psychiatry*, **22**, 411–19.

Lecrubier, Y., Boyer, P., Turjanski, S., & Rein, W. (1997). Amisulpride versus imipramine and placebo in dysthymia and major depression. Amisulpride Study Group. *Journal of Affective Disorders*, **43**, 95–103.

Lepola, U., Koponen, H., & Leinonen, E. (1996). A naturalistic 6-year follow-up study of patients with panic disorder. *Acta Psychiatrica Scandinavica*, **93**, 181–3.

Leone, N.F. (1982). Response of borderline patients to loxapine and chlorpromazine. *Journal of Clinical Psychiatry*, **43**, 148–50.

Lesser, I.M., Rubin, R.T., Pecknold, J.C. et al. (1988). Secondary depression in panic disorder and agoraphobia, I: Frequency, severity, and response to treatment. *Archives of General Psychiatry*, **45**, 437–43.

Liebowitz, M.R. (1993). Depression with anxiety and atypical depression. *Journal of Clinical Psychiatry*, **54**[Suppl. 2], 10–14.

Liebowitz, M.R., Quitkin, F.M., Stewart, J.W. et al. (1985). Affects of panic attacks on treatment of atypical depressions. *Psychopharmacology Bulletin*, **21**, 558–61.

Liebowitz, M.R., Hollander, E., Schneier, F. et al. (1990). Anxiety and depression: discrete diagnostic entities? *Journal of Clinical Psychopharmacology*, **10**[Suppl. 3], 61S–6S.

Linehan, M.M. (1993). *Cognitive-Behavioral Treatment of Borderline Personality Disorder*. New York, Guilford Press.

Linehan, M.M. (1995). Combining pharmacotherapy with psychotherapy for substance abusers with borderline personality disorder: strategies for enhancing compliance. *NIDA Research Monographs*, **150**, 129–42.

Linehan, M.M., Hubert, A.E., Suarez, A., Douglas, A., & Heard, H.L. (1991). Cognitive-behavioral treatment of chronically parasuicidal borderline patients. *Archives of General Psychiatry*, **48**, 1060–4.

Lipper, S., Davidson, J.R.T., Grady, T.A. et al. (1986). Preliminary study of carbamazepine in posttraumatic stress disorder. *Psychosomatics*, **27**, 849–54.

Loranger, A.W., Lenzenweger, M.F., Gartner, A.F. et al. (1991). Trait-state artifacts and the diagnosis of personality disorders. *Archives of General Psychiatry*, **48**, 720–8.

Lydiard, R.B. (1991). Co-existing depression and anxiety: special diagnostic and treatment issues. *Journal of Clinical Psychiatry*, **52**[Suppl. 6], 48–54.

Lydiard, R.B. & Ballenger, J.C. (1987). Antidepressants in panic disorder and agoraphobia. *Journal of Affective Disorders*, **13**, 153–68.

Lydiard, R.B., Laraia, M.T., Ballenger, J.C., & Howell, E.F. (1987). Emergence of depressive symptoms in patients receiving alprazolam for panic disorder. *American Journal of Psychiatry*, **144**, 644–65.

McDougle, C.J. (1997). Update on pharmacologic management of OCD: agents and augmentation. *Journal of Clinical Psychiatry*, **58**[Suppl. 12], 11–17.

MacEwan, W.G. & Remick, R.A. (1988). Treatment-resistant depression: a clinical perspective. *Canadian Journal of Psychiatry*, **33**, 788–92.

McGrath, P.J., Nunes, E.V., Stewart, J.W. et al. (1996). Imipramine treatment of alcoholics with primary depression: A placebo-controlled clinical trial. *Archives of General Psychiatry*, **53**, 232–40.

McLellan, A.T., Grissom, G.R., Zanis, D., Randall, M., Brill, P., & O'Brien, C.P. (1997). Problem-service 'matching' in addiction treatment: a prospective study in 4 programs. *Archives of General Psychiatry*, **54**, 730–5.

Madden, J.S. (1991). Alcohol and depression. *British Journal of Hospital Medicine*, **50**, 261–3.

Markowitz, J.C., Moran, M.E., Kocsis, J.H., & Frances, A.J. (1992). Prevalence and comorbidity of dysthymic disorder among psychiatric outpatients. *Journal of Affective Disorders*, **24**, 63–71.

Marshall, R.D., Schneier, F.R., Fallon, B.A. et al. (1998). An open trial of paroxetine in patients with noncombat-related, chronic posttraumatic stress disorder. *Journal of Clinical Psychopharmacology*, **18**, 10–18.

Marin, D.B., Kocsis, J.H., Frances, A.J., & Parides, M. (1994). Desipramine for treatment of 'pure dythymia' versus 'double depression'. *American Journal of Psychiatry*, **151**, 1079–80.

Markovitz, P. & Wagner, S. (1995). Venlafaxine in the treatment of borderline personality disorder. *Psychopharmacology Bulletin*, **31**, 773–7.

Markovitz, P.J., Calabrese, J.R., Schulz, S.C., & Meltzer, H.Y. (1991). Fluoxetine in borderline and schizotypal personality disorder. *American Journal of Psychiatry*, **148**, 1064–7.

Markowitz, J.C., Moran, M.E., Kocsis, J.H. et al. (1992). Prevalence and comorbidity of dysthymic disorders among psychiatric outpatients. *Journal of Affective Disorders*, **24**, 63–71.

Mason, B.J., Kocsis, J.H., Ritvo, C.E., & Cutler, R.B. (1996). A double-blind placebo controlled trial of desipramine for primary alcohol dependence stratified on the presence or absence of major depression. *Journal of the American Medical Association*, **275**, 761–7.

Mavissakalian, M. & Perel, J. (1994). Imipramine doses and plasma-level-response relationships in panic disorder with agoraphobia. *American Journal of Psychiatry*, **152**, 673–82.

Meredith, L.S., Sherbourne, C.D., Jackson, C.A., Camp, P., & Wells, K.B. (1997). Treatment typically provided for comorbid anxiety disorder. *Archives of Family Medicine*, **6**, 231–7.

Merikangas, K.R. & Gelernter, C.S. (1990). Comorbidity for alcoholism and depression. *Psychiatric Clinics of North America*, **13**, 613–32.

Merikangas, K.R., Angst, J., Eaton, W. et al. (1996). Comorbidity and boundaries of affective disorders with anxiety disorders and substance misuse: results of an international task force. *British Journal of Psychiatry*, Suppl. Jun(30), 58–67.

Miller, I.W., Norman, W., & Dow, M. (1986). Psychosocial characteristics of 'double depression'. *American Journal of Psychiatry*, **143**, 1042–4.

Millon, T. & Kotik-Harper, D. (1995). The relationship of depression to disorders of personality. In *Handbook of Depression*, ed. E.E. Beckham & W.R. Leber, pp. 107–46. New York: Guilford Press.

Modigh, K., Westberg, P., & Eriksson, E. (1992). Superiority of clomipramine over imipramine in the treatment of panic disorder: a placebo-controlled trial. *Journal of Clinical Psychopharmacology*, **12**, 251–61.

Moras, K. & Barlow, D. (1992). Definitions of secondary depression: effects on comorbidity and outcome in anxiety disorders. *Psychopharmacology Bulletin*, **28**, 27–33.

Naranjo, C.A., Kadlec, K.E., Sanhueza, P., Woodley-Remus, D., & Sellers, E.M. (1990). Fluoxetine differentially alters alcohol intake and other consummatory behaviors. *Clinical Pharmacology and Therapeutics*, **47**, 490–8.

Neale, M.C. & Kendler, K.S. (1995). Models of comorbidity for multifactorial disorders. *Ammerican Journal of Human Genetics*, **57**, 935–53.

Nelson, M.R. & Dunner, D.L. (1995). Clinical and differential diagnostic aspects of treatment-resistant depression. *Journal of Psychiatric Research*, **29**, 43–50.

Nelson, J.C., Mazure, C.M., & Jatlow, P.I. (1994). Characteristics of desipramine-refractory depression. *Journal of Clinical Psychiatry*, **55**, 12–19.

Nierenberg, A.A. & McColl, R.D. (1996). Management options for refractory depression. *American Journal of Medicine*, **101**, 45S–52S.

Nobler, M.S., Devanand, D.P., Kim, M.K. et al. (1996). Fluoxetine treatment of dysthymia in the elderly. *Archives of General Psychiatry*, **53**, 777–84.

Norden, M.J. (1989). Fluoxetine in borderline personality disorder. *Progress in Neuropsychopharmacology and Biological Psychiatry*, **13**, 885–93.

Noyes, R.L. (1990). The comorbidity and mortality of panic disorder. *Psychiatric Medicine*, **8**, 4166.

Noyes, R., Reich, J., Christiansen, J., Suelzer, M., Pfohl, B., & Coryell, W.A. (1990). Outcome of panic disorders: relationship to diagnostic subtypes and comorbidity. *Archives of General Psychiatry*, **47**, 809–18.

Nunes, E., Quitkin, F.M., Brady, R., & Stewart, J.W. (1991). Imipramine treatment of methadone maintenance patients with affective disorder and illicit drug use. *American Journal of Psychiatry*, **148**, 667–9.

Nunes, E.V., McGrath, P.J., Quitkin, F.M. et al. (1995). Imipramine treatment of cocaine abuse: Possible boundaries of efficacy. *Drug and Alcohol Dependency*, **39**, 185–95.

Nunes, E.V., Deliyannides, D., Donovan, S., & McGrath, P.J. (1996). The management of treatment resistance in depressed patients with substance use disorders. *Psychiatric Clinics of North America*, **19**, 311–27.

Nutt, D. (1997). Management of patients with depression associated with anxiety symptoms. *Journal of Clinical Psychiatry*, **58**[Suppl. 8], 11–16.

O'Malley, S.S., Jaffee, A., Chang, G. et al. (1996). Six-month follow-up of naltrexone and psychotherapy for alcohol dependence. *Archives of General Psychiatry*, **53**, 217–24.

Ormel, J., Koeter, M.W., van der Brink, W., & van de Willige, G. (1991). Recognition, management, and course of anxiety and depression in general practice. *Archives of General Psychiatry*, **48**, 700–6.

Otto, M.W. & Gould, R.A. (1996). Maximizing treatment outcome for panic disorder: cognitive-behavioral strategies. *Challenges in Clinical Practice: Pharmacological and Psychosocial Strategies*, ed. M.H. Pollack, M.W. Otto, & J.F. Rosenbaum, pp. 113–40. New York, NY: Guilford Press.

Parsons, B., Quitkin, F.M., McGrath, P.J. et al. (1989). Phenelzine, imipramine, and placebo in borderline patients meeting criteria for atypical depression. *Psychopharmacology Bulletin*, **25**, 524–34.

Patience, D.A., McGuire, R.J., Scott, A.I., & Freeman, C.P. (1995). The Edinburgh Primary Care

Depression Study: personality disorder and outcome. *British Journal of Psychiatry*, **167**, 324–30.

Pepper, C.M., Klein, D.M., Anderson, R.L., Riso, L.P., Ouimette, P.C., & Lizardi, H. (1995). DSM-III-R axis II comorbidity in dysthymia and major depression. *American Journal of Psychiatry*, **152**, 239–47.

Perry, J.C. (1992). Problems and considerations in the valid assessment of personality disorders. *American Journal of Psychiatry*, **149**, 1645–53.

Perse, T.L., Greist, J.H., Jefferson, W., Rosenfeld, R., & Dar, R. (1987). Fluvoxamine treatment of obsessive-compulsive disorder. *American Journal of Psychiatry*, **144**, 1543–8.

Peselow, E.D., Sanfilipo, M.P., Fieve, R.R., & Gulbenkian, G. (1994). Personality traits during depression and after clinical recovery. *British Journal of Psychiatry*, **164**, 349–54.

Petrakis, I.L., Carroll, K., Gordon, L., Cushing, G., & Rounsaville, B. (1994). Fluoxetine treatment for dually diagnosed methadone maintained opioid addicts: A pilot study. *Journal of Addictive Diseases*, **13**, 27–34.

Pfohl, B., Stangl, D., & Zimmerman, M. (1984). The implications of DSM-III personality disorders for patients with major depression. *Journal of Affective Disorders*, **7**, 309–18.

Pilkonis, P.A. & Frank, E. (1988). Personality pathology in recurrent depression: nature, prevalence, and relationship to treatment response. *American Journal of Psychiatry*, **145**, 435–41.

Pohl, R., Yergani, V.K., & Balon, R. (1988). The jitteriness syndrome in panic disorder patients treated with antidepressants. *Journal of Clinical Psychiatry*, **49**, 100–4.

Pollack, M.H. (1987). Clonazepam: A review of open clinical trials. *Journal of Clinical Psychiatry*, **48**[Suppl. 10], 12–14.

Pollack, M.H. & Smoller, J.W. (1996). Pharmacological approaches to treatment-resistant panic disorder. In *Challenges in Clinical Practice: Pharmacological and Psychosocial Strategies*, ed. M.H. Pollack, M.W. Otto, & J.F. Rosenbaum, pp. 89–112. New York, NY: Guilford Press.

Pollack, M.H., Worthington, J.J. III, Otto, M.W. et al. (1996). Venlafaxine for panic disorder: results from a double-blind, placebo-controlled study. *Psychopharmacology Bulletin*, **32**, 667–70.

Pollice, C., Kaye, W.H., Greeno, C.G., & Weltzin, T.E. (1997). Relationship of depression, anxiety, and obsessionality to state of illness in anorexia nervosa. *International Journal of Eating Disorders*, **21**, 367–76.

Popper, C.W. (1997). Antidepressants in the treatment of attention-deficit/hyperactivity disorder. *Journal of Clinical Psychiatry*, **58**[Suppl. 14], 14–29.

Primeau, F., Fontaine, R., & Beauclair, L. (1990). Valproic acid and panic disorder. *Canadian Journal of Psychiatry*, **35**, 248–50.

Quinton, D., Gulliver, L., & Rutter, M. (1995). A 15–20 year follow-up of adult psychiatric patients. Psychiatric disorder and social functioning. *British Journal of Psychiatry*, **167**, 315–23.

Rauch, S.L., Baer, L., & Jenike, M. (1996). Treatment-resistant obsessive-compulsive disorder: practical strategies for management. In *Challenges in Clinical Practice: Pharmacological and Psychosocial Strategies*, ed. M.H. Pollack, M.W. Otto, & J.F. Rosenbaum, pp. 201–18. New York, NY: Guilford Press.

Regier, D.A., Farmer, M.E., Rae, D.S. et al. (1990). Comorbidity of mental disorders with alcohol and other drug abuse: results from the Epidemiological Catchment Area (ECA) Study. *Journal of the American Medical Association,* **264**, 2511–18.

Reich, J.H. & Green, A.I. (1991). Effect of personality disorders on outcome of treatment. *Journal of Nervous and Mental Diseases,* **179**, 74–82.

Reich, J.H. & Vasile, R.G. (1983). Effect of personality disorders on the treatment outcome of Axis I conditions. An update. *Journal of Nervous and Mental Diseases,* **181**, 475–84.

Reich, J., Noyes, R., Hirschfeld, R., Coryell, W., & O'Gorman, T. (1987). State and personality in depressed and panic patients. *American Journal of Psychiatry,* **144**, 181–7.

Reich, J., Warshaw, M., Peterson, M. et al. (1993). Comorbidity of panic and major depressive disorder. *Journal of Psychiatric Research,* **27**[Suppl. 1], 23–33.

Remick, R.A., Sadovnick, A.D., Lam, R.W., Zis, A.P., & Yee, I.M. (1996). Major depression, minor depression, and double depression: are they distinct clinical entities? *American Journal of Medical Genetics,* **67**, 347–53.

Reyntjens, A., Goelders, Y.G., Hoppenbrouwers, M.J.A., & Bussche, G.V. (1986). Thymostenic effects of ritanserin (R 55667), a centrally acting serotonin S2 blocker. *Drug Development Research* 8, 205–11.

Rickels, R. & Schweizer, E. (1993). The treatment of generalized anxiety disorder in patients with depressive symptomatology. *Journal of Clinical Psychiatry,* **54**[Suppl.], 20–3.

Rickels, R., Downing, R., Schweizer, E., & Hassman, H. (1993). Antidepressants for the treatment of generalized anxiety disorder. *Archives of General Psychiatry,* **50**, 884–95.

Robins, L.N., Locke, B.Z., & Regier, D.A. (1991). An overview of psychiatric disorders in America. In *Psychiatric Disorders in America: The Epidemiologic Catchment Area Study,* ed. L.N. Robins & D.A. Regier, pp. 328–66. New York: Free Press.

Rohde, P., Lewinsohn, P.M., & Seeley, J.R. (1991). Comorbidity of unipolar depression. II. Comorbidity with other mental disorders in adolescents and adults. *Journal of Abnormal Psychology,* **100**, 214–22.

Roose, S.P., Glassman, A.H., Walsh, B.T. et al. (1986). Tricyclic nonresponders: phenomenology and treatment. *American Journal of Psychiatry,* **143**, 345–84.

Rosenbaum, J.F., Fava, M., Nierenberg, A.A. et al. (1995). Treatment-resistant mood disorders. In *Treatment of Psychiatric Disorders,* 2nd edn, ed. G.O. Gabbard, pp. 1275–328. Washington DC: American Psychiatric Press.

Roth, A., Ostroff, R.B., & Hoffman, R.I. (1996). Naltrexone as a treatment for repetitive self-injurious behavior: an open-label trial. *Journal of Clinical Psychiatry,* **57**, 233–7.

Rousanville, B.J., Kosten, T.R., Weissman, M.M. et al. (1986). Prognostic significance of psychopathology in treated opiate addicts: a 2.5 year follow-up study. *Archives of General Psychiatry,* **43**, 739–45.

Rousanville, B.J., Dolinsky, Z.S., Babor, T.F. et al. (1987). Psychopathology as a predictor of treatment outcome in alcoholics. *Archives of General Psychiatry,* **44**, 505–13.

Salzman, C., Wolfson, A.N., Schatzberg, A. et al. (1995). Effect of fluoxetine on anger in symptomatic volunteers with borderline personality disorder. *Journal of Clinical Psychopharmacology,* **15**, 23–9.

Sanderson, W.C., Beck, A.T., & Beck, J. (1990). Syndrome comorbidity in patients with major depression or dysthymia: prevalence and temporal relationships. *American Journal of Psychiatry*, **147**, 1025–8.

Sanderson, W.C., Wetzler, S., Beck, A.T., & Betz, F. (1992). Prevalence of personality disorders in patients with major depression and dysthymia. *Psychiatry Research*, **42**, 93–9.

Sartorius, N., Ustun, T.B., Lecrubier, Y., & Wittchen, H.U. (1996). Depression comorbid with anxiety: results from the WHO study on psychological disorders in primary health care. *British Journal of Psychiatry*, Suppl. June(30), 38–43.

Sato, T., Sakado, K., Sato, S., & Morikawa, T. (1994). Cluster A personality disorder: a marker of worse treatment outcome of major depression? *Psychiatry Research*, **53**, 153–9.

Schottenfeld, R.S., Pakes, J.R., Oliveto, A., Ziedonis, D., & Kosten, T.R. (1997). Buprenorphine vs. methadone maintenance treatment for concurrent opioid dependence and cocaine abuse. *Archives of General Psychiatry*, **54**, 713–20.

Schuckit, M.A., Tipp, J.E., Bergman, M., Reich, W., Hesselbrock, V.M., & Smith, T.L. (1997). Comparison of induced and independent major depressive disorders in 2,945 alcoholics. *American Journal of Psychiatry*, **154**, 948–57.

Sharma, V., Mazmanian, D., Persad, E., & Kueneman, K. (1995). A comparison of comorbid patterns in treatment-resistant unipolar and bipolar depression. *Canadian Journal of Psychiatry*, **40**, 270–4.

Shea, M.T., Glass, D., Pilkonis, P.A., Watkins, J., & Docherty, J.P. (1987). Frequency and implications of personality disorders in a sample of depressed outpatients. *Journal of Personality Disorders*, **1**, 27–42.

Shea, M.T., Pilkonis, P.A., Beckham, E. et al. (1990). Personality disorders and treatment outcome in the NIMH treatment of depression collaborative research program. *American Journal of Psychiatry*, **147**, 711–18.

Shea, M.T., Widiger, T.A., & Klein, M.H. (1992). Comorbidity of personality disorders and depression: implications for treatment. *Journal of Consulting and Clinical Psychology*, **60**, 857–68.

Shear, M.K., Pilkonis, P.A., Cloitre, M., & Leon, A.C. (1994). Cognitive behavioral treatment compared with nonprescriptive treatment of panic disorder. *Archives of General Psychiatry*, **51**, 305–401.

Sherbourne, C.D. & Wells, K.B. (1997). Course of depression in patients with comorbid anxiety disorders. *Journal of Affective Disorders*, **43**, 245–50.

Sherbourne, C.D., Hays, R.D., Wells, K.B., Rogers, W., & Burnam, M.A. (1993). Prevalence of comorbid alcohol disorder and consumption in medically ill and depressed patients. *Archives of Family Medicine*, **2**, 1142–50.

Shestatzky, M., Greenberg, D., & Lerer, B. (1988). A controlled trial of phenelzine in posttraumatic stress disorder. *Psychiatry Research*, **24**, 149–55.

Soloff, P.H., George, A., Nathan, R.S., Schulz, P.M., & Perel, J.M. (1986). Paradoxical effects of amitriptyline in borderline patients. *American Journal of Psychiatry*, **143**, 1603–5.

Soloff, P.H., George, A., Nathan, R.S. et al. (1989). Amitriptyline versus haloperidol in borderlines: final outcomes and predictors of response. *Journal of Clinical Psychopharmacology*, **9**, 238–46.

Soloff, P.H., Cornelius, J.R., George, A. et al. (1993). Efficacy of phenelzine and haloperidol in borderline personality disorder. *Archives of General Psychiatry*, **50**, 377–85.

Sotsky, S.M., Glass, D.R., Shea, T. et al. (1991). Patient predictors of response to psychotherapy and pharmacotherapy: findings in the NIMH Treatment of Depression Collaborative Research Program. *American Journal of Psychiatry*, **148**, 997–1008.

Spencer, T., Biederman, J., Wilens, T., Harding, M., O'Donnell, D., & Griffin, S. (1996). Pharmacotherapy of attention-deficit hyperactivity disorder across the life cycle. *Journal of the American Academy of Child and Adolescent Psychiatry*, **35**, 409–32.

Sramek, J.J., Tansman, M., Suri, A. et al. (1996). Efficacy of buspirone in generalized anxiety disorder with coexisting mild depressive symptoms. *Journal of Clinical Psychiatry*, **57**, 287–91.

Stavrakaki, C. & Vargo, B. (1986). The relationship of anxiety and depression: a review of the literature. *British Journal of Psychiatry*, **149**, 7–16.

Steffens, D.C., Hays, J.C., George, L.K., Krishnan, K.R., & Blazer, D.G. (1996). Sociodemographic and clinical correlates of number of previous depressive episodes in the depressed elderly. *Journal of Affective Disorders*, **8**, 99–106.

Stein, M.B., Tancer, M.E., & Uhde, T.W. (1990). Major depression in patients with panic disorder: Factors associated with course and recurrence. *Journal of Affective Disorders*, **19**, 287–96.

Stuart, S., Simons, A.D., Thase, M.E., & Pilkonis, P. (1992). Are personality assessments valid in acute major depression ? *Journal of Affective Disorders*, **24**, 281–90.

Sullivan, P.F., Joyce, P.R., & Mulder, R.T. (1994). Borderline personality disorder in major depression. *Journal of Nervous and Mental Diseases*, **182**, 508–16.

Teicher, M.H., Glod, C.A., Aaronson, S.T. et al. (1989). Open assessment of the safety and efficacy of thioridazine in the treatment of patients with borderline personality disorder. *Psychopharmacology Bulletin*, **25**, 535–49.

Thase, M.E., Fava, M., Halbreich, U. et al. (1996). A placebo-controlled, randomized clinical trial comparing sertraline and imipramine for the treatment of dysthymia. *Archives of General Psychiatry*, **53**, 777–84.

Thase, M.E. & Howland, R. (1994). Refractory depression: relevance of psychosocial factors and therapies. *Psychiatric Annals*, **24**, 232–40.

Thase, M.E. (1996). The role of Axis II comorbidity in the management of patients with treatment-resistant depression. *Psychiatric Clinics of North America*, **19**, 287–309.

Thase, M.E., Triveldi, M.H., & Rush, A.J. (1995). MAOIs in the contemporary treatment of depression. *Neuropsychopharmacology*, **12**, 185–219.

Thompson, L.W., Gallagher, D., & Czirr, R. (1988). Personality disorder and outcome in the treatment of late-life depression. *Journal of Geriatric Psychiatry*, **21**, 133–53.

Tiffon, L., Coplan, J.D., Papp, L.A., & Gorman, J.M. (1994). Augmentation strategies with tricyclic or fluoxetine treatment in seven partially responsive panic disorder patients. *Journal of Clinical Psychiatry*, **55**, 66–9.

Titievsky, J., Seco, G., Barranco, M. et al. (1982). Doxepin as adjunctive therapy for depressed methadone maintenance patients: a double-blind study. *Journal of Clinical Psychiatry*, **43**, 454–6.

Tollefson, G.D., Souetre, E., Thomander, L., & Potvin, J.H. (1993). Comorbid anxious signs and symptoms in major depression: impact on functional work capacity and comparative treatment outcomes. *International Clinical Psychopharmacology*, **8**, 281–93.

Tome, M.B., Cloninger, C.R., Watson, J.P., & Isaac, M.T. (1997). Serotonergic autoreceptor blockade in the reduction of antidepressant latency: personality variables and response to paxil and pindolol. *Journal of Affective Disorders*, **44**, 101–9.

Tyrer, P., Casey, P., & Gall, J. (1983). Relationship between neurosis and personality disorder. *British Journal of Psychiatry*, **142**, 404–8.

Vallejo, J., Gastro, O., Catalan, R., & Salamero, M. (1987). Double-blind study of imipramine versus phenelzine in melancholias and dysthymic disorders. *British Journal of Psychiatry*, **151**, 639–51.

Vallejo, J., Olivares, J., Marcos, T., Bulbena, A., & Menchon, J. (1992). Clomipramine versus phenelzine in obsessive-compulsive disorder: a controlled trial. *British Journal of Psychiatry*, **161**, 665–70.

van der Kolk, B.A., Dreyfuss, D., Michaels, M. et al. (1994). Fluoxetine in posttraumatic stress disorder. *Journal of Clinical Psychiatry*, **55**, 517–52.

van der Kolk, B.A. (1983). Psychopharmacological issues in posttraumatic stress disorder. *Hospital and Community Psychiatry*, **34**, 683–91.

Vanelle, J.M., Attar-Levy, D., Poirier, M.F., Bouhassira, M., Blin, P., & Olie, J.P. (1997). Controlled efficacy study of fluoxetine in dysthymia. *British Journal of Psychiatry*, **170**, 345–50.

Van Valkenburg, C., Akiskal, H.S., Puzantian, V., & Rosenthal, T. (1984). Anxious depressions: Clinical, family history, and naturalistic outcome – comparisons for persons with panic and major depressive disorders. *Journal of Affective Disorders*, **6**, 627–82.

van Vliet, I.M., den Boer, J.A., & Westenberg, H.G.M. (1994). Psychopharmacological treatment of social phobia: a double-blind, placebo-controlled study with fluvoxamine. *Psychopharmacology*, **115**, 128–34.

Versiani, M. (1994). Pharmacotherapy of dysthymia: a controlled study with imipramine, moclobemide, or placebo. *Neuropsychopharmacology*, **10**(3S), 298.

Versiani, M., Nardi, A.E., Mundim, D., Alves, A.B., Liebowitz, M.R., & Amren, R. (1992). Pharmacotherapy of social phobia: a controlled study with moclobemide and phenelzine. *British Journal of Psychiatry*, **161**, 353–60.

Vine, R.G., & Steingart, A.B. (1994). Personality disorder in the elderly depressed. *Canadian Journal of Psychiatry*, **39**, 392–8.

Vollrath, M. & Angst, J. (1989). Outcome of panic and depression in a seven-year follow-up: results of the Zurich study. *Acta Psychiatrica Scandinavica*, **80**, 591–6.

Volpicelli, J.R., Rhines, K.C., Rhines, J.S., Volpicelli, L.A., Alterman, A.I., & O'Brien, C.P. (1997). Naltrexone and alcohol dependence: role of subject compliance. *Archives of General Psychiatry*, **54**, 737–42.

Volpicelli, J.R., Alterman, A.I., Hyashida, M., & O'Brien, C.P. (1992). Naltrexone in the treatment of alcohol dependence. *Archives of General Psychiatry*, **49**, 876–80.

Volpicelli, J.R., Rhines, K.C., Rhines, J.S., Volpicelli, L.A., Alterman, A.I., & O'Brien, C.P. (1997). Naltrexone and alcohol dependence: role of subject compliance. *Archives of General Psychiatry*, **54**, 737–42.

Walsh, B.T. & Devlin, M.J. (1995). Psychopharmacology of anorexia nervosa, bulimia nervosa, and binge eating. In *Psychopharmacology: The Fourth Generation of Progress*, ed. F.E. Bloom & D.J. Kupfer, pp. 1581–9. New York: Raven Press.

Walsh, B.T., Wilson, G.T., Loeb, K.L. et al. (1997). Medication and psychotherapy in the treatment of bulimia nervosa. *American Journal of Psychiatry*, **154**, 523–31.

Weiss, R. (1988). Relapse to cocaine abuse after initiating desipramine treatment. *Journal of the American Medical Association*, **260**, 2545–6.

Weissman, M.M. & Myers, J.K. (1980). Clinical depression in alcoholism. *American Journal of Psychiatry*, **137**, 372–3.

Weissman, M.M., Prusoff, B.A., & Klerman, G.L. (1978). Personality and prediction of long-term outcome of depression. *American Journal of Psychiatry*, **135**, 797–800.

Weissman, M.M., Bland, R.C., Canino, G.J. et al. (1996). Cross-national epidemiology of major depression and bipolar disorder. *Journal of the American Medical Association*, **276**, 293–9.

Wells, K.B., Burnam, A., Rogers, W., Hays, R., & Camp, P. (1992). The course of depression in adult outpatients: results from the medical outcomes study. *Archives of General Psychiatry*, **49**, 788–94.

Westen, D. (1997). Assessing personality disorders. *American Journal of Psychiatry*, **154**, 895–903.

Wetzler, S. & Katz, M.M. (1989). Problems with the differentiation of anxiety and depression. *Journal of Psychiatric Research*, **23**, 1–12.

Winokur, G., Black, D.W., & Nasrallah, A. (1988). Depressions secondary to other psychiatric disorders and medical illnesses. *American Journal of Psychiatry*, **145**, 233–7.

Wolf, M.E., Alavi, A., & Mosnaim, A.D. (1988). Posttraumatic stress disorder in Vietnam veterans: clinical and EEG findings; possible therapeutic effects of carbamazepine. *Biological Psychiatry*, **23**, 642–4.

Woody, G.E., O'Brien, B.P., & Rickels, K. (1975). Depression and anxiety in heroin addicts: a placebo controlled study of doxepin in combination with methadone. *American Journal of Psychiatry*, **132**, 447–50.

Woody, G.E., McLellan, A.T., Luborsky, L. et al. (1984). Psychiatric severity as a predictor of benefits from psychotherapy: the Penn-VA study. *American Journal of Psychiatry*, **141**, 1172–7.

Worthington, J., Fava, M., Agustin, C. et al. (1996). Consumption of alcohol, nicotine, and caffeine among depressed outpatients: relationship with response to treatment. *Psychosomatics*, **37**, 518–22.

Zajecka, J.M. (1996). The effect of nefazodone on comorbid anxiety symptoms associated with depression: experience in family practice and psychiatric outpatient settings. *Journal of Clinical Psychiatry*, **57**[Suppl. 2], 10–14.

Zajecka, J.M. & Ross, J.S. (1995). Management of comorbid anxiety and depression. *Journal of Clinical Psychiatry*, **56**[Suppl. 2], 10–13.

Zimmerman, M. & Coryell, W. (1989). DSM-III personality disorder diagnoses in a nonpatient sample. *Archives of General Psychiatry*, **46**, 682–9.

Zimmerman, M., Coryell, W., Pfohl, B., Corenthal, C., & Stangl, D. (1986). ECT response in depressed patients with and without a DSM-III personality disorder. *American Journal of Psychiatry*, **143**, 1030–2.

Zimmerman, M., Pfohl, B., Coryell, W., Stangl, D., & Corenthal, C. (1988). Diagnosing personality disorder in depressed patients. A comparison of patient and informant interviews. *Archives of General Psychiatry*, **45**, 733–7.

Zuckerman, D.M., Prusoff, B.A., Weissman, M.M., & Padian, N.S. (1980). Personality as a predictor of psychotherapy and pharmacology outcome for depressed outpatients. *Journal of Consulting and Clinical Psychology*, **48**, 730–5.

# 20

# Suicide in treatment-refractory depression

Jan Fawcett and Stanley G. Harris, Sr

## Introduction

Depression in certain types of individuals carry an increased risk of suicide, and the longer they go unsuccessfully treated, the greater the risk becomes. Treatment-resistant depression (trd) which for this discussion signifies a form of depression that does not readily fully respond to treatment, leaves its victim in continual suffering and vulnerable to a full relapse, with associated increased suicide risk. Treatment-refractory depression (TRD) is used to define a type of depression that for all intents and purposes shows no response to a series of adequately delivered treatments, leaving its victim to suffer the severe symptoms and disability of a full episode, as well as both depression related and realistic hopelessness. In the context of untreated high risk factors and increasing despair, as treatment after treatment fails to help, it is no mystery that either form accentuates the risk of suicide inherent in a high risk individual.

What forms of trd/TRD carry a high risk of suicide? One of the most common forms of trd/TRD is that with comorbid severe psychic anxiety (Fawcett et al., 1990). A number of studies have shown that comorbid anxiety symptoms such as panic attacks, phobias, and obsessional symptoms have poor treatment outcomes compared to uncomplicated depression, both in terms of requiring more treatment courses, and more use of multiple medications to attain response, with partial response (trd) as a common outcome, and a related higher rate of relapse (Clayton et al., 1991). Prospective studies of suicidal outcomes in a cohort of predominantly inpatients, have shown that, while suicidal ideation, hopelessness, and prior suicidal attempts are correlated with a suicidal outcome over 1 year of follow-up, that severe psychic anxiety, panic attacks, and global insomnia as well as severe anhedonia, were correlates of suicide within the first year after clinical assessment, while the communication of suicidal thoughts and prior suicide attempts correlated only with suicide in 2–10 years from the time of assessment (Fawcett et al., 1990).

Further study of specific suicide cases (see pattern case review below) point to the presence of a ruminative form of anxiety, often thought to be obsessional because of its repetitive quality, but ego syntonic, unlike most obsessional thoughts. Frequently, the topics of worry seem like normal, even realistic worries, but the persistent recurrence of the thoughts become constant, and the feeling of anxiety associated with them is at a level of intensity much greater than everyday worry. The patient becomes tortured by intense anxiety associated with a repetitive fearful thought. At times, one can find a delusional idea is driving this anxious rumination. The constant repetition of this increasingly fearful idea becomes inescapable torture for the patient, true psychic pain, from which the idea that the only escape is death seems a logical conclusion. This can advance to a clearly agitated state, but need not do so to result in suicide, especially in the presence of a depressive delusion (often not obvious) driving the intensity of the anxiety. This pattern is very commonly observed in inpatients prior to suicide in a recent study of 15 records of patients who committed suicide while hospitalized or within a week of hospital discharge (Busch et al., 1993). In the inpatient cases, severe episodes of associated agitation were observed during the week prior to suicide in 85% of cases studied, in the context that 65% of the patients studied denied suicidal intent as their last communication before their suicide. Similar patterns can be observed in outpatients, but the presence of underlying psychotic depressive delusions are often hidden by the banality or perceived 'normality' of the worry generated. The level of agitation is usually not as severe as that observed in inpatients (based on hospital staff notes), possibly because the level of observations is less intense in the outpatient situation (often based on periodic outpatient treatment notes rather than 24-hour staff notes of patient's behavior – see illustrative case pattern presentations below). Sometimes the only indication of the severity of the recurrent anxiety is the recorded occurrence of panic attacks, or limited symptom panic attacks.

The aggressive treatment of this anxiety with potent, short-acting benzodiazepines (except in some borderline patients who may experience disinhibition or dissociation, resulting in an increase of impulsive self-destructive behaviors) can reduce acute suicide risk so that antidepressant therapy can have the required time to relieve the depressive symptoms. Neuroleptics are also necessary in the case of suspected depressive delusions, unless severity of suicidal risk suggests that emergency hospitalization and ECT is indicated. This is frequently the case when full-blown depressive delusions emerge from a state of ruminative anxiety, and there is poor response to anxiolytic medications. Our study of these cases of suicide both in and out of the hospital have indicated the importance of looking at short-term or acute predictors of suicide and separating this assessment conceptually from long-term or chronic risk factors, since they seem very different and carry very different implications for clinical decision-making.

The same prospective study of suicide in patients with major affective disorder has identified some features which correlate with high risk for suicide in the long term. Suicide ideation and past suicide attempts were in this category, though the risk for a completed suicide decreased significantly after three attempts (Fawcett et al., 1987; Murphy et al., 1979). Other 'chronic high risk' features were a history of the abuse of alcohol and one other substance ('double abuse') and the one significant psychosocial factor 'not having a child under 18 in the home' was associated with significantly higher risk. These were considered 'chronic risk factors' in that they did not correlate with suicide after 1 year of the clinical assessment (Thies-Flechtner et al., 1996). It seems important to consider both chronic and acute risk factors in the assessment of suicide risk, especially when deciding on intervention strategies and tactics.

## Some typical patterns in suicide

Studies of nearly 100 inpatient suicide records and approximately 30 outpatient suicide cases suggest four 'typical clinical patterns' (Muller-Oerlinghausen et al., 1996). Illustrative case vignettes will be presented to emphasize these observed patterns. These patterns are not by any means exhaustive, but may be a useful beginning for the clinician treating various forms of treatment-resistant or refractory depression to be able to recognize.

### The anxiety-agitation (with unrecognized psychosis) pattern
Case #1

A 34-year-old tool and die maker consulted his family physician after having injured his leg at work. He reports that he was under extreme stress because of demand for his services, working 12-hour days, 6 days a week. He complained of difficulty sleeping for 2 weeks since his injury. The patient was referred for an orthopedic consultation and treated with a benzodiazepine sleep medication. He was seen 2 weeks later after his orthopedic consultation, which resulted in a recommendation for minor surgery in the next week. He continued to complain of difficulty sleeping, and mentioned to his physician that he may have made an error in filling out his part of the temporary disability form that the physician had signed on the first visit. He was told not to worry about this. However, his physician noted depressed affect, and outlook, and started the patient on fluoxetine, 20 mg per day. Three weeks later the patient still complained of poor sleep and appeared depressed. The fluoxetine was increased to 40 mg daily. Two months later the patient had recovered from the minor surgery but seemed more depressed. His wife accompanied him expressing concern about continued insomnia, described fears by the patient that his job would not be available when he tried to return to work (despite the prior demand for his services) and vague suicidal thoughts expressed by the patient. The patient denied suicidal thoughts when queried by the physician, and agreed to the physician's demand that he give up his guns at home to his brother-in-law. The patient again raised concern about his disability form, asking his physician if he could have violated some law by filling it out incorrectly. The patient was reassured that his disability was established beyond doubt. Because of his failure to improve, the patient was begun on nefazodone, 200 mg per day and fluoxetine was discontinued. Another type of sleep medication, chloral hydrate 1.0 g qhs, was prescribed. Two weeks later the patient continued depressed and sleep was unimproved, though he denied suicidal thoughts. Because of the lack of improvement, the primary physician referred the patient to a psychiatrist for evaluation the next week. The psychiatric evaluation was done reviewing the history with the patient and his wife. The examination noted the presence of significant anxiety, but no evidence of delusions or hallucinations. Suicidal thoughts or impulses were denied. A diagnosis of Major Depression, with severe anxiety, was made. Nefazodone was increased to 400 mg to relieve the patient's anxiety, and to effect an antidepressant response and the patient was scheduled to return in 1 week. The patient hanged himself 5 days later.

This patient appears to have manifested a depression unresponsive to an initial course of fluoxetine, which worsened with the patient developing an anxious depressive rumination which appeared to become a delusional ruminative thought that he would be punished as a criminal for making what he believed to be an error in his temporary disability application, despite the fact that it had not been called into question. The doubt initially was expressed as a worry and dismissed with reassurance by his physician. It appears that the doubt became a conviction that he would be punished for a criminal error resulting in discernable anxiety and worsening of the depression, despite increased treatment efforts. The psychiatrist inquired about psychosis and suicidal thoughts which were denied by the patient, but could see that the patient was manifesting significant anxiety. Unfortunately, the history of verbalized suicidal thoughts about 1 month prior to the examination was not communicated to the psychiatrist. In retrospect, a more aggressive attempt to define the thoughts underlying the patient's visible anxiety with the patient and his spouse may have yielded information about the patient's anxious ruminations and perhaps the psychotic delusion that was driving them to the point of terror and sufficient psychic pain and desperation to lead to suicide. This case resembles a pattern which we have seen repeated in many cases. The ruminative anxiety is noted, but its underlying content and severity, as well as its psychotic basis was unexplored and undiscovered.

This presentation of recurrent panic attacks, ruminative (often called 'obsessional' anxiety and worry), accompanying depression in a more subtle form has been recognized in studying the less intensive records of outpatients who ultimately committed suicide while in treatment. These cases are disturbingly difficult to recognize prospectively. I believe this does argue for taking recurrent anxiety, worry, and panic attacks in patients struggling with depression very seriously, and considering the use of directed anxiolytic treatment. By directed, I mean a focus on the description and the severity–duration of the anxiety, and attention to treating to a point where it is not a prominent factor in the patient's experience.

## The depression, substance abuse, interpersonal loss, impulsive pattern
Case #2

A 43-year-old professor with a past history of alcohol, and marijuana abuse is treated for a major depression, developing in the context of job problems and marital strife. In response to increasing job pressures, the patient has begun abusing alcohol and marijuana, leading to marital quarrels, angry outbursts, and finally marital separations. The patient's depression shows a pattern of periods of improvement, punctuated by relapses, resulting in several medication changes, each with limited periods of benefit. The patient overdoses with a non-lethal antidepressant after failing to get his wife to move back with him and threatening to shoot himself. After seeing that the patient is hospitalized, his wife files for divorce, with resulting depression, rage, and pleading on the part of the husband. In a joint session with the patient's therapist, he agrees to stop abusing alcohol and marijuana, and agrees to a period of separation while he proves he is able to change. He again became depressed when she refused to return to him, attacked her verbally, and again threatened to shoot himself. When friends stop by to check on him at his wife's request, he assures them that he was merely trying to 'scare her' into returning. Later, it became evident to the patient that his wife had filed for divorce. The patient assures his therapist that he is sure his wife will drop the divorce, resumes drinking upon returning home, calls his wife pleading for her to return. She refuses, expressing concern for her own safety. The patient does not show up for work, and is found dead at his home, having shot himself.

The patient manifests relapsing depression, associated with alcohol and marijuana abuse, along with a long history of impulsive behavior, episodes of irritability associated with his depression, inability to soothe himself, and inability to tolerate separation from a wife he abused. When faced with sustained separation he could not reverse with denial and threats, he drank heavily and shot himself. These patients are particularly difficult to treat. They have periods of short-lived improvement in their depression, but are unable to negotiate a relationship, falling back on intimidation, threats, demands, and impulsive suicide gestures, which eventually exhausts their partner, leading to a separation, which they cannot tolerate. In some cases, if the spouse is unable to maintain the separation, but later declares an intent to leave, a murder–suicide can result. The problem is one of depression occurring in the context of a pattern of impulsive behavior associated with a multiple substance abuse history and current substance abuse (alcohol and marijuana in this case). The time of risk is greatest during 6 months of the patient's perception that the relationship is lost. This period of time is sometimes difficult to determine. In another case, a middle-aged salesman with a history of past alcohol abuse, after finding out that his wife who had divorced him 2 years before, had remarried, drank heavily, then shot himself while his treating psychiatrist was on vacation. While the divorce had occurred 2 years before, the patient had maintained intermittent communication with his former wife, even if only to disagree over financial matters, she had recently remarried and was on her honeymoon when he took his life.

Retrospectively considered, this patient could have suffered from a bipolar type II disorder, with recent periods of moderate mixed mania, being somewhat obscured by concomitant drinking. On the other hand, Murphy has well documented that suicide in alcoholic patients occur in those who manifest major depression, and in the context of an interpersonal loss within six months of the loss (Murphy et al., 1979). Both of these diagnostic possibilities are important to consider, since the time of high risk is at least somewhat indicated by a knowledgable therapist who is in touch with the patient's perception of loss, who may be able to anticipate the period of increased risk with the patient, and help them with working through and more intensive contacts (the need was actively denied by the patient in this case, and unchallenged by the therapist). On the other hand, if a diagnosis of bipolar disorder can be made, there may be a rationale for the addition of lithium carbonate to a patient's pharmacological treatment. A recently published prospective treatment study (Thies-Flechtner et al., 1996) and other studies point to the possibility that lithium therapy may reduce the risk of both suicide attempts and completed suicides in bipolar patients (Muller-Oerling-hausen, 1998; Muller-Oerlinghausen et al., 1996). Although it requires more study, lithium carbonate may have the effect of reducing the risk of impulsive suicide in non-bipolar patients with histories of recurrent depression and impulsive traits. Since suicide risk is so difficult to assess and to intervene against acutely, these types of diagnostic and treatment issues though subtle need to be considered and expanded on when treating patients known to be at high chronic risk who could become acutely suicidal.

## The borderline-depressive patient with impending separation
Case #3

The patient is an 18-year-old female inpatient who has had three past hospitalizations beginning at age 14. Her past hospitalizations were precipitated by suicide threats in one instance, cutting her wrist in the second and a suicide gesture consisting of being found in bed with a towel knotted around her neck by her mother. The current admission was precipitated by her threatening a young woman with a knife at the doorway of her apartment. She plunged the large knife into the woman's apartment door while screaming that she would kill her if she continued to try to take her former boyfriend (after the boyfriend had broken off the relationship with the patient). Hours after her admission, she broke a small mirror in her room and carved the boys initials into her abdomen. The patient was treated with an SSRI antidepressant with little change. She was very demanding of staff attention, either threatening to 'rip the face off' a female staff member or wrapping a towel around her neck in her bathroom while nude when she was aware she was being checked by male staff. She was on one-to-one for most of her initial week in the hospital, and continued to be sexually provocative with both male and female staff. An attempt was made to shorten her periods of one-to-one supervision after each episode of self-destructive acting out, when it became evident that her acting out was increasing in frequency.

By the third week she seemed less provocative and demanding. Her managed care company reviewer raised questions about the usefulness of inpatient care at this point. A staffing meeting was held after a meeting with the patient and her parents. A decision was made to recommend care in a day program at another hospital, with the idea being that the patient would live at home and commute daily for treatment. The patient and her parents agreed with this plan and a discharge date was set. The patient presented that night with a self-inflicted cut of her left forearm and a notable crease around her neck which the patient claimed resulted from long shoe strings from her Doc Martin boots. The patient was placed on risk precautions and the shoe laces were removed. She seemed to settle down and stabilize over the next 48 hours and was taken off precautions. Her acute depression seemed to lift as she talked about looking forward to seeing a friend at the day treatment program. Although the patient looked preoccupied at times, her behavior normalized. She was given a brief pass to go shopping with her mother. She returned from the pass talking about wanting to be discharged. Her discharge was again scheduled. She was noted to appear 'thoughtful' at times but her behavior was otherwise appropriate. She attended a group meeting where she and others discussed their future plans. She excused herself from the group to lie down before a planned activity.

When her room was checked a few minutes later, the patient was found with a knotted bedsheet thrown over the bathroom door and tied around her neck, with a chair on its side next to her. The patient was in coma and had no palpable heart rate. She was resuscitated with CPR, but never regained consciousness and died in the medical intensive care unit 5 days later.

This case represents a recurring theme, seen in patients with clear borderline behavior pattern histories combined with affective symptoms which wax and wane over time. Many of these patients show poor responses to initial antidepressant medication treatment. The staff and physician are in a bind with these cases, since one-to-one supervision seems to reinforce regressive, acting out, and self destructive behavior patterns, yet one-to-one supervision is the only effective way to prevent a serious suicidal behavior, even if the patient does not necessarily intend to die from the gesture. In this case, the patient's hospital stay was extended by a suicide gesture, and the patient's final gesture was fatal. In this theme, the attempts or gestures that may prove fatal seem to occur without obvious behavioral warnings just prior to a planned discharge or even after a discharge or transfer plan has been discussed with the patient.

It is speculated, based on the available clinical evidence (from chart notes) in these cases that these patients become anxious at the anticipation of a change, and utilize the hanging or self-asphyxiation attempts as both a neurotic effort to deal with the anxiety of the anticipated separation and a ploy to stave it off.

How can such a suicide be prevented? If hospitalization can be avoided in favor of a day program or can be used only acutely, the risk may be reduced over all. Medication with low dose high potency neuroleptics (perphenezine, fluphenazine, and more recently resperidone or olanzepine) in many cases help these patients to avoid a loss of control which seems associated with an inner disintegration in response of separation. The use of anticonvulsants such as divalproex or gabapentin may also reduce anxiety and impulsive behavior. Antidepressants are sometimes problematic because of the waxing and waning of depressive mood and its mixture with anger and irritability. One must be careful not to miss an atypical bipolar disorder with associated mixed or dysphoric agitated states. Finally, it would seem that, when changes are planned, the patient's anxiety and proneness to act out should be defied in planning for the patient's safety and in helping the patient to anticipate, perhaps through guided fantasy, their possible acting out in an attempt to substitute verbalization of impulses for acting out.

## The totally treatment-refractory patient, in which suicide is precipitated by series of losses
Case #4

After a number of hospitalizations, he met a young woman who was also a patient receiving treatment for a chronic severe mental illness. They married and had a child within the first year. This initially positive turn of events did not prevent the recurrence of the patient's depression, nor the necessity for his hospitalization. Having no benefit from high dose tricyclic medications, two SSRI antidepressants, augmentation with lithium, T3 (triiodothyronine), combined antidepressants, and stimulants, produced only short lasting minor improvement. High dose MAOI, with lithium, then dexedrine augmentation failed after a failed series of 13 bilateral ECT treatments. This involved repeated hospitalizations for suicidal impulses and medical complications of his treatment. During the 2 years of these treatment efforts after his marriage, major schisms arose in the marriage, as the limitations of both partners interacted with what had become a treatment-refractory depression (TRD). He was again hospitalized and after the failure of yet another MAOI in high doses (120 mg/day) and augmented with dextroamphetamine 20 mg bid, with minimal results, another course of 15 bilateral ECT was attempted. The result was a partial response and the patient was transferred to a day hospital program. The patient's marriage further deteriorated, with divorce proceedings and disputes over his access to his son resulting. After 2 months while the patient seemed to lose ground despite added antidepressants, he made a decision to leave his residential placement and to return to his condominium apartment. When he returned, he found his wife and child, as well as all the furniture gone, and an empty apartment. Without calling anyone, he jumped 30 stories to his death.

Reviewing this case provides little basis for improving the outcome. Virtually every treatment with a potential to help depression, including psychosocial therapies, residential and day hospital support in addition to the spectrum of psychopharmacology for treatment-refractory depression, and two courses of ECT failed to deflect this patients down hill course. We must accept the fact that there are patients we are not yet able to help, and we must continue to labor to advance the effectiveness of available treatments to reach these refractory cases. It is customary to review our successes not our therapeutic failures. We should learn from our failures, because the same scenarios are likely to present in clinical practice, even if the odds are that the situation will present to a different clinician. An effective treatment for this patient's chronic, severe depression would have probably saved his life. We must not be complacent concerning the adequacy of available treatment. We need to develop more effective treatments, particularly for both treatment-resistant and treatment-refractory patients. This is the reason for this collection of chapters. There is much left to be done in this field.

It is always possible that the next treatment course will help, no matter how many previous failures there have been. How do we motivate the patient to continue, in the face of both depression induced hopelessness, a realistic series of treatment failures, and our own demoralization as nothing seems to help? It is when we give up that we allow the patient to give up. A new idea, a consultation with a colleague who might see the patient from a different perspective, even a tapered transfer of care (not a dump – but a chance for a fresh perspective from someone who brings the hopefulness of a new start – if such an angel can be found to help) may help avert a suicide. As long as the patient is alive, there is a chance for recovery.

Expertise in the treatment of resistant depression is a skill that every practicing clinician should develop. Treatment of refractory depression is an activity that every clinician may not want to pursue. The risk of suicide is substantial in a significant proportion of these patients. The treatment that is necessary may be unconventional, and may be of higher risk than conventional treatments. There is the risk of being blamed for the use of unconventional treatments if they are not successful or if they lead to serious, and even not so serious side effects.

To be sued for 'causing' worsening in a patient with refractory depression when treatments were administered competently and with full explanation and consent to a desperate patient is a highly demoralizing experience. Yet, there is this risk in a situation where there is frustration with prior failures, side effects, mixed with the use of unconventional and even controversial treatments. In such cases, very careful explanations and consent procedures should be documented with both the patient and the significant other(s) (double or multiple consent). Success can be held out as a possibility – hope can be offered, but everyone must acknowledge the justification for the proposed treatment, and the possibility that it may not succeed. It must always be emphasized that if the chosen treatment course is not successful, there are always other choices which may be. Realistic hopefulness without falsely high expectations of a quick 'cure' must be conveyed to our patients.

In a recent film on depression, 'Dead Blue,' author William Styron, used the phrase, 'condemned to life' to describe the suffering of the depressed, hopeless individual. It is this psychic pain combined with no hope of recovery that many patients with treatment-refractory depression experience that leads to the 'logic of suicide' as a desired outcome. This is what the clinician is up against. Recognition of this state, reducing psychic pain by recognizing and treating comorbid anxiety, conveying realistic hopefulness, and increasing the effectiveness of antidepressant therapies can save and restore lives. We must not be complacent about the effectiveness of currently available treatment, but continue to work toward improving the clinical assessment of patients and improving the effectiveness, and integration of psychopharmacologic and psychosocial treatments.

## REFERENCES

Busch, K.A., Clark, D.C., Fawcett, J., & Kravitz, H.M. (1993). Clinical features of inpatient suicide. *Psychiatric Annals*, **23**(5), 256–62.

Clayton, P.J., Grove, W.M., Coryell, W., Keller, M., Hirschfeld, R., & Fawcett, J. (1991). Follow-up and family study of anxious depression. *American Journal of Psychiatry*, **148**(11), 1512–17.

Fawcett, J., Scheftner, W., Clark, D., Hedeker, D., Gibbons, R., & Coryell, W. (1987). Clinical predictors of suicide in patients with major affective disorders: a controlled prospective study. *American Journal of Psychiatry*, **144**(1), 35–40.

Fawcett, J., Sheftner, W.A., Fogg, L. et al. (1990). Time-related predictors of suicide in major affective disorder. *American Journal of Psychiatry*, **147**(9), 1189–94.

Muller-Oerlinghausen, B. (1998). Treatment of suicidal patients. *New England Journal of Medicine*, **338**(4), 262.

Muller-Oerlinghausen, B., Wolf, T., Ahrends, B. et al. (1996). Mortality of patients who dropped out from regular lithium prophylaxis: a collaborative study by the International Group for the Study of Lithium-treated inpatients (IGSLI). *Acta Psychiatrica Scandinavica*, **94**(5), 344–7.

Murphy, G.E., Armstrong, J.W., Hermele, S.L., Fischer, J.R., & Clendenin, W.W. (1979). Suicide and alcoholism. Interpersonal loss confirmed as a predictor. *Archives of General Psychiatry*, **36**(1), 65–9.

Thies-Flechtner, K., Muller-Oerlinghausen, B., Seibert, W., Walther, A., & Greil, W. (1996). Effect of prophylactic treatment on suicide risk in patients with major affective disorders. Data from a randomized prospecive trial. *Pharmacopsychiatry*, **29**(3), 103–7.

**Part V**

# Economic and ethical issues

# 21

# The economic impact of treatment non-response in major depressive disorders

Jeffrey S. McCombs, Glen L. Stimmel, Rita L. Hui, and T. Jeffrey White

## Introduction

Major depressive disorders (MDD) impose a heavy toll on the US economy. Greenberg et al. (1993) estimate the economic burden of depression in 1990 at $44 billion due to the direct health care costs to treat depression ($12.4 billion), mortality cost due to suicide ($7.5 billion), and morbidity costs due to increased absenteeism and reduced productivity at work ($23.8 billion). Specific data on the components of aggregate costs are also available in the literature: reduced work place productivity and disability (Mintz, et al., 1992; Conti & Burton, 1994; Von Korff, et al., 1992; Broadhead, et al., 1990); increased mortality due to suicides (Barraclough, et al., 1974: Brent et al., 1988); and direct medical care costs (Wells et al., 1989; Katon & Sullivan, 1990).

Aggregate cost-of-illness data are an important first step in guiding society in determining how best to allocate scarce health-care resources between competing needs. Depression is an disorder which requires the attention of the US health-care system based on the data quoted above. However, much more detailed data are required to justify the allocation of additional resources to the treatment of depression. Specifically, data are needed on the frequency of, and cost associated with, suboptimal treatment outcomes. This is the focus of this chapter. Other chapters in this text present data on the effectiveness of alternative strategies for the re-treatment of patients who fail to respond to their initial course of therapy. If non-response to available therapies is found to be common and costly, then the deployment of alternative strategies for treating treatment-resistant depression may be economically justified.

## Treatment outcomes in depression: available data on frequency and costs

Patient responses to initial therapy for major depressive disorders (MDD) fall into four basic outcome categories. While this chapter focuses on the economic impact of treatment non-response, it is important that the reader understands the frequency and health-care costs associated with all four treatment outcome categories. In addition, the cost of treatment non-response is best measured relative to the costs experienced by patients who succeed on their initial course of therapy.

## Unrecognized depression

Many MDD patients who engage the health-care system to treat their depression are not recognized as depressed patients by their care givers. For example, Wells et al. (1989) found that only half of 650 patients with a current depressive disorder were properly diagnosed by non-mental health specialists. Katon et al. (1990) screened 767 patients with high primary care utilization profiles for possible depression. Over 44% of these patients were classified as possibly depressed, a rate far in excess of the 6-month prevalence rate of 1–3% estimated by Myers et al. (1984). Katon and his colleagues completed psychiatric interviews with 119 of these patients and found 24% to have a current episode of major depression and 68% to have had a lifetime history of major depression. Nearly half of the patients interviewed by the psychiatrist (47%) were evaluated as requiring drug therapy. However, only 45% of these patients had received antidepressant therapy in the previous 12 months (unrecognized depression).

Unrecognized depression is a major cost factor for the US health-care system due to its frequency and to the health-care demands of these patients. The disproportional representation of unrecognized depressed patients in the high utilization sample studied by Katon et al. (1990) suggests that these patients frequently seek symptomatic relief from their primary care physician. Controlling for diagnosis and severity, Verbosky et al. (1993) found that hospitalized patients with depression require significantly longer hospital stays than non-depressed patients. In this study, patients with untreated depression had significantly longer stays relative to patients whose depression was treated. Interestingly, much of the direct health-care costs associated with unrecognized depression are not included in most aggregate cost-of-depression calculations.

## Patients with side effects from drug therapy

Treated MDD patients typically receive pharmacological interventions as first line therapy, possibly in conjunction with cognitive mental health services. However, given the side-effect profiles of most older antidepressants, some patients may be unable or unwilling to tolerate the side effects of their prescribed therapy, resulting in a switch in therapies or a withdrawal from treatment.

Montgomery et al. (1994) reviewed 42 published, randomized, controlled clinical trials comparing the selective serotonin reuptake inhibitors (SSRIs) with tricyclic antidepressants (TCAs). Treatment was discontinued due to side effects in 14.9% of SSRI patients and 19% of TCA patients. However, discontinuation rates experienced in a clinical trial may be significantly lower than rates experienced in real-world clinical practice. For example, Simon et al. (1996) found that approximately 27% of patients treated with a TCA as initial therapy required a change in therapy within 1 month due to side effects, while the rate for fluoxetine, an SSRI, was 9%.

### Treatment-resistant depression

Patients failing to respond to an adequate trial of antidepressant therapy (treatment-resistant depression) may either: (i) be withdrawn from treatment, (ii) have their initial therapy augmented with a second antidepressant or antipsychotic medication, or (iii) be switched to an alternative antidepressant. As with side-effects, data on the frequency of treatment-resistant depression are summarized by Montgomery et al. (1994). Discontinuation rates due to lack of efficacy for SSRIs ranged between 6% in head-to-head trials with TCAs and 7.1% in placebo-controlled trials. The corresponding rates for TCAs were 5.1% and 6.3%. However, the total discontinuation rates summarized by Montgomery et al. (1994) for TCAs (24.1%) are significantly below TCA discontinuation rates of 45% reported by Simon et al. (1996).

### Treatment successes

The goal of pharmacological treatment of depression is to reduce the symptoms and functional impairment of the patient. According to accepted treatment guidelines (AHCPR, 1993), successful drug therapy requires a 4–9 month course of uninterrupted drug therapy at a dose adequate to treat the depression. Due to the side-effect profile of some antidepressants, allowances are made for dose titration. Switches in therapy may be required due to side effects or lack of efficacy, and the efficacy of treating side effects and non-responsive patients has been discussed above.

The deviation in the above rates for side effects and treatment non-response in the clinical trials and real world practices clearly demonstrate that efficacy rates derived from randomized clinical trails may significantly overstate the treatment's effectiveness in real world clinical practice. For example, most clinical trials of alternative antidepressants report efficacy rates of 60–80%. Real world effectiveness rates appear to be much lower. For example, in the California Medicaid (Medi-Cal) program, nearly 80% of patients treated for depression failed to complete 6 months of uninterrupted drug therapy at minimum therapeutic doses (McCombs et al., 1990). Thompson et al. (1996) considered the costs associated with six categories of outcomes for depressed patients treated with an SSRI: early discontinuations (19.1%), augmentation/switching (20.3%), upward titration (25.9%), partial compliance (20.9%), compliance for 3 months (10.7%) and other

(3.6%). Patients who withdraw from therapy due to side effects are likely to fall into the early discontinuation group and switchers. Patients experiencing efficacy problems are more likely to augment their initial therapy or switch medications.

Data on the health-care costs associated specifically with treatment-resistant depression or switching/withdrawal due to side effects of antidepressant therapy are not available and must be inferred from other studies. For example, McCombs et al. (1990) found interrupted or terminated therapy to increase total health care costs by over $1000 per patient in the first post-treatment year relative to patients who completed therapy. No attempt was made to differentiate side-effect patients from treatment non-response. Thompson et al. (1996) found the switching/augmentation population experienced an additional $4197 in total health-care costs in the 1 year post-treatment period relative to 3-month compliers. Patients who discontinued therapy early experienced additional costs of $2217 relative to compliers.

## Background

The data for this analysis were derived from the Medicaid program in California (Medi-Cal) which finances a wide range of health-care services for the poor and disabled, including outpatient prescription drugs. The Medi-Cal program generates a longitudinal research database for a random 5% sample of all recipients for as long as the sample recipient is eligible. This database provides patient-level demographic data combined with a summary of each claim for covered services paid on behalf of the recipient. Data include type of service, date of service, amount billed, amount paid, and units (days) of service. Prescription drug claims identify the specific product dispensed, quantity, strength and the date the prescription was filled. Prescription drugs are provided under Medi-Cal subject to a $1 copayment by the recipient, although anecdotal information suggests that the copayment is not routinely collected by the pharmacy. Data for this analysis were drawn from the period January 1987 to July 1996.

Medi-Cal costs in the pre- and post-treatment periods were partitioned by type of service. The amount paid by Medi-Cal understate total payments incurred by elderly and disabled Medi-Cal recipients who are dually eligible for Medicare which becomes the primary payer for these patients. The gap between Medi-Cal payments and total payments for institutional care was bridged by multiplying days of hospital, and skilled nursing facility (SNF) and intermediate care facility (ICF) days by per diem cost estimates for these services. Hospital days were assigned a cost of $979 per day (California's Medical Assistance Program, 1995), while SNF and ICF costs per day were valued at $270 (Health Care Financing Administration, 1996). To assure consistency, hospital and nursing home costs were estimated for all patients in the study, not just the Medicare eligible. In addition, the Medi-Cal cost for ambulatory services covered under Part B of Medicare were used to estimate total ambulatory care costs in both the pre-treatment and post-treatment periods for all patients over 65 years of age. Actual Medi-Cal expenditures were used for patients under age 65. All reported non-institutional expenditures were adjusted to 1994 dollars using historical Medi-Cal specific rates of fee schedule adjustments by type of service.

Diagnostic data were rarely recorded by providers on their Medi-Cal payment claim This precluded any attempt to limit the analyses to MDD-specific services. However, conducting this analysis using total health-care costs may provide a more accurate estimate of the impact of adequate dose and duration of therapy given the effects of depression on disability days, functional status, well-being, and the consumption of health services related to other illnesses. For example, Broad-head et al. (1990) found that MDD increased the risk of disability by a factor of 4.78 and increased the number of disability days by 51%. Hays et al. (1995) found patients with depressive symptoms to be comparable to or worse off in terms of functioning and wellbeing than patients with eight major chronic medical conditions. Finally, Verbosky et al. (1993) found that depression increased the average length of hospital stays by 10 days even after controlling for primary diagnosis and severity of illness.

## Inclusion and exclusion criteria

The study population was selected from patients using antidepressants between 1987 to mid-1996. Hence, by definition, unrecognized depressed patient are not included in this study. A total of 1648 new patient-episodes of antidepressant therapy were identified as potential study observations. Episodes of therapy were included in the analysis if: (i) more than one year of post-treatment data were available, and the patient was (ii) between 18 and 100 years of age and (iii) not institutionalized in a nursing home within 30 days of the time therapy was initiated.

New patient-episodes of antidepressant therapy were excluded from this sample for the following reasons: (i) The patient's paid claims included a recorded diagnosis of schizophrenia, mania, bipolar depression, dementia, chronic or transient organic psychotic conditions, or a drug history which included mood-stabilizing medications, the use of an antipsychotic medication prior to the treatment episode, or the use of an MAO inhibitor or two different antidepressant medications as initial therapy; (ii) The patient's paid claims include a gap in all paid claims in excess of three months which may indicate a temporary loss of eligibility for patients under the age of 65; (iii) The patient consumed more than

**Table 21.1.** Potential study population by initial therapy

| Type of initial therapy | Minimum therapeutic dose specification | Final study population: ($N=1235$) |
|---|---|---|
| Tricyclics with MDD diagnosis | | 970 |
| Imipramine | 75 mg/day | 176 |
| Amitriptyline/Perphenazine | 75 mg/day | 144 |
| Amitriptyline | 75 mg/day | 333 |
| Desipramine | 75 mg/day | 114 |
| Protriptyline | 20 mg/day | 7 |
| Nortriptyline | 40 mg/day | 196 |
| Heterocyclics | | 311 |
| Trazodone | 150 mg/day | 308 |
| Bupropion | 255 mg/day | 3 |
| Paroxetine | 20 mg/day | 97 |
| Sertraline | 50 mg/day | 130 |
| Fluoxetine | 10 mg/day | 140 |

(Initial $N=1648$)

$1000 in 'other' services in the 6 months prior to the treatment episode, or more than $2000 in such services in the 1 year post-treatment period; (iv) No diagnosis of MDD (ICD-9 296.2, 296.3) for patients taking TCAs or heterocyclic antidepressants; and (v) The patient consumed more than 120 days of acute hospital care or more than $100 000 in ambulatory care in the post-treatment period, or more than $50 000 in ambulatory care use in the 6-month period immediately prior to the initiation of antidepressant therapy.

## Definition of adequate dose and duration of therapy

The key for identifying patients who are non-responsive to antidepressant therapy is first to identify patients who achieved an adequate course of therapy. The costs of non-response will be measured relative to the costs patterns achieved by patients with an adequate course of therapy in terms of dose and duration.

The guidelines for the treatment of depression developed by the Agency for Health Care Policy Research (AHCPR, 1993) were used as a basis for setting minimum therapeutic dose specifications for the analysis. The minimum dose requirements are listed in Table 21.1 for each drug included in this study. AHCPR guidelines specify that antidepressant drug therapy should continue for between 4 and 9 months. For this analysis, the duration of therapy required for 'completed' treatment was set at 180 days or 6 months.

Adequate dose and duration was established using two methods. The first method was applied separately to the stream of prescription data available for the patient's initial antidepressant and to each added medication. This approach calculated the total milligrams of medication dispensed for each prescription (doses dispensed × strength) which was then divided by the calculated number of days between fill dates. The resulting estimate of average daily dose was then divided by the minimum therapeutic daily dose specified in Table 21.1 for the medication dispensed to derive the relative effective dose achieved for each prescription filled. A patient was considered to have achieved a minimum therapeutic dose for the first initial or added prescription filled if the estimated effective dose exceeded 0.5, or 50% of the drug's minimum therapeutic dose. The second prescription was deemed therapeutic if the estimated effective dose exceeded 0.75. Each subsequent prescription was deemed therapeutic if the calculated effective dose exceeded 0.9, thus allowing for limited early and late refills.

The number of therapeutic days achieved on the initial antidepressant dispensed was obtained by adding the number of days covered by each prescription until the effective dose drops below target levels, thus allowing for dose titration. If a second medication was used prior to 45 days from the last refill of the initial prescription, the therapeutic days achieved on subsequent medications were included allowing for titration. If a gap in excess of 45 days has occurred, the number of therapeutic days was limited to that achieved on the preceding drug. A separate count of therapeutic days achieved on added medications was also undertaken using the same criteria, regardless of any gap that may have transpired between medications, as a measure of treatment completion with secondary medications.

The method outlined above may not represent an accurate count of therapeutic days because of early refills, or augmentation and titration of the initial prescription with the same medication at a different strength. Therefore, a second method of calculating therapeutic days was developed which divides the total milligrams of medication dispensed (regardless of strength) by the total days covered by all prescriptions for a single medication, accounting for overlapping coverage and breaks in coverage in excess of 15 days. As before, this aggregate calculation of average daily dose was divided by the minimum daily therapeutic dose specified in the AHCPR guidelines to derive the relative effective dose achieved. If this value exceeded 0.9, then the entire period covered by the prescription(s) was identified as therapeutic. Similar calculations were undertaken for the first two added medications if the patient changed the medication used.

## Statistical methods

Multivariate ordinary least-squares (OLS) regression analyses were used to investigate the impact of the patient's drug use profile on health-care costs. All models

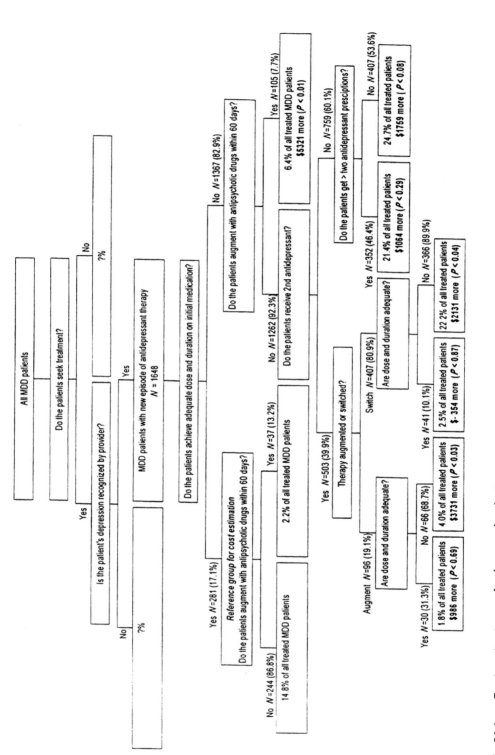

Fig. 21.1.    Treatment outcomes for depressed patients.

included the following independent variables: age, gender, urban or rural residence, number of prior episodes of antidepressant drug therapy, year in which treatment was initiated (time trend), prior use of health-care, including the use of psychiatrists, psychologists and mental health centers, diagnostic mix and drug profile in the pretreatment period, including whether or not the patient used a single pharmacy for all prescriptions.

## Drug therapy outcomes and associated costs

The antidepressant drug therapy outcomes achieved by newly treated Medi-Cal patients are depicted in Fig. 21.1. It is important to note that this study does not supply any new information on the rate at which MDD patients seek medical care for their illness, or the likelihood that the health-care professional treating the patient will correctly diagnose and treat the MDD.

An adequate course of therapy on the initial antidepressant therapy prescribed was achieved by 281 patients, or 17.1% of all treated patients. Thirty-seven of these patients (13.2%) augmented their initial antidepressant with an antipsychotic within 60 days of the start of treatment. The combined group of 281 patients completing their initial therapy will serve as the index population against which the costs of all other categories of drug therapy outcomes will be compared.

Nearly 83% of newly treated MDD patients did not achieve an adequate course of therapy on their initial medication. One hundred and five of these patients (7.7%) augmented their initial antidepressant therapy with an antipsychotic medication and are likely to have experienced a lack of efficacy of their initial antidepressant medication (treatment-resistant depression). This class of treatment-resistant patients were estimated to cost $5321 ($P < 0.01$) more in total health-care in the first post-treatment year than patients who achieved an adequate course of therapy on their initial medication. The bulk of the increased costs were accounted for by hospital care ($1514, $P < 0.01$) and nursing home care ($2185, $P < 0.01$)(see Table 21.2).

Patients who did not complete their initial course of therapy and did not augment therapy with an antipsychotic medication (1262 patients) fall into two groups: 39.9% added a second antidepressant to their drug regimen ($n = 503$), while 60.1% terminated therapy without adding a second antidepressant ($n = 759$). For patients adding a second antidepressant, only 96 patients (19.1%) continued to purchase their original antidepressant at least once after adding the second antidepressant medication (augmentation). This pattern of antidepressant use is also consistent with treatment-resistant depression.

Over 31% of patients who augmented their initial antidepressant therapy with a second antidepressant medication succeeded in achieving an adequate course of

**Table 21.2.** Estimated cost differences by outcome category (patients with adequate initial therapy as comparison group)

| Outcome category | Part B | Drugs | Hospital | LTC | Other | Net Rx | Total |
|---|---|---|---|---|---|---|---|
| Augmented with antipsychotic $n=105$ | $1596 ($P<0.11$) | -$31 ($P<0.92$) | $1514 ($P<0.01$) | $2185 ($P<0.01$) | $58 ($P<0.62$) | $5352 ($P<0.01$) | $5321 ($P<0.01$) |
| Augmented with second AD: Adequate therapy $n=30$ | $386 ($P<0.82$) | $367 ($P<0.44$) | -$362 ($P<0.70$) | $291 ($P<0.78$) | $303 ($P<0.13$) | $619 ($P<0.79$) | $986 ($P<0.69$) |
| Augmented with second AD: Inadequate therapy $n=66$ | $2658 ($P<0.03$) | -$25 ($P<0.95$) | $315 ($P<0.63$) | $929 ($P<0.21$) | -$56 ($P<0.69$) | $3756 ($P<0.03$) | $3731 ($P<0.03$) |
| Switched to second AD: Adequate therapy $n=41$ | $304 ($P<0.84$) | $220 ($P<0.60$) | -$324 ($P<0.69$) | -$436 ($P<0.63$) | -$118 ($P<0.49$) | -$574 ($P<0.78$) | -$354 ($P<0.87$) |
| Switched to second AD: Inadequate therapy $n=366$ | $1626 ($P<0.02$) | -$192 ($P<0.33$) | $551 ($P<0.15$) | $123 ($P<0.78$) | $23 ($P<0.78$) | $2323 ($P<0.02$) | $2131 ($P<0.04$) |
| Terminated therapy: < 3 prescriptions $n=407$ | $1825 ($P<0.01$) | -$329 ($P<0.09$) | -$113 ($P<0.76$) | $512 ($P<0.22$) | -$137 ($P<0.78$) | $2088 ($P<0.02$) | $1759 ($P<0.08$) |
| Terminated therapy: 3 + prescriptions $n=352$ | $468 ($P<0.50$) | -$314 ($P<0.12$) | $292 ($P<0.45$) | $654 ($P<0.13$) | -$36 ($P<0.67$) | $1379 ($P<0.15$) | $1064 ($P<0.29$) |

therapy. This 'delayed' completion of an adequate course of therapy was associated with higher costs of $986, though this estimate is not statistically different relative to completers of initial therapy. However, patients who augmented their initial course of antidepressant therapy but failed to achieve adequate dose and duration were found to experience significantly higher costs of $3731 ($P < 0.02$), primarily due to higher costs for ambulatory (Part B) services. This pattern of increased ambulatory cost is unlike that consumed by treatment-resistant patients who augmented their drug regimen with an antipsychotic medication. These latter patients consumed more hospital and nursing home care (Table 21.2).

The majority of patients who added a second antidepressant ($n = 407$, 80.9%) discontinued their initial medication (switchers). This pattern of use could indicate either side effect or efficacy problems. Switchers who achieved adequate dose and duration on their second antidepressant medication exhibited health-care use patterns which were very similar to patients who achieved an adequate course of therapy on their initial medication. However, as with patients who augmented therapy with a second antidepressant, failing to achieve an adequate course of therapy after switching to a second medication increased total costs by $2131 ($P < 0.04$), primarily due to higher costs for ambulatory services ($1626, $P < 0.02$).

Over 60% of all newly treated MDD patients fail to achieve an adequate course of therapy on their initial medication and do not augment their initial therapy with an antipsychotic medication terminate therapy without augmenting their drug regimen with a second antidepressant ($n = 759$). This population was broken down into two groups depending on the number of prescriptions filled for the initial antidepressant. Over 53% of these patients filled no more than two prescriptions for their initial antidepressant. Thompson et al., (1996) found these patients used more health-care services than patients who completed an adequate course of therapy on their initial medication. This was also the case here. Early termination of antidepressant therapy was associated with higher total costs relative to completers ($1759), but this difference was not statistically significant ($P < 0.08$). However, early quitters were more costly than patients who filled three or more prescriptions for their initial antidepressant ($1064, $P < 0.29$). This latter group of patients may have experienced efficacy problems with their initial antidepressant, whereas early terminations of antidepressant therapy may have been due to side effects which tend to appear early in the antidepressant treatment episode.

## Clinical applications

Practicing clinicians can take away two important messages from these results. First, just over 21% of newly treated MDD patients achieve an adequate course of antidepressant therapy in terms of dose and duration: 17.1% on their initial medication and an additional 4.3% after the addition of a second antidepressant (14.1% of those who added a second antidepressant). This nearly 80% 'failure' rate is even more perplexing as the patients studied here were Medicaid recipients who received their medications at minimal out-of-pocket cost.

Second, the failure to achieve an adequate course of therapy is a costly outcome to the health-care system. Patients who fail to achieve an adequate course of antidepressant therapy in spite of having added an antipsychotic or second antidepressant to their drug regimen were estimated to increase cost by between $2000 and $5200 in the first post-treatment year relative to patients who successfully complete their initial course of therapy.

Much more attention must be paid to ensuring that newly treated MDD patients achieve this goal, either through better selection of the initial medication used, more careful attention to dose and titration to avoid side effects or more aggressive therapy in terms of augmentation or the addition of or switching to a second antidepressant. These data also suggest that the costs of more aggressive treatment of MDD patients may be offset by reductions in total health-care costs if such efforts are successful. The answer to this question is beyond the scope of this analysis.

## REFERENCES

Agency for Health Care Policy and Research (AHCPR) (1993). Depression in primary care: Detection, diagnosis and treatment. Quick Reference Guide for Clinicians (No.5). Public Health Service, US Department of Health and Human Services. AHCPR Publication No. 93-0552.

Barraclough, B., Bunch, J., & Nelson, B. (1974). A hundred cases of suicide: Clinical aspects. *British Journal of Psychiatry*, **125**, 355–74.

Brent, D.A., Kupfer, D.J., Bromet, E.J. et al. (1988). The assessment and treatment of patients at risk for suicide. In *Review of Psychiatry*, vol. 7, Washington DC: American Psychiatric Press.

Broadhead, W.E., Blazer, D.G., George, L.K., & Tse, C.K. (1990). Depression, disability days, and days lost from work in a prospective epidemiologic survey. *Journal of the American Medical Association*, **264**(19), 2524–8.

California's Medical Assistance Program (1995). *Annual Statistical Report: Calendar Year 1994*. Medical Care Statistics Section, Department of Health Services.

Conti, D.J. & Burton, W.N. (1994). The economic impact of depression in a workplace. *Journal of Occupational Medicine*, **36**, 983–8.

Greenberg, P.E., Stiglin, L.E., Finkelstein, S.N., & Berndt, E.R. (1993). The economic burden of depression in 1990. *Journal of Clinical Psychiatry*, **54**(11), 405–18.

Hays, R.D., Wells, K.B., Sherbourne, C.D., Rogers, W., & Spritzer, K. (1995). Functioning and well-being outcomes of patients with depression compared with chronic general medical illnesses. *Archives of General Psychiatry*, **52**, 11–19.

Health Care Financing Administration (1996). Medicare and Medicaid Statistical Supplement. *Health Care Financing Review*, **17**(Suppl.), 278 (Table 38).

Katon, W. & Sullivan, M.D. (1990). Depression and chronic medical illness. *Journal of Clinical Psychiatry*, **51**(6, Suppl.), 3–11.

Katon, W., Von Korff, M., Lin, E. et al. (1990). Distressed high utilizers of medical care: DSM-III-R diagnoses and treatment needs. *General Hospital Psychiatry*, **12**, 355–62.

McCombs, J.S., Nichol, M.B., Stimmel, G.L., Sclar, D.A., Beasley, C.M., & Gross, L.S. (1990). The cost of antidepressant drug therapy failure: A study of antidepressant use patterns in a Medicaid population. *Journal of Clinical Psychiatry*, **51**(Suppl.), 60–9.

Mintz, J., Mintz, L.I., Arruda, M.J., & Hwang, S.S. (1992). Treatments of depression and the functional capacity to work. *Archives of General Psychiatry*, **49**, 761–8.

Montgomery, S.A., Henry, J., McDonald, G. et al. (1994). Selective serotonin reuptake inhibitors: meta-analysis of discontinuation rates. *International Clinical Psychopharmacology*, **9**, 47–53.

Myers, J.K., Weissman, M.M., Tischler, G.L. et al. (1984). Six-month prevalence of psychiatric disorders in three communities. *Archives of General Psychiatry*, **41**, 959–67.

Simon, G.E., Von Korff, M., Heiligenstein, J.H. et al. (1996). Initial antidepressant choice in primary care. *Journal of the American Medical Association*, **275**(24), 1897–902.

Thompson, D., Buesching, D., Gregor, K.J., & Oster, G. (1996). Patterns of antidepressant use and their relation to costs of care. *American Journal of Managed Care*, **2**(9), 1239–46.

Verbosky, L.A., Franco, K.N., & Zrull, J.P. (1993). The relationship between depression and length of stay in the general hospital patient. *Journal of Clinical Psychiatry*, **54**(5), 177–81.

Von Korff, M., Ormel, J., Katon, W., & Lin, E.H. (1992). Disability and depression among high utilizers of health care. *Archives of General Psychiatry*, **49**, 91–100.

Wells, K.B., Hays, R.D., Burnam, M.A., Rogers, W., Greenfield, S., & Ware, J.E. (1989). Detection of depressive disorder for patients receiving prepaid or fee-for-service care: Results from the Medical Outcomes Study. *Journal of the American Medical Association*, **262**(23), 3298–303.

# 22

# Ethical issues in research and treatment of patients with mood disorders

Paul Root Wolpe and Arthur Caplan

## Introduction

Patients with mood disorders pose ethical challenges for both the clinicians who treat them and the researchers who study them. Although many of those challenges are similar to those posed by other patients with mental illnesses, there are characteristics of mood disorders that present unique problems for issues of informed consent, competence, treatment plan adherence, and so on. Mood disorders may weaken a patient's capacity to make autonomous, informed decisions, and so impose a special moral duty on those who care for them or who involve them in research.

The field of bioethics has achieved consensus about the centrality of a few basic ethical principles and values which have been articulated by physicians, professional organizations, legislatures, and the courts over the last 40 years. Respect for the self determination and dignity of all patients, the need for free, uncoerced informed consent, the importance of patient confidentiality, the right to treatment, truthfulness in all dealings with patients and their families, and equity in the selection of research subjects and the distribution of any risk associated with research form the modern foundations of clinical and research ethics. While these values and principles apply to all patient populations, they have special implications in psychiatric populations.

## Clinical issues

Patients with mood disorders present special ethical problems for the clinician. Depressed patients are often indecisive or resistant to treatment, which raises the dilemma of when to consider such resistance a reasonable refusal of consent and when the resistance is a product of the illness itself. Treatment decisions must balance the effectiveness of a treatment against its potential side effects. A clinician may need to advise patients on the wisdom of using neuroleptics when already suffering from tardive dyskenesia, or may need to take the role of advocate for a treatment that has become stigmatized in the popular mind (e.g. ECT, psychosurgery). Advocacy requires that a special effort be made to honestly and lucidly explain the risks and benefits associated with treatment while remaining open to the possibility that the patient may choose to reject the best available form of care.

Mood disorders, like many psychiatric illnesses, often provoke a variety of crises in the lives of patients, from loss of relationships and employment to self-destructive behavior and suicidality. In addition, new health-care systems can restrict the available formulary of physicians and mandate treatment strategies at odds with best clinical judgment. Clinicians must be sure that patient decisions about treatment are not coerced or hasty, that patients are given the opportunity to reconsider decisions they have made once treatment has been started or a decision has been made not to start, and that patients are aware of all useful treatment modalities even if they are not readily available to them due to limits of insurance or ability to pay.

Decisions about initiating treatment are often followed by problems with adherence to the treatment plan. Agreements reached by physicians with mood disorder patients may often later be abrogated by the patient. Patients in the aftermath of a manic episode may agree to notify the physician when they feel the first signs of entering another manic phase, yet fail to do so in the often pleasant early stages of mania. Similarly, the clinician may have an understanding with the patient about treatment – agreeing to undergo ECT when she gets manic, for example – only to have her refuse when the manic episode is under way. Many patients also agree to allow the physician to involve family members in their care, only to withdraw permission when impaired.

Generally, decisions made when competency is clearly present ought to be accorded more force than decisions made when competency is impaired or absent. Patients and their families should know that clinicians will, when in doubt about a patient's wishes or consent, follow the therapeutic course that they sincerely believe to be in the patient's best interest. Physicians, however, have a moral obligation not to use the impaired capacity of the patient to undertake a treatment that the patient declined when competent, even if it is believed by the physician to be in the best interest of the patient.

Finally, there are a number of vulnerable populations that compound the ethical problems confronting the clinician when dealing with patients with mood disorders. Pregnant patients present a significant therapeutic challenge for the physician. The physician must consider both the health of the patient and the fetus, whether assessing the impact of drugs or assessing the impact of a mother's refusal to be medicated. Recent court decisions have upheld a competent pregnant woman's right to make decisions regarding her health-care even if it might negatively impact the fetus. The physician treating an incompetent patient may be held legally accountable to protect her from the consequences of her incompetent behavior as it impacts on both her and the fetus.

Similarly vexing problems confront the treatment of other vulnerable populations, such as pediatric populations, the elderly, institutionalized patients (especially the involuntarily institutionalized), the poor and homeless, and the comorbid patient. Clinicians and researchers working with those with mood disorders should be aware that many institutions recommend the appointment of patient advocates or subject consent monitors when dealing with these vulnerable populations. However, the ethical problems most common to mood-disordered patients revolve around the difficult issues of capacity and informed consent.

## Informed consent and capacity

The doctrine of informed consent is a both an ethical and a legal concept, which, by the early 1970s, had been established as the cornerstone safeguard in both clinical settings and in human subjects' research. A prerequisite of informed consent is the ability to understand and rationally manipulate information in order to make a reasonable judgment about a treatment or about participation in research. This notion draws from the well-established legal principle of 'competence' (developed in relation to the ability to draw a will and make contracts) to set a minimum threshold for the ability of a patient to participate in a valid informed consent process. The notion of legal competency presumes some sort of judicial process of review in order to determine whether a person's abilities have fallen below this threshold.

Competence, as a legal term, has problems when applied to a clinical setting. A person may not have been judged legally impaired or incompetent but may still have obvious and serious limits with respect to decision-making. In addition, the ability to make decisions may wax and wane depending upon any number of factors and circumstances. Therefore, bioethicists prefer the more robust term capacity, which describes the fact that a person may have the ability to make certain kinds of decisions (what they will wear, whether to take PRN pain medication) but not others (choice of psychotropic medication, whether to participate in a clinical research trial). The mere fact that an individual has been diagnosed with a psychiatric disorder does not imply that he or she lacks any decision-making capacity concerning research, standard medical treatment, or any other life decision (Sullivan & Younger, 1995). Even an individual who is 'incompetent' with respect to, for example, his or her financial affairs, is not necessarily so incapacitated that he or she cannot make a decision about how much medication can comfortably be tolerated. Similarly, a patient can be judged incompetent to make a major decision, such as whether to have a dangerous or innovative surgery, and still be competent to decide on less risky medical procedures.

## Assessing capacity

Capacity is traditionally assessed by an evaluation of the person's cognitive capabilities, that is, their ability to understand. Capacity is a property of an individual, determined by an assessor's personal normative standard. In other words, determination of capacity is a value judgment that varies from situation to situation (Caplan, 1992). Though competence is best judged by continual observation over a period of time (Fulbrook, 1994), psychiatrists are often called upon to determine competence after a single evaluation. Also, in psychiatric illnesses, evaluations can be made more difficult by the cyclical nature of symptoms. In schizophrenia, for example, psychosis is episodic and cognitive deficits can be subtle; in mood disorders as well, simple legal competence may not be enough of an assurance of comprehension and voluntariness.

Unfortunately, no agreed-upon standard for assessing competence is accepted by the psychiatric profession. There is surprisingly little in the psychiatric literature that actually directs psychiatrists on how to clinically determine competency, outside of appealing to clinical judgment. Therefore, the discussion of competence in the psychiatric literature has tended to use as its guidepost the standards that are found in law and operationalized in the courts (Grisso & Appelbaum, 1995; Appelbaum & Grisso, 1988; Roth et al., 1977, 1982). Court standards of competence, however, tend to be clinically vague and inconsistent, while competence determination in clinical settings must be geared towards the particular kind of decision that needs to be made. This precludes single-test evaluations. Roth et al. (1977, p. 283) write:

The search for a single test of competency is a search for a Holy Grail. Unless it is recognized that there is no magical definition of competency to make decisions about treatment, the search for an acceptable test will never end.

This often leads to highly subjective assessment; Grisso and Appelbaum (1995), for example, found that different standards used by clinicians affected the identity and proportion of those considered competent, that different groups were identified as impaired depending on the measures used, and the proportion of impaired subjects increased when using multiple or compound standards.

An additional problem with legally derived standards is that they refer to matters of degree, yet provide no way of measuring the quantities involved or of deciding on a cutoff. Understanding, for example, is a matter of degree, yet it is possible to make up a test of understanding, and a criterion for grading the test, so that almost everyone will pass or everyone will fail (Baron, 1994). The law tends to assume that some 'natural' test and criterion exist, but anyone experienced with test design or psychological measurement will realize that such natural criteria typically cannot be found (e.g. Flavell, 1971).

Appelbaum and his colleagues (Appelbaum & Roth, 1982; Appelbaum & Grisso, 1988; Appelbaum, 1996) have developed the most cited formulation of the legal standard for competence. They highlight four standards most commonly used by the courts and by those writing about competence:

### The ability to communicate a choice

Patients must be able to communicate, to maintain stable communication at the time of implementation of a procedure, and not rapidly and repeatedly alter their consent. They must be able and willing to participate in decision-making. Their verbal communication must be consistent with their actions (e.g. not declining venipuncture as they roll up their sleeve).

### The ability to understand information relevant to the decision about treatment

This is the most widely accepted criterion for competency. In terms of abilities, it involves the cognitive capacity to understand issues, a memory for words, phrases, ideas, and sequencing of information, and the ability to comprehend the facts as they are given. Operationally, it means knowledge of such things as risks and benefits, likelihood of success or failure of a treatment, recognition that there is a choice to make and the consequences of choosing, and available alternative options.

### The ability to appreciate the significance for one's own situation of the information disclosed about the illness and possible treatments

A patient may understand facts, in terms of being able to paraphrase them and answer questions about them, without having the reflective ability to understand their implications for their own future. The patient may deny that they are ill, for example. The patient should be able to demonstrate a realistic evaluation of his or her own situation and the potential consequences of various options on that situation.

### The ability to manipulate the information rationally

Patients should be able not only to memorize or paraphrase information, but to use logical processes to compare risks and benefits. Where appreciating information is an issue of values, rationally manipulating information is a matter of weighing information.

All four components focus primarily on issues of understanding, as the law uses cognitive ability as its standard. The capacity to understand, however, should not be conflated with the capacity to make a sound judgment. The emphasis on 'capacity to understand' in the law has influenced both bioethics and psychiatric evaluations, and has enabled, and even encouraged, ethicists and clinicians to avoid difficult questions about the nature and quality of judgment. Questions of judgment are more difficult than questions about understanding, because they go more directly to the decision-making process itself.

## Judgment and mood disorders

The fact that capacity for judgment is not the same as capacity for understanding is most obvious in the case of mood disorders. While clinically depressed patients, for example, often can recall and describe medical facts in great detail, standard texts in the field still assume that significant depression impairs a patient's ability to make certain kinds of decisions (Beauchamp & Childress, 1994; Loewy, 1989; Kaplan & Sadock, 1995). Loewy (1992, p. 1068) states it baldly: 'Almost all professionals feel that depression adversely affects decision-making ability.' Appelbaum (1996, p. 245) also states that 'depressed patients typically are assumed to be impaired in their ability to appreciate the potential value of treatment, because of the hopelessness that so often accompanies the disorder.' Depressed patients often have difficulty making a clear decision, either equivocating or feeling guilt afterward for decisions they have made (Helmchen, 1981).

Yet, the exact nature of the deficit involved in depression is hard to detect, and so clinicians often miss impairments of judgment in depressed populations (Gutheil & Bursztajn, 1986). Sullivan and Younger (1995) write that the clinical evaluation of the effect of depression on a patient's capacity to make medical decisions is difficult because

(i) depression is easily seen as a 'reasonable' response to serious medical illness, (ii) depression produces more subtle distortions of decision making than delirium or psychosis (i.e. preserving the understanding of medical facts while impairing the appreciation of their personal importance), and (iii) a diagnosis of major depression is neither necessary nor sufficient for determining that the patient's medical decision making is impaired.

Howe et al. (1991) suggest that, while depressed patients retain their capacity to reason, their logic is distorted. They tend to make characteristic errors such as focusing on negative feedback and ignoring positive feedback, or being certain, due to hopelessness, that they will inevitably fall into the 10% for whom a particular treatment fails. Lee and Ganzini (1992) add other distortions, such as a sense of worthlessness, which may make the patient believe that they should not be cured because they are a burden on others; apathy and poor motivation which may result in seeing invasive or painful procedures as intolerable; and anger and paranoia, which may impair development of a trusting relationship to care-givers.

If it is true that judgment tends to be distorted in depressed patients, then it is important that clinicians and researchers take it into account when considering informed consent in depressed subjects. Howe et al. (1991) suggests that the severely depressed are more fortunate in this sense than the less impaired, because those with lesser impairment may be presumed to be competent when they are not. Yet, there is also the danger that patients with mood disorders will be seen as lacking decision-making capacity simply because they are affectively impaired. The clinician is obligated to balance the need to determine if capacity is impaired and the obligation to protect patient autonomy.

## Surrogate decision-making

Among patients with mood disorders, then, there are cases where decision-making capacity is impaired to the point at which others must take over the decision-making role for the patient. Surrogacy refers to the transfer of decision-making powers to another, often (but not always) a family member, who makes decisions they feel are in the best interest of the patient. Substituted judgment differs from surrogacy in that it refers to the attempt to determine what the patient him or herself would have wanted were they able to make the decision.

Though there are cases where patients are too impaired to make decisions regarding their care, every effort should be made to include the patient in the decision-making process to the degree possible. For example, refusal by a mildly impaired subject to engage in a procedure in a situation without serious health consequences should be respected, even if the patient is not considered legally competent. Federal regulations for research on the cognitively impaired suggest the same; the policy of the Clinical Center of the National Institutes of Health (NIH) states that 'consent of impaired subjects is necessary but is not sufficient' for involvement in research, suggesting that impaired subjects should be consulted and their wishes not to participate respected. If there are surrogates who must engage in the official consent process, researchers must be satisfied by obtaining a 'substituted judgment' – the belief that the subject would consent to the research if he or she were not impaired.

There is relatively little literature which examines the ability of surrogates to act on behalf of patients involved in research. The studies which do exist in the area of surrogate decision making for end of life care decisions among the elderly suggest that merely being a family member does not mean that a person is in a useful position to articulate a patient's preferences or values. Clinicians must both establish the nature of the relationship between a family member and a potential subject or patient and also make every effort to educate and empower the surrogate to act on the patient's behalf. When the patient has expressed previous wishes, preferences, or values, these must be taken very seriously by surrogates. When there has been no prior expression of values or opinions, then surrogates must base their decision-making on what they believe to be in the patient's best interest. If patients are in a position to be questioned about their wishes concerning choice of a surrogate to represent them, then they should be consulted. Every effort should also be made to debrief patients and their surrogates in order to insure that the surrogate has truly acted and will continue to act in accordance with the patient's or subject's wishes and preferences.

# Research issues

## Research with the mentally impaired

The history of mental illness research includes sincere attempts to find a cure or treatment for psychiatric disorders, and also many instances of the mentally ill being used as convenient, powerless subjects for a variety of ethically problematic experiments. Flagrant abuses occurred as recently as the middle of the twentieth century, when the Federal Committee on Medical Research funded influenza research conducted in psychiatric institutions. The combination of the history of abuse, and the activism of patient rights organizations, have at times created a climate where doing even ethically faultless research has been controversial.

Modern attempts to protect vulnerable subjects in research settings trace back to the 1946 and the Nuremberg Code, developed in the wake of the Nuremberg Doctors' Trial. Twenty physicians and three Nazi administrative officials were tried for the unethical medical experiments on concentration camp inmates, including a number selected because they were mentally ill. The Nuremberg Code established many modern principles, including that subjects should be competent, that experiments be performed first on animals and reflect a knowledge of the natural history of the disease under study, that experiments result in a good for society not attainable by other means, and that the informed consent of the subject is an absolute, inviolate requirement for research participation. It should be noted that The Code places the responsibility for the ethical design and competent application of the experimental protocol squarely on the shoulders of the researcher (Shamoo & Irving, 1993; Caplan, 1992).

Since then, there have been numerous attempts to update and refine The Code, and a number of scandals – such as the Tuskegee Syphilis Study, the Willowbrook study and the Brooklyn Jewish Hospital cancer study of the 1960s and 1970s – have highlighted and reinforced the need to establish strong guidelines to assure ethical human subjects' research. The result has been a significant amount of federal regulation establishing safeguards for federally funded human subjects' research, especially among vulnerable populations.

While medical researchers have accepted, if not always enthusiastically embraced, the stringent mechanisms set up to insure subject protection in the United

States, psychiatric researchers (and some lay advocates) have been singularly vocal in arguing that existing informed consent safeguards (whatever they were at the moment) were sufficient to safeguard subjects, and that further regulation was not needed. An article in *Psychiatric Annals* in 1976, for example, argued that legal and medical perspectives on informed consent were

> fundamentally incompatible – particularly in the area of the mentally disabled, where appreciation of the concept of informed consent is well on its way to paralyzing research and treatment (Chayet, 1976).

Some advocates for the mentally ill also have argued that any special protections would be stigmatizing and would erode patient autonomy, and thus further contribute to the powerlessness and distrust experienced by the mentally ill.

Such resistance is one reason that federal regulation does not treat the mentally ill as a vulnerable group worthy of explicit, legal protections. In contrast to other vulnerable populations such as children, prisoners, and pregnant women, the sole specific protection offered to the mentally disabled and mentally incapacitated is the charge that Institutional Review Boards should be aware of the vulnerable nature of the mentally ill. This ambiguity has left the issue of ethical participation of incapacitated adults in research unsettled, not only for the mentally ill, but also for those who become incapacitated secondary to a medical condition or an iatrogenic incident, as well as unconscious emergency room patients (Wolpe & Merz, 1997).

## Concerns about psychiatric research

While there have certainly been significant improvements in the quality of human subjects' protections among psychiatric patients involved in medical research, many clinicians and patient advocacy groups still voice concern about the nature and scope of current research. Some worry that too much non-therapeutic research is being conducted, and others, that subjects with severe chronic mental illness are involved in studies which use inactive placebos or require 'washout' periods. The debate about the morality of research with subjects who are mentally ill divides researchers, clinicians, patients, and advocates for the mentally ill into two camps. One argues that the protections which already exist – informed consent and local peer review by institutional review boards (IRBs) – are sufficient, and that the creation of special regulations may inhibit useful and important research and further stigmatize subjects. Others believe that special protections for the mentally ill involved in research are necessary and long overdue, and worry that an increasingly competitive and privately funded research climate is one in which the interests of the mentally ill require increased protection.

There is also disagreement about the kinds of research that ought be done. Some psychiatric research is conducted in an atmosphere which is potentially coercive, such as when patients are involuntarily institutionalized or undergoing court-ordered treatment for substance abuse or in response to criminal behavior. To some, the vulnerability produced by limits in competency, societal stigma, and the potentially coercive pressures of psychiatric treatment renders immoral any research that does not directly benefit the patient. Others are willing to allow a significant amount of research involving risk as long as there is adequate subject or surrogate informed consent, thorough peer review, adequate supervision of the research process, and careful debriefing of the parties involved.

## Institutionalized populations

Institutionalized populations are particularly vulnerable to coercion and manipulation, and so draw the special attention of ethicists and regulators. Institutionalized populations tend to be used disproportionately because of their convenience, and so some argue that they should not be used for research purposes at all (Levine, 1996). However, participation in research may have beneficial effects for the patient, both therapeutically, in terms of self-worth, and in increased interaction with health-care providers. The compromise that has been generally agreed upon is that institutionalized populations who lack capacity to consent should only be subjected to experiments from which they might derive some benefit, which are minimally risky and that are directly related to their conditions. Those capable of consent should only be approached about experiments for which there is minimal risk (itself an ambiguous concept, but beyond the scope of this chapter, see Levine, 1986).

## Drug-free, 'washout' studies, and placebo research

In May, 1994, the Office for the Prevention of Research Risks (OPRR) of NIH reported on complaints against schizophrenia researchers at UCLA from subjects who had participated in studies of fluphenazine decanoate, an antipsychotic medication. The study had followed a 'washout' strategy, where the subject is maintained in a drug-free state for a period to establish a baseline level of functioning. The UCLA study's purpose was to identify predictors of successful functioning without antipsychotics.

Subjects first underwent a 1-year, fixed dose study in which they received injections every 2 weeks. Those willing to continue entered a second, randomized, double-blind and placebo-controlled study of the same dose of fluphenazine. After 12 weeks the two groups crossed over, with those subjects who had received active medication now getting placebo, and vice versa. After another 12 weeks, stable subjects entered a withdrawal protocol, where medications were stopped and subjects were followed for at least a year or until they experienced an exacerbation or relapse. During this period, one subject experienced a severe relapse and threatened to kill his parents, at one point approaching his mother with a carving knife.

The ethical problems with the schizophrenia washout studies are equally applicable to subjects with mood disorders. The ethical objections include questions about the basic morality of washout studies, with their high likelihood of relapse and subject suffering, inadequate monitoring of patient relapse, the use of standard rather than individualized doses of medication, and the nature of the informed consent process.

Some critics of the washout studies argue that drug-free trials should never be permitted, because a basic aim is to induce patient relapse, with all the suffering that entails. The *Declaration of Helsinki* requires that every subject, including controls, be 'assured of the best proven diagnostic and therapeutic method' available. Being removed from medication for research purposes may not fulfill this requirement. Advocates of washout studies, on the other hand, argue that all experimentation entails risk, and that, with careful monitoring, the risk of relapse is no greater than that taken by subjects in other research protocols. Additionally, given the side effects and limitations of current psychotropic medications, determining who can remain drug-free and stable could be of great benefit to patients themselves.

These concerns raise an ethical question at the heart of all placebo research – is it ever ethical to deny patients treatments that are known to be effective in the pursuit of research goals, even laudable ones, especially when, as in the case of patients with schizophrenia or clinical depression, the results of placebo are likely to cause significant discomfort or harm in a percentage of subjects? One way to answer this question is to insist that placebo studies be done only when there is no other way to acquire information of vital importance for subjects with particular ailments and conditions.

It is generally agreed upon by bioethicists that, if a placebo is to be used, the subjects must stand some chance of therapeutic benefit from the study, unless they are themselves competent enough to accept the risks entailed by the use of placebo. Placebo trials that involve washout phases should be conducted only under the strict supervision of an independent data monitoring board which can report any adverse outcomes or reactions to the investigator, the subjects of the study, and the appropriate institutional review board (Caplan, 1998).

# REFERENCES

Appelbaum, P.S. (1996). Patients competence to consent to neurobiological research. *Accountability in Research*, **4**, 241–5.

Appelbaum, P.S. & Grisso, T. (1988). 'Assessing patients' capacities to consent to treatment. *New England Journal of Medicine*, **319**, 1635–8.

Appelbaum, P.S. & Roth, L.H. (1982). Competency to consent to research: a psychiatric overview. *Archives of General Psychiatry*, **39**, 951–8.

Baron, J. (1994). *Thinking and Deciding. 2nd edn*. New York, NY: Cambridge University Press.

Beauchamp, T.L. & Childress, J.F. (1994). *Principles of Biomedical Ethics*. New York, NY: Oxford University Press.

Caplan, A.L. (1992). *If I Were A Rich Man Could I Buy a Pancreas? and Other Essays On the Ethics of Health Care*. Bloomington, IN: Indiana University Press.

Caplan, A.L. (1998). *Am I My Brothers Keeper?* Bloomington, IN: Indiana University Press.

Chayet, N.L. (1976). Informed consent of the mentally disabled: a failing fiction. *Psychiatric Annals*, **6** (6), 82–9.

Flavell, J.H. (1971). Stage-related properties of cognitive development. *Cognitive Psychology*, **2**, 421–53.

Fulbrook, P. (1994). Assessing mental competence of patients and relatives. *Journal of Advanced Nursing*, **20** (3), 457–61.

Grisso, T. & Appelbaum, P.S. (1995). Comparison of standards for assessing patients' capacities to make treatment decisions. *The American Journal of Psychiatry*, **152**, 1033–7.

Gutheil, T.G. & Bursztajn, H. (1986). Clinician's guidelines for assessing subtle forms of patient incompetency in legal settings. *American Journal of Psychiatry*, **143**, 1021–3.

Helmchen, H. (1981). Problems of informed consent for clinical trials in psychiatry. *Controlled Clinical Trials*, **1**, 435–40.

Howe, E.G., Gordon, D.S., & Valentin, M. (1991). Medical determination (and preservation) of decision-making capacity. *Law, Medicine and Health Care*, **19**, 27–33.

Kaplan, H.I. & Sadock, B.J. (1995). Geriatric psychiatry. In *Comprehensive Textbook of Psychiatry/VI*, 6th edn. Vol. VI. Baltimore, MD: Williams & Wilkins.

Lee, M.A. & Ganzini, L. (1992). Depression in the elderly: effect on patient attitudes toward life-sustaining therapy. *Journal of the American Geriatrics Society*, **40**, 983–8.

Levine, R.J. (1986). *Ethics and the Regulation of Clinical Research, 2nd edn*. Baltimore, MD: Urban & Schwarzenberg.

Levine, R.J. (1996). Proposed regulations for research involving those institutionalized as mentally infirm: a consideration of their relevance in 1996. *IRB*, **18**, (5) 1–5.

Loewy, E.H. (1989). *Textbook of Medical Ethics*. New York, NY: Plenum Publishing.

Loewy, E.H. (1992). Of depression, anecdote, and prejudice: a confession. *Journal of the American Geriatrics Society*, **40**, 1068–74.

Roth, L.H., Meisel, A., & Lidz, C.W. (1977). Tests of competency to consent in treatment. *American Journal of Psychiatry*, **164** (3), 279–84.

Roth, L.H., Lidz, C.W., Meisel, A. et al. (1982). Competency to decide about treatment or research: an overview of some empirical data. *International Journal of Law and Psychiatry*, **5**, 29–50.

Shamoo, A.E. & Irving, D.E. (1993). Accountability in research using persons with mental illness. *Accountability in Research*, **3**, 1–17.

Sullivan, M. & Younger, S. (1995). Depression, competence, and the right to refuse lifesaving medical treatment. *American Journal of Psychiatry*, **151**, 971–8.

Wolpe, P.R. & Merz, J.F. (1997). Hospital ERs on front line in informed consent debate. *Forum for Applied Research and Public Policy*, **12**(3), 127–31.

# Index

Printed in the United States
105187LV00005BA/119-122/A

9 780521 041812